MW01064185

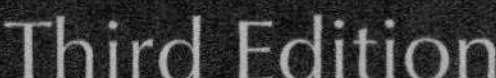

Third Edition

MEDICAL TERMINOLOGY

A LIVING LANGUAGE

Bonnie F. Fremgen, PhD

Suzanne S. Frucht, PhD
Associate Professor Emeritus
Northwest Missouri State University
Maryville, MO

Boston • Columbus • Indianapolis • New York • San Francisco
Amsterdam • Cape Town • Dubai • London • Madrid • Milan • Munich • Paris • Montréal • Toronto
Delhi • Mexico City • São Paulo • Sydney • Hong Kong • Seoul • Singapore • Taipei • Tokyo

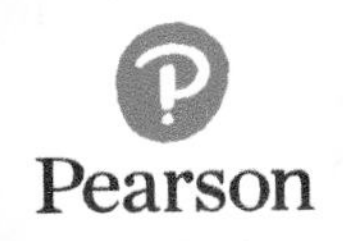

Pearson

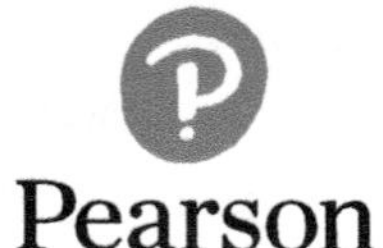

330 Hudson Street, New York, NY 10013
Hardcover ISBN 10: 0-13-448066-X
Hardcover ISBN 13: 978-0-13448066-4
1 16

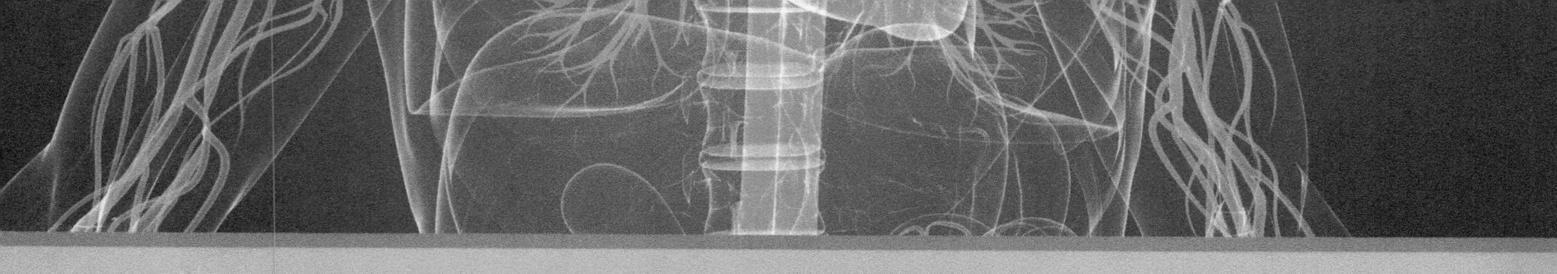

Welcome!

Welcome to the fascinating study of medical language—a vital part of your preparation for a career as a health professional. We are glad that you have joined us. Throughout your career, in a variety of settings, you will use medical terminology to communicate with co-workers and patients. Employing a carefully constructed learning system, ***Medical Terminology: A Living Language*** has helped thousands of readers gain a successful grasp of medical language within a real-world context.

In developing this book we had six goals in mind:

1. To provide a clear introduction to the basic rules of using word parts to form medical terms.
2. To use phonetic pronunciations that will help you easily pronounce terms by spelling out the word part according to the way it sounds.
3. To help you understand medical terminology within the context of the human body systems. Realizing that this book is designed for a terminology course and not an anatomy & physiology course, we have aimed to stick to only the basics.
4. To help you develop a full range of Latin and Greek word parts used to build medical terms so that you will be able to interpret unfamiliar terms you encounter in the future.
5. To help you visualize medical language with an abundance of real-life photographs and accurate illustrations.
6. To provide you with a wealth of practice applications at the end of each chapter to help you review and master the content as you go along.

Please turn the page to get a visual glimpse of what makes this book an ideal guide to your exploration of medical terminology.

Streamlined Content

Fourteen chapters and only the most essential anatomy & physiology coverage makes this book a perfect mid-sized fit for students new to medical terminology.

Chapter-Opening Page Spreads

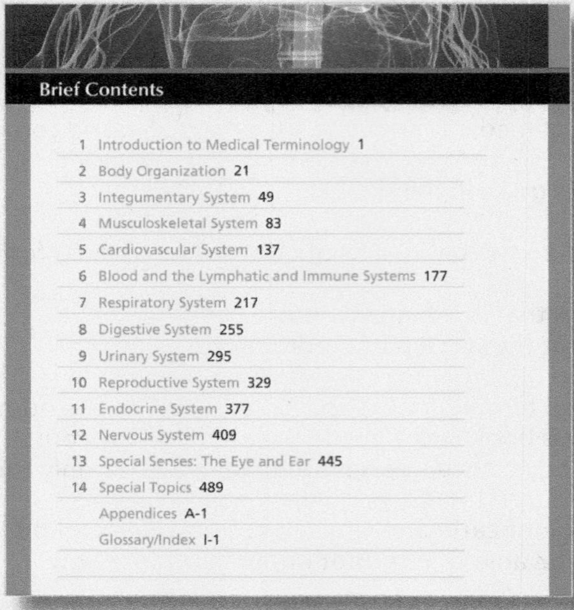

Brief Contents

"At a Glance" and "Illustrated" pages begin each chapter, providing a quick, visual snapshot of what's covered.

Key Terms and Pronunciations

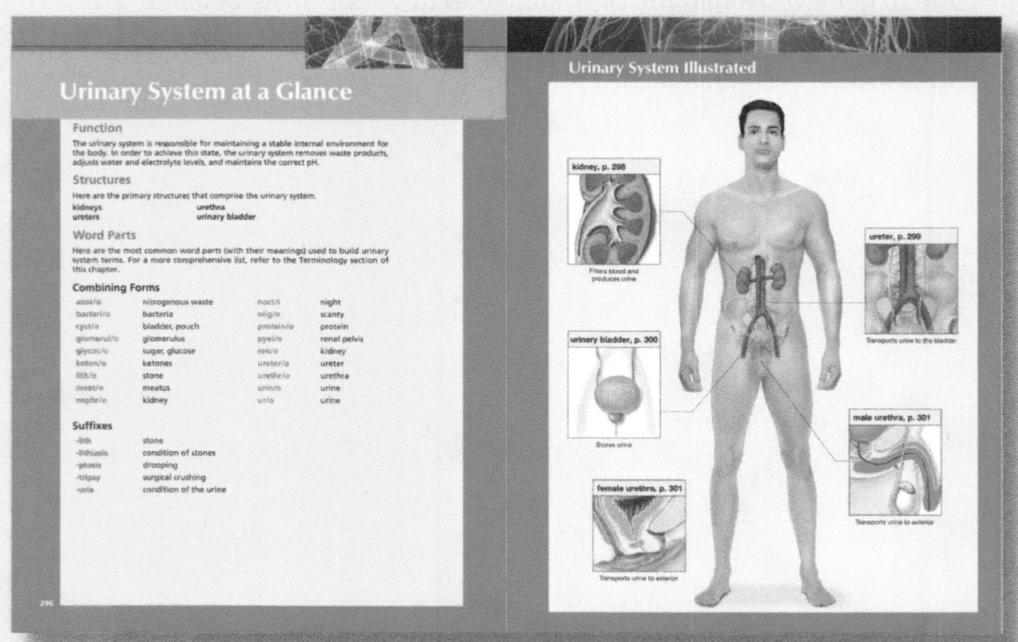

Urinary System at a Glance

Function

The urinary system is responsible for maintaining a stable internal environment for the body. In order to achieve this state, the urinary system removes waste products, adjusts water and electrolyte levels, and maintains the correct pH.

Structures

Here are the primary structures that comprise the urinary system.

kidneys — urethra
ureters — urinary bladder

Word Parts

Here are the most common word parts (with their meanings) used to build urinary system terms. For a more comprehensive list, refer to the Terminology section of this chapter.

Combining Forms

azot/o	nitrogenous waste	noct/i	night
bacteri/o	bacteria	olig/o	scanty
cyst/o	bladder, pouch	protein/o	protein
glomerul/o	glomerulus	pyel/o	renal pelvis
glycos/o	sugar, glucose	ren/o	kidney
keton/o	ketones	ureter/o	ureter
lith/o	stone	urethr/o	urethra
meat/o	meatus	urin/o	urine
nephr/o	kidney	ur/o	urine

Suffixes

-lith	stone
-lithiasis	condition of stones
-ptosis	drooping
-tripsy	surgical crushing
-uria	condition of the urine

296

Every subsection starts with a list of key terms and pronunciations for those words that will be covered in that section. This sets the stage for comprehension and mastery.

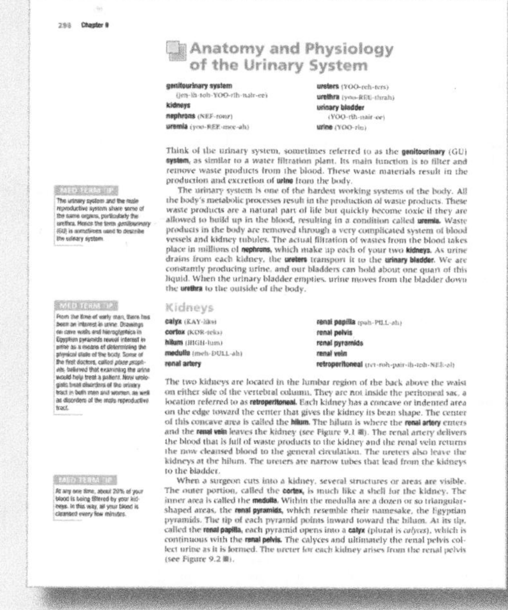

298 Chapter 9

Anatomy and Physiology of the Urinary System

genitourinary system (jen-ih-toh-YOO-rih-nair-ee)
kidneys
nephrons (NEF-ronz)
uremia (yoo-REE-mee-ah)
ureters (YOO-reh-ters)
urethra (yoo-REE-thrah)
urinary bladder (YOO-rih-nair-ee)
urine (YOO-rin)

Think of the urinary system, sometimes referred to as the **genitourinary** (GU) **system**, as similar to a water filtration plant. Its main function is to filter and remove waste products from the blood. These waste materials result in the production and excretion of **urine** from the body.

The urinary system is one of the hardest working systems of the body. All the body's metabolic processes result in the production of waste products. These waste products are a natural part of life but quickly become toxic if they are allowed to build up in the blood, resulting in a condition called **uremia**. Waste products in the body are removed through a very complicated system of blood vessels and kidney tubules. The actual filtration of wastes from the blood takes place in millions of **nephrons**, which make up each of your two **kidneys**. As urine drains from each kidney, the **ureters** transport it to the **urinary bladder**. We are constantly producing urine, and our bladders can hold about one quart of this liquid. When the urinary bladder empties, urine moves from the bladder down the **urethra** to the outside of the body.

MED TERM TIP

The urinary system and the male reproductive system share some of the same organs, particularly the urethra. Hence the term *genitourinary* (GU) is sometimes used to describe the urinary system.

Kidneys

calyx (KAY-liks)
cortex (KOR-teks)
hilum (HIGH-lum)
medulla (meh-DULL-ah)
renal artery
renal papilla (pah-PILL-ah)
renal pelvis
renal pyramids
renal vein
retroperitoneal (ret-roh-pair-ih-toh-NEE-al)

The two kidneys are located in the lumbar region of the back above the waist on either side of the vertebral column. They are not inside the peritoneal sac, a location referred to as **retroperitoneal**. Each kidney has a concave or indented area on the edge toward the center that gives the kidney its bean shape. The center of this concave area is called the **hilum**. The hilum is where the **renal artery** enters and the **renal vein** leaves the kidney (see Figure 9.1 ■). The renal artery delivers the blood that is full of waste products to the kidney and the renal vein returns the now cleansed blood to the general circulation. The ureters also leave the kidneys at the hilum. The ureters are narrow tubes that lead from the kidneys to the bladder.

When a surgeon cuts into a kidney, several structures or areas are visible. The outer portion, called the **cortex**, is much like a shell for the kidney. The inner area is called the **medulla**. Within the medulla are a dozen or so triangular-shaped areas, the **renal pyramids**, which resemble their namesake, the Egyptian pyramids. The tip of each pyramid points inward toward the hilum. At its tip, called the **renal papilla**, each pyramid opens into a **calyx** (plural is *calyces*), which is continuous with the **renal pelvis**. The calyces and ultimately the renal pelvis collect urine as it is formed. The ureter for each kidney arises from the renal pelvis (see Figure 9.2 ■).

MED TERM TIP

From the time of early man, there has been an interest in urine. Drawings on cave walls and hieroglyphics in Egyptian pyramids reveal interest in urine as a means of determining the physical state of the body. Some of the first doctors, called *pisse prophets*, believed that examining the urine would help treat a patient. Now urologists treat disorders of the urinary tract in both men and women, as well as disorders of the male reproductive tract.

MED TERM TIP

At any one time, about 20% of your blood is being filtered by your kidneys. In this way, all your blood is cleansed every few minutes.

Med Term Tips

This popular feature offers tidbits of noteworthy information about medical terms that engage learners.

Medically-Accurate Illustrations

Concepts come to life with vibrant, clear, consistent, and scientifically precise images.

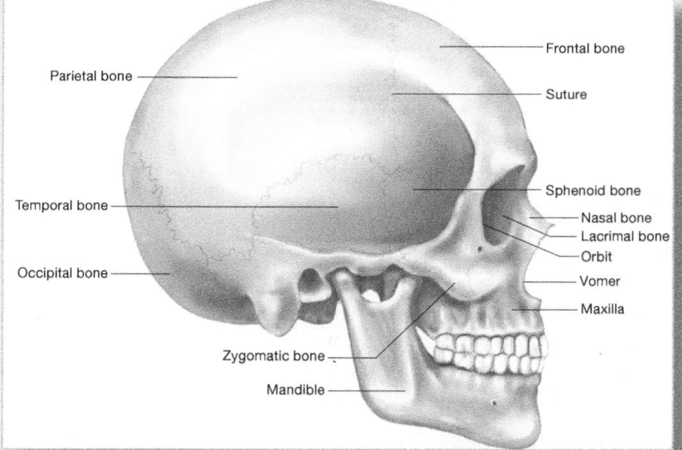

Word Tables

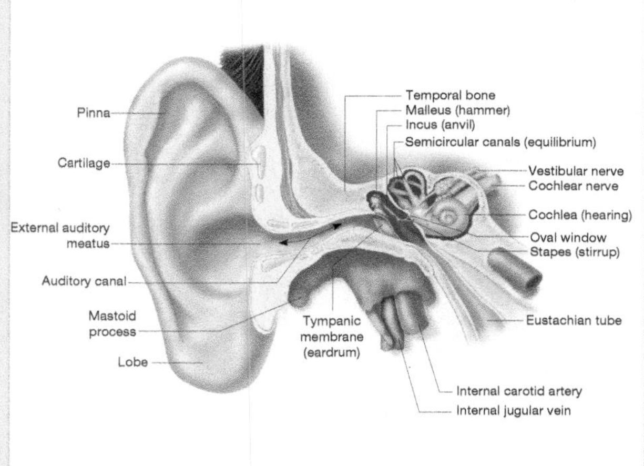

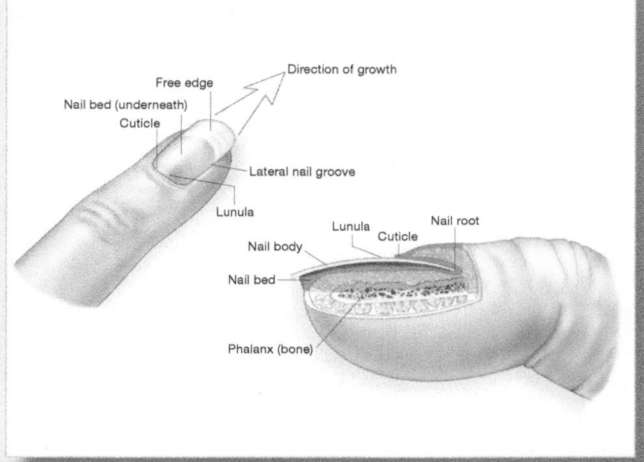

Study lists are categorized and presented in a clear, logical, color-coded format that eases the learning process.

Workbook Sections

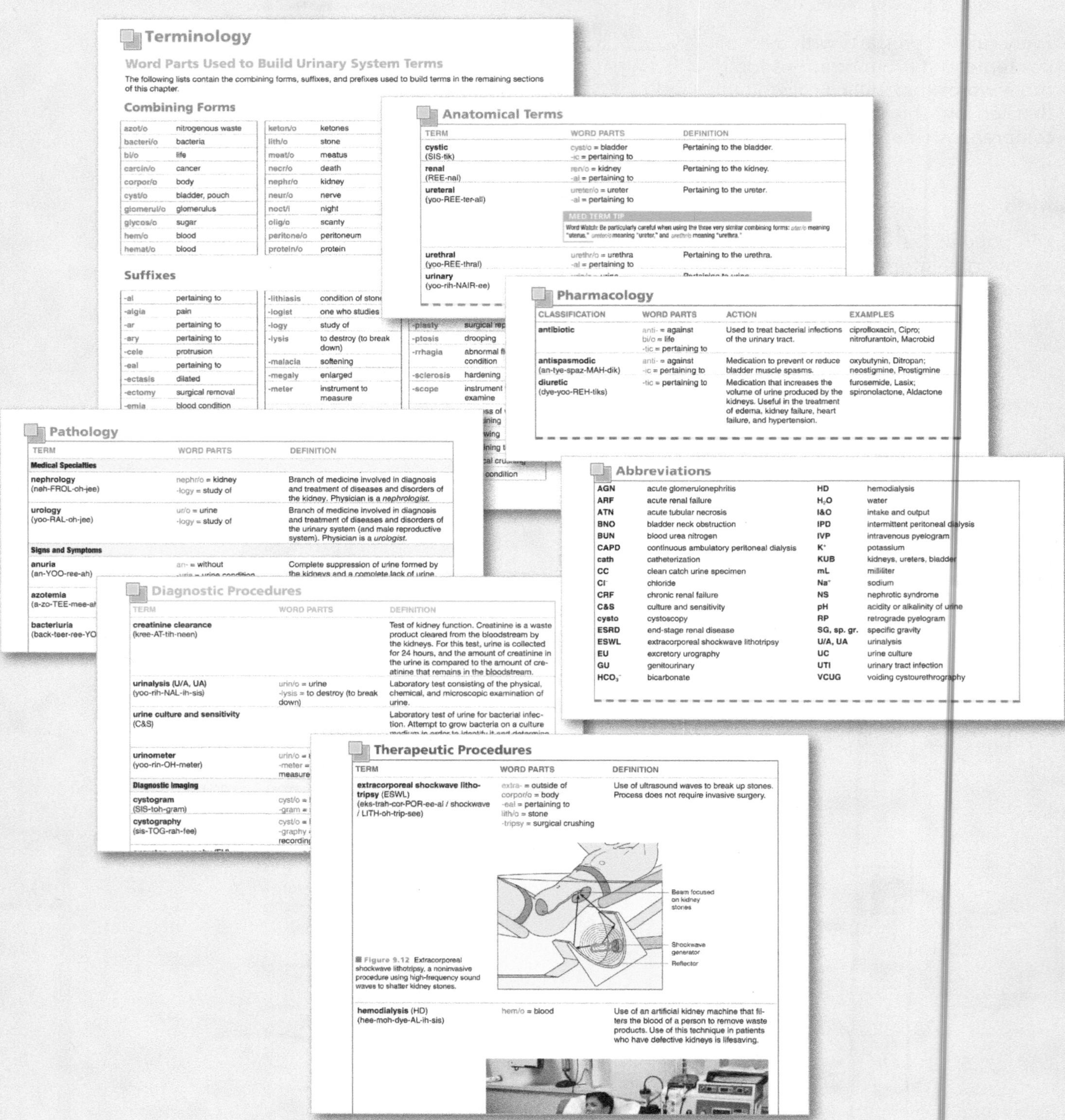

Terminology

Word Parts Used to Build Urinary System Terms

The following lists contain the combining forms, suffixes, and prefixes used to build terms in the remaining sections of this chapter.

Combining Forms

azot/o	nitrogenous waste	keton/o	ketones
bacteri/o	bacteria	lith/o	stone
bi/o	life	meat/o	meatus
carcin/o	cancer	necr/o	death
corpor/o	body	nephr/o	kidney
cyst/o	bladder, pouch	neur/o	nerve
glomerul/o	glomerulus	noct/i	night
glycos/o	sugar	olig/o	scanty
hem/o	blood	peritone/o	peritoneum
hemat/o	blood	protein/o	protein

Suffixes

-al	pertaining to	-lithiasis	condition of stone		
-algia	pain	-logist	one who studies		
-ar	pertaining to	-logy	study of	-plasty	surgical rep
-ary	pertaining to	-lysis	to destroy (to break down)	-ptosis	drooping
-cele	protrusion			-rrhagia	abnormal fl
-eal	pertaining to	-malacia	softening		condition
-ectasis	dilated	-megaly	enlarged	-sclerosis	hardening
-ectomy	surgical removal	-meter	instrument to measure	-scope	instrument examine
-emia	blood condition				

Anatomical Terms

TERM	WORD PARTS	DEFINITION
cystic (SIS-tik)	cyst/o = bladder -ic = pertaining to	Pertaining to the bladder.
renal (REE-nal)	ren/o = kidney -al = pertaining to	Pertaining to the kidney.
ureteral (yoo-REE-ter-all)	ureter/o = ureter -al = pertaining to	Pertaining to the ureter.
urethral (yoo-REE-thral)	urethr/o = urethra -al = pertaining to	Pertaining to the urethra.
urinary (yoo-rih-NAIR-ee)		

MED TERM TIP

Word Watch: Be particularly careful when using the three very similar combining forms: uter/o meaning "uterus," ureter/o meaning "ureter," and urethr/o meaning "urethra."

Pharmacology

CLASSIFICATION	WORD PARTS	ACTION	EXAMPLES
antibiotic	anti- = against bi/o = life -tic = pertaining to	Used to treat bacterial infections of the urinary tract.	ciprofloxacin, Cipro; nitrofurantoin, Macrobid
antispasmodic (an-tye-spaz-MAH-dik)	anti- = against -ic = pertaining to	Medication to prevent or reduce bladder muscle spasms.	oxybutynin, Ditropan; neostigmine, Prostigmine
diuretic (dye-yoo-REH-tiks)	-tic = pertaining to	Medication that increases the volume of urine produced by the kidneys. Useful in the treatment of edema, kidney failure, heart failure, and hypertension.	furosemide, Lasix; spironolactone, Aldactone

Pathology

TERM	WORD PARTS	DEFINITION
Medical Specialties		
nephrology (neh-FROL-oh-jee)	nephr/o = kidney -logy = study of	Branch of medicine involved in diagnosis and treatment of diseases and disorders of the kidney. Physician is a *nephrologist*.
urology (yoo-RAL-oh-jee)	ur/o = urine -logy = study of	Branch of medicine involved in diagnosis and treatment of diseases and disorders of the urinary system (and male reproductive system). Physician is a *urologist*.
Signs and Symptoms		
anuria (an-YOO-ree-ah)	an- = without	Complete suppression of urine formed by the kidneys and a complete lack of urine
azotemia (a-zo-TEE-mee-a		
bacteriuria (back-teer-ree-YO		

Abbreviations

AGN	acute glomerulonephritis	HD	hemodialysis
ARF	acute renal failure	H_2O	water
ATN	acute tubular necrosis	I&O	intake and output
BNO	bladder neck obstruction	IPD	intermittent peritoneal dialysis
BUN	blood urea nitrogen	IVP	intravenous pyelogram
CAPD	continuous ambulatory peritoneal dialysis	K^+	potassium
cath	catheterization	KUB	kidneys, ureters, bladder
CC	clean catch urine specimen	mL	milliliter
Cl^-	chloride	Na^+	sodium
CRF	chronic renal failure	NS	nephrotic syndrome
C&S	culture and sensitivity	pH	acidity or alkalinity of urine
cysto	cystoscopy	RP	retrograde pyelogram
ESRD	end-stage renal disease	SG, sp. gr.	specific gravity
ESWL	extracorporeal shockwave lithotripsy	U/A, UA	urinalysis
EU	excretory urography	UC	urine culture
GU	genitourinary	UTI	urinary tract infection
HCO_3^-	bicarbonate	VCUG	voiding cystourethrography

Diagnostic Procedures

TERM	WORD PARTS	DEFINITION
creatinine clearance (kree-AT-tih-neen)		Test of kidney function. Creatinine is a waste product cleared from the bloodstream by the kidneys. For this test, urine is collected for 24 hours, and the amount of creatinine in the urine is compared to the amount of creatinine that remains in the bloodstream.
urinalysis (U/A, UA) (yoo-rih-NAL-ih-sis)	urin/o = urine -lysis = to destroy (to break down)	Laboratory test consisting of the physical, chemical, and microscopic examination of urine.
urine culture and sensitivity (C&S)		Laboratory test of urine for bacterial infection. Attempt to grow bacteria on a culture
urinometer (yoo-rin-OH-meter)	urin/o = -meter = measure	
Diagnostic Imaging		
cystogram (SIS-toh-gram)	cyst/o = -gram =	
cystography (sis-TOG-rah-fee)	cyst/o = -graphy = recording	

Therapeutic Procedures

TERM	WORD PARTS	DEFINITION
extracorporeal shockwave lithotripsy (ESWL) (eks-trah-cor-POR-ee-al / shockwave / LITH-oh-trip-see)	extra- = outside of corpor/o = body -eal = pertaining to lith/o = stone -tripsy = surgical crushing	Use of ultrasound waves to break up stones. Process does not require invasive surgery.
hemodialysis (HD) (hee-moh-dye-AL-ih-sis)	hem/o = blood	Use of an artificial kidney machine that filters the blood of a person to remove waste products. Use of this technique in patients who have defective kidneys is lifesaving.

Figure 9.12 Extracorporeal shockwave lithotripsy, a noninvasive procedure using high-frequency sound waves to shatter kidney stones.

A wide array of exercises at the end of each chapter serve as a fun and challenging study review. Here are some examples:

Labeling Exercises—A visual challenge to reinforce students' grasp of anatomy & physiology concepts.

Medical Record Analysis—Exercises that challenge students to read examples of real medical records and then to apply their medical terminology knowledge in answering related questions.

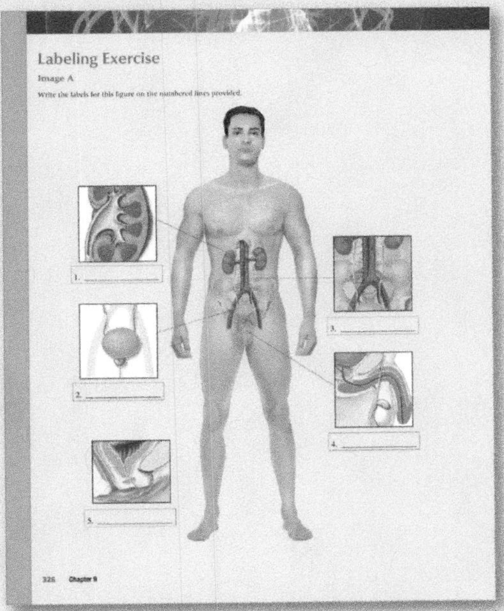

Labeling Exercise

Image A

Write the labels for this figure on the numbered lines provided.

1. ______
2. ______
3. ______
4. ______
5. ______

326 Chapter 9

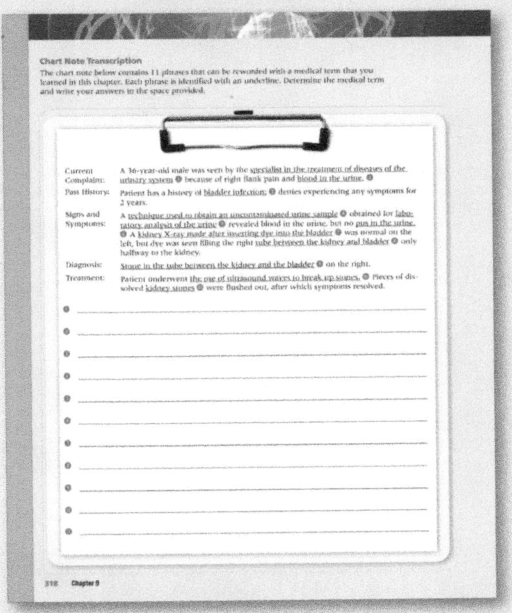

Chart Note Transcription

The chart note below contains 11 phrases that can be reworded with a medical term that you learned in this chapter. Each phrase is identified with an underline. Determine the medical term and write your answers in the space provided.

Current Complaint:	A 36-year-old male was seen by the specialist in the treatment of diseases of the urinary system ❶ because of right flank pain and blood in the urine. ❷
Past History:	Patient has a history of bladder infection; ❸ denies experiencing any symptoms for 2 years.
Signs and Symptoms:	A technique used to obtain an uncontaminated urine sample ❹ obtained for laboratory analysis of the urine ❺ revealed blood in the urine, but no pus in the urine. ❻ A kidney X-ray made after inserting dye into the bladder ❼ was normal on the left, but dye was seen filling the right tube between the kidney and bladder ❽ only halfway to the kidney.
Diagnosis:	Stone in the tube between the kidney and the bladder ❾ on the right.
Treatment:	Patient underwent the use of ultrasound waves to break up stones. ❿ Pieces of dissolved kidney stones ⓫ were flushed out, after which symptoms resolved.

❶ ______
❷ ______
❸ ______
❹ ______
❺ ______
❻ ______
❼ ______
❽ ______
❾ ______
❿ ______
⓫ ______

318 Chapter 9

Case Study—Scenarios that use critical thinking questions to help students develop a firmer understanding of the terminology in context.

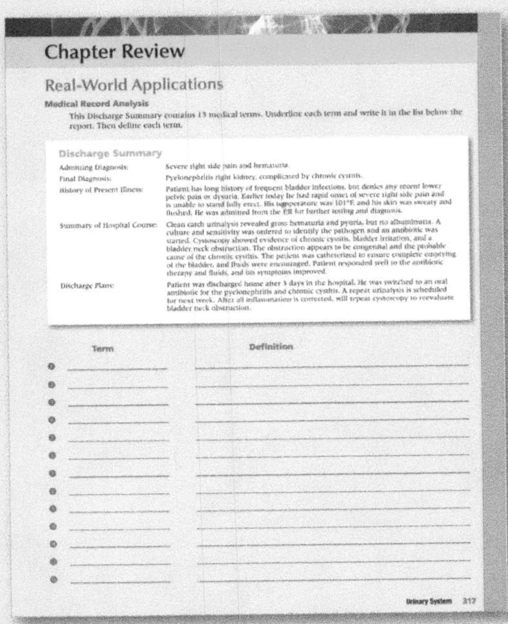

Chapter Review

Real-World Applications

Medical Record Analysis

This Discharge Summary contains 13 medical terms. Underline each term and write it in the list below the report. Then define each term.

Discharge Summary

Admitting Diagnosis:	Severe right side pain and hematuria.
Final Diagnosis:	Pyelonephritis right kidney, complicated by chronic cystitis.
History of Present Illness:	Patient has long history of frequent bladder infections, but denies any recent lower pelvic pain or dysuria. Earlier today he had rapid onset of severe right side pain and is unable to stand fully erect. His temperature was 101°F, and his skin was sweaty and flushed. He was admitted from the ER for further testing and diagnosis.
Summary of Hospital Course:	Clean catch urinalysis revealed gross hematuria and pyuria, but no albuminuria. A culture and sensitivity was ordered to identify the pathogen and an antibiotic was started. Cystoscopy showed evidence of chronic cystitis, bladder irritation, and a bladder neck obstruction. The obstruction appears to be congenital and the probable cause of the chronic cystitis. The patient was catheterized to ensure complete emptying of the bladder, and fluids were encouraged. Patient responded well to the antibiotic therapy and fluids, and his symptoms improved.
Discharge Plans:	Patient was discharged home after 3 days in the hospital. He was switched to an oral antibiotic for the pyelonephritis and chronic cystitis. A repeat urinalysis is scheduled for next week. After all inflammation is corrected, will repeat cystoscopy to reevaluate bladder neck obstruction.

	Term	Definition
❶	______	______
❷	______	______
❸	______	______
❹	______	______
❺	______	______
❻	______	______
❼	______	______
❽	______	______
❾	______	______
❿	______	______
⓫	______	______
⓬	______	______
⓭	______	______

Urinary System 317

Chart Note Transcription—Slice-of-real-life exercise that asks students to replace lay terms in a medical chart with the proper medical term.

Case Study

Below is a case study presentation of a patient with a condition discussed in this chapter. Read the case study and answer the questions below. Some questions will ask for information not included within this chapter. Use your text, a medical dictionary, or any other reference material you choose to answer these questions.

A 32-year-old female is seen in the urologist's office because of a fever, chills, and generalized fatigue. She also reported urgency, frequency, dysuria, and hematuria. In addition, she noticed that her urine was cloudy with a fishy odor. The physician ordered the following tests: a clean catch specimen for a U/A, a urine C&S, and a KUB. The U/A revealed pyuria, bacteriuria, and a slightly acidic pH. A common type of bacteria was grown in the culture. X-rays reveal acute pyelonephritis resulting from cystitis, which has spread up to the kidney from the bladder. The patient was placed on an antibiotic and encouraged to "push fluids" by drinking 2L of water a day.

(Gina Smith/Shutterstock)

Questions

1. This patient has two urinary system infections in different locations; name them. Which one caused the other and how?
2. List and define each of the patient's presenting symptoms in your own words.
3. What diagnostic tests did the urologist order? Describe them in your own words.
4. Explain the results of each diagnostic test in your own words.
5. What were the physician's treatment instructions for this patient? Explain the purpose of each treatment.
6. Describe the normal appearance of urine.

Preface

Since the first edition of ***Medical Terminology: A Living Language*** was

published it has been noted for its "clean" and logical format that promotes learning. In this revised edition, we have built upon this strength by enhancing many features to make this text an ideal choice for semester-or quarter-length courses.

Features of this Edition

This new fifth edition contains features that facilitate student mastery, while maintaining the best aspects of previous editions. Each chapter is arranged in a similar format and the content is organized with an emphasis on maintaining consistency and accuracy. All terms have been evaluated to ensure they remain in current use and reflect the newest technologies and procedures.

We have revised ***Medical Terminology: A Living Language*** so that it provides for an even more valuable teaching and learning experience. Here are the enhancements we have made:

- The Terminology section includes a comprehensive list of all combining forms, suffixes, and prefixes used to build terms in the remaining sections of the chapter.
- The Signs and Symptoms subsection within the Pathology table contains disease-related terms grouped by organ. This allows terms to be categorized into smaller groups, therefore making learning easier.
- Improved three-column format in the word building sections allows for the term (with pronunciation and/or abbreviation), word parts (if appropriate), and definitions to be displayed. The Pharmacology table also includes word parts in a new fourth column.
- The Anatomical Terms section includes anatomical terms as well as adjective forms of organs.
- Color-coded word parts—red combining forms, blue suffixes, and green prefixes allow for quick recognition throughout the book.
- The Real World Applications section now contains three critical thinking activities (Medical Record Analysis, Chart Note Transcription, and a new Case Study) to allow readers to apply their knowledge to real world situations.

Organization of the Book

Introductory Chapter

Chapter 1 contains information necessary for an understanding of how medical terms are formed. This includes learning about word roots, combining forms, prefixes, and suffixes, and general rules for building medical terms. Readers will also learn about terminology for medical records and the different health care settings. Chapter 2 presents terminology relating to the body organization, including organs and body systems. Here readers will first encounter word building tables, a feature found in each remaining chapter that lists medical terms and their respective word parts.

Anatomy and Physiology Chapters

Chapters 3 through 13 are organized by body system. Each chapter begins with a System

At A Glance which lists combining forms, prefixes, and/or suffixes with their meanings and is followed by System Illustrated overview of the organs in the system. The anatomy and physiology section is divided into the various components of the system, and each subsection begins with a list of key medical terms accompanied by a pronunciation guide. Key terms are boldfaced the first time they appear in the narrative. The Terminology section of each chapter begins with a list of all word parts used within the chapter. For ease of learning, the medical terms are divided into five separate sections: anatomical terms, pathology, diagnostic procedures, therapeutic procedures, and pharmacology. The word parts used to build terms are highlighted within each table. An abbreviations section then follows to complete the chapter.

Special Topics Chapter

Chapter 14 contains timely information and appropriate medical terms relevant to the following medical specialties: pharmacology, mental health, diagnostic imaging, rehabilitation services, surgery, and oncology. Knowledge of these topics is necessary for the well-rounded health care worker.

Appendices

The appendices contain helpful reference lists of word parts and definitions. This information is intended for quick access. There are three word part/definition appendices: Word Parts Arranged Alphabetically and Defined, Word Parts Arranged Alphabetically by Definition and Abbreviations. All of the key terms appear again in the glossary/index at the end of the text.

Supplemental Resources

The chapters and appendices are comprehensive and current, offering content and practices needed to prepare for your next steps in the health science learning continuum. However, the health care environment is rapidly changing, particularly diagnostic and treatment practices and procedures. Additionally, recording and reporting procedures and reimbursement requirements are continuously being revised with new medical terminology introduced. To stay current, additional resources should be explored and accessed to supplement the content and enhance the activities presented. Examine medical and dental dictionaries and multimedia resources, interpret technical materials, journals, fact sheets, newsletters and professional association materials, and government agencies that set new standards and guidelines related to health care and investigate electronic media with appropriate supervision.

Bonnie F. Fremgen

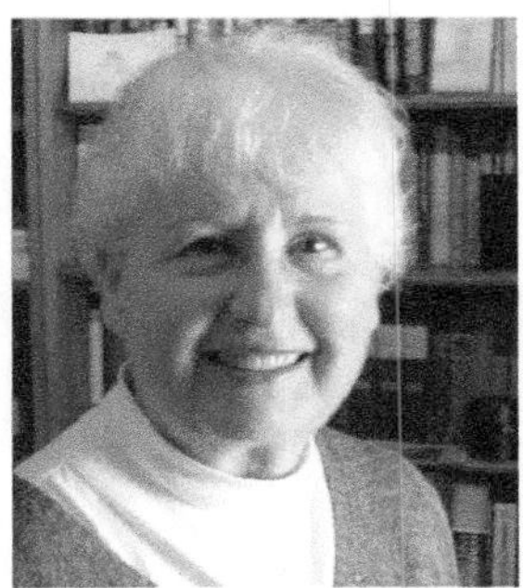

Bonnie F. Fremgen is a former associate dean of the Allied Health Program at Robert Morris College. She has taught medical law and ethics courses as well as clinical and administrative topics. In addition, she has served as an advisor for students' career planning. She has broad interests and experiences in the health care field, including hospitals, nursing homes, and physicians' offices.

Dr. Fremgen holds a nursing degree as well as a master's in health care administration. She received her PhD from the College of Education at the University of Illinois. She has performed postdoctoral studies in Medical Law at Loyola University Law School in Chicago. She has authored five textbooks with Pearson.

Suzanne S. Frucht

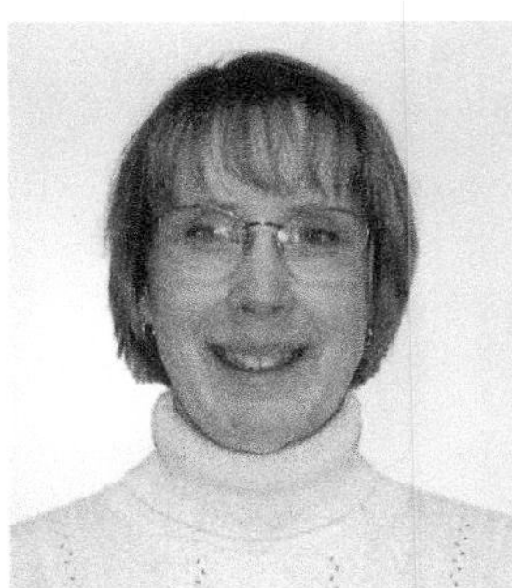

Suzanne S. Frucht is an Associate Professor Emeritus of Anatomy and Physiology at Northwest Missouri State University (NWMSU). She holds baccalaureate degrees in biological sciences and physical therapy from Indiana University, an MS in biological sciences at NWMSU, and a PhD in molecular biology and biochemistry from the University of Missouri-Kansas City.

For 14 years she worked full-time as a physical therapist in various health care settings, including acute care hospitals, extended care facilities, and home health. Based on her educational and clinical experience she was invited to teach medical terminology part-time in 1988 and became a full-time faculty member three years later as she discovered her love for the challenge of teaching. She taught a variety of courses including medical terminology, human anatomy, human physiology, and animal anatomy and physiology. She received the Governor's Award for Excellence in Teaching in 2003. After retiring from teaching in 2008, she continues to be active in student learning through writing medical terminology texts and anatomy and physiology laboratory manuals.

About the Illustrators

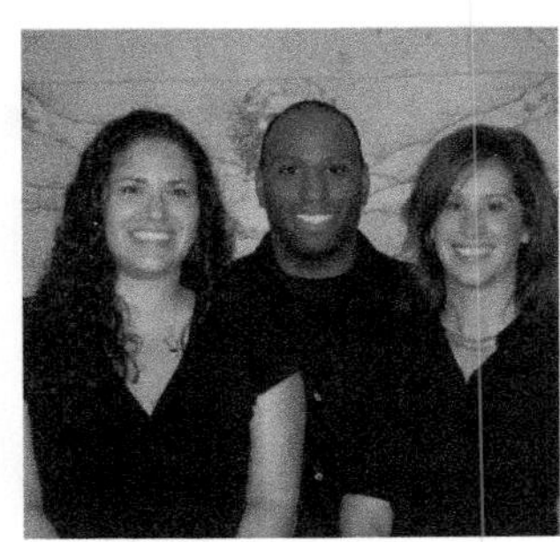

Marcelo Oliver is president and founder of Body Scientific International LLC. He holds an MFA degree in Medical and Biological Illustration from University of Michigan. For the past 15 years, his passion has been to condense complex anatomical information into visual education tools for students, patients, and medical professionals. For seven years he worked as a medical illustrator and creative director developing anatomical charts used for student and patient education. In the years that followed, he created educational and marketing tools for medical device companies prior to founding Body Scientific International, LLC.

Body Scientific's lead artists in this publication were medical illustrators Liana Bauman and Katie Burgess. Both hold an Master of Science degrees in Biomedical Visualization degree from the University of Illinois at Chicago. Their contribution in the publication was key in the creation and editing of artwork throughout.

Dr. Pam Besser Ph.D

Contents

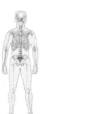

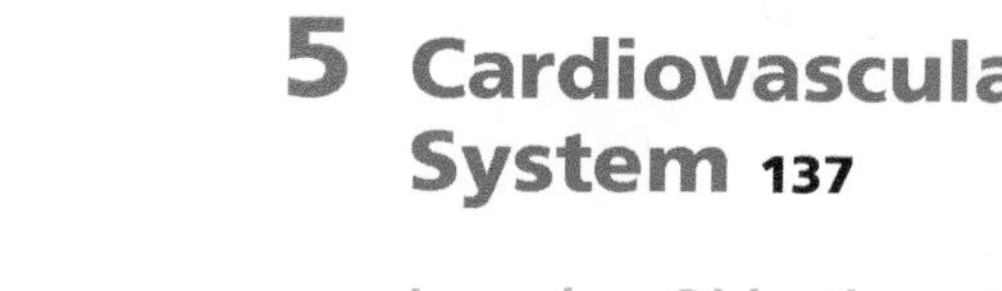

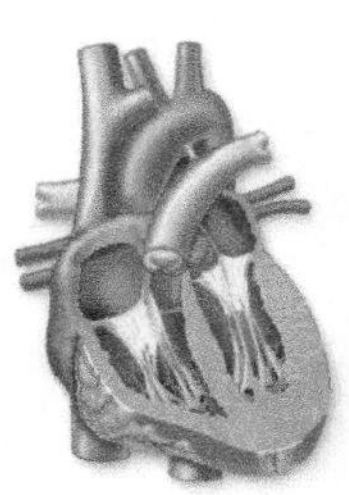

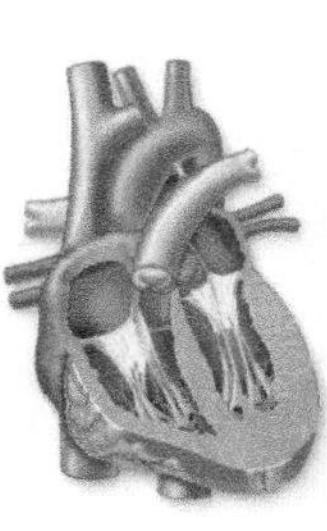

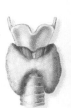

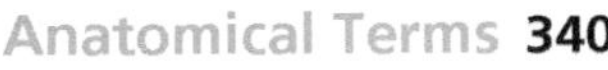

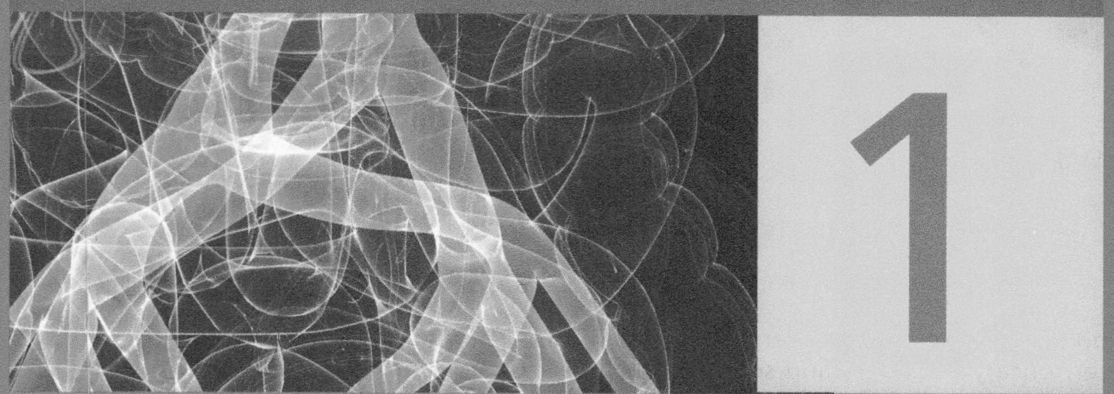

1

INTRODUCTION TO MEDICAL TERMINOLOGY

Learning Objectives

Upon completion of this chapter, you will be able to

- Discuss the four parts of medical terms.
- Recognize word roots and combining forms.
- Identify the most common prefixes and suffixes.
- Define word building and describe a strategy for translating medical terms.
- State the importance of correct spelling of medical terms.
- State the rules for determining singular and plural endings.
- Discuss the importance of using caution with abbreviations.
- Recognize the documents found in a medical record.
- Recognize the different healthcare settings.
- Understand the importance of confidentiality.
- Understand reporting and recording medical information.
- Review health care teams.

Medical Terminology at a Glance

Learning medical terminology can initially seem like studying a strange new language. However, once you understand some of the basic rules about how medical terms are formed using word building, it will become much like piecing together a puzzle. The general guidelines for forming words; an understanding of word roots, combining forms, prefixes, and suffixes; pronunciation; and spelling are discussed in this chapter. In addition, "Med Term Tips" are sprinkled throughout to assist in clarifying some of the material. New medical terms discussed in each section are listed separately at the beginning of the section, and each chapter contains numerous pathological, diagnostic, treatment, and surgical terms. You can use these lists as an additional study tool for previewing and reviewing terms.

Understanding medical terms requires you being able to put words together or build words from their parts. It is impossible to memorize thousands of medical terms; however, once you understand the basics, you can distinguish the meaning of medical terms by analyzing their prefixes, suffixes, and word roots. Remember that there will always be some exceptions to every rule, and medical terminology is no different. We attempt to point out these exceptions where they exist. Most medical terms, however, do follow the general rule that there is a **word root** or fundamental meaning for the word, a **prefix** and a **suffix** that modify the meaning of the word root, and sometimes a **combining vowel** to connect other word parts. You will be amazed at the seemingly difficult words you will be able to build and understand when you follow the simple steps in word building (see Figure 1.1 ■).

You have likely spent time with a medical or dental specialist in the past. As you begin to study medical and dental terminology and phrases, use your prior knowledge and experiences from those visits to recall how these terms were used. Also think about how you learned to use word parts and combining phrases in English language arts, mathematics, and science coursework. The process is much the same for medical terminology. But remember, that while it is essential to master medical terminology, it is also important that you are able to translate the terminology into language that patients and clients can understand.

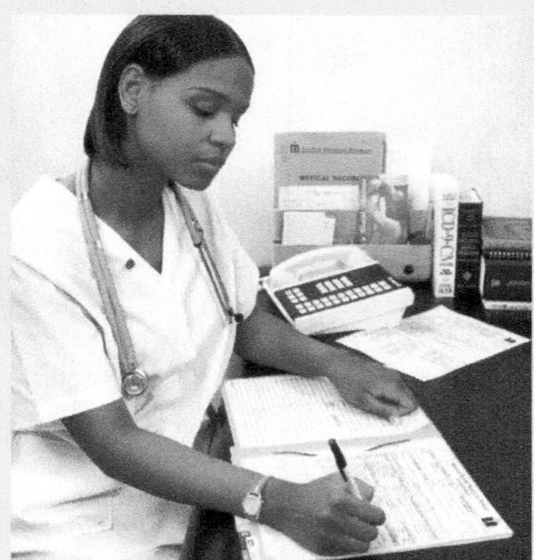

■ **Figure 1.1** Nurse completing a patient report. Healthcare workers use medical terminology in order to accurately and efficiently communicate patient information to each other.

Building Medical Terms from Word Parts

Four different word parts or elements can be used to construct medical terms:

1. The **word root** is the foundation of the word.	**cardi**ogram = record of the heart
2. A **prefix** is at the beginning of the word.	**peri**cardium = around the heart
3. A **suffix** is at the end of the word.	card**itis** = inflammation of the heart
4. The **combining vowel** is a vowel (usually *o*) that links the word root to another word root or a suffix.	cardi**o**my**o**pathy = disease of the heart muscle

MED TERM TIP

Medical terms are built from word parts:

Word Building Part	Example (Meaning)
1. Word root	*cardi* (heart)
2. Prefix	*peri-* (around)
3. Suffix	*-itis* (inflammation)

When these components are put together, the word *pericarditis* is formed, meaning inflammation around the heart.

The following sections on word roots, combining vowels and forms, prefixes, and suffixes will consider each of these word parts in more detail and present examples of some of those most commonly used. Medical terms must be appropriate for the health science scenario; spelled, written, and pronounced correctly. Breaking words into parts will help with pronunciation.

Word Roots

The word root is the foundation of a medical term and provides the general meaning of the word. The word root often indicates the body system or part of the body being discussed, such as *cardi* for heart. At other times the word root may be an action. For example, the word root *cis* means to cut (as in incision).

A term may have more than one word root. For example, **osteoarthritis** (oss-tee-oh-ar-THRY-tis) combines the word root *oste* meaning bone and *arthr* meaning the joints. When the suffix *-itis*, meaning inflammation, is added, we have the entire word, meaning an inflammation involving bone at the joints.

Combining Vowel/Form

To make it possible to pronounce long medical terms with ease and to combine several word parts, a combining vowel is used. This is most often the vowel *o*. Combining vowels are utilized in two places: between a word root and a suffix or between two word roots.

To decide whether or not to use a combining vowel between a word root and a suffix, first look at the suffix. If it begins with a vowel, do not use the combining vowel. If, however, the suffix begins with a consonant, then use a combining vowel. For example: To combine *arthr* with *-scope* will require a combining vowel: **arthroscope** (AR-throh-scope). But to combine *arthr* with *-itis* does not require a combining vowel: **arthritis** (ar-THRY-tis).

The combining vowel is typically kept between two word roots, even if the second word root begins with a vowel. For example, in forming the term **gastroenteritis** (gas-troh-en-ter-EYE-tis) the combining vowel is kept between the two word roots *gastr* and *enter* (gastrenteritis is incorrect). As you can tell from pronouncing these two terms, the combining vowel makes the pronunciation easier.

When writing a word root by itself, its **combining form** is typically used. This consists of the word root and its combining vowel written in a word root/vowel form, for example, *cardi/o*. Since it is often simpler to pronounce word roots when they appear in their combining form, this format is used throughout this text.

MED TERM TIP

Remember to break down every word into its components (prefix, word root/combining form, and suffix) when learning medical terminology. Do not try to memorize every medical term. Instead, figure out how the word is formed from its components. In a short time you will be able to do this automatically when seeing a new term.

Common Combining Forms

Some commonly used word roots in their combining form, their meaning, and examples of their use follow. Review the examples to observe when a combining vowel was kept and when it was dropped according to the rules presented on the preceding page.

COMBINING FORM	MEANING	EXAMPLE (DEFINITION)
aden/o	gland	adenopathy (gland disease)
carcin/o	cancer	carcinoma (cancerous tumor)
cardi/o	heart	cardiac (pertaining to the heart)
chem/o	chemical	chemotherapy (treatment with chemicals)
cis/o	to cut	incision (process of cutting into)
dermat/o	skin	dermatology (study of the skin)
enter/o	small intestine	enteric (pertaining to the small intestine)
gastr/o	stomach	gastric (pertaining to the stomach)
gynec/o	female	gynecology (study of females)
hemat/o	blood	hematic (pertaining to the blood)
hydr/o	water	hydrocele (protrusion of water [in the scrotum])
immun/o	immunity	immunology (study of immunity)
laryng/o	voice box	laryngeal (pertaining to the voice box)
nephr/o	kidney	nephromegaly (enlarged kidney)
neur/o	nerve	neural (pertaining to a nerve)
ophthalm/o	eye	ophthalmic (pertaining to the eye)
ot/o	ear	otic (pertaining to the ear)
path/o	disease	pathology (study of disease)
pulmon/o	lung	pulmonary (pertaining to the lungs)
rhin/o	nose	rhinoplasty (surgical repair of the nose)

Prefixes

A new medical term is formed when a prefix is added to the front of the term. Prefixes frequently give information about the location of an organ, the number of parts, or the time (frequency). For example, the prefix *bi-* stands for two of something, such as **bilateral** (bye-LAH-ter-al), meaning to have two sides. However, not every term will have a prefix.

Common Prefixes

Some of the more common prefixes, their meanings, and examples of their use follow. When written by themselves, prefixes are followed by a hyphen.

PREFIX	MEANING	EXAMPLE (DEFINITION)
a-	without, away from	aphasia (without speech)
an-	without	anoxia (without oxygen)
ante-	before, in front of	antepartum (before birth)
anti-	against	antibiotic (against life)
auto-	self	autograft (a graft from one's own body)
brady-	slow	bradycardia (slow heartbeat)
contra-	against	contraception (against conception)
de-	without	depigmentation (without pigment)
dys-	painful, difficult, abnormal	dyspnea (difficulty breathing)
endo-	within, inner	endoscope (instrument to view within)
epi-	upon, over	epigastric (upon or over the stomach)
eso-	inward	esotropia (inward turning)
eu-	normal, good	eupnea (normal breathing)
ex-	external, outward	exostosis (condition of external bone)
exo-	outward	exotropia (outward turning)
extra-	outside of	extracorporeal (outside of the body)
hetero-	different	heterograft (graft [like a skin graft] from another species)
homo-	same	homograft (graft [like a skin graft] from the same species)
hydro-	water	hydrotherapy (water therapy)
hyper-	over, above	hypertrophy (overdevelopment)
hypo-	under, below	hypodermic (under the skin)
in-	not; inward	infertility (not fertile); inhalation (to breathe in)
inter-	among, between	intervertebral (between the vertebrae)
intra-	within, inside	intravenous (inside, within a vein)
macro-	large	macrotia (having large ears)
micro-	small	microtia (having small ears)
myo-	to shut	myopia (to shut eyes/squint)
neo-	new	neonatology (study of the newborn)
pan-	all	pansinusitis (inflammation of all the sinuses)
para-	beside, near; abnormal; two like parts of a pair	paranasal (beside the nose); paresthesia (abnormal sensation); paraplegia (paralysis of two like parts of a pair/the legs)
per-	through	percutaneous (through the skin)
peri-	around	pericardial (around the heart)
post-	after	postpartum (after birth)
pre-	before, in front of	preoperative (before a surgical operation)
pro-	before	prolactin (before milk)
pseudo-	false	pseudocyesis (false pregnancy)

MED TERM TIP

Be very careful with prefixes; many have similar spellings but very different meanings. For example:

anti- means "against"; *ante-* means "before"

inter- means "between"; *intra-* means "inside"

per- means "through"; *peri-* means "around"

PREFIX	MEANING	EXAMPLE (DEFINITION)
retro-	backward, behind	retroperitoneal (behind the peritoneum)
sub-	below, under	subcutaneous (under, below the skin)
supra-	above	suprapubic (above the pubic bone)
tachy-	rapid, fast	tachycardia (fast heartbeat)
trans-	through, across	transurethral (across the urethra)
ultra-	beyond, excess	ultrasound (high-frequency sound waves)
un-	not	unconscious (not conscious)

Number Prefixes

Some common prefixes pertaining to the number of items or measurement, their meanings, and examples of their use follow.

PREFIX	MEANING	EXAMPLE (DEFINITION)
bi-	two	bilateral (two sides)
hemi-	half	hemiplegia (paralysis of one side/half of the body)
mono-	one	monoplegia (paralysis of one extremity)
multi-	many	multigravida (woman pregnant more than once)
nulli-	none	nulligravida (woman with no pregnancies)
poly-	many	polyuria (large amounts of urine)
primi-	first	primigravida (first pregnancy)
quadri-	four	quadriplegia (paralysis of all four limbs)
semi-	partial, half	semiconscious (partially conscious)
tetra-	four	tetraplegia (paralysis of all four limbs)
tri-	three	triceps (muscle with three heads)

Suffixes

A suffix is attached to the end of a word to add meaning, such as a condition, disease, or procedure. For example, the suffix *-itis,* meaning inflammation, when added to *cardi-* forms the new word **carditis** (car-DYE-tis), meaning inflammation of the heart. Every medical term *must* have a suffix. Most often the suffix is added to a word root, as in carditis above; however, terms can also be built from a suffix added directly to a prefix, without a word root. For example, the term **dystrophy** (DIS-troh-fee), meaning abnormal development, is built from the prefix *dys-* (meaning abnormal) and the suffix *-trophy* (meaning development).

MED TERM TIP

Remember, if a suffix begins with a vowel, the combining vowel is dropped; for example, *mastitis* rather than *mast**o**itis.*

Common Suffixes

Some common suffixes, their meanings, and examples of their use follow. When written by themselves, suffixes are preceded by a hyphen.

SUFFIX	MEANING	EXAMPLE (DEFINITION)
-algia	pain	gastralgia (stomach pain)
-cele	hernia, protrusion	cystocele (protrusion of the bladder)

SUFFIX	MEANING	EXAMPLE (DEFINITION)
-cyte	cell	erythrocyte (red cell)
-dynia	pain	cardiodynia (heart pain)
-ectasis	dilation	bronchiectasis (dilated bronchi)
-gen	that which produces	pathogen (that which produces disease)
-genesis	produces, generates	spermatogenesis (produces sperm)
-genic	producing, produced by	carcinogenic (producing cancer)
-ia	state, condition	bradycardia (condition of slow heart)
-iasis	abnormal condition	lithiasis (abnormal condition of stones)
-iatry	medical treatment	podiatry (medical treatment for the foot)
-ism	state of	hypothyroidism (state of low thyroid)
-itis	inflammation	dermatitis (inflammation of skin)
-logist	one who studies	cardiologist (one who studies the heart)
-logy	study of	cardiology (study of the heart)
-lysis	destruction	hemolysis (blood destruction)
-lytic	destruction	thrombolytic (clot destruction)
-malacia	abnormal softening	chondromalacia (abnormal cartilage softening)
-megaly	enlargement, large	cardiomegaly (enlarged heart)
-oid	resembling	fibroid (resembling fibers)
-oma	tumor, mass, swelling	carcinoma (cancerous tumor)
-osis	abnormal condition	cyanosis (abnormal condition of being blue)
-pathy	disease	myopathy (muscle disease)
-phobia	fear	photophobia (fear of light)
-plasia	development, growth	hyperplasia (excessive development)
-plasm	formation, development	neoplasm (new formation)
-ptosis	drooping	blepharoptosis (drooping eyelid)
-rrhage	excessive, abnormal flow	hemorrhage (excessive bleeding)
-rrhagia	abnormal flow condition	cystorrhagia (abnormal flow from the bladder)
-rrhea	discharge, flow	rhinorrhea (discharge from the nose)
-rrhexis	rupture	hysterorrhexis (ruptured uterus)
-sclerosis	hardening	arteriosclerosis (hardening of an artery)
-stenosis	narrowing	angiostenosis (narrowing of a vessel)
-therapy	treatment	chemotherapy (treatment with chemicals)
-trophy	nourishment, development	hypertrophy (excessive development)
-ule	small	venule (small vein)

Adjective Suffixes

The following suffixes are used to convert a word root into an adjective. These suffixes usually are translated as *pertaining to.*

SUFFIX	MEANING	EXAMPLE (DEFINITION)
-ac	pertaining to	cardiac (pertaining to the heart)
-al	pertaining to	duodenal (pertaining to the duodenum)
-an	pertaining to	ovarian (pertaining to the ovary)
-ar	pertaining to	ventricular (pertaining to a ventricle)
-ary	pertaining to	pulmonary (pertaining to the lungs)
-atic	pertaining to	lymphatic (pertaining to lymph)
-eal	pertaining to	esophageal (pertaining to the esophagus)
-iac	pertaining to	chondriac (pertaining to cartilage)
-ic	pertaining to	gastric (pertaining to the stomach)
-ile	pertaining to	penile (pertaining to the penis)
-ine	pertaining to	uterine (pertaining to the uterus)
-ior	pertaining to	superior (pertaining to above)
-nic	pertaining to	embryonic (pertaining to an embryo)
-ory	pertaining to	auditory (pertaining to hearing)
-ose	pertaining to	adipose (pertaining to fat)
-ous	pertaining to	intravenous (pertaining to within a vein)
-tic	pertaining to	acoustic (pertaining to hearing)

Surgical Suffixes

The following suffixes indicate surgical procedures.

MED TERM TIP

Surgical suffixes have very specific meanings:

-otomy means "to cut into"
-ostomy means "to create a new opening"
-ectomy means "to cut out" or "remove"

SUFFIX	MEANING	EXAMPLE (DEFINITION)
-centesis	puncture to withdraw fluid	arthrocentesis (puncture to withdraw fluid from a joint)
-ectomy	surgical removal	gastrectomy (surgically remove the stomach)
-ostomy	surgically create an opening	colostomy (surgically create an opening for the colon [through the abdominal wall])
-otomy	cutting into	thoracotomy (cutting into the chest)
-pexy	surgical fixation	nephropexy (surgical fixation of a kidney)
-plasty	surgical repair	dermatoplasty (surgical repair of the skin)
-rrhaphy	suture	myorrhaphy (suture together muscle)

Procedural Suffixes

The following suffixes indicate procedural processes or instruments.

SUFFIX	MEANING	EXAMPLE (DEFINITION)
-gram	record or picture	electrocardiogram (record of heart's electricity)
-graph	instrument for recording	electrocardiograph (instrument for recording the heart's electrical activity)

SUFFIX	MEANING	EXAMPLE (DEFINITION)
-graphy	process of recording	electrocardiography (process of recording the heart's electrical activity)
-meter	instrument for measuring	audiometer (instrument to measure hearing)
-metry	process of measuring	audiometry (process of measuring hearing)
-scope	instrument for viewing	gastroscope (instrument to view stomach)
-scopy	process of visually examining	gastroscopy (process of visually examining the stomach)

Word Building

Word building consists of putting together two or more word elements to form a variety of terms. Prefixes and suffixes may be added to a combining form to create a new descriptive term. For example, adding the prefix *hypo-* (meaning below) and the suffix *-ic* (meaning pertaining to) to the combining form *derm/o* (meaning skin) forms **hypodermic** (high-poh-DER-mik), pertaining to below the skin.

Interpreting Medical Terms

The following strategy is a reliable method for puzzling out the meaning of an unfamiliar medical term.

STEP	EXAMPLE
1. Divide the term into its word parts.	gastr/o/enter/o/logy
2. Define each word part.	**gastr** = stomach **o** = combining vowel, no meaning **enter** = small intestine **o** = combining vowel, no meaning **-logy** = study
3. Combine the meaning of the word parts.	stomach, small intestine, study of

MED TERM TIP

To gain a quick understanding of a term, it may be helpful to you to read from the end of the word (or the suffix) back to the beginning (the prefix), and then pick up the word root. For example, *pericarditis* reads inflammation (*-itis*) surrounding (*peri-*) the heart (*cardi/o*).

Pronunciation

You will hear different pronunciations for the same terms depending on where people were born or educated. As long as it is clear which term people are discussing, differing pronunciations are acceptable. Some people are difficult to understand over the telephone or on a transcription tape. If you have any doubt about a term being discussed, ask for the term to be spelled. For example, it is often difficult to hear the difference between the terms **abduction** and **adduction**. However, since the terms refer to opposite directions of movement, it is very important to double-check if there is any question about which term was used.

Each new term in this text is introduced in boldface type, with the phonetic or "sounds like" pronunciation in parentheses immediately following. The part of the word that should receive the greatest emphasis during pronunciation appears in capital letters: for example, **pericarditis** (per-ih-car-DYE-tis).

Spelling

> **MED TERM TIP**
>
> If you have any doubt about the meaning or spelling of a word, look it up in your medical dictionary. Even experienced medical personnel still need to look up a few words.

Although you will hear differing pronunciations of the same term, there will be only one correct spelling. If you have any doubt about the spelling of a term or of its meaning, always look it up in a medical dictionary. If only one letter of the word is changed, it could make a critical difference for the patient. For example, imagine the problem that could arise if you note for insurance purposes that a portion of a patient's **ileum,** or small intestine, was removed when in reality he had surgery for removal of a piece of his **ilium,** or hip bone.

Some words have the same beginning sounds but are spelled differently. Examples include:

Sounds like *si*

psy	**psychiatry** (sigh-KIGH-ah-tree)
cy	**cytology** (sigh-TALL-oh-gee)

Sounds like *dis*

dys	**dyspepsia** (dis-PEP-see-ah)
dis	**dislocation** (dis-low-KAY-shun)

Singular and Plural Endings

Many medical terms originate from Greek and Latin words. The rules for forming the singular and plural forms of some words follow the rules of these languages rather than English. For example, the heart has a left atrium and a right atrium for a total of two *atria,* not two *atriums.* Other words, such as *virus* and *viruses,* are changed from singular to plural by following English rules. Each medical term needs to be considered individually when changing from the singular to the plural form. The following examples illustrate how to form plurals.

Words ending in	Singular	Plural
-a	vertebra	vertebrae
-ax	thorax	thoraces
-ex or -ix	appendix	appendices
-is	metastasis	metastases
-ma	sarcoma	sarcomata
-nx	phalanx	phalanges
-on	ganglion	ganglia
-us	nucleus	nuclei
-um	ovum	ova
-y	biopsy	biopsies

Abbreviations and Acronyms

Abbreviations are commonly used in the medical profession as a way of saving time. However, some abbreviations can be confusing, such as *SM* for simple mastectomy and *sm* for small. Use of the incorrect abbreviation can result in problems for a patient, as well as with insurance records and processing. An acronym is formed by using the first letter of several words combined. Acronyms can be identified since they are pronounced as a word such as ROM (range of motion). As with abbreviations the acronyms are replete throughout health care to create a more concise method of recording and reporting medical information. If you have any concern that you will confuse someone by using an abbreviation or acronym, spell out the word instead. It is never acceptable to use made-up abbreviations. All types of healthcare facilities will have a list of approved abbreviations, and it is extremely important that you become familiar with this list and follow it closely.

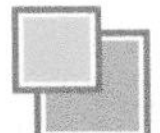

The Medical Record

The **medical record** or chart documents the details of a patient's hospital stay. Each healthcare professional who has contact with the patient in any capacity completes the appropriate report of that contact and adds it to the medical chart. This results in a permanent physical record of the patient's day-to-day condition, when and what services he or she received, and the response to treatment. Each institution adopts a specific format for each document and its location within the chart. This is necessary because each healthcare professional must be able to locate quickly and efficiently the information he or she needs in order to provide proper care for the patient. The medical record is also a legal document. Therefore, it is essential that all chart components be completely filled out and signed. Each page must contain the proper patient identification information: the patient's name, age, gender, physician, admission date, and identification number.

While the patient is still in the hospital, a unit clerk is usually responsible for placing documents in the proper place. After discharge, the medical records department ensures that all documents are present, complete, signed, and in the correct order. If a person is readmitted, especially for the same diagnosis, parts of this previous chart can be pulled and added to the current chart for reference (see Figure 1.2 ■). Physicians' offices and other outpatient care providers such as clinics and therapists also maintain a medical record detailing each patient's visit to their facility.

The digital revolution has impacted health care with the introduction and increasing use of the **Electronic Health Record EHR**, also referred to as the Electronic Medical Record (EMR). In 2000 the Institute of Medicine (IOM) reported that almost 100,000 people each year die from medical errors. It is believed that many of these errors can be corrected with the use of EHRs. Today nearly every aspect of health care is being impacted by the use of electronic recording and reporting. EHRs are defined as a longitudinal electronic record of patient health information generated by one or more encounters in any care delivery setting. The EHR is a confidential and legal document. Unauthorized personnel do not have the privilege of reading, recording or sharing information on the document. With your supervisor investigate a sample EHR to see what information is included and identify the medical terminology abbreviations and acronyms used for recording the information.

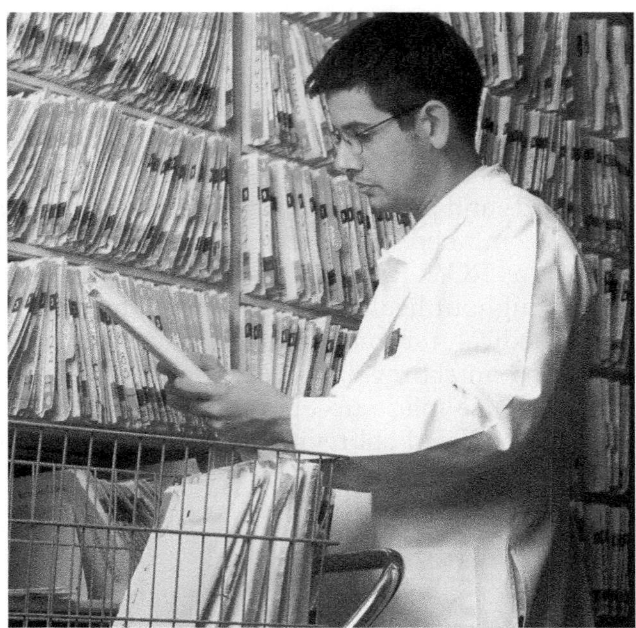

Figure 1.2 Health information professionals maintain accurate, orderly, and permanent patient records. Medical records are securely stored and available for future reference.

History and Physical—Written or dictated by admitting physician; details patient's history, results of physician's examination, initial diagnoses, and physician's plan of treatment

Physician's Orders—Complete list of care, medications, tests, and treatments physician orders for patient

Nurse's Notes—Record of patient's care throughout the day; includes vital signs, treatment specifics, patient's response to treatment, and patient's condition

Physician's Progress Notes—Physician's daily record of patient's condition, results of physician's examinations, summary of test results, updated assessment and diagnoses, and further plans for patient's care

Consultation Reports—Reports given by specialists whom physician has asked to evaluate patient

Ancillary Reports—Reports from various treatments and therapies patient has received, such as rehabilitation, social services, or respiratory therapy

Diagnostic Reports—Results of diagnostic tests performed on patient, principally from clinical lab (e.g., blood tests) and medical imaging (e.g., X-rays and ultrasound)

Informed Consent—Document voluntarily signed by patient or a responsible party that clearly describes purpose, methods, procedures, benefits, and risks of a diagnostic or treatment procedure

Operative Report—Report from surgeon detailing an operation; includes pre- and postoperative diagnosis, specific details of surgical procedure itself, and how patient tolerated procedure

Anesthesiologist's Report—Relates details regarding substances (such as medications and fluids) given to patient, patient's response to anesthesia, and vital signs during surgery

Pathologist's Report—Report given by pathologist who studies tissue removed from patient (e.g., bone marrow, blood, or tissue biopsy)

Discharge Summary—Comprehensive outline of patient's entire hospital stay; includes condition at time of admission, admitting diagnosis, test results, treatments and patient's response, final diagnosis, and follow-up plans

Healthcare Settings

The use of medical terminology is widespread. It provides healthcare professionals with a precise and efficient method of communicating very specific patient information to one another, regardless of whether they are in the same type of facility (see Figure 1.3 ■). Descriptions follow of the different types of settings where medical terminology is used.

Acute Care or General Hospitals—Provide services to diagnose (laboratory, diagnostic imaging) and treat (surgery, medications, therapy) diseases for a short period of time; in addition, they usually provide emergency and obstetrical care

Specialty Care Hospitals—Provide care for very specific types of diseases; for example, a psychiatric hospital

Nursing Homes or Long-Term Care Facilities—Provide long-term care for patients needing extra time to recover from illness or injury before returning home, or for persons who can no longer care for themselves

Ambulatory Care Centers, Surgical Centers, or Outpatient Clinics—Provide services not requiring overnight hospitalization; services range from simple surgeries to diagnostic testing or therapy

Physicians' Offices—Provide diagnostic and treatment services in a private office setting

Health Maintenance Organization (HMO)—Provides wide range of services by a group of primary-care physicians, specialists, and other healthcare professionals in a prepaid system

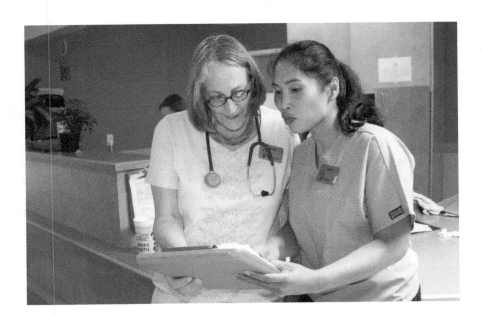

■ **Figure 1.3** A nurse and medical assistant review a patient's chart and plan his or her daily care.

Home Health Care—Provides nursing, therapy, personal care, or housekeeping services in patient's own home

Rehabilitation Centers—Provide intensive physical and occupational therapy; includes inpatient and outpatient treatment

Hospices—Provide supportive treatment to terminally ill patients and their families

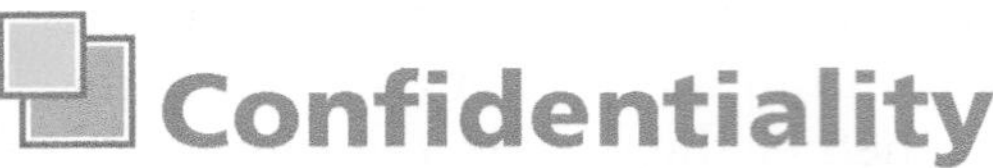

Confidentiality

Anyone working with medical terminology and involved in the medical profession must have a firm understanding of confidentiality. Any information or record relating to a patient must be considered privileged. This means that you have a moral and legal responsibility to keep all information about the patient confidential. If you are asked to supply documentation relating to a patient, the proper authorization form must be signed by the patient. Give only the specific information that the patient has authorized. The Health Insurance Portability and Accountability Act of 1996 (HIPAA) set federal standards providing patients with more protection of their medical records and health information, better access to their own records, and greater control over how their health information is used and to whom it is disclosed.

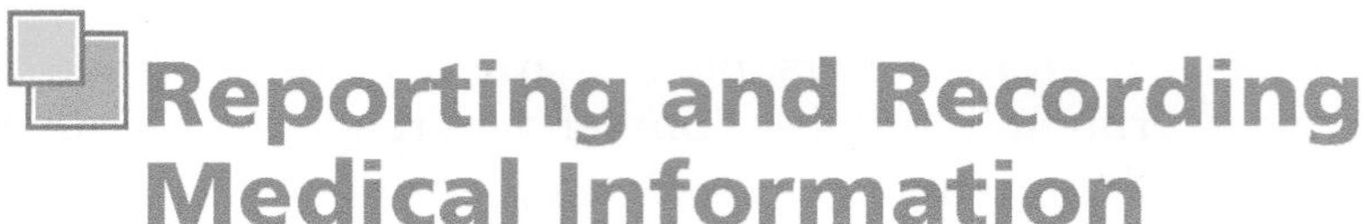

Reporting and Recording Medical Information

Medical information is often shared with a variety of health care providers. This information describes the patients' status and accurate reporting can affect the outcomes. For the best results possible, the information and ideas must be expressed, accurately, clearly and concisely to ensure that diagnosis and treatment is appropriate and beneficial to the recipient. To achieve this goal, as noted in this chapter, abbreviations such as 'sm' or EMR and acronyms such as PET scan are used for data reporting. It is important to be familiar with the many medical abbreviations and acronyms commonly used in health care practices.

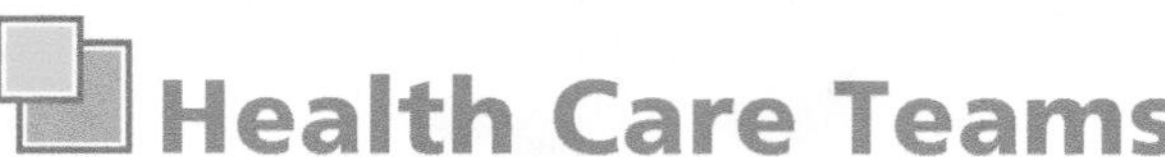

Health Care Teams

Research, prevention, diagnosis and treatment are all part of providing health care. Due to the scope of each process or procedure, practitioners with particular specialties must have the ability to cooperate, contribute, and collaborate as a team to ensure optimum care and treatment. From assistive personnel to the most highly prepared professional, each has a role in providing quality health care from research to uncover new diagnostics, practices and treatments to those that have direct contact with patients. To ensure the best outcome for those seeking care each team member must be competent in their role and participate as needed within their defined "scope of practice."

Chapter Review

Practice Exercises

A. Complete the Statement

1. The combination of a word root and the combining vowel is called a(n) ______________________.
2. The vowel that connects two word roots or a suffix with a word root is usually a(n) ______________________.
3. A word part used at the end of a word root to change the meaning of the word is called a(n) ______________________.
4. A(n) ______________________ is used at the beginning of a word to indicate number, location, or time.
5. Although the pronunciation of medical terms may differ slightly from one person to another, the ______________________ must never change.
6. The four components of a medical term are ______________________, ______________________, ______________________, and ______________________.

B. Terminology Matching

Match each definition to its term.

1. _______ Provides services for a short period of time
2. _______ Complete outline of a patient's entire hospital stay
3. _______ Describes purpose, methods, benefits, and risks of procedure
4. _______ Contains updated assessment, diagnoses, and further plans for care
5. _______ Provides supportive care to terminally ill patients and families
6. _______ Written by the admitting physician
7. _______ Reports results from study of tissue removed from the patient
8. _______ Written by the surgeon
9. _______ Provides services not requiring overnight hospital stay
10. _______ Report given by a specialist
11. _______ Record of a patient's care through the day
12. _______ Clinical lab and medical imaging reports
13. _______ Provides intensive physical and occupational therapy
14. _______ Report of treatment/therapy the patient received
15. _______ Provides care for patients who need more time to recover

a. rehabilitation center
b. nurse's notes
c. ancillary report
d. hospice
e. discharge summary
f. physician's progress notes
g. ambulatory care center
h. diagnostic report
i. long-term care facility
j. informed consent
k. history and physical
l. acute care hospital
m. pathologist's report
n. consultation report
o. operative report

C. Define the Suffix

1. -plasty ____________
2. -stenosis ____________
3. -itis ____________
4. -al ____________
5. -algia ____________
6. -otomy ____________
7. -megaly ____________
8. -ectomy ____________
9. -rrhage ____________
10. -centesis ____________
11. -gram ____________
12. -ac ____________
13. -malacia ____________
14. -ism ____________
15. -rrhaphy ____________
16. -ostomy ____________
17. -pexy ____________
18. -rrhea ____________
19. -scopy ____________
20. -oma ____________

D. Combining Form and Suffix Practice

Join a combining form and a suffix to form words with the following meanings.

1. study of lungs ____________
2. pain relating to a nerve ____________
3. nose discharge or flow ____________
4. abnormal softening of a kidney ____________
5. enlarged heart ____________
6. cutting into the stomach ____________
7. inflammation of the skin ____________
8. surgical removal of the voice box ____________
9. surgical repair of a joint ____________
10. gland disease ____________

E. Name That Prefix

1. within, inside ____________
2. large ____________
3. before, in front of ____________
4. around ____________
5. new ____________

6. without ______________________________

7. half ______________________________

8. painful, difficult ______________________________

9. above ______________________________

10. over, above ______________________________

11. many ______________________________

12. slow ______________________________

13. self ______________________________

14. across ______________________________

15. two ______________________________

F. Prefix Practice

Circle the prefixes in the following terms and define in the space provided.

1. tachycardia ______________________________
2. pseudocyesis ______________________________
3. hypoglycemia ______________________________
4. intercostal ______________________________
5. eupnea ______________________________
6. postoperative ______________________________
7. monoplegia ______________________________
8. subcutaneous ______________________________

G. Make It Plural

Change the following singular terms to plural terms.

1. metastasis ______________________________
2. ovum ______________________________
3. diverticulum ______________________________
4. atrium ______________________________
5. diagnosis ______________________________
6. vertebra ______________________________

H. Name That Term

Use the suffix -ology to write a term for each medical specialty.

1. heart ______________________________
2. stomach ______________________________
3. skin ______________________________
4. eye ______________________________
5. immunity ______________________________
6. kidney ______________________________
7. blood ______________________________
8. female ______________________________

9. nerve ______

10. disease ______

I. Abbreviations, Acronyms, and Medical Terms

Using a separate sheet of paper, re-write the paragraph using abbreviations, acronyms, and medical terms for more concise and effective recording and reporting.

As the patient enters the office you must ask her to complete and sign the Health Information Portability Accountability Act (HIPAA) Confidentiality form before seeing the physician. The physician has now completed an examination to determine the cause of the patients' complaint; stomach pain (gastralgia) in a small area in the lower right side. The physician enters the initial diagnostic information; inflammation of the appendix (appendicitis), into the Electronic Medical Record (EMR).

J. Building Medical Terms

Build a medical term by combining the word parts requested in each question.

For example, use the combining form for *spleen* with the suffix meaning *enlargement* to form a word meaning *enlargement of the spleen* (answer: *splenomegaly*).

1. combining form for *heart* ______
   suffix meaning *abnormal softening* ______
   ______ term meaning *softening of the heart*
2. word root form for *stomach* ______
   suffix meaning *to surgically create an opening* ______
   ______ term meaning *creating an opening into the stomach*
3. combining form for *nose* ______
   suffix meaning *surgical repair* ______
   ______ term meaning *surgical repair of the nose*
4. prefix meaning *over, above* ______
   suffix meaning *nourishment, development* ______
   ______ term meaning *overdevelopment*
5. combining form meaning *disease* ______
   suffix meaning *the study of* ______
   ______ term meaning *the study of disease*
6. word root meaning *gland* ______
   suffix for *tumor/mass* ______
   ______ term meaning *gland tumor or mass*
7. combining form meaning *stomach* ______
   combining form meaning *small intestine* ______
   suffix meaning *study of* ______
   ______ term meaning *study of stomach and small intestine*
8. word root meaning *ear* ______
   suffix meaning *inflammation* ______
   ______ term meaning *ear inflammation*
9. prefix meaning *water* ______
   suffix meaning *treatment* ______
   ______ term meaning *water treatment*
10. combining form meaning *cancer* ______
    suffix meaning *that which produces* ______
    ______ term meaning *that which produces cancer*

K. Write it out

SIDS____

CAT____

SCHIP____

RAD____

PET____

L. Define the Combining Form

1. aden/o ____
2. carcin/o ____
3. cardi/o ____
4. chem/o ____
5. cis/o ____
6. dermat/o ____
7. enter/o ____
8. gastr/o ____
9. gynec/o ____
10. hemat/o ____
11. hydr/o ____
12. immun/o ____
13. laryng/o ____
14. path/o ____
15. nephr/o ____
16. neur/o ____
17. ophthalm/o ____
18. ot/o ____
19. pulmon/o ____
20. rhin/o ____

M. Phonetic Practice

Use phonetic writing examples to aid in pronunciation of each word. With a partner, practice pronunciation using your phonetic examples.

Confidentiality____

Epithelium____

Appendicitis____

Physician____

Anesthesiologist____

Diagnosis____

N. Prior Knowledge

Using prior knowledge and experiences, list four medical or dental terms used by the office team during your visit(s).

1. ____

2. ____

3. ____

4. ____

O. Teamwork

In order for a team to function well, it is important to build relationships with all of your teammates. One way to develop a relationship is to find common bonds. For example, you and another team member might both enjoy playing soccer. Or, you might both have brothers or sisters. Or, you might both play the guitar. Discovering common bonds helps you understand the other person so you can work together successfully as a team.

In teams of four, identify at least five common bonds among you. How would the things you all have in common help you function better as a team? Work together to create a description of your team's dynamics. What are your strengths? What are your weaknesses? Present your team to the class and explain why it's essential to be able to contribute and collaborate as part of a team.

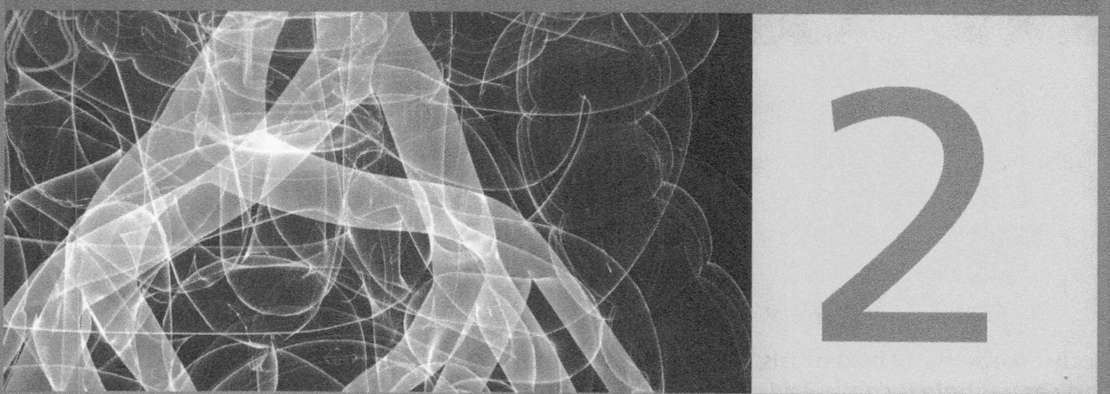

BODY ORGANIZATION

Learning Objectives

Upon completion of this chapter, you will be able to

- Recognize the combining forms introduced in this chapter.
- Correctly spell and pronounce medical terms and anatomical structures relating to body structure.
- Discuss the organization of the body in terms of cells, tissues, organs, and systems.
- Describe the common features of cells.
- Define the four types of tissues.
- List the major organs found in the 12 organ systems.
- Describe the anatomical position.
- Define the body planes.
- Identify regions of the body.
- Define directional and positional terms.
- List the body cavities and their contents.
- Locate and describe the nine anatomical and four clinical divisions of the abdomen.
- Build body organization medical terms from word parts.
- Interpret abbreviations associated with body organization.

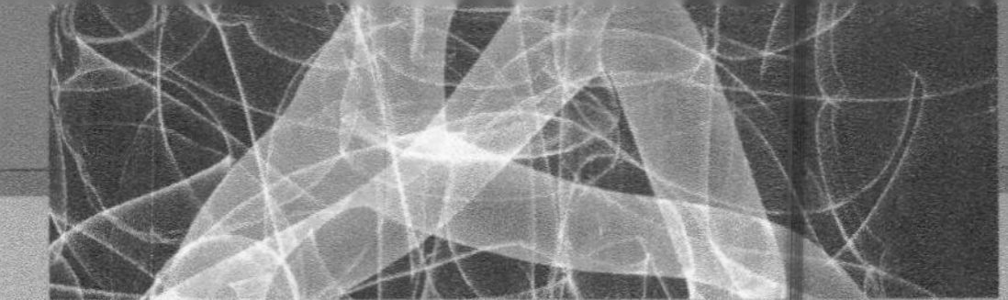

Body Organization at a Glance

Arrangement

The body is organized into levels; each is built from the one below it. In other words, the body as a whole is composed of systems, a system is composed of organs, an organ is composed of tissues, and tissues are composed of cells.

Levels

cells tissues organs systems body

Word Parts

Presented here are some of the more common combining forms used to build body organizational terms. For a list of the prefixes and suffixes used, refer to the Terminology section of this chapter.

Combining Forms

abdomin/o	abdomen
adip/o	fat
anter/o	front
brachi/o	arm
cardi/o	heart
caud/o	tail
cephal/o	head
cervic/o	neck
chondr/o	cartilage
crani/o	skull
crin/o	to secrete
crur/o	leg
cyt/o	cell
dermat/o	skin
dist/o	away from
dors/o	back of body
enter/o	small intestine
epitheli/o	epithelium
gastr/o	stomach
glute/o	buttock
gynec/o	woman
hemat/o	blood
hist/o	tissue
immun/o	protection
infer/o	below
laryng/o	larynx
later/o	side
lumb/o	loin
lymph/o	lymph
medi/o	middle
muscul/o	muscles
nephr/o	kidney
neur/o	nerve
ophthalm/o	eye
ot/o	ear
pelv/o	pelvis
peritone/o	peritoneum
pleur/o	pleura
poster/o	back
proct/o	rectum and anus
proxim/o	near to
pub/o	genital region
pulmon/o	lung
rhin/o	nose
spin/o	spine
super/o	above
thorac/o	chest
ur/o	urine
vascul/o	blood vessel
ventr/o	belly
vertebr/o	vertebra
viscer/o	internal organ

Body Organization Illustrated

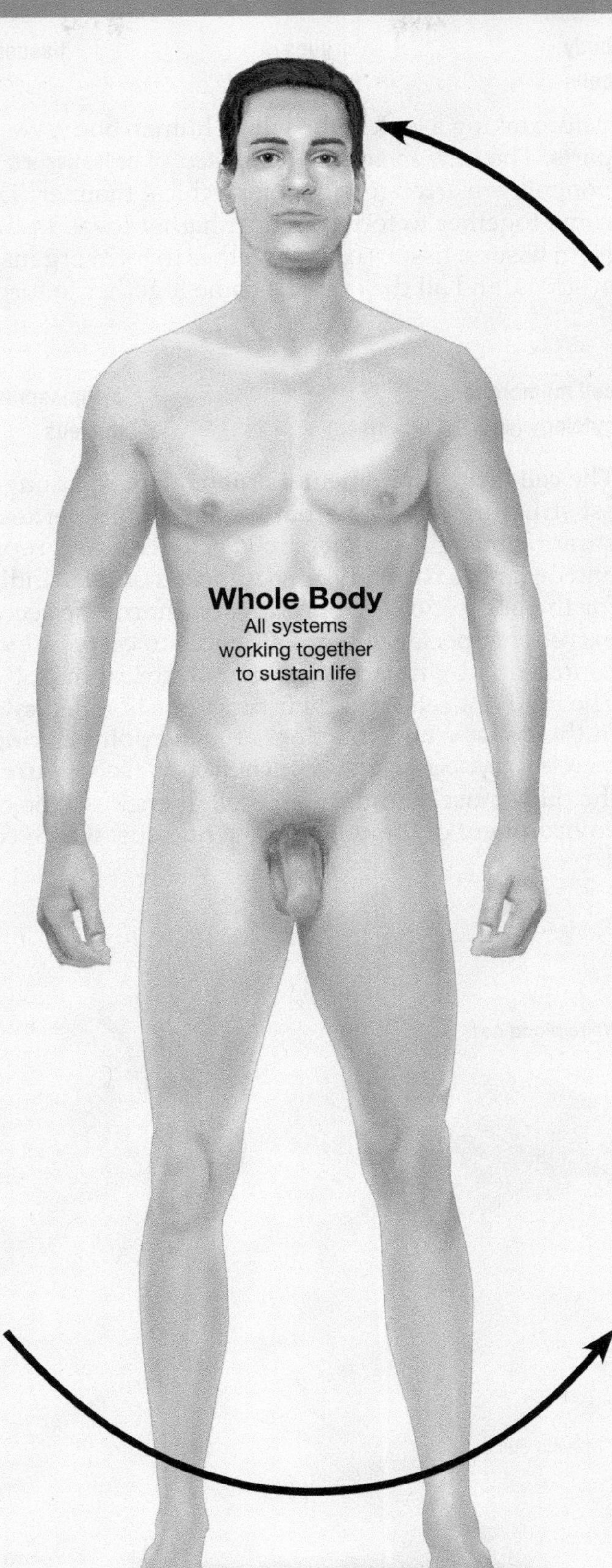

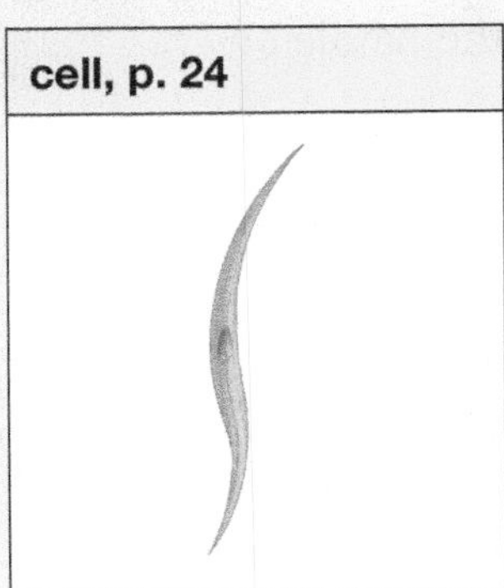

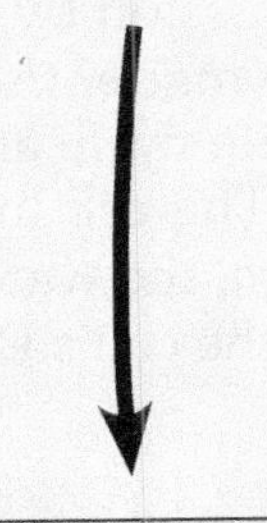

Basic unit of life

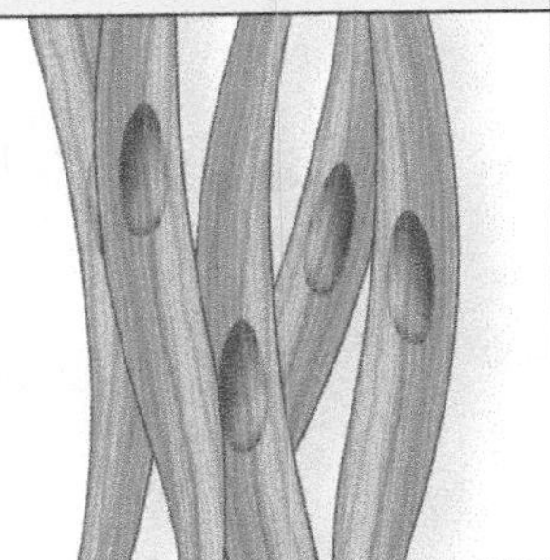

Group of identical cells working together

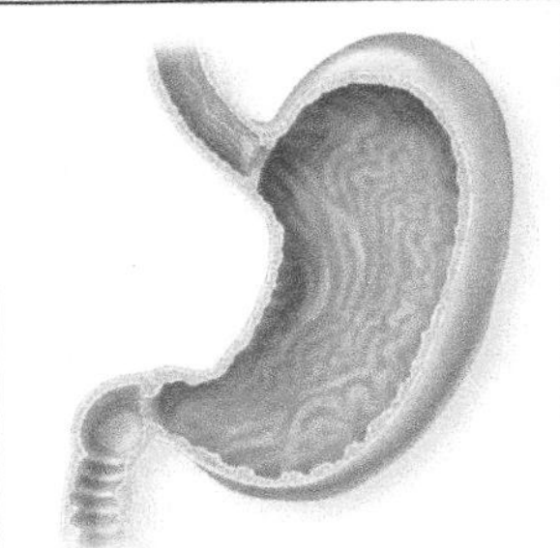

Composed of two or more types of tissue

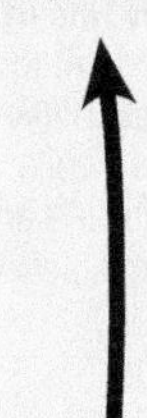

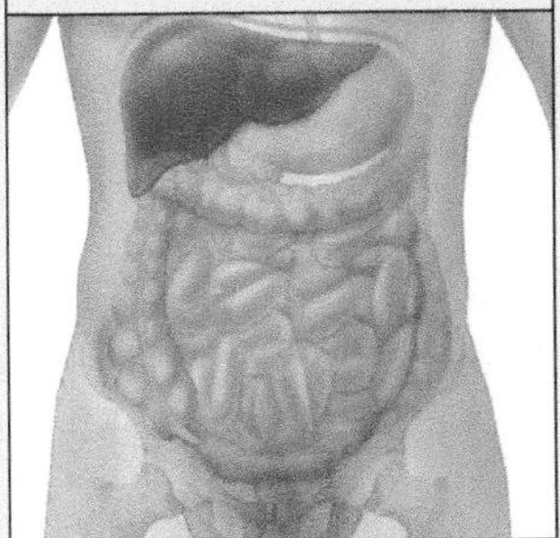

Collection of organs working together

Levels of Body Organization

body **cells** **organs** **systems** **tissues**

Before taking a look at the whole human body, we need to examine its component parts. The human **body** is composed of **cells, tissues, organs,** and **systems.** These components are arranged in a hierarchical manner. That is, parts from a lower level come together to form the next higher level. In that way, cells come together to form tissues, tissues come together to form organs, organs come together to form systems, and all the systems come together to form the whole body.

Cells

cell membrane
cytology (sigh-TALL-oh-jee)
cytoplasm (SIGH-toh-plazm)
nucleus

The cell is the fundamental unit of all living things. That is to say, it is the smallest structure of a body that has all the properties of being alive: responding to stimuli, engaging in metabolic activities, and reproducing itself. All the tissues and organs in the body are composed of cells. Individual cells perform functions for the body such as reproduction, hormone secretion, energy production, and excretion. Special cells are also able to carry out very specific functions, such as contraction by muscle cells and electrical impulse transmission by nerve cells. The study of cells and their functions is called **cytology.** No matter the difference in their shape and function, at some point during their life cycle all cells have a **nucleus, cytoplasm,** and a **cell membrane** (see Figure 2.1 ■). The cell membrane is the outermost boundary of a cell. It encloses the cytoplasm, the watery internal environment of the cell, and the nucleus, which contains the cell's DNA.

MED TERM TIP

Cells were first seen by Robert Hooke over 300 years ago. To him, the rectangular shapes looked like prison cells, so he named them cells. It was a common practice for early anatomists to name an organ solely on its appearance.

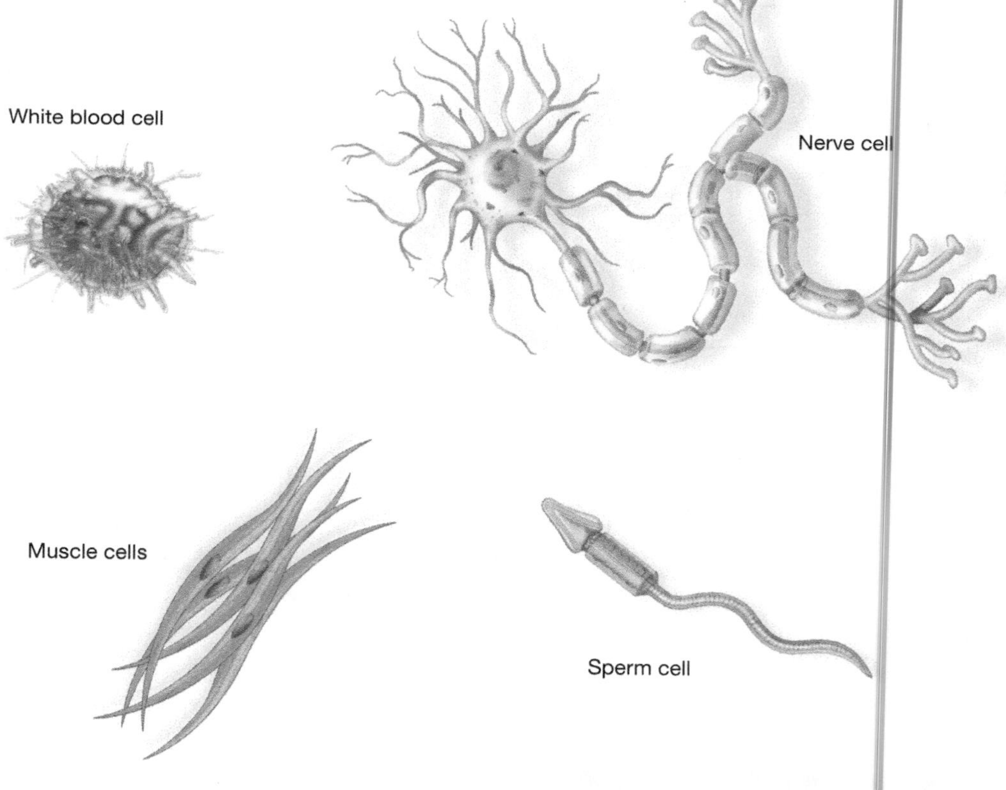

■ **Figure 2.1** Examples of four different types of cells from the body. Although each cell has a cell membrane, nucleus, and cytoplasm, each has a unique shape depending on its location and function.

Tissues

connective tissue
epithelial tissue (ep-ih-THEE-lee-al)
histology (hiss-TALL-oh-jee)
muscle tissue
nervous tissue

Histology is the study of tissue. A tissue is formed when like cells are grouped together and function together to perform a specific activity. The body has four types of tissue: **muscle tissue, epithelial tissue, connective tissue,** and **nervous tissue** (see Figure 2.2 ■).

Muscle Tissue

cardiac muscle
smooth muscle
muscle fibers
skeletal muscle

Muscle tissue produces movement in the body through contraction, or shortening in length, and is composed of individual muscle cells called **muscle fibers.** Muscle tissue forms one of three basic types of muscles: **skeletal muscle, smooth muscle,** or **cardiac muscle.** Skeletal muscle is attached to bone. Smooth muscle is found in internal organs such as the intestine, uterus, and blood vessels. Cardiac muscle is found only in the heart.

Epithelial Tissue

epithelium (ep-ih-THEE-lee-um)

Epithelial tissue, or **epithelium,** is found throughout the body and is composed of close-packed cells that form the covering for and lining of body structures. For example, both the top layer of skin and the lining of the stomach are epithelial tissue (see Figure 2.2). In addition to forming a protective barrier, epithelial tissue may be specialized to absorb substances (such as nutrients from the intestine), secrete substances (such as sweat glands), or excrete wastes (such as the kidney tubules).

MED TERM TIP

The term *epithelium* comes from the prefix *epi-* meaning "on top of" and the combining form *theli/o* meaning "nipple" (referring to any projection from the surface).

Connective Tissue

adipose (ADD-ih-pohs)
bone
cartilage (CAR-tih-lij)
tendons

Connective tissue is the supporting and protecting tissue in body structures. Because connective tissue performs many different functions depending on its location, it appears in many different forms so that each is able to perform the task required at that location. For example, **bone** provides structural support for the whole body. **Cartilage** is the shock absorber in joints. **Tendons** tightly connect skeletal muscles to bones. **Adipose** provides protective padding around body structures (see Figure 2.2).

Nervous Tissue

brain
nerves
neurons
spinal cord

Nervous tissue is composed of cells called **neurons** (see Figure 2.2). This tissue forms the **brain, spinal cord,** and a network of **nerves** throughout the entire body, allowing for the conduction of electrical impulses to send information between the brain and the rest of the body.

Figure 2.2 The appearance of different types of tissues—muscle, epithelial, nervous, connective—and their location within the body.

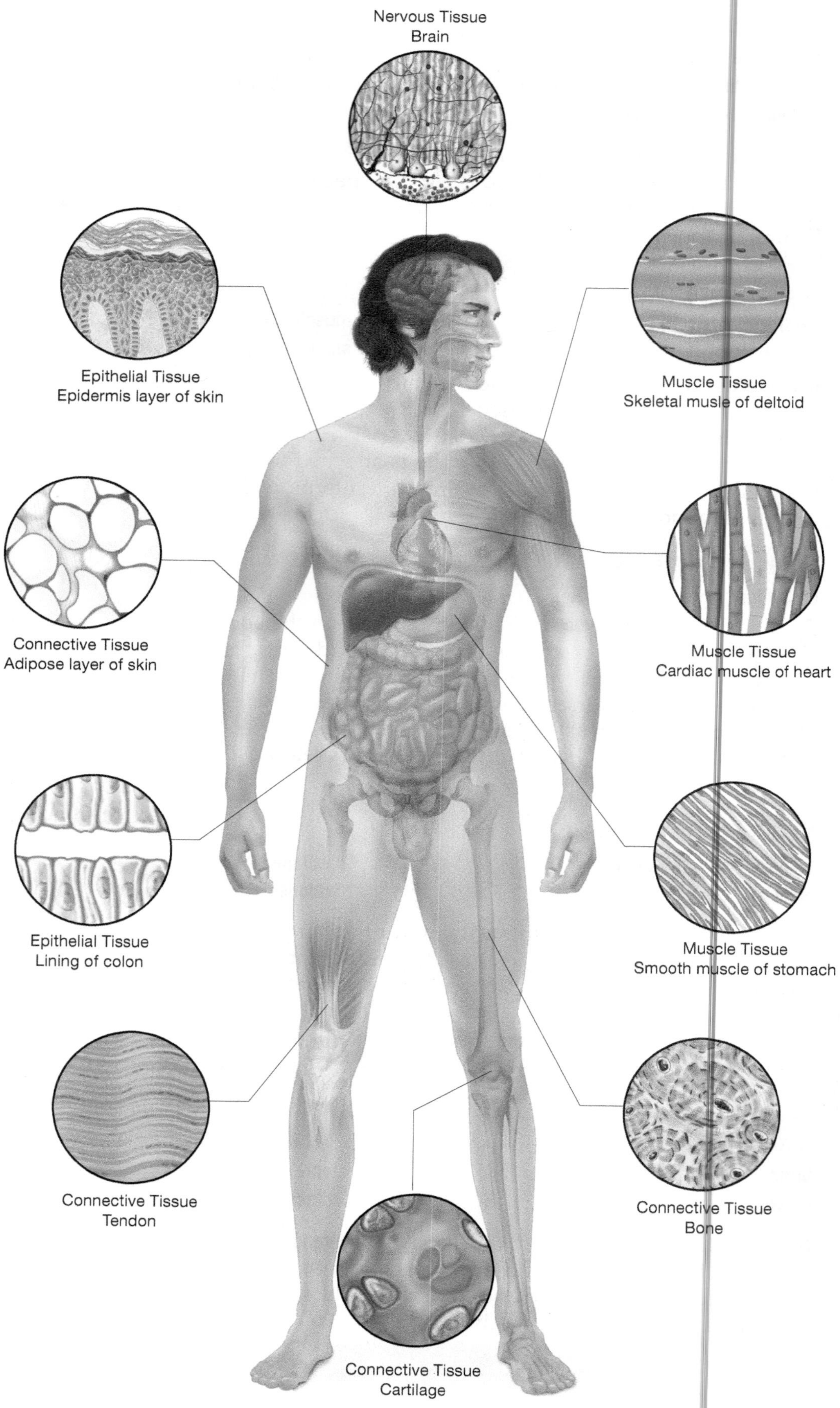

Nervous Tissue
Brain

Epithelial Tissue
Epidermis layer of skin

Muscle Tissue
Skeletal musle of deltoid

Connective Tissue
Adipose layer of skin

Muscle Tissue
Cardiac muscle of heart

Epithelial Tissue
Lining of colon

Muscle Tissue
Smooth muscle of stomach

Connective Tissue
Tendon

Connective Tissue
Bone

Connective Tissue
Cartilage

Organs and Systems

Organs are composed of several different types of tissue that work as a unit to perform special functions. For example, the stomach contains smooth muscle tissue, nervous tissue, and epithelial tissue that allow it to contract to mix food with digestive juices.

A system is composed of several organs working in a coordinated manner to perform a complex function or functions. To continue our example, the stomach plus the other digestive system organs—the oral cavity, esophagus, liver, pancreas, small intestine, and colon—work together to ingest, digest, and absorb our food.

Table 2.1 ■ presents the organ systems that are discussed in this text along with the major organs found in each system, the system functions, and the medical specialties that treat conditions of that system.

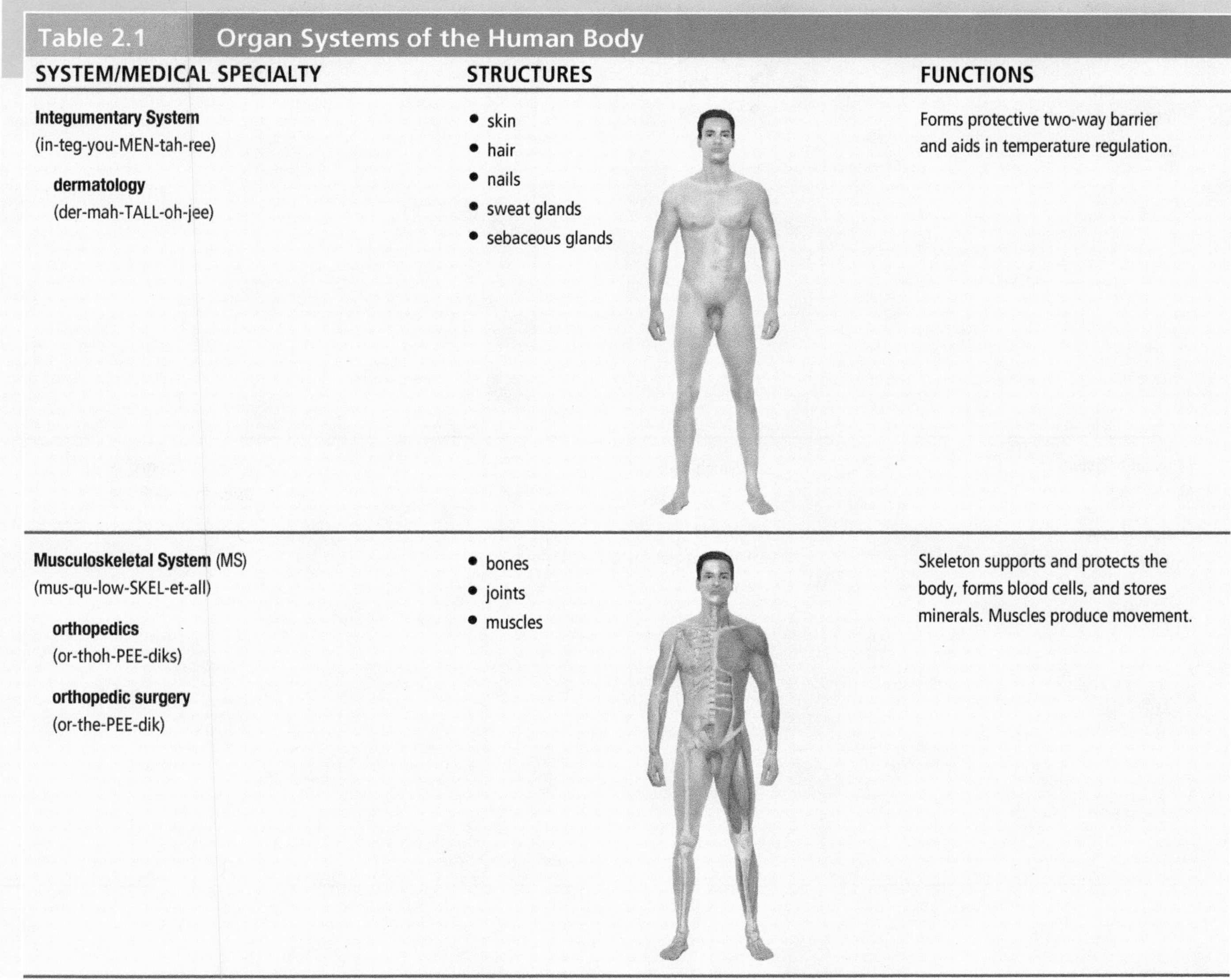

Table 2.1 Organ Systems of the Human Body

SYSTEM/MEDICAL SPECIALTY	STRUCTURES	FUNCTIONS
Integumentary System (in-teg-you-MEN-tah-ree) **dermatology** (der-mah-TALL-oh-jee)	• skin • hair • nails • sweat glands • sebaceous glands	Forms protective two-way barrier and aids in temperature regulation.
Musculoskeletal System (MS) (mus-qu-low-SKEL-et-all) **orthopedics** (or-thoh-PEE-diks) **orthopedic surgery** (or-the-PEE-dik)	• bones • joints • muscles	Skeleton supports and protects the body, forms blood cells, and stores minerals. Muscles produce movement.

Table 2.1 Organ Systems of the Human Body (continued)

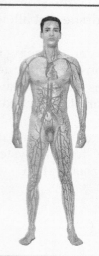

SYSTEM/MEDICAL SPECIALTY	STRUCTURES	FUNCTIONS
Cardiovascular System (CV) (car-dee-oh-VAS-kew-lar) **cardiology** (car-dee-ALL-oh-jee)	• heart • arteries • veins	Pumps blood throughout the entire body to transport nutrients, oxygen, and wastes.
Blood (Hematic System) (he-MAT-tik) **hematology** (hee-mah-TALL-oh-jee)	• plasma • erythrocytes • leukocytes • platelets	Transports oxygen, protects against pathogens, and controls bleeding.
Lymphatic System (lim-FAT-ik) **immunology** (im-yoo-NALL-oh-jee)	• lymph nodes • lymphatic vessels • spleen • thymus gland • tonsils 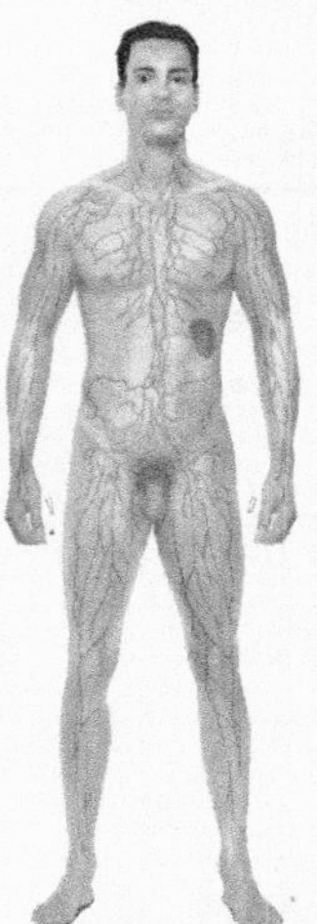	Protects the body from disease and invasion from pathogens.

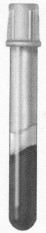

Table 2.1 Organ Systems of the Human Body (continued)

SYSTEM/MEDICAL SPECIALTY	STRUCTURES		FUNCTIONS
Respiratory System **otorhinolaryngology** (ENT) (oh-toh-rye-noh- lair-ing-GALL-oh-jee) **pulmonology** (pull-mon-ALL-oh-jee) **thoracic surgery** (tho-RASS-ik)	• nasal cavity • pharynx • larynx • trachea • bronchial tubes • lungs	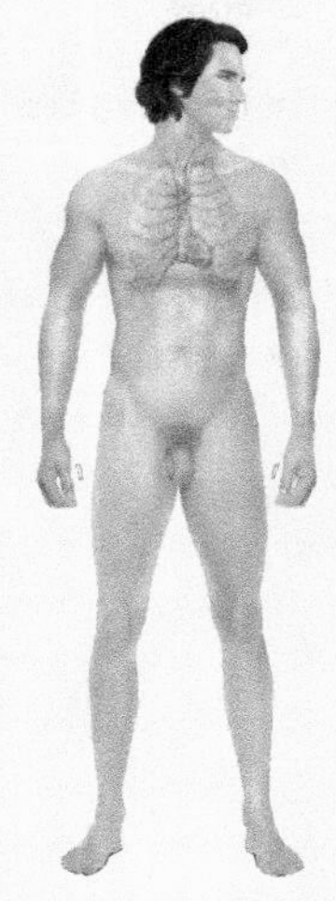	Obtains oxygen and removes carbon dioxide from the body.
Digestive or **Gastrointestinal System** (GI) **gastroenterology** (gas-troh-en-ter-ALL-oh-jee) **proctology** (prok-TOL-oh-jee)	• oral cavity • pharynx • esophagus • stomach • small intestine • colon • liver • gallbladder • pancreas • salivary glands	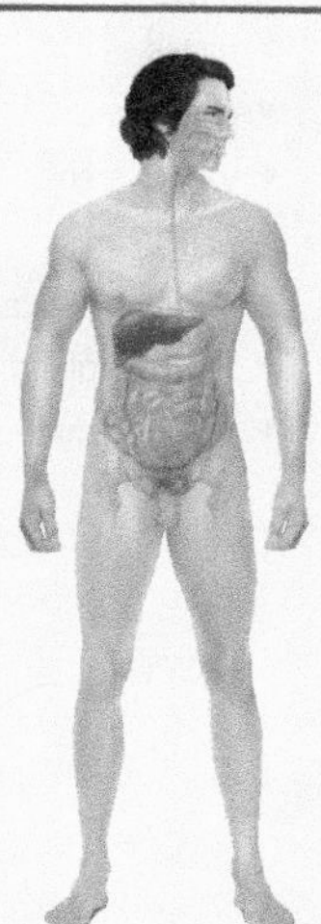	Ingests, digests, and absorbs nutrients for the body.
Urinary System (YOO-rih-nair-ee) **nephrology** (neh-FROL-oh-jee) **urology** (yoo-RALL-oh-jee)	• kidneys • ureters • urinary bladder • urethra	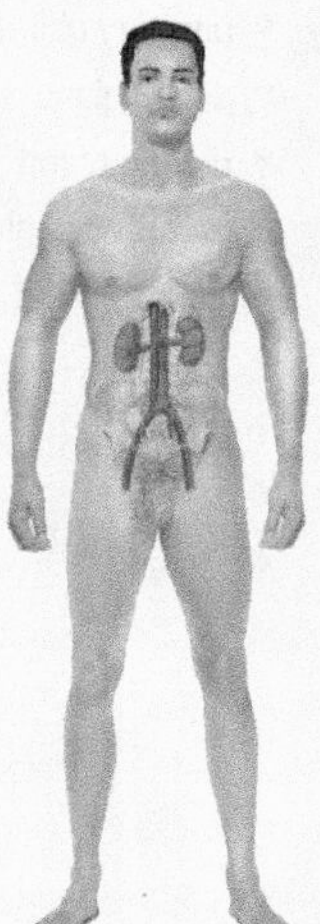	Filters waste products out of the blood and removes them from the body.

Table 2.1 Organ Systems of the Human Body (continued)

SYSTEM/MEDICAL SPECIALTY	STRUCTURES	FUNCTIONS
Female Reproductive System **gynecology** (GYN) (gigh-neh-KOL- oh-jee) **obstetrics** (OB) (ob-STET-riks)	• ovary • fallopian tubes • uterus • vagina • vulva • breasts	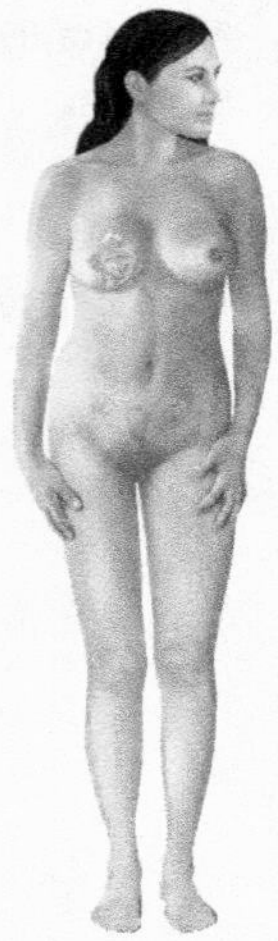 Produces eggs for reproduction and provides place for growing baby.
Male Reproductive System **urology** (yoo-RALL-oh-jee)	• testes • epididymis • vas deferens • penis • seminal vesicles • prostate gland • bulbourethral gland	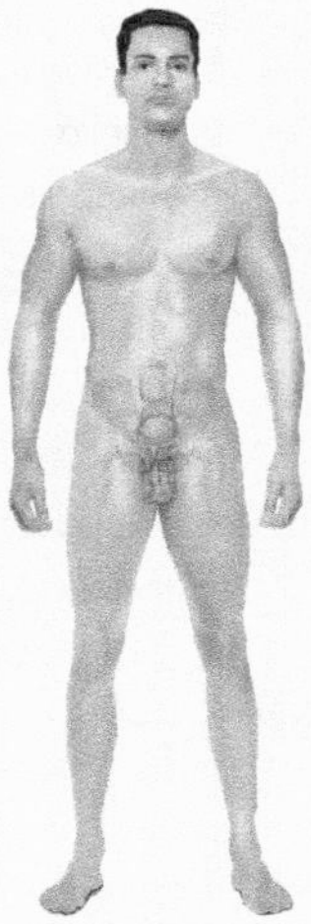 Produces sperm for reproduction.
Endocrine System (EN-doh-krin) **endocrinology** (en-doh-krin-ALL-oh-jee)	• pituitary gland • pineal gland • thyroid gland • parathyroid glands • thymus gland • adrenal glands • pancreas • ovaries • testes	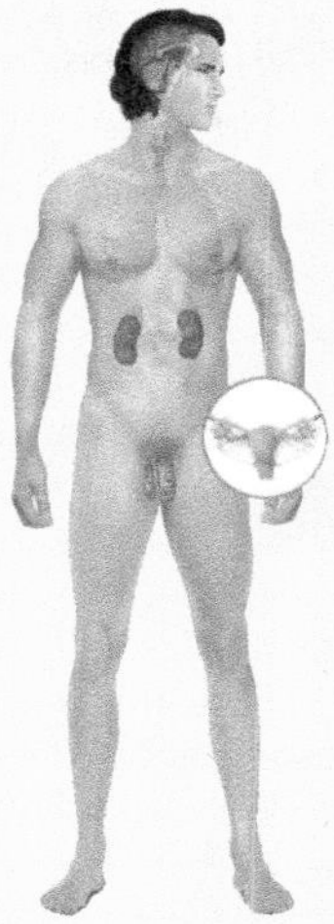 Regulates metabolic activities of the body.

Table 2.1 Organization Systems of the Human Body (continued)

SYSTEM/MEDICAL SPECIALTY	STRUCTURES	FUNCTIONS
Nervous System **neurology** (noo-RAL-oh-jee) **neurosurgery** (noo-roh-SIR-jer-ee)	• brain • spinal cord • nerves	Receives sensory information and coordinates the body's response.
Special Senses **ophthalmology** (off-thal-MALL-oh-jee)	• eye	Vision
otorhinolaryngology (ENT) (oh-toh-rye-noh-lair- ing-GALL-oh-jee)	• ear	Hearing and balance

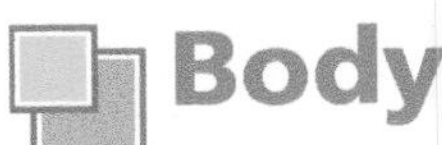

Body

anatomical position

As seen from the previous sections, the body is the sum of all the systems, organs, tissues, and cells found in it. It is important to learn the anatomical terminology that applies to the body as a whole in order to correctly identify specific locations and directions when dealing with patients. The **anatomical position** is used when describing the positions and relationships of structures in the human body. A body in the anatomical position is standing erect with the arms at the sides of the body, the palms of the hands facing forward, and the eyes looking straight ahead. In addition, the legs are parallel with the feet, and the toes are pointing forward (see Figure 2.3 ■). For descriptive purposes the assumption is always that the person is in the anatomical position even if the body or parts of the body are in any other position.

Body Planes

coronal plane (kor-RONE-al)
coronal section
cross-section
frontal plane
frontal section
horizontal plane
longitudinal section
median plane
sagittal plane (SAJ-ih-tal)
sagittal section
transverse plane
transverse section

The terminology for body planes is used to assist medical personnel in describing the body and its parts. To understand body planes, imagine cuts slicing through the body at various angles. This imaginary slicing allows us to use more specific language when describing parts of the body. These body planes, illustrated in Figure 2.4 ■, include the following:

1. **Sagittal plane:** This vertical plane runs lengthwise from front to back and divides the body or any of its parts into right and left portions. The right and left sides do not have to be equal. If the sagittal plane passes through the middle of the body, thus dividing it into equal right and left halves, it is called a **midsagittal** or **median plane.** A cut along the sagittal plane yields a **sagittal section** view of the inside of the body.

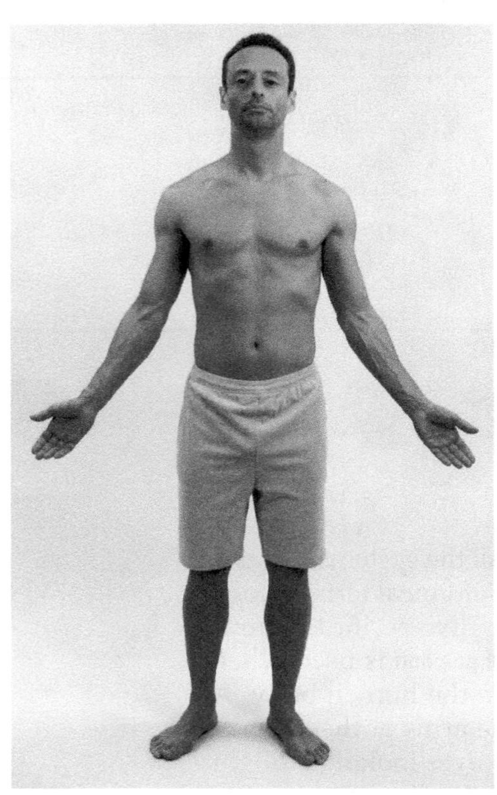

■ Figure 2.3 The anatomical position: standing erect, gazing straight ahead, arms down at sides, palms facing forward, fingers extended, legs together, and toes pointing forward.

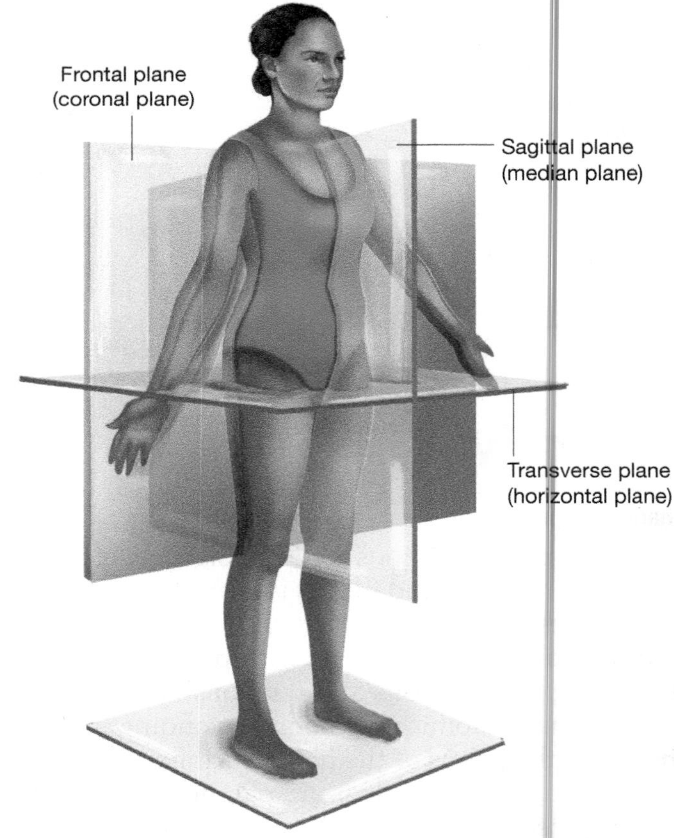

■ Figure 2.4 The planes of the body. The sagittal plane is vertical from front to back, the frontal plane is vertical from left to right, and the transverse plane is horizontal.

2. **Frontal plane:** The frontal, or **coronal plane,** divides the body into front and back portions; a vertical lengthwise plane is running from side to side. A cut along the frontal plane yields a **frontal** or **coronal section** view of the inside of the body.
3. **Transverse plane:** The transverse, or **horizontal plane,** is a crosswise plane that runs parallel to the ground. This imaginary cut would divide the body or its parts into upper and lower portions. A cut along the transverse plane yields a **transverse section** view of the inside of the body.

The terms **cross-section** and **longitudinal section** are frequently used to describe internal views of structures. A longitudinal section is produced by a lengthwise slice along the long axis of a structure. A cross-section view is produced by a slice perpendicular to the long axis of the structure.

Body Regions

abdominal region (ab-DOM-ih-nal)
brachial region (BRAY-kee-all)
cephalic region (she-FAL-ik)
cervical region (SER-vih-kal)
crural region (KREW-ral)
dorsum (DOOR-sum)
gluteal region (GLOO-tee-all)
lower extremities
pelvic region (PELL-vik)
pubic region (PEW-bik)
thoracic region (tho-RASS-ik)
trunk
upper extremities
vertebral region (VER-tee-bral)

The body is divided into large regions that can easily be identified externally. The **cephalic region** is the entire head. The neck is the **cervical region** and connects the head to the **trunk** (the torso). The trunk is further subdivided into different anterior and posterior regions. The anterior side consists of the **thoracic** (the chest), **abdominal, pelvic,** and **pubic** (genital) **regions.** The posterior side consists of the **dorsum** (the back), **vertebral region,** and **gluteal** (buttock) **region.** The **upper extremities** (UE) and **lower extremities** (LE) are attached to the trunk. The upper extremities or **brachial regions** are the arms. The lower extremities or **crural regions** are the legs. See Figure 2.5 ■ to locate each region on the body.

MED TERM TIP

As you learn medical terminology, it is important that you remember not to use common phrases and terms any longer. Many people commonly use the term *stomach* (an organ) when they actually mean *abdomen* (a body region).

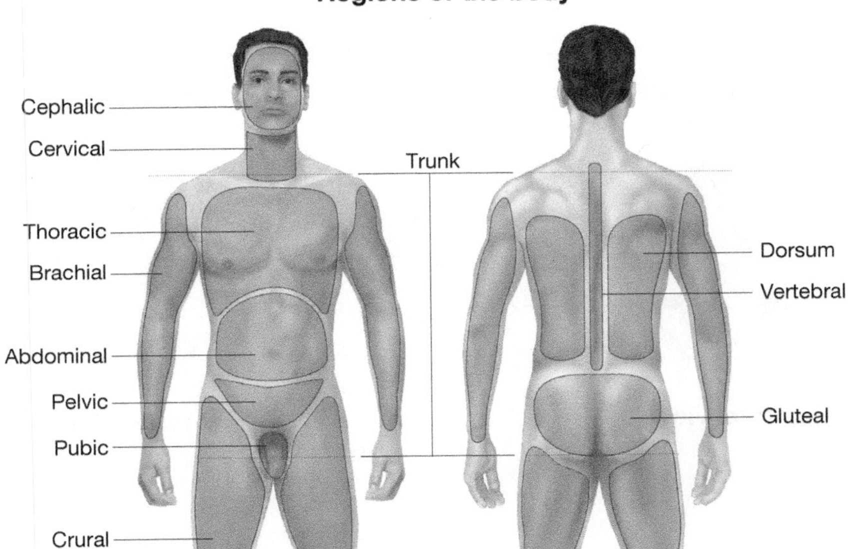

■ **Figure 2.5** Anterior and posterior views of the body illustrating the location of various body regions.

Body Cavities

abdominal cavity
abdominopelvic cavity (ab-dom-ih-noh-PELL-vik)
cranial cavity (KRAY-nee-al)
diaphragm (DYE-ah-fram)
mediastinum (mee-dee-ass-TYE-num)
parietal layer (pah-RYE-eh-tal)
parietal peritoneum
parietal pleura
pelvic cavity
pericardial cavity (pair-ih-CAR-dee-al)
peritoneum (pair-ih-toh-NEE-um)
pleura (PLOO-rah)
pleural cavity (PLOO-ral)
spinal cavity
thoracic cavity
viscera (VISS-er-ah)
visceral layer (VISS-er-al)
visceral peritoneum
visceral pleura

The body is not a solid structure; it has many open spaces or cavities. The cavities are part of the normal body structure and are illustrated in Figure 2.6 ■. We can divide the body into four major cavities—two dorsal cavities and two ventral cavities.

The dorsal cavities include the **cranial cavity,** containing the brain, and the **spinal cavity,** containing the spinal cord.

The ventral cavities include the **thoracic cavity** and the **abdominopelvic cavity.** The thoracic cavity contains the two lungs and a central region between them called the **mediastinum.** The heart, aorta, esophagus, trachea, and thymus gland are some of the structures located in the mediastinum. There is an actual physical wall between the thoracic cavity and the abdominopelvic cavity called the **diaphragm.** The diaphragm is a muscle used for breathing. The abdominopelvic cavity is generally subdivided into a superior **abdominal cavity** and an inferior **pelvic cavity.** The organs of the digestive, excretory, and reproductive systems are located in

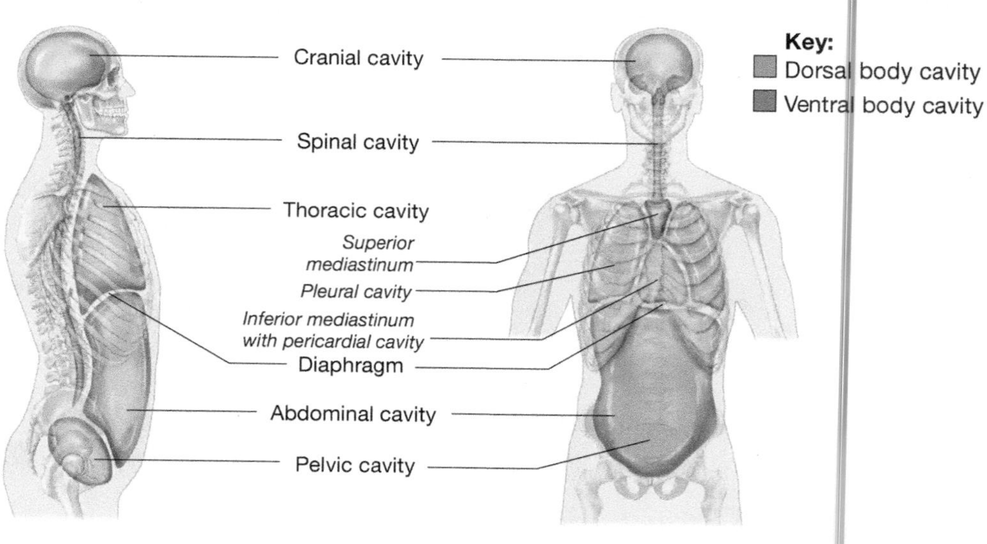

■ **Figure 2.6** The dorsal (orange) and ventral (purple) body cavities.

these cavities. The organs within the ventral cavities are referred to as a group as the internal organs or **viscera.** Table 2.2 ■ describes the body cavities and their major organs.

All of the cavities are lined by, and the viscera are encased in, a two-layer membrane called the **pleura** in the thoracic cavity and the **peritoneum** in the abdominopelvic cavity. The outer layer that lines the cavities is called the **parietal layer** (i.e., **parietal pleura** and **parietal peritoneum**), and the inner layer that encases the viscera is called the **visceral layer** (i.e., **visceral pleura** and **visceral peritoneum**).

Within the thoracic cavity, the pleura is subdivided, forming the **pleural cavity,** containing the lungs, and the **pericardial cavity,** containing the heart. The larger abdominopelvic cavity is usually subdivided into regions so different areas can be precisely referred to. Two different methods of subdividing this cavity are used: the anatomical divisions and the clinical divisions. Choose a method partly on personal preference and partly on which system best describes the patient's condition. See Table 2.3 ■ for a description of these methods for dividing the abdominopelvic cavity.

MED TERM TIP

The kidneys are the only major abdominopelvic organ located outside the sac formed by the peritoneum. Because they are found behind this sac, their position is referred to as *retroperitoneal* (retro- = behind; peritone/o = peritoneum; -al = pertaining to).

Directional and Positional Terms

Directional terms assist medical personnel in discussing the position or location of a patient's complaint. Directional or positional terms also help to describe one process, organ, or system as it relates to another. Table 2.4 ■ presents commonly used terms for describing the position of the body or its parts. They are listed in pairs that have opposite meanings; for example, superior versus inferior, anterior versus posterior, medial versus lateral, proximal versus distal, superficial versus deep, and supine versus prone. Directional terms are illustrated in Figure 2.7 ■.

MED TERM TIP

Remember when using location or direction terms, it is assumed that the patient is in the anatomical position unless otherwise noted.

Table 2.2 Body Cavities and Their Major Organs

CAVITY	MAJOR ORGANS
Dorsal cavities	
Cranial cavity	Brain
Spinal cavity	Spinal cord
Ventral cavities	
Thoracic cavity	Pleural cavity: lungs Pericardial cavity: heart Mediastinum: heart, esophagus, trachea, thymus gland, aorta
Abdominopelvic cavity	
Abdominal cavity	Stomach, spleen, liver, gallbladder, pancreas, and portions of the small intestines and colon
Pelvic cavity	Urinary bladder, ureters, urethra, and portions of the small intestines and colon *Female:* uterus, ovaries, fallopian tubes, vagina *Male:* prostate gland, seminal vesicles, portion of the vas deferens

Table 2.3 Methods of Subdividing the Abdominopelvic Cavity

Anatomical Divisions of the Abdomen

- **Right hypochondriac** (high-poh-KON-dree-ak): Right lateral region of upper row beneath the lower ribs
- **Epigastric** (ep-ih-GAS-trik): Middle area of upper row above the stomach
- **Left hypochondriac:** Left lateral region of the upper row beneath the lower ribs
- **Right lumbar:** Right lateral region of the middle row at the waist
- **Umbilical** (um-BILL-ih-kal): Central area over the navel
- **Left lumbar:** Left lateral region of the middle row at the waist
- **Right iliac** (ILL-ee-ak): Right lateral region of the lower row at the groin
- **Hypogastric** (high-poh-GAS-trik): Middle region of the lower row beneath the navel
- **Left iliac:** Left lateral region of the lower row at the groin

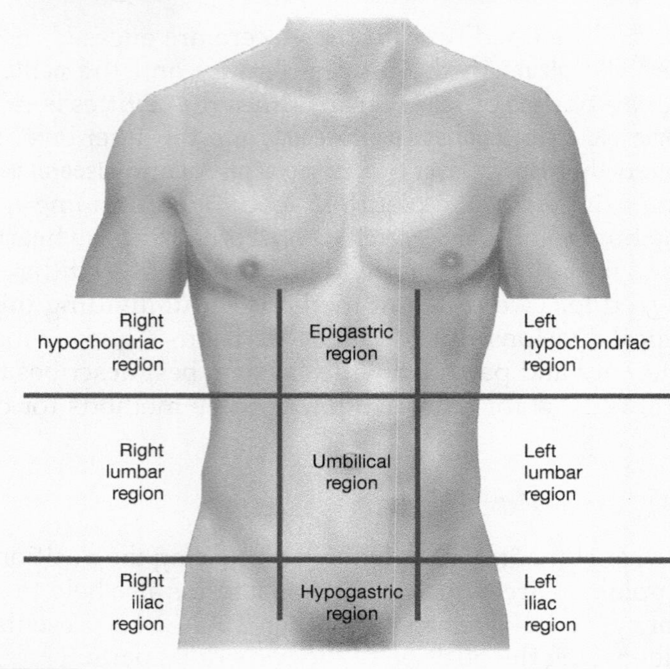

MED TERM TIP

To visualize the nine anatomical divisions, imagine a tic-tac-toe diagram over this region.

MED TERM TIP

The term *hypochondriac,* literally meaning "under the cartilage" (of the ribs), has come to refer to a person who believes he or she is sick when there is no obvious cause for illness. These patients commonly complain of aches and pains in the hypochondriac region.

Clinical Divisions of the Abdomen

- **Right upper quadrant (RUQ):** Contains majority of liver, gallbladder, small portion of pancreas, right kidney, small intestines, and colon
- **Right lower quadrant (RLQ):** Contains small intestines and colon, right ovary and fallopian tube, appendix, and right ureter
- **Left upper quadrant (LUQ):** Contains small portion of liver, spleen, stomach, majority of pancreas, left kidney, small intestines, and colon
- **Left lower quadrant (LLQ):** Contains small intestines and colon, left ovary and fallopian tube, and left ureter
- Midline organs: uterus, bladder, prostate gland

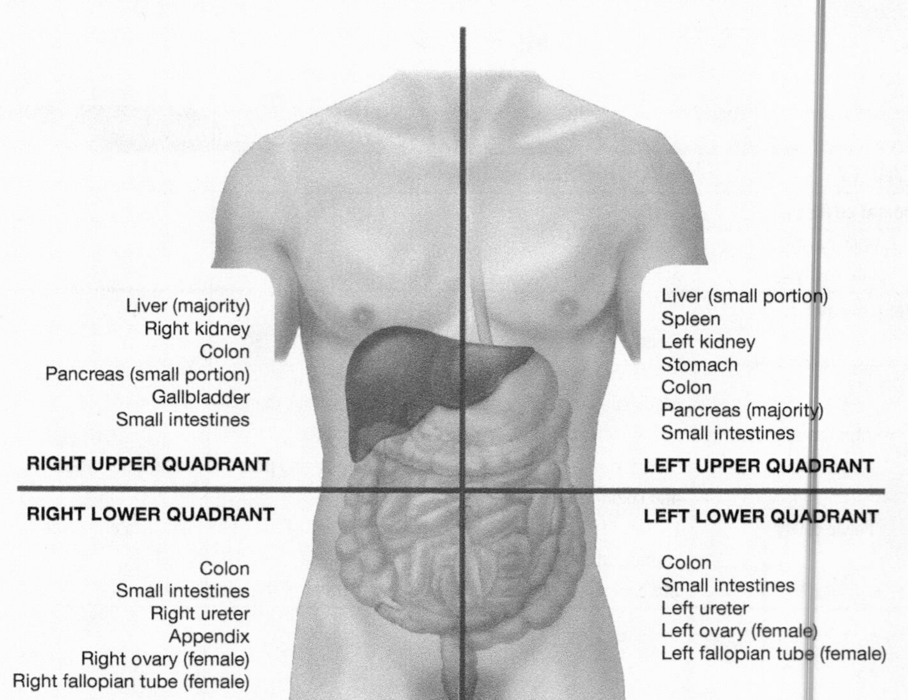

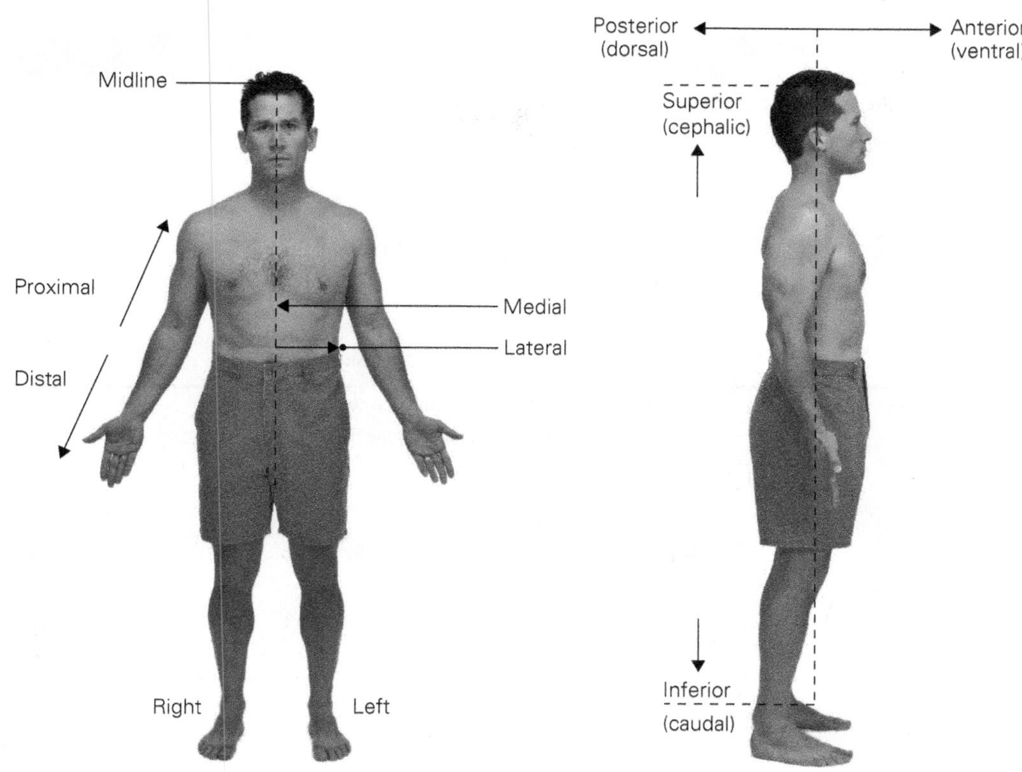

■ **Figure 2.7** Anterior and lateral views of the body illustrating directional terms.

Table 2.4	Terms for Describing Body Position
superior (soo-PEE-ree-or) or **cephalic** (seh-FAL-ik)	More toward the head, or above another structure. *Example:* The adrenal glands are superior to the kidneys.
inferior (in-FEE-ree-or) or **caudal** (KAWD-al)	More toward the feet or tail, or below another structure. *Example:* The intestine is inferior to the heart.
anterior (an-TEE-ree-or) or **ventral** (VEN-tral)	More toward the front or belly-side of the body. *Example:* The navel is located on the anterior surface of the body.
posterior (poss-TEE-ree-or) or **dorsal** (DOR-sal)	More toward the back or spinal cord side of the body. *Example:* The posterior wall of the right kidney was excised.
medial (MEE-dee-al)	Refers to the middle or near the middle of the body or the structure. *Example:* The heart is medially located in the chest cavity.
lateral (lat) (LAT-er-al)	Refers to the side. *Example:* The ovaries are located lateral to the uterus.
proximal (PROK-sim-al)	Located nearer to the point of attachment to the body. *Example:* In the anatomical position, the elbow is proximal to the hand.
distal (DISS-tal)	Located farther away from the point of attachment to the body. *Example:* The hand is distal to the elbow.
apex (AY-peks)	Tip or summit of an organ. *Example:* We hear the heart beat by listening over the apex of the heart.
base	Bottom or lower part of an organ. *Example:* On the X-ray, a fracture was noted at the base of the skull.
superficial	More toward the surface of the body. *Example:* The cut was superficial.
deep	Further away from the surface of the body. *Example:* An incision into an abdominal organ is a deep incision.

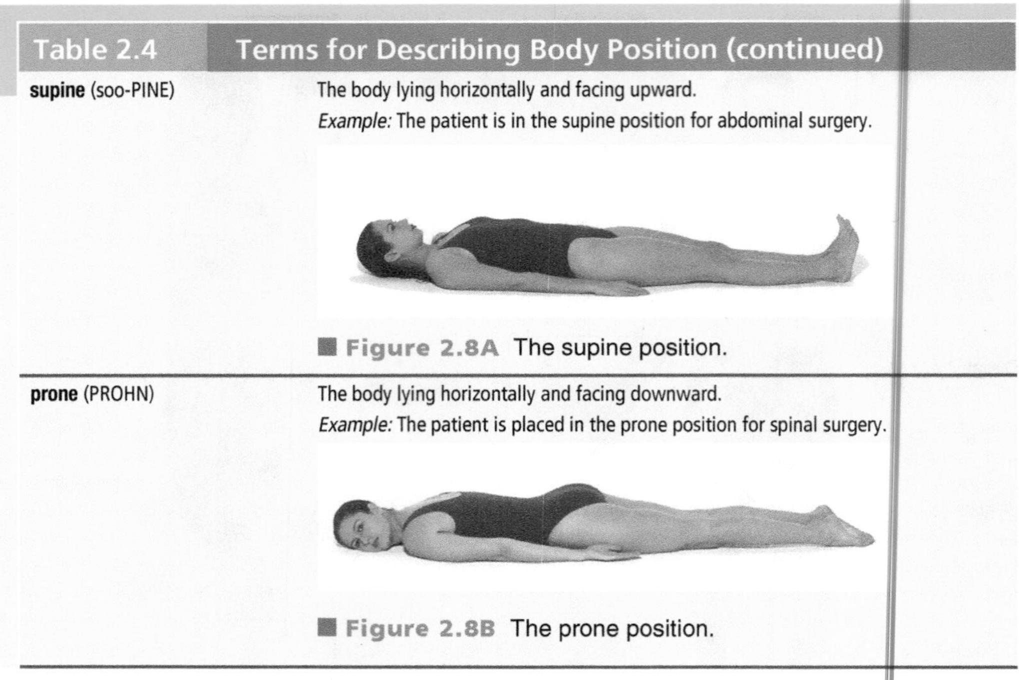

Table 2.4	Terms for Describing Body Position (continued)
supine (soo-PINE)	The body lying horizontally and facing upward. *Example:* The patient is in the supine position for abdominal surgery. ■ Figure 2.8A The supine position.
prone (PROHN)	The body lying horizontally and facing downward. *Example:* The patient is placed in the prone position for spinal surgery. ■ Figure 2.8B The prone position.

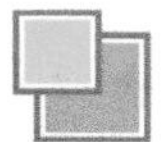

Terminology

The following lists contain the suffixes and prefixes used to build terms in the remaining section of this chapter. The combining forms were introduced earlier in this chapter.

Suffixes

-ac	pertaining to
-al	pertaining to
-ar	pertaining to
-ary	pertaining to
-atic	pertaining to
-iac	pertaining to
-ic	pertaining to
-ior	pertaining to
-logy	study of
-ose	resembling

Prefixes

endo-	within
epi-	above
hypo-	under
peri-	around
retro-	behind

The terms below, introduced in this chapter, are built directly from word parts following the rules given earlier. Review these terms in order to begin to familiarize yourself with how medical terms are built.

Anatomical Terms

TERM	WORD PARTS	DEFINITION
abdominal	abdomin/o = abdomen -al = pertaining to	pertaining to the abdomen
adipose	adip/o = fat -ose = resembling	resembling fat
anterior	anter/o = front -ior = pertaining to	pertaining to the front
brachial	brachi/o = arm -al = pertaining to	pertaining to the arm
cardiac	cardi/o = heart -ac = pertaining to	pertaining to the heart
cardiology	cardi/o = heart -logy = study of	study of the heart
cardiovascular	cardi/o = heart vascul/o = blood vessel -ar = pertaining to	pertaining to the heart and blood vessels
caudal	caud/o = tail -al = pertaining to	pertaining to the tail
cephalic	cephal/o = head -ic = pertaining to	pertaining to the head
cervical	cervic/o = neck -al = pertaining to	pertaining to the neck
cranial	crani/o = skull -al = pertaining to	pertaining to the skull
crural	crur/o = leg -al = pertaining to	pertaining to the leg
cytology	cyt/o = cell -logy = study of	study of the cell
dermatology	dermat/o = skin -logy = study of	study of the skin
distal	dist/o = away from -al = pertaining to	pertaining to away from
dorsal	dors/o = back of body -al = pertaining to	pertaining to the back of body
endocrinology	endo- = within crin/o = to secrete -logy = study of	study of secreting within [endocrine system]
epigastric	epi- = above gastr/o = stomach -ic = pertaining to	pertaining to above the stomach
epithelial	epitheli/o = epithelium -al = pertaining to	pertaining to the epithelium

Anatomical Terms *(continued)*

TERM	WORD PARTS	DEFINITION
gastroenterology	gastr/o = stomach enter/o = small intestine -logy = study of	study of the stomach and small intestine
gluteal	glute/o = buttock -al = pertaining to	pertaining to the buttocks
gynecology	gynec/o = woman -logy = study of	study of women
hematic	hemat/o = blood -ic = pertaining to	pertaining to the blood
hematology	hemat/o = blood -logy = study of	study of the blood
histology	hist/o = tissue -logy = study of	study of tissue
hypochondriac	hypo- = under chondr/o = cartilage -iac = pertaining to	pertaining to under the cartilage
hypogastric	hypo- = under gastr/o = stomach -ic = pertaining to	pertaining to under the stomach
immunology	immun/o = protection -logy = study of	study of protection [immune system]
inferior	infer/o = below -ior = pertaining to	pertaining to below
lateral	later/o = side -al = pertaining to	pertaining to the side
lumbar	lumb/o = loin -ar = pertaining to	pertaining to the loin [side and back between ribs and pelvic bones]
lymphatic	lymph/o = lymph -atic = pertaining to	pertaining to lymph
medial	medi/o = middle -al = pertaining to	pertaining to the middle
muscular	muscul/o = muscles -ar = pertaining to	pertaining to muscles
nephrology	nephr/o = kidney -logy = study of	study of the kidney
neurology	neur/o = nerve -logy = study of	study of nerves
ophthalmology	ophthalm/o = eye -logy = study of	study of the eye
otorhinolaryngology	ot/o = ear rhin/o = nose laryng/o = larynx -logy = study of	study of ear, nose, and larynx
pelvic	pelv/o = pelvis -ic = pertaining to	pertaining to the pelvis
peritoneal	peritone/o = peritoneum -al = pertaining to	pertaining to the peritoneum

Anatomical Terms *(continued)*

TERM	WORD PARTS	DEFINITION
pleural	pleur/o = pleura -al = pertaining to	pertaining to the pleura
posterior	poster/o = back -ior = pertaining to	pertaining to the back
proctology	proct/o = rectum and anus -logy = study of	study of the rectum and anus
proximal	proxim/o = near to -al = pertaining to	pertaining to near to
pubic	pub/o = genital region -ic = pertaining to	pertaining to the genital region
pulmonology	pulmon/o = lung -logy = study of	study of the lungs
spinal	spin/o = spine -al = pertaining to	pertaining to the spine
superior	super/o = above -ior = pertaining to	pertaining to above
thoracic	thorac/o = chest -ic = pertaining to	pertaining to the chest
urology	ur/o = urine -logy = study of	study of urine
ventral	ventr/o = belly -al = pertaining to	pertaining to the belly [side]
vertebral	vertebr/o = vertebra -al = pertaining to	pertaining to the vertebrae
visceral	viscer/o = internal organ -al = pertaining to	pertaining to internal organs

Abbreviations

AP	anteroposterior
CV	cardiovascular
ENT	ear, nose, and throat
GI	gastrointestinal
GYN	gynecology
lat	lateral
LE	lower extremity
LLQ	left lower quadrant
LUQ	left upper quadrant
MS	musculoskeletal
OB	obstetrics
PA	posteroanterior
RLQ	right lower quadrant
RUQ	right upper quadrant
UE	upper extremity

Chapter Review

Practice Exercises

A. Complete the Statement

1. The levels of organization of the body in order from smallest to largest are: ______________________, ______________________, ______________________, ______________________, ______________________.

2. No matter its shape, all cells have a ______________________, ______________________, and ______________________.

3. ______________________ is the study of tissue.

4. ______________________ tissue lines internal organs and serves as a covering for the skin.

5. In the ______________________ position the body is standing erect with arms at sides and palms facing forward.

6. The ______________________ quadrant of the abdomen contains the appendix.

7. The dorsal cavities are the ______________________ cavity and the ______________________ cavity.

8. There are ______________________ anatomical divisions in the abdominal cavity.

9. The ______________________ region of the abdominal cavity is located in the right lower lateral region near the groin.

10. Within the thoracic cavity the lungs are found in the ______________________ cavity and the heart is found in the ______________________ cavity.

B. Body Plane Matching

Match each body plane to its definition.

1. _______ frontal plane
2. _______ sagittal plane
3. _______ transverse plane

a. divides the body into right and left
b. divides the body into upper and lower
c. divides the body into anterior and posterior

C. Prefix Practice

Circle the prefixes in the following terms and define in the space provided.

1. epigastric ____
2. pericardium ____
3. hypochondriac ____
4. retroperitoneal ____

D. Terminology Matching

Match each term to its definition.

1. _______ distal
2. _______ prone
3. _______ lateral
4. _______ inferior
5. _______ deep
6. _______ apex
7. _______ base
8. _______ posterior
9. _______ superficial
10. _______ supine
11. _______ anterior
12. _______ medial
13. _______ proximal
14. _______ superior

a. away from the surface
b. toward the surface
c. located closer to point of attachment to the body
d. caudal
e. tip or summit of an organ
f. lying face down
g. cephalic
h. ventral
i. dorsal
j. lying face up
k. to the side
l. middle
m. bottom or lower part of an organ
n. located further away from point of attachment to the body

E. What's the Abbreviation?

1. musculoskeletal ______________________________
2. lateral ______________________________
3. right upper quadrant ______________________________
4. cardiovascular ______________________________
5. gastrointestinal ______________________________
6. anteroposterior ______________________________
7. obstetrics ______________________________
8. left lower quadrant ______________________________

F. Build a Medical Term

Build terms for each expression using the correct prefixes, suffixes, and combining forms.

1. pertaining to spinal cord side ______
2. pertaining to the chest ______
3. pertaining to above ______
4. pertaining to the tail ______
5. pertaining to internal organs ______
6. pertaining to the side ______
7. pertaining to away from ______
8. pertaining to nerves ______
9. study of the lungs ______
10. pertaining to the muscles ______
11. pertaining to the belly side ______
12. pertaining to the front ______
13. pertaining to the head ______
14. pertaining to the middle ______

G. Define the Combining Form

1. viscer/o ______
2. poster/o ______
3. abdomin/o ______
4. thorac/o ______
5. medi/o ______
6. ventr/o ______
7. anter/o ______
8. hist/o ______
9. epitheli/o ______
10. crani/o ______
11. cyt/o ______
12. proxim/o ______
13. cephal/o ______

H. Organ System and Function Challenge

For each organ listed below, identify the name of the system it belongs to and then match it to its function.

	Organ	System		
1.	_______ skin	____________________	a.	supports the body
2.	_______ heart	____________________	b.	provides place for growing baby
3.	_______ stomach	____________________	c.	filters waste products from blood
4.	_______ uterus	____________________	d.	provides two-way barrier
5.	_______ bones	____________________	e.	produces movement
6.	_______ lungs	____________________	f.	produces sperm
7.	_______ kidney	____________________	g.	ingest, digest, absorb nutrients
8.	_______ testes	____________________	h.	coordinates body's response
9.	_______ brain	____________________	i.	pumps blood through blood vessels
10.	_______ muscles	____________________	j.	obtains oxygen

I. Body Region Practice

For each term below, write the corresponding body region.

1. head ____________________
2. genitals ____________________
3. leg ____________________
4. buttocks ____________________
5. neck ____________________
6. arm ____________________
7. back ____________________
8. chest ____________________

J. Terminology Matching

Match each organ to its body cavity.

1. _______ gallbladder	a.	right upper quadrant
2. _______ appendix	b.	left upper quadrant
3. _______ urinary bladder	c.	right lower quadrant
4. _______ small intestines	d.	left lower quadrant
5. _______ right kidney	e.	all quadrants
6. _______ left ovary	f.	midline structure
7. _______ stomach		
8. _______ colon		
9. _______ right ureter		
10. _______ pancreas (majority)		

K. Fill in the Blank

cardiology	otorhinolaryngology	urology	gynecology
ophthalmology	gastroenterology	dermatology	orthopedics

1. John is a musician who plays an electric bass guitar and is experiencing difficulty in hearing soft voices. He would consult a physician in ______________________.
2. Ruth is a stock trader with the Chicago Board of Trade. She has had a pounding and racing heartbeat. She would consult a physician specializing in ______________________.
3. Mary Ann is experiencing excessive bleeding from the uterus. She would consult a ______________________ doctor.
4. José has fractured his wrist in a fall. He would be seen for an examination by a physician in ______________________.
5. A physician who performs eye exams specializes in the field of ______________________.
6. When her daughter had repeated bladder infections, Mrs. Cortez sought the opinion of a specialist in ______________________.
7. Martha could not get rid of a persistent skin rash with over-the-counter creams. She decided to make an appointment with a specialist in ______________________.
8. After reviewing his X-ray, the specialist in ______________________ informed Mr. Sparks that he had a stomach ulcer.

Labeling Exercise

Image A

1. Write the labels for this figure on the numbered lines provided.

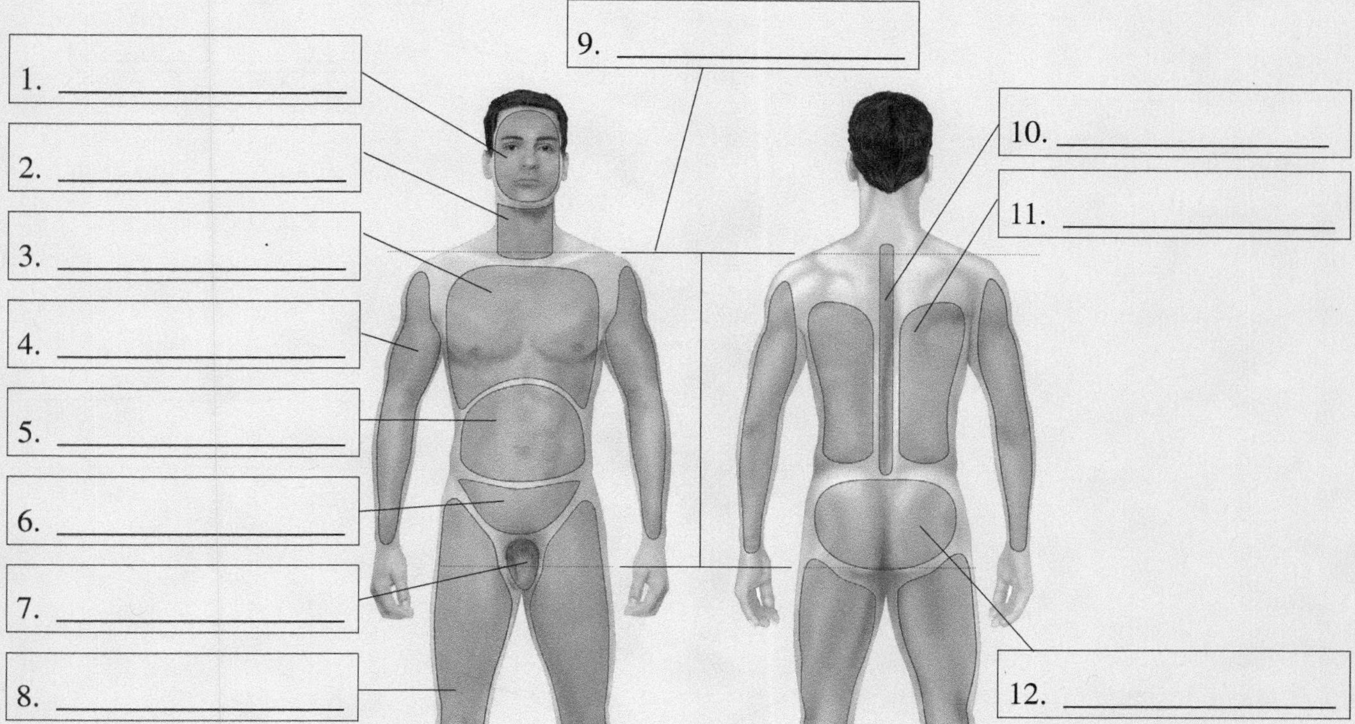

Image B

2. Write the labels for this figure on the numbered lines provided.

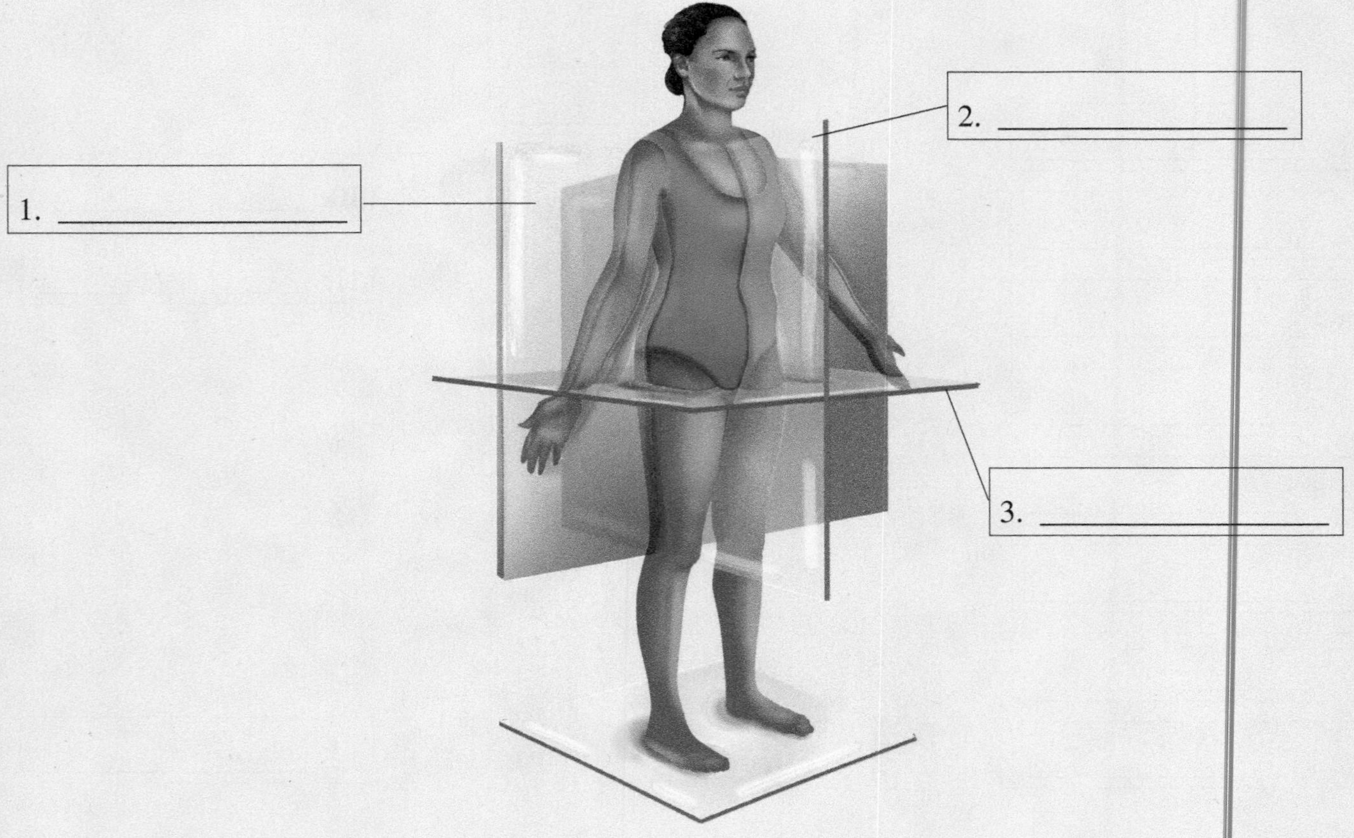

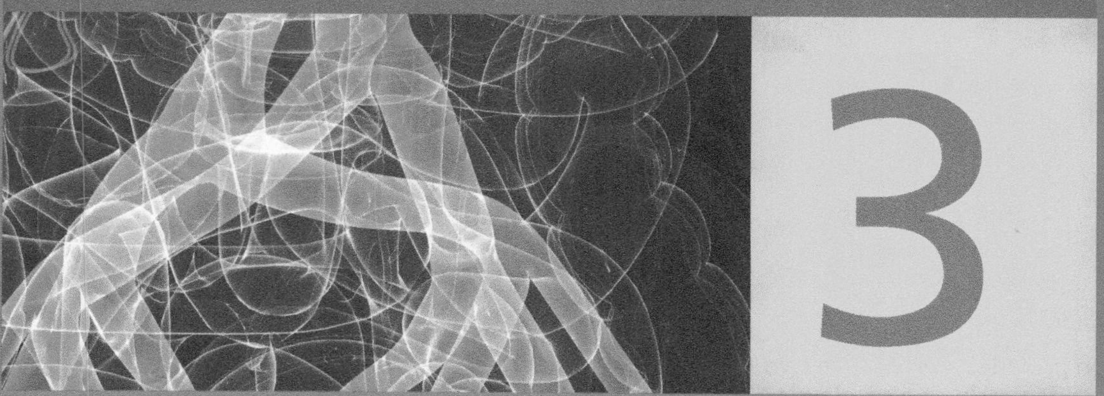

3

INTEGUMENTARY SYSTEM

Learning Objectives

Upon completion of this chapter, you will be able to

- Identify and define the combining forms, prefixes, and suffixes introduced in this chapter.
- Correctly spell and pronounce medical terms and major anatomical structures relating to the integumentary system.
- List and describe the three layers of skin and their functions.
- List and describe the four purposes of the skin.
- List and describe the accessory organs of the skin.
- Identify and define integumentary system anatomical terms.
- Identify and define selected integumentary system pathology terms.
- Identify and define selected integumentary system diagnostic procedures.
- Identify and define selected integumentary system therapeutic procedures.
- Identify and define selected medications relating to the integumentary system.
- Define selected abbreviations associated with the integumentary system.

Integumentary System at a Glance

Function

The skin provides a protective two-way barrier between our internal environment and the outside world. It also plays an important role in temperature regulation, houses sensory receptors to detect the environment around us, and secretes important fluids.

Structures

Here are the primary structures that comprise the integumentary system.

skin **hair** **nails** **sebaceous glands** **sweat glands**

Word Parts

Here are the most common word parts (with their meanings) used to build integumentary system terms. For a more comprehensive list, refer to the Terminology section of this chapter.

Combining Forms

albin/o	white	melan/o	black
bi/o	life	myc/o	fungus
cry/o	cold	necr/o	death
cutane/o	skin	onych/o	nail
cyan/o	blue	pedicul/o	lice
derm/o	skin	phot/o	light
dermat/o	skin	py/o	pus
diaphor/o	profuse sweating	rhytid/o	wrinkle
electr/o	electricity	scler/o	hard
erythr/o	red	seb/o	oil
hidr/o	sweat	trich/o	hair
ichthy/o	scaly, dry	ungu/o	nail
kerat/o	hard, horny	vesic/o	bladder
leuk/o	white	xer/o	dry
lip/o	fat		

Suffixes

-derma	skin condition
-opsy	view of
-tome	instrument used to cut

Prefixes

allo-	other, different from usual
xeno-	strange, foreign

Integumentary System Illustrated

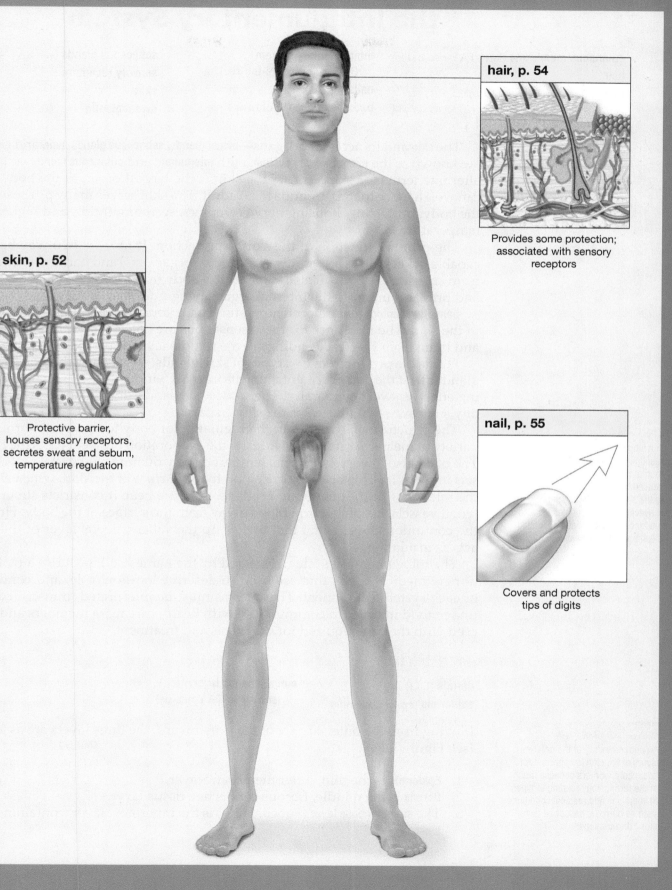

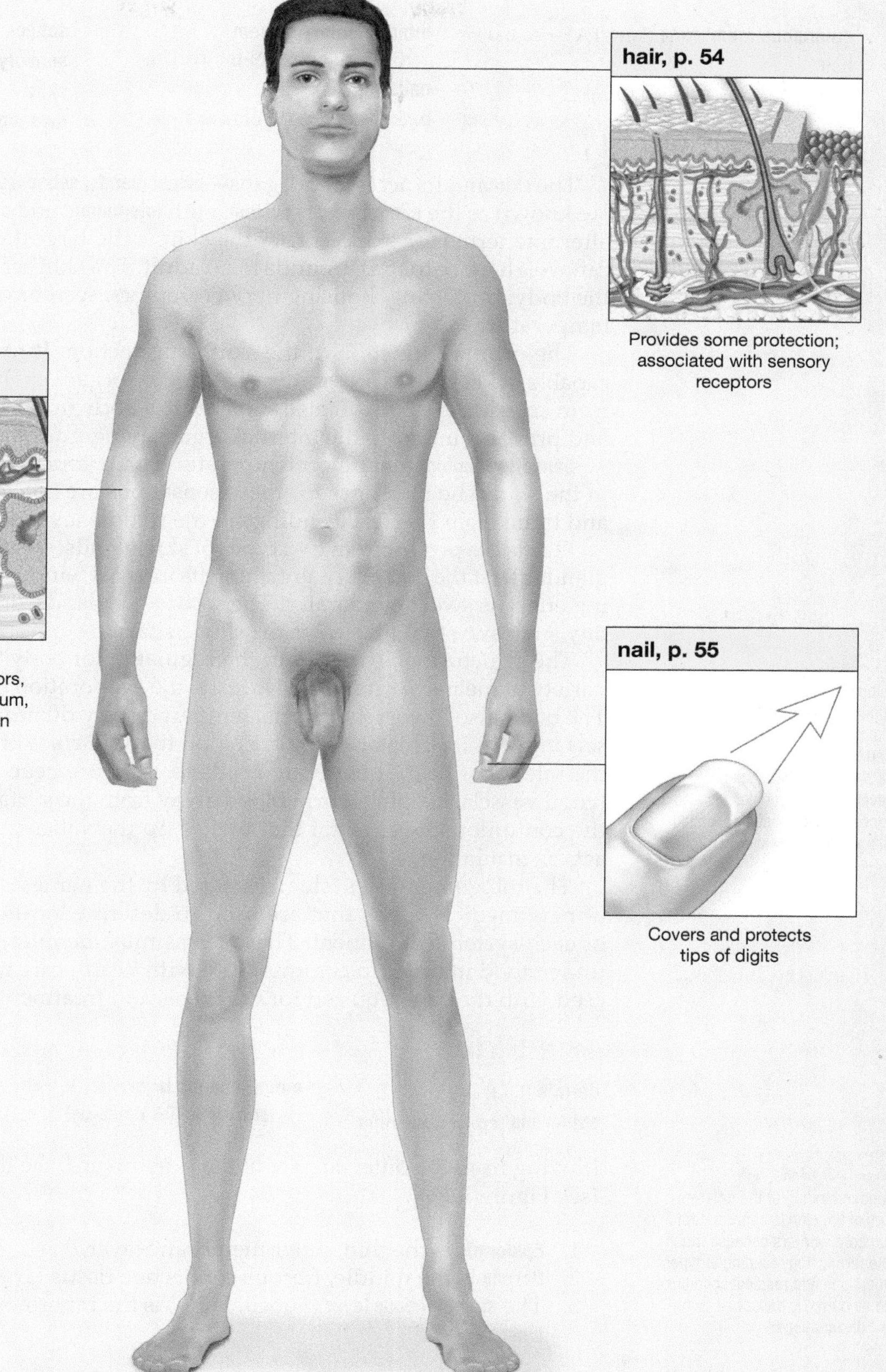

Anatomy and Physiology of the Integumentary System

cutaneous membrane (kew-TAY-nee-us)
hair
integument (in-TEG-you-mint)
integumentary system (in-teg-you-MEN-tah-ree)
nails
pathogens (PATH-oh-jenz)
sebaceous glands (see-BAY-shus)
sensory receptors
skin
sweat glands

The **skin** and its accessory organs—**sweat glands, sebaceous glands, hair,** and **nails**—are known as the **integumentary system,** with **integument** and **cutaneous membrane** being alternate terms for skin. In fact, the skin is the largest organ of the body and can weigh more than 20 pounds in an adult. The skin serves many purposes for the body: protecting, housing nerve receptors, secreting fluids, and regulating temperature.

The primary function of the skin is protection. It forms a two-way barrier capable of keeping **pathogens** (disease-causing organisms) and harmful chemicals from entering the body. It also stops critical body fluids from escaping the body and prevents injury to the internal organs lying underneath the skin.

Sensory receptors that detect temperature, pain, touch, and pressure are located in the skin. The messages for these sensations are conveyed to the spinal cord and brain from the nerve endings in the middle layer of the skin.

Fluids are produced in two types of skin glands: sweat and sebaceous. Sweat glands assist the body in maintaining its internal temperature by creating a cooling effect as sweat evaporates. The sebaceous glands, or oil glands, produce an oily substance that lubricates the skin surface.

MED TERM TIP

Flushing of the skin, a normal response to an increase in environmental temperature or to a fever, is caused by an increased blood flow to the skin of the face and neck. However, in some people, it is also a response to embarrassment called blushing and is not easily controlled.

The structure of skin aids in the regulation of body temperature through a variety of means. As noted previously, the evaporation of sweat cools the body. The body also lowers its internal temperature by dilating superficial blood vessels in the skin. This brings more blood to the surface of the skin, which allows the release of heat. If the body needs to conserve heat, it constricts superficial blood vessels, keeping warm blood away from the surface of the body. Finally, the continuous layer of fat that makes up the subcutaneous layer of the skin acts as insulation.

The integumentary system, as noted by the name itself, includes a plethora of new medical terms that are used to describe location, role, and condition of each system component. These terms must be interpreted, transcribed and understood in order to communicate with health care team members and proceed with the care required for diagnosis and treatment.

The Skin

dermis (DER-mis)
epidermis (ep-ih-DER-mis)
subcutaneous layer (sub-kyoo-TAY-nee-us)

MED TERM TIP

An understanding of the different layers of the skin is important for healthcare workers because much of the terminology relating to types of injections and medical conditions, such as burns, is described using these designations.

Moving from the outer surface of the skin inward, the three layers are as follows (see Figure 3.1 ■):

1. **Epidermis** is the thin, outer membrane layer.
2. **Dermis** is the middle, fibrous connective tissue layer.
3. The **subcutaneous layer** (Subcu, Subq) is the innermost layer, containing fatty tissue.

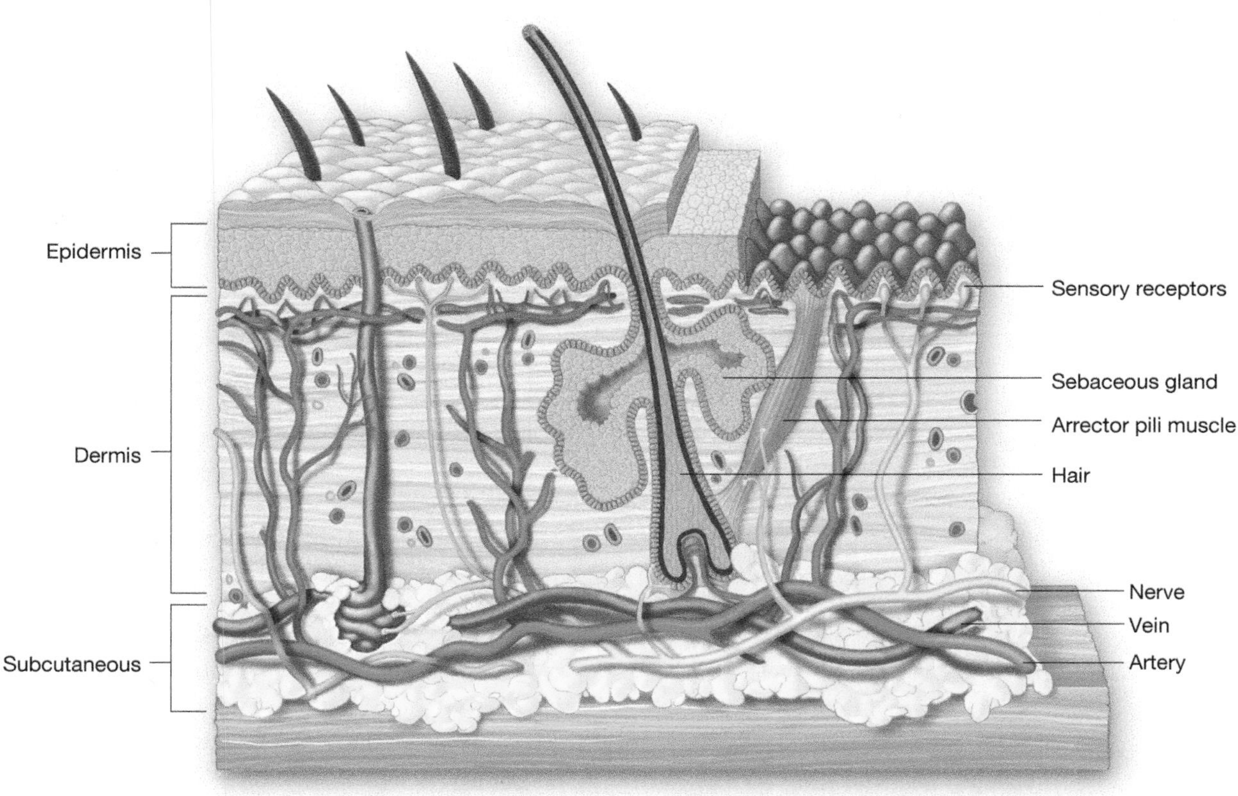

■ Figure 3.1 Skin structure, including the three layers of the skin and the accessory organs: sweat gland, sebaceous gland, and hair.

Epidermis

basal layer (BAY-sal)
keratin (KAIR-ah-tin)
melanin (MEL-ah-nin)
melanocytes (mel-AN-oh-sights)
stratified squamous epithelium (STRAT-ih-fyde / SKWAY-mus / ep-ih-THEE-lee-um)

The epidermis is composed of **stratified squamous epithelium** (see Figure 3.2 ■). This type of epithelial tissue consists of flat scale-like cells arranged in overlapping layers or strata. The epidermis does not have a blood supply or any connective tissue, so it is dependent for nourishment on the deeper layers of skin.

The deepest layer within the epidermis is called the **basal layer.** Cells in this layer continually grow and multiply. New cells that are forming push the old cells toward the outer layer of the epidermis. During this process the cells shrink, die, and become filled with a hard protein called **keratin.** These dead, overlapping, keratinized cells allow the skin to act as an effective barrier to infection and also make it waterproof.

The basal layer also contains special cells called **melanocytes,** which produce the black pigment **melanin.** Not only is this pigment responsible for the color of the skin, but it also protects against damage from the ultraviolet rays of the sun. This damage may be in the form of leatherlike skin and wrinkles, which are not hazardous, or it may be one of several forms of skin cancer. Dark-skinned people have more melanin and are generally less likely to get wrinkles or skin cancer.

MED TERM TIP

We lose 30,000-50,000 old, dead skin cells per minute and replace them with new, younger cells. In fact, because of this process, the epidermis is completely replaced every 25 days.

MED TERM TIP

A suntan can be thought of as a protective response to the rays of the sun. However, when the melanin in the skin is not able to absorb all the rays of the sun, the skin burns and DNA may be permanently and dangerously damaged.

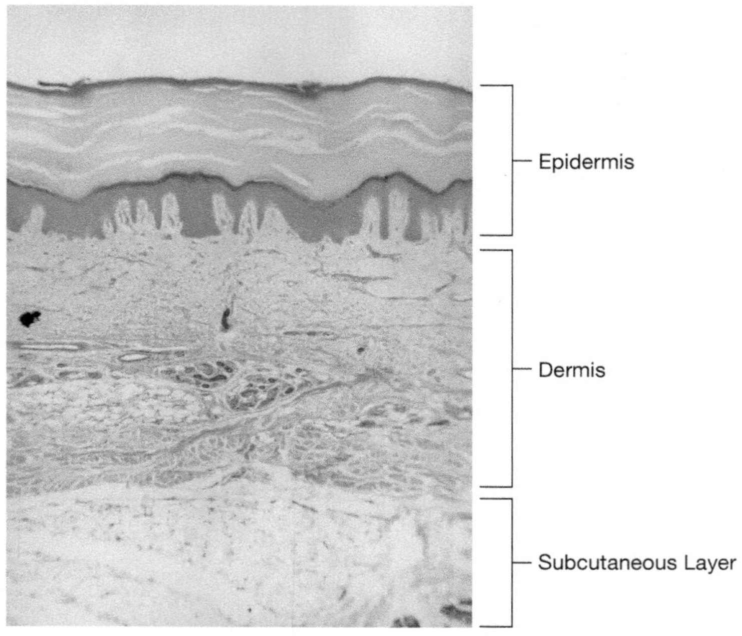

■ **Figure 3.2** Photomicrograph showing the three layers of the skin. *(Jubal Harshaw/Shutterstock)*

Dermis

collagen fibers (KOL-ah-jen)
corium (KOH-ree-um)

MED TERM TIP

Ridges formed in the dermis of our fingertips are what give each of us unique fingerprints. These do not change during a person's lifetime and so are a reliable means of identification. In fact, fingerprints are still visible on Egyptian mummies.

The dermis, also referred to as the **corium,** is the middle layer of skin, located between the epidermis and the subcutaneous layer (see Figure 3.2 ■). Its name means "true skin." Unlike the thinner epidermis, the dermis is living tissue with a very good blood supply. The dermis itself is composed of connective tissue and **collagen fibers.** Collagen fibers are made from a strong, fibrous protein present in connective tissue, forming a flexible "glue" that gives connective tissue its strength. The dermis houses hair follicles, sweat glands, sebaceous glands, blood vessels, lymph vessels, sensory receptors, nerve fibers, and muscle fibers.

Subcutaneous Layer

hypodermis (high-poh-DER-mis)
lipocytes (LIP-oh-sights)

The third and deepest layer of the skin is the subcutaneous layer, also called the **hypodermis.** This layer of tissue, composed of fat cells called **lipocytes,** protects the deeper tissues of the body and acts as insulation for heat and cold. (see Figure 3.2)

Accessory Organs

The accessory organs of the skin are the anatomical structures located within the dermis, including the hair, nails, sebaceous glands, and sweat glands.

Hair

arrector pili (ah-REK-tor / pee-lie)
hair follicle (FALL-ikl)
hair root
hair shaft

MED TERM TIP

Our hair turns gray as part of the normal aging process when we no longer produce melanin.

The fibers that make up hair are composed of the protein keratin, the same hard protein material that fills the cells of the epidermis. The process of hair formation is much like the process of growth in the epidermal layer of the skin. The deeper cells in the **hair root** force older keratinized cells to move upward, forming the **hair shaft.** The hair shaft grows toward the skin surface within the **hair follicle.** Melanin gives hair its color. Sebaceous glands release oil directly into the hair follicle. Each hair has a small slip of smooth muscle attached to it called the **arrector pili** muscle (see Figure 3.3 ■). When this muscle contracts the hair shaft stands up and results in "goose bumps."

Nails

cuticle (KEW-tikl)
free edge
nail root
lunula (LOO-nyoo-lah)
nail bed
nail body

Nails are a flat plate of keratin called the **nail body** that covers the ends of fingers and toes. The nail body is connected to the tissue underneath by the **nail bed.** Nails grow longer from the **nail root,** which is found at the base of the nail and is covered and protected by the soft tissue **cuticle.** The **free edge** is the exposed edge that is trimmed when nails become too long. The light-colored half-moon area at the base of the nail is the **lunula** (see Figure 3.4 ■).

MED TERM TIP

Because of its rich blood supply and light color, the nail bed is an excellent place to check patients for low oxygen levels in their blood. Deoxygenated blood is a very dark purple-red and gives skin a bluish tinge called *cyanosis.*

Sebaceous Glands

sebum

Sebaceous glands, found in the dermis, secrete the oil **sebum,** which lubricates the hair and skin, thereby helping to prevent drying and cracking. These glands secrete sebum directly into hair follicles, rather than a duct (see Figure 3.1 ■). Secretion from the sebaceous glands increases during adolescence, playing a role in the development of acne. Sebum secretion begins to diminish as age increases. A loss of sebum in old age, along with sun exposure, can account for wrinkles and dry skin.

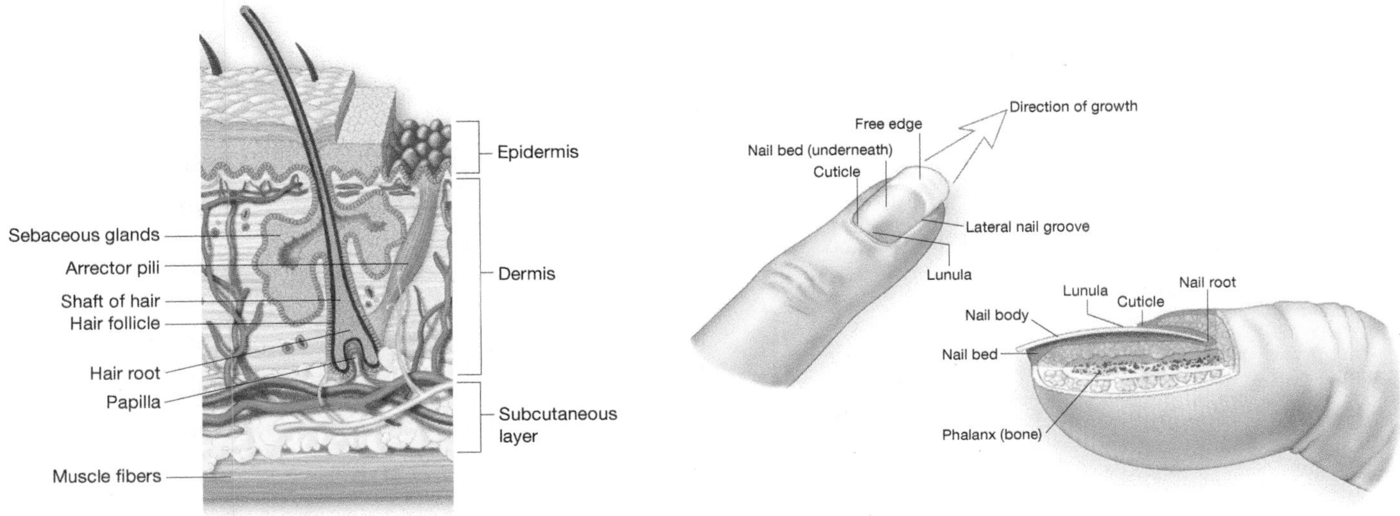

■ **Figure 3.3** Structure of a hair and its associated sebaceous gland.

■ **Figure 3.4** External and internal structures of nails.

Sweat Glands

apocrine glands (APP-oh-krin)
perspiration
sudoriferous glands (sue-doh-RIF-er-us)
sweat duct
sweat pore

About 2 million sweat glands, also called **sudoriferous glands,** are found throughout the body. These highly coiled glands are located in the dermis. Sweat travels to the surface of the skin in a **sweat duct.** The surface opening of a sweat duct is called a **sweat pore** (see Figure 3.1 ■).

Sweat glands function to cool the body as sweat evaporates. Sweat or **perspiration** contains a small amount of waste product but is normally colorless and odorless. However, there are sweat glands called **apocrine glands** in the pubic and underarm areas that secrete a thicker sweat, which can produce an odor when it comes into contact with bacteria on the skin. This is what we recognize as body odor.

MED TERM TIP

Word Watch: Be careful when using *hydro-* meaning "water" and *hidr/o* meaning "sweat."

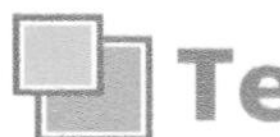

Terminology

Word Parts Used to Build Integumentary System Terms

The following lists contain the combining forms, suffixes, and prefixes used to build terms in the remaining sections of this chapter.

Combining Forms

albin/o	white
angi/o	vessel
bas/o	the base
bi/o	life
carcin/o	cancer
chem/o	chemical
cis/o	to cut
cry/o	cold
cutane/o	skin
cyan/o	blue
cyt/o	cell
derm/o	skin
dermat/o	skin
diaphor/o	profuse sweating
electr/o	electricity
erythr/o	red
esthesi/o	feeling
hem/o	blood
hidr/o	sweat
ichthy/o	scaly, dry
kerat/o	hard, horny
leuk/o	white
lip/o	fat
melan/o	black
myc/o	fungus
necr/o	death
onych/o	nail
pedicul/o	lice
phot/o	light
py/o	pus
rhytid/o	wrinkle
sarc/o	flesh
scler/o	hard
seb/o	oil
system/o	system
trich/o	hair
ungu/o	nail
vesic/o	bladder
xer/o	dry

Suffixes

-al	pertaining to
-derma	skin condition
-ectomy	surgical removal
-emia	blood condition
-ia	state, condition
-ic	pertaining to
-ism	state of

-itis	inflammation
-logy	study of
-malacia	softening
-oma	mass
-opsy	to view
-osis	abnormal condition

-ous	pertaining to
-phagia	eating
-plasty	surgical repair
-rrhea	discharge
-tic	pertaining to
-tome	instrument to cut
-ule	small

Prefixes

allo-	other
an-	without
anti-	against
auto-	self

de-	without
epi-	upon
hyper-	excessive
hypo-	under

intra-	within
para-	beside
sub-	under
xeno-	strange, foreign

Anatomical Terms

TERM	WORD PARTS	DEFINITION
cutaneous (kyoo-TAY-nee-us)	cutane/o = skin -ous = pertaining to	pertaining to the skin
dermal (DER-mal)	derm/o = skin -al = pertaining to	pertaining to the skin
epidermal (ep-ih-DER-mal)	epi- = upon derm/o = skin -al = pertaining to	pertaining to upon the skin
hypodermic (high-poh-DER-mik)	hypo- = under derm/o = skin -ic = pertaining to	pertaining to under the skin
intradermal (in-trah-DER-mal)	intra- = within derm/o = skin -al = pertaining to	pertaining to within the skin
subcutaneous (sub-kyoo-TAY-nee-us)	sub- = under cutane/o = skin -ous = pertaining to	pertaining to under the skin
ungual (UNG-gwal)	ungu/o = nail -al = pertaining to	pertaining to the nails

Pathology

TERM	WORD PARTS	DEFINITION
Medical Specialties		
dermatology (Derm, derm) (der-mah-TALL-oh-jee)	dermat/o = skin -logy = study of	Branch of medicine involving diagnosis and treatment of conditions and diseases of the integumentary system. Physician is a *dermatologist.*
plastic surgery		Surgical specialty involved in repair, reconstruction, or improvement of body structures such as the skin that are damaged, missing, or misshapen. Physician is a *plastic surgeon.*
Signs and Symptoms		
abrasion (ah-BRAY-zhun)		A scraping away of the skin surface by friction.
anhidrosis (an-hi-DROH-sis)	an- = without hidr/o = sweat -osis = abnormal condition	Abnormal condition of no sweat.
comedo (KOM-ee-do)		Collection of hardened sebum in hair follicle. Also called a *blackhead.*
contusion		Injury caused by a blow to the body; causes swelling, pain, and bruising. The skin is not broken.
cyanosis (sigh-ah-NOH-sis)	cyan/o = blue -osis = abnormal condition	Bluish tint to the skin caused by deoxygenated blood.
■ **Figure 3.5** A cyanotic infant. Note the bluish tinge to the skin around the lips, chin, and nose. *(St. Bartholomew's Hospital, London/Photo Researchers, Inc.)*	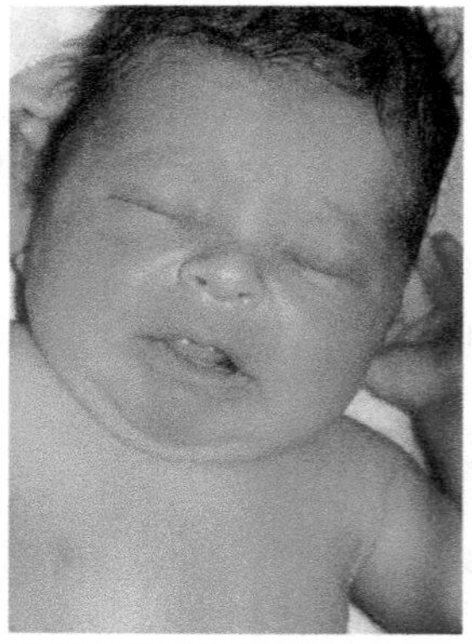	
cyst (SIST)	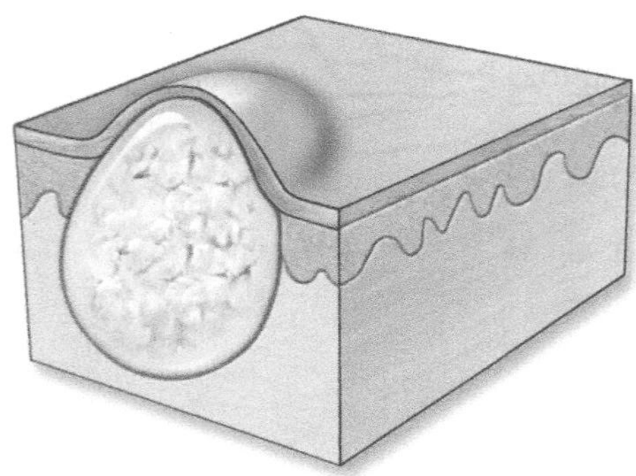	Fluid-filled sac under the skin.
■ **Figure 3.6** Cyst.		

Pathology *(continued)*

TERM	WORD PARTS	DEFINITION
depigmentation (dee-pig-men-TAY-shun)	de- = without	Loss of normal skin color or pigment.
diaphoresis (dye-ah-for-REE-sis)	diaphor/o = profuse sweating	Profuse sweating.
ecchymosis (ek-ih-MOH-sis)	-osis = abnormal condition	Skin discoloration caused by blood collecting under the skin following blunt trauma to the skin. A bruise.

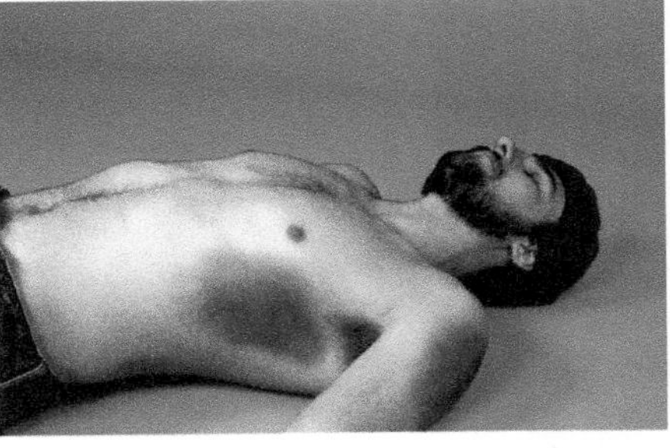

■ **Figure 3.7** Male lying supine with large ecchymosis on lateral rib cage and shoulder.

TERM	WORD PARTS	DEFINITION
erythema (er-ih-THEE-mah)	erythr/o = red hem/o = blood	Redness or flushing of the skin.
erythroderma (eh-rith-roh-DER-mah)	erythr/o = red -derma = skin condition	The condition of having reddened or flushed skin.
eschar (ES-kar)		A thick layer of dead tissue and tissue fluid that develops over a deep burn area.
fissure (FISH-er)		Crack-like lesion or groove on the skin.

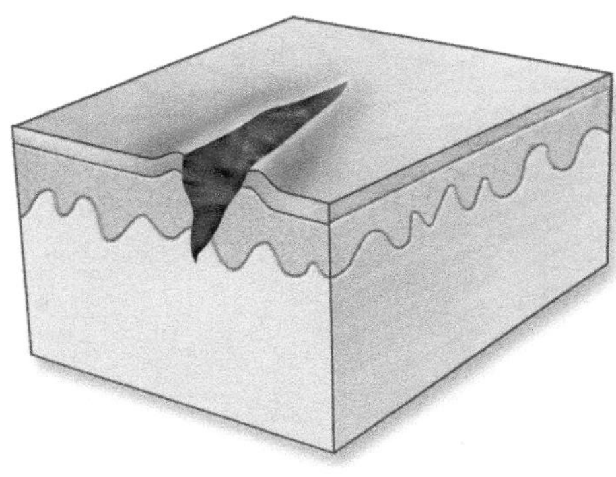

■ **Figure 3.8** Fissure.

TERM	WORD PARTS	DEFINITION
hirsutism (HER-soot-izm)		Excessive hair growth over the body.
hyperemia (high-per-EE-mee-ah)	hyper- = excessive -emia = blood condition	Redness of the skin due to increased blood flow.
hyperhidrosis (high-per-hi-DROH-sis)	hyper- = excessive hidr/o = sweat -osis = abnormal condition	Abnormal condition of excessive sweat.
hyperpigmentation (high-per-pig-men-TAY-shun)	hyper- = excessive	Abnormal amount of pigmentation in the skin.
ichthyoderma (ick-thee-oh-DER-mah)	ichthy/o = scaly, dry -derma = skin condition	The condition of having scaly and dry skin.

Pathology *(continued)*

TERM	WORD PARTS	DEFINITION
lesion (LEE-shun)		A general term for a wound, injury, or abnormality.
leukoderma (loo-koh-DER-mah)	leuk/o = white -derma = skin condition	Having skin that appears white because the normal skin pigment is absent. May be all the skin or just in some areas.
lipoma (lip-OH-mah)	lip/o = fat -oma = mass	Fatty mass.
macule (MACK-yool)	-ule = small	Flat, discolored area that is flush with the skin surface. An example would be a freckle or a birthmark.
■ **Figure 3.9** Macule.		
necrosis (neh-KROH-sis)	necr/o = death -osis = abnormal condition	Abnormal condition of death.
nevus (NEV-us)		Pigmented skin blemish, birthmark, or mole. Usually benign but may become cancerous.
nodule (NOD-yool)	-ule = small	Firm, solid mass of cells in the skin larger than 0.5 cm in diameter.
■ **Figure 3.10** Nodule.		
onychomalacia (on-ih-koh-mah-LAY-she-ah)	onych/o = nail -malacia = softening	Softening of the nails.
pallor (PAL-or)		Abnormal paleness of the skin.

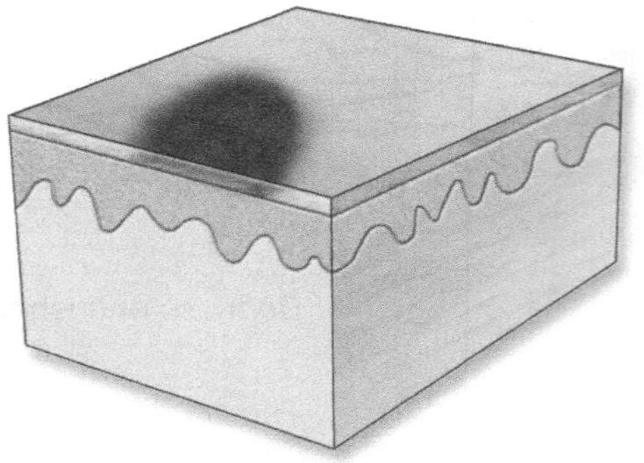

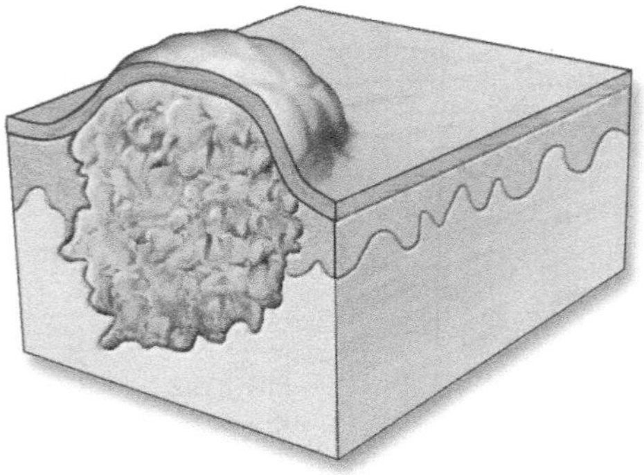

Pathology *(continued)*

TERM	WORD PARTS	DEFINITION
papule (PAP-yool) 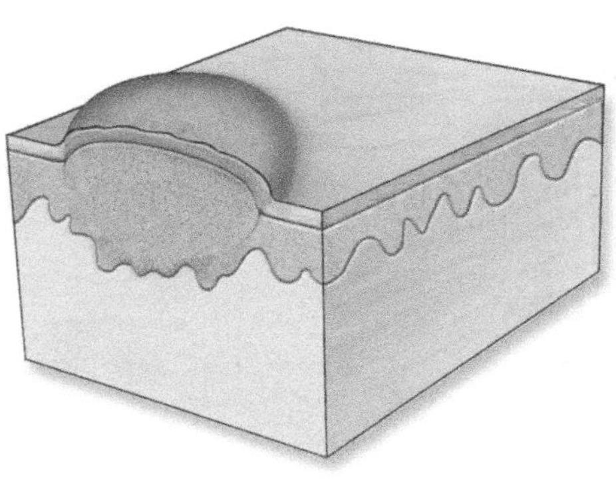 ■ **Figure 3.11** Papule.	-ule = small	Small, solid, circular raised spot on the surface of the skin less than 0.5 cm in diameter.
petechiae (peh-TEE-kee-eye)  ■ **Figure 3.12** Petechiae, pinpoint skin hemorrhages. *(Custom Medical Stock)*		Pinpoint purple or red spots from minute hemorrhages under the skin.
photosensitivity (foh-toh-sen-sih-TIH-vih-tee)	phot/o = light	Condition in which the skin reacts abnormally when exposed to light, such as the ultraviolet (UV) rays of the sun.
pruritus (proo-RIGH-tus)		Severe itching.
purpura (PER-pew-rah) 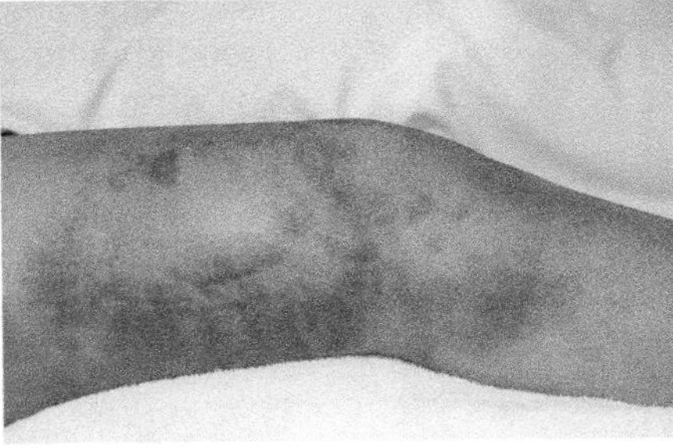 ■ **Figure 3.13** Purpura, hemorrhaging into the skin due to fragile blood vessels.		Hemorrhages into the skin due to fragile blood vessels. Commonly seen in older adults. **MED TERM TIP** *Purpura* comes from the Latin word for "purple," which refers to the color of these pinpoint hemorrhages.
purulent (PYUR-yoo-lent)		Containing pus or an infection that is producing pus. Pus consists of dead bacteria, white blood cells, and tissue debris.

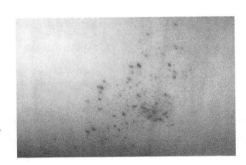

Pathology (continued)

TERM	WORD PARTS	DEFINITION
pustule (PUS-tyool)	-ule = small	Raised spot on the skin containing pus.

■ Figure 3.14 Pustule.

TERM	WORD PARTS	DEFINITION
pyoderma (pye-oh-DER-mah)	py/o = pus -derma = skin condition	The presence of pus on or in the layers of skin. A sign of a bacterial infection.
scleroderma (sklair-ah-DER-mah)	scler/o = hard -derma = skin condition	A condition in which the skin has lost its elasticity and become hardened.
seborrhea (seb-or-EE-ah)	seb/o = oil -rrhea = discharge	Oily discharge.
suppurative (SUP-pure-a-tiv)		Containing or producing pus.
ulcer (ULL-ser)		Open sore or lesion in skin or mucous membrane.

■ Figure 3.15 Ulcer.

TERM	WORD PARTS	DEFINITION
urticaria (er-tih-KAY-ree-ah)		Also called *hives;* a skin eruption of pale reddish wheals with severe itching. Usually associated with food allergy, stress, or drug reactions.
vesicle (VESS-ikl)	vesic/o = bladder	A blister; small, fluid-filled raised spot on the skin.

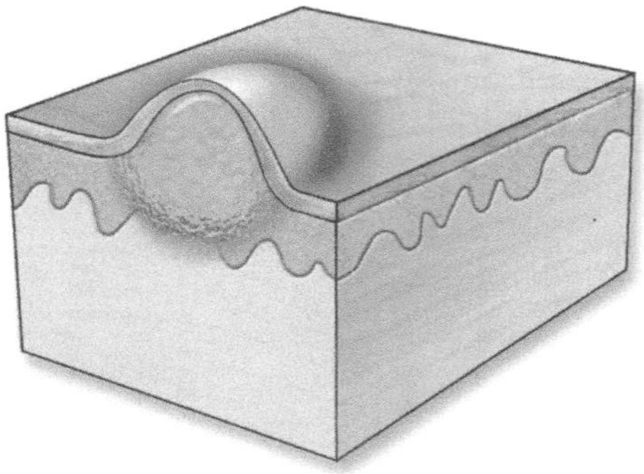

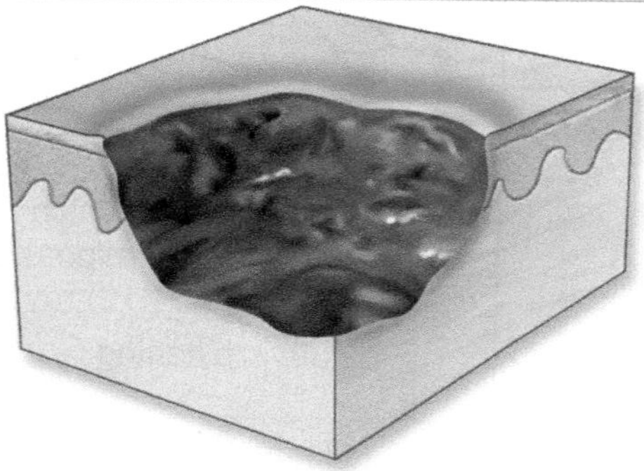

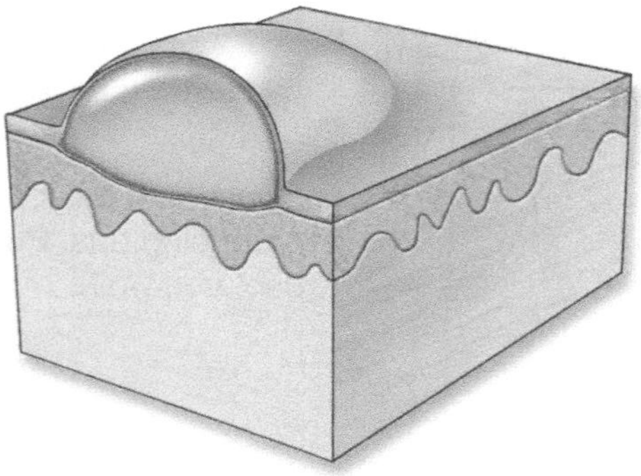

■ Figure 3.16 Vesicle.

Pathology *(continued)*

TERM	WORD PARTS	DEFINITION
wheal (WEEL)		Small, round, swollen area on the skin; typically seen in allergic skin reactions such as *hives* and usually accompanied by urticaria.

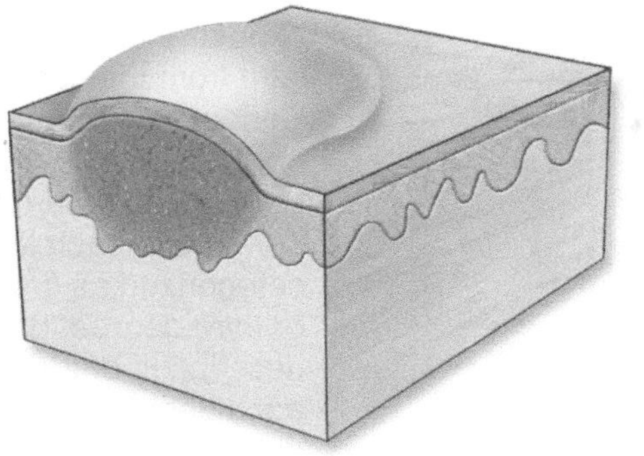

■ **Figure 3.17** Wheal.

TERM	WORD PARTS	DEFINITION
xeroderma (zee-roh-DER-mah)	xer/o = dry -derma = skin condition	Condition in which the skin is abnormally dry.
Skin		
abscess (AB-sess)		A collection of pus in the skin.
acne (ACK-nee)		Inflammatory disease of the sebaceous glands and hair follicles resulting in papules and pustules.
acne rosacea (ACK-nee roh-ZAY-she-ah)		Chronic form of acne seen in adults involving redness, tiny pimples, and broken blood vessels, primarily on the nose and cheeks.
acne vulgaris (ACK-nee vul-GAY-ris)		Common form of acne seen in teenagers. Characterized by comedo, papules, and pustules.
albinism (al-BIH-nizm)	albin/o = white -ism = state of	A genetic condition in which the body is unable to make melanin. Characterized by white hair and skin and red pupils due to the lack of pigment. The person with albinism is called an *albino.*
basal cell carcinoma (BCC) (BAY-sal / sell / kar-sin-NOH-ma)	bas/o = the base -al = pertaining to carcin/o = cancer -oma = tumor	Cancerous tumor of the basal cell layer of the epidermis. A frequent type of skin cancer that rarely metastasizes or spreads. These cancers can arise on sun-exposed skin.

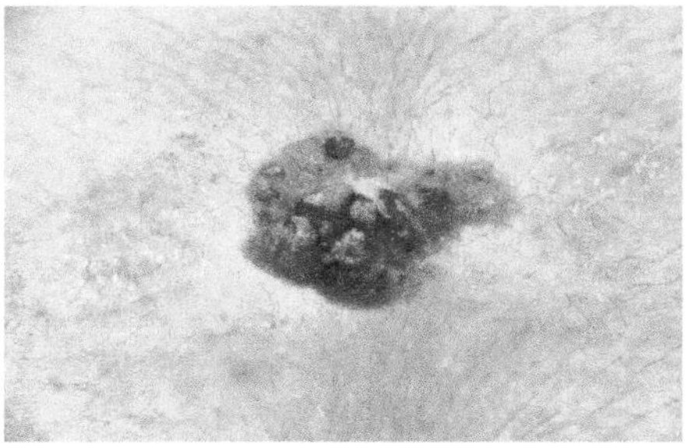

■ **Figure 3.18** Basal cell carcinoma, a frequent type of skin cancer that rarely metastasizes. *(Bob Craig/CDC)*

Pathology (continued)

TERM	WORD PARTS	DEFINITION
burn		Damage to the skin that can result from exposure to open fire, electricity, ultraviolet light from the sun, or caustic chemicals. Seriousness depends on the amount of body surface involved and the depth of the burn as determined by the amount of damage to each layer. Skin and burns are categorized as first degree, second degree, or third degree. See Figure 3.19 ■ for a description of the damage associated with each degree of burn. Extent of a burn is estimated using the Rule of Nines (see Figure 3.20 ■).

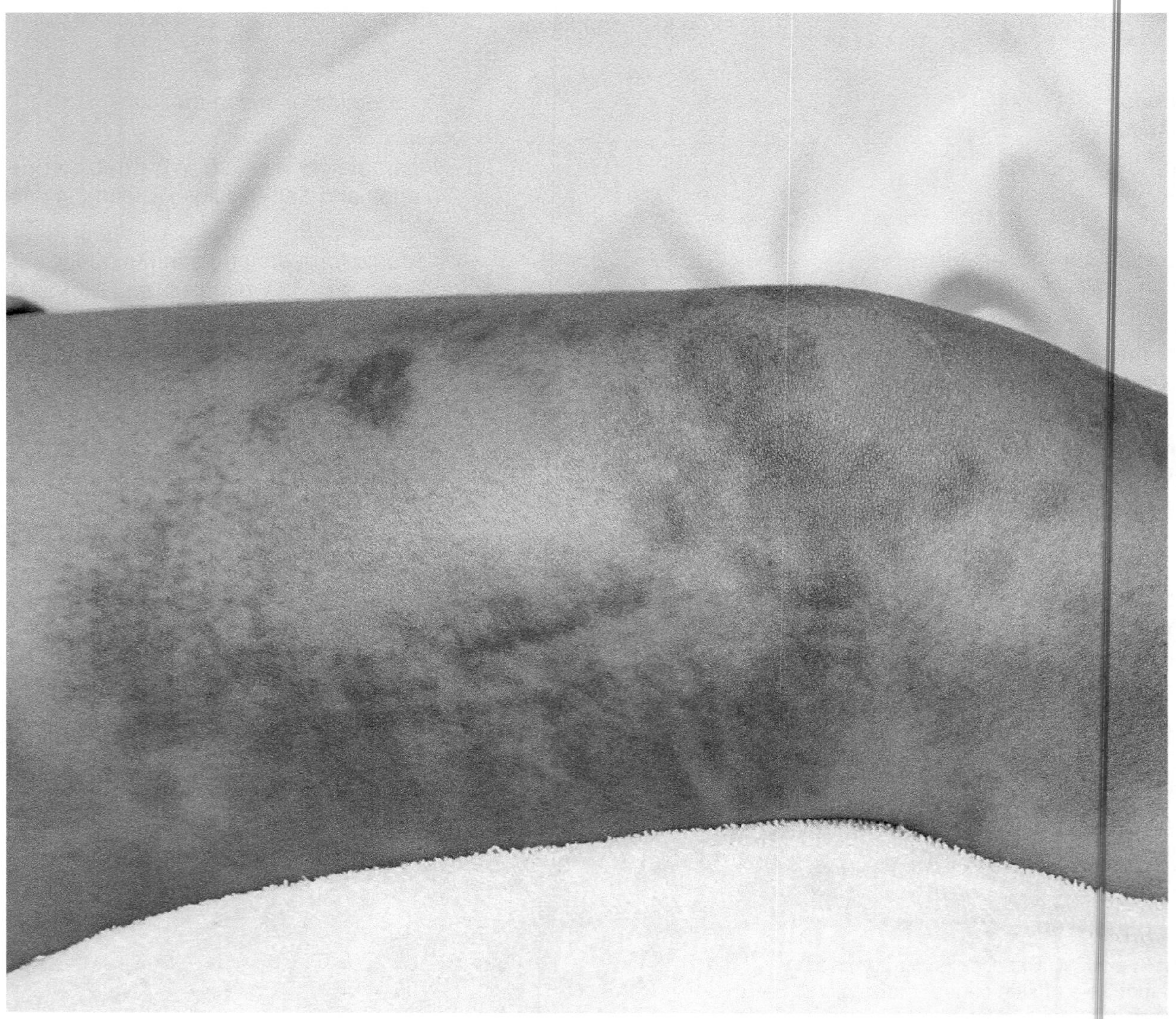

■ **Figure 3.19** Comparison of the level of skin damage as a result of the three different degrees of burns.

Pathology *(continued)*

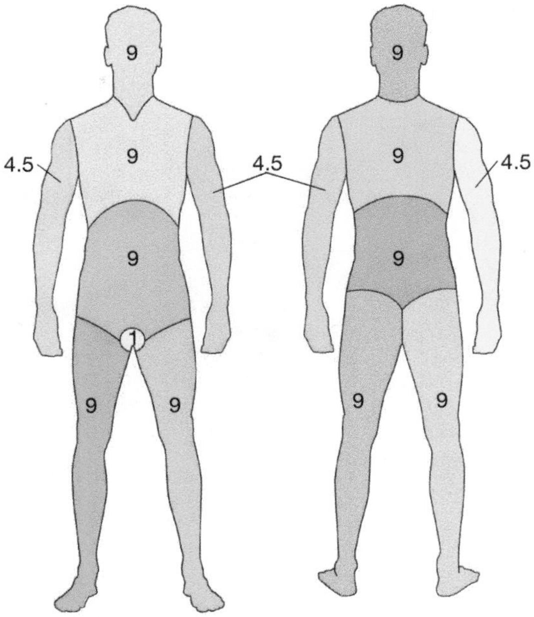

■ **Figure 3.20** Rule of Nines. A method for determining percentage of body burned. Each different-colored section represents a percentage of the body surface. All sections added together will equal 100%.

TERM	WORD PARTS	DEFINITION
cellulitis (sell-you-LYE-tis)	-itis = inflammation	A diffuse, acute infection and inflammation of the connective tissue found in the skin.
cicatrix (SICK-ah-trix)		A scar.
decubitus ulcer (decub) (dee-KYOO-bih-tus)	MED TERM TIP: *Decubitus* comes from the Latin word *decumbo,* meaning "lying down," which leads to the use of the term for a bedsore or pressure sore.	Open sore caused by pressure over bony prominences cutting off the blood flow to the overlying skin. These can appear in bedridden patients who lie in one position too long and can be difficult to heal. Also called *bedsore* or *pressure sore.*
dermatitis (der-mah-TYE-tis)	dermat/o = skin -itis = inflammation	Inflammation of the skin.
dermatosis (der-mah-TOH-sis)	dermat/o = skin -osis = abnormal condition	A general term indicating the presence of an abnormal skin condition.
dry gangrene (GANG-green)		Late stages of gangrene characterized by the affected area becoming dried, blackened, and shriveled; referred to as *mummified.*
eczema (EK-zeh-mah)		Superficial dermatitis of unknown cause accompanied by redness, vesicles, itching, and crusting.
gangrene (GANG-green)		Tissue necrosis usually due to deficient blood supply.
ichthyosis (ick-thee-OH-sis)	ichthy/o = scaly, dry -osis = abnormal condition	Condition in which the skin becomes dry, scaly, and keratinized.

Pathology *(continued)*

TERM	WORD PARTS	DEFINITION
impetigo (im-peh-TYE-goh)		A highly infectious bacterial infection of the skin with pustules that rupture and become crusted over.
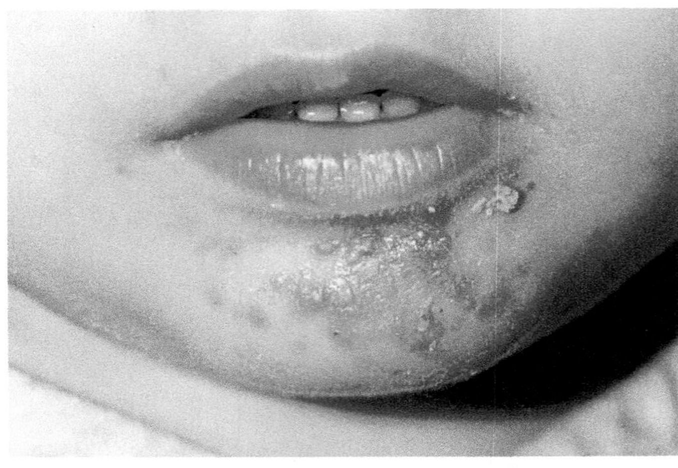 ■ **Figure 3.21** Impetigo, a highly contagious bacterial infection. *(Dr. Jason L. Smith)*		
Kaposi's sarcoma (KAP-oh-seez / sar-KOH-mah)	sarc/o = flesh -oma = tumor	Form of skin cancer frequently seen in acquired immunodeficiency syndrome (AIDS) patients. Consists of brownish-purple papules that spread from the skin and metastasize to internal organs.
keloid (KEE-loyd)		Formation of a raised and thickened hypertrophic scar after an injury or surgery.
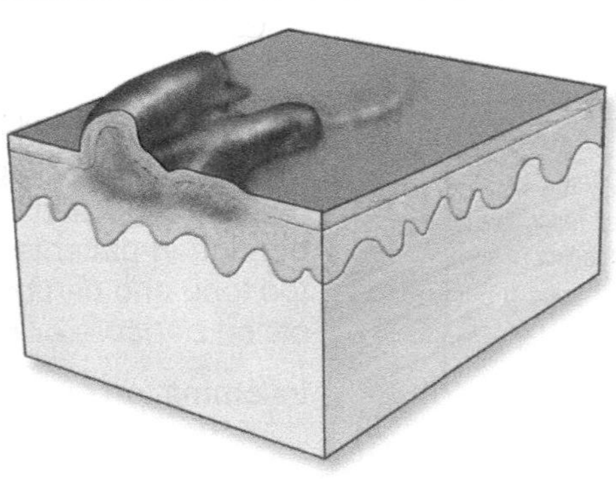 ■ **Figure 3.22** Keloid.		
keratosis (kair-ah-TOH-sis)	kerat/o = hard, horny -osis = abnormal condition	Term for any skin condition involving an overgrowth and thickening of the epidermis layer.
laceration		A torn or jagged wound; incorrectly used to describe a cut.
malignant melanoma (MM) (mah-LIG-nant / mel-a-NOH-ma)	melan/o = black -oma = tumor	Dangerous form of skin cancer caused by an uncontrolled growth of melanocytes. May quickly metastasize or spread to internal organs.
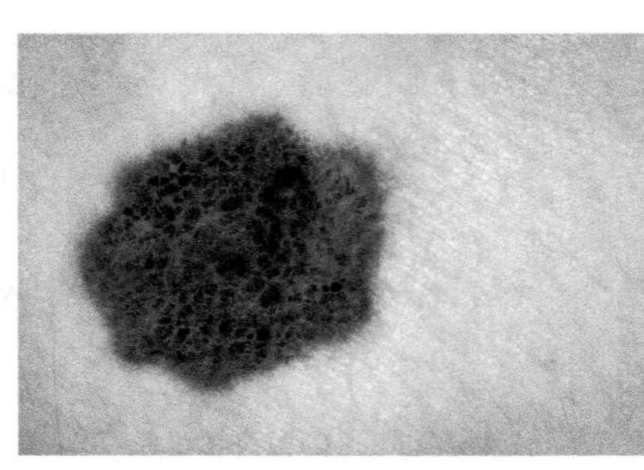 ■ **Figure 3.23** Malignant melanoma. This photograph demonstrates the highly characteristic color of this tumor.		

Pathology *(continued)*

TERM	WORD PARTS	DEFINITION
pediculosis (peh-dik-you-LOH-sis)	pedicul/o = lice -osis = abnormal condition	Infestation with lice. The eggs laid by the lice are called nits and cling tightly to hair.
psoriasis (soh-RYE-ah-sis) ■ Figure 3.24 Psoriasis. This photograph demonstrates the characteristic white skin patches of this condition. *(kenxro/Shutterstock)*		Chronic inflammatory condition consisting of papules forming "silvery scale" patches with circular borders.
rubella (roo-BELL-ah)		Contagious viral skin infection. Commonly called *German measles.*
scabies (SKAY-bees)		Contagious skin disease caused by an egg-laying mite that burrows through the skin and causes redness and intense itching; often seen in children.
sebaceous cyst (see-BAY-shus / SIST)	seb/o = oil	Sac under the skin filled with sebum or oil from a sebaceous gland. This can grow to a large size and may need to be excised.
squamous cell carcinoma (SCC) (SKWAY-mus / sell / kar-sih-NOH-mah) ■ Figure 3.25 Squamous cell carcinoma.	carcin/o = cancer -oma = tumor 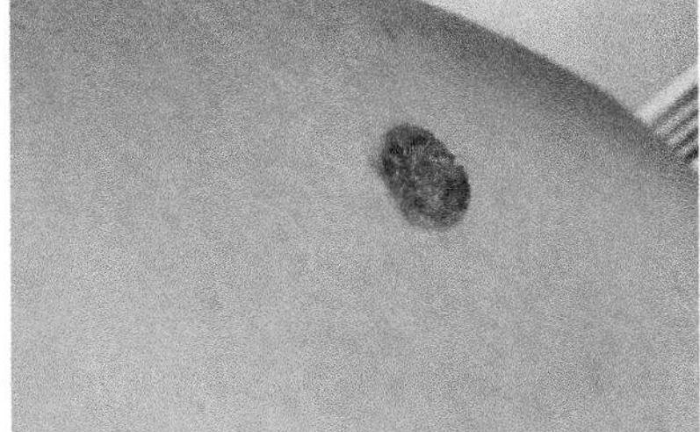	Cancer of the epidermis layer of skin that may invade deeper tissue and metastasize. Often begins as a sore that does not heal.

Pathology *(continued)*

TERM	WORD PARTS	DEFINITION
strawberry hemangioma (hee-man-jee-OH-ma)	hem/o = blood angi/o = vessel -oma = tumor	Congenital collection of dilated blood vessels causing a red birthmark that fades a few months after birth.
systemic lupus erythematosus (SLE) (sis-TEM-ik / LOO-pus / air-ih-them-ah-TOH-sis)	system/o = system -ic = pertaining to erythr/o = red	Chronic disease of the connective tissue that injures the skin, joints, kidneys, nervous system, and mucous membranes. This is an autoimmune condition meaning that the body's own immune system attacks normal tissue of the body. May produce a characteristic red, scaly butterfly rash across the cheeks and nose.
tinea (TIN-ee-ah)		Fungal skin disease resulting in itching, scaling lesions.
tinea capitis (TIN-ee-ah / CAP-it-is)	*capitis* is the Latin term for the head	Fungal infection of the scalp. Commonly called *ringworm.*
tinea pedis (TIN-ee-ah / PED-is)	*pedis* is the Latin term for the foot	Fungal infection of the foot. Commonly called *athlete's foot.*
varicella (vair-ih-SELL-ah)		Contagious viral skin infection. Commonly called *chickenpox.*
verruca (ver-ROO-kah)		Commonly called *warts;* a benign growth caused by a virus. Has a rough surface that is removed by chemicals and/or laser therapy.

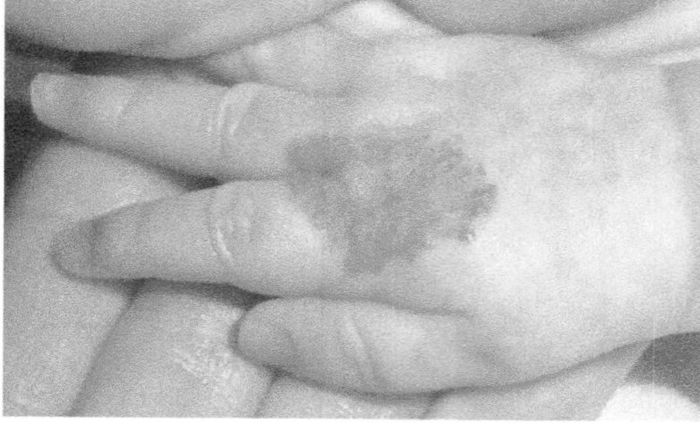

■ Figure 3.26 Strawberry hemangioma, a birthmark caused by a collection of blood vessels in the skin. *(H.C. Robinson/Science Photo Library/Photo Researchers)*

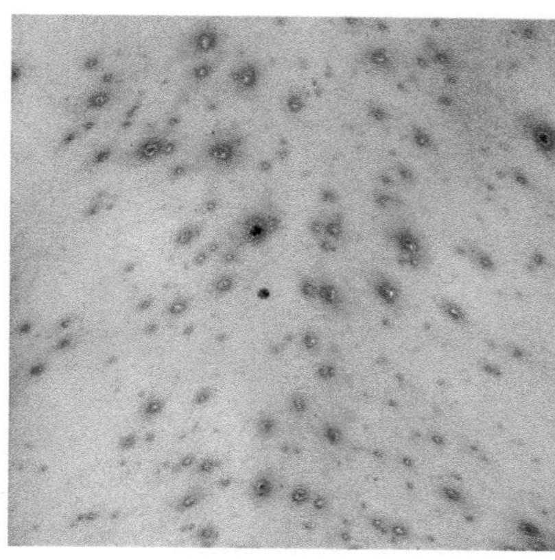

■ Figure 3.27 Varicella or chickenpox, a viral skin infection. In this photograph, the rash is beginning to form scabs.

Pathology *(continued)*

TERM	WORD PARTS	DEFINITION
vitiligo (vit-ill-EYE-go)		Disappearance of pigment from the skin in patches, causing a milk-white appearance. Also called *leukoderma.*
wet gangrene (GANG-green)		An area of gangrene that becomes secondarily infected by pus-producing bacteria.
Hair		
alopecia (al-oh-PEE-she-ah)		Absence or loss of hair, especially of the head. Commonly called *baldness.*
carbuncle (CAR-bung-kl)		Furuncle involving several hair follicles.
furuncle (FOO-rung-kl)		Bacterial infection of a hair follicle. Characterized by redness, pain, and swelling. Also called a *boil.*
trichomycosis (trik-oh-my-KOH-sis)	trich/o = hair myc/o = fungus -osis = abnormal condition	Abnormal condition of hair fungus.
Nails		
onychia (oh-NICK-ee-ah)	onych/o = nail -ia = state, condition	Infected nail bed.
onychomycosis (on-ih-koh-my-KOH-sis)	onych/o = nail myc/o = fungus -osis = abnormal condition	Abnormal condition of nail fungus.
onychophagia (on-ih-koh-FAY-jee-ah)	onych/o = nail -phagia = eating	Nail eating (nail biting).
paronychia (pair-oh-NICK-ee-ah)	para- = beside onych/o = nail -ia = state, condition	Infection of the skin fold around a nail.

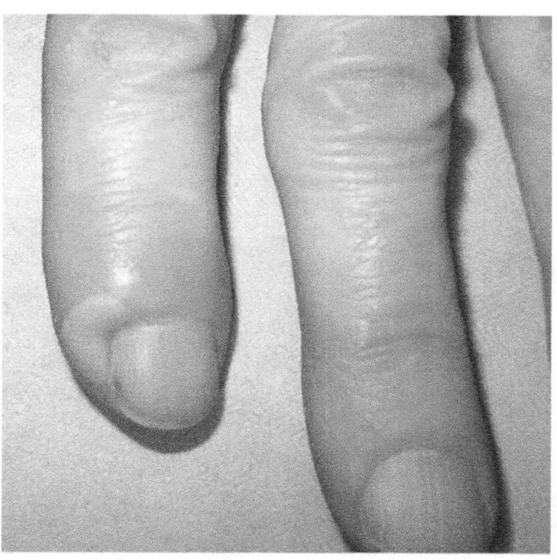

■ **Figure 3.28** Paronychia.
(Local Images Inc.)

Diagnostic Procedures

TERM	WORD PARTS	DEFINITION
Clinical Laboratory Tests		
culture and sensitivity (C&S)		Laboratory test that grows a colony of bacteria removed from an infected area in order to identify the specific infecting bacteria and then determine its sensitivity to a variety of antibiotics.
Biopsy Procedures		
biopsy (BX, bx) (BYE-op-see) MED TERM TIP Word Watch: Be careful when using *bi-* meaning "two" and *bi/o* meaning "life."	bi/o = life -opsy = to view	Piece of tissue removed by syringe and needle, knife, punch, or brush to examine under a microscope. Used to aid in diagnosis.
exfoliative cytology (ex-FOH-lee-ah-tiv / sigh-TALL-oh-jee)	cyt/o = cell -logy = study of	Scraping cells from tissue and then examining them under a microscope.
frozen section (FS)		Thin piece of tissue cut from a frozen specimen for rapid examination under a microscope.
fungal scrapings	-al = pertaining to	Scrapings, taken with a curette or scraper, of tissue from lesions are placed on a growth medium and examined under a microscope to identify fungal growth.

Therapeutic Procedures

TERM	WORD PARTS	DEFINITION
Skin Grafting		
allograft (AL-oh-graft)	allo- = other	Skin graft from one person to another; donor is usually a cadaver. Also called *homograft* (homo = same).
autograft (AW-toh-graft)	auto- = self	Skin graft from a person's own body.
dermatome (DER-mah-tohm)	derm/o = skin -tome = instrument to cut	Instrument for cutting the skin or thin transplants of skin.

■ **Figure 3.29** A freshly applied autograft. Note that the donor skin has been perforated so that it can be stretched to cover a larger burned area. *(Courtesy of Dr. William Dominic, Community Regional Medical Center)*

Therapeutic Procedures *(continued)*

TERM	WORD PARTS	DEFINITION
dermatoplasty (DER-mah-toh-plas-tee)	dermat/o = skin -plasty = surgical repair	Skin grafting; transplantation of skin.
skin graft (SG)		Transfer of skin from a normal area to cover another site. Used to treat burn victims and after some surgical procedures. Also called *dermatoplasty.*
xenograft (ZEN-oh-graft)	xeno- = strange, foreign	Skin graft from an animal of another species (usually a pig) to a human. Also called *heterograft* (hetero- = other).
Surgical Procedures		
cauterization (kaw-ter-ih-ZAY-shun)		Destruction of tissue by using caustic chemicals, electric currents, heat, or by freezing.
cryosurgery (cry-oh-SER-jer-ee)	cry/o = cold	Use of extreme cold to freeze and destroy tissue.
curettage (koo-REH-tahz)		Removal of superficial skin lesions with a curette (surgical instrument shaped like a spoon) or scraper.
debridement (de-BREED-mint)		Removal of foreign material and dead or damaged tissue from a wound.
electrocautery (ee-leck-troh-KAW-teh-ree)	electr/o = electricity	To destroy tissue with an electric current.
incision and drainage (I&D)	cis/o = to cut	Making an incision to create an opening for the drainage of material such as pus.
onychectomy (on-ee-KECK-toh-mee)	onych/o = nail -ectomy = surgical removal	Removal of a nail.
Plastic Surgery Procedures		
chemabrasion (kee-moh-BRAY-zhun)	chem/o = chemical	Abrasion using chemicals. Also called a *chemical peel.*
dermabrasion (DERM-ah-bray-shun)	derm/o = skin	Abrasion or rubbing using wire brushes or sandpaper. Performed to remove acne scars, tattoos, and scar tissue.
laser therapy		Removal of skin lesions and birthmarks using a laser beam that emits intense heat and power at a close range. The laser converts frequencies of light into one small, powerful beam.
liposuction (LIP-oh-suck-shun)	lip/o = fat	Removal of fat beneath the skin by means of suction.
rhytidectomy (rit-ih-DECK-toh-mee)	rhytid/o = wrinkle -ectomy = surgical removal	Surgical removal of excess skin to eliminate wrinkles. Commonly referred to as a *face lift.*

Pharmacology

CLASSIFICATION	WORD PARTS	ACTION	EXAMPLES
anesthetic (an-es-THET-tic)	an- = without esthesi/o = feeling -ic = pertaining to	Applied to the skin to deaden pain.	lidocaine, Xylocaine; procaine, Novocain
antibiotic (an-tye-bye-AW-tic)	anti- = against bi/o = life -tic = pertaining to	Kill bacteria causing skin infections.	bacitracin/neomycin/polymixinB, Neosporin ointment
antifungal (an-tye-FUNG-all)	anti- = against -al = pertaining to	Kill fungi infecting the skin.	miconazole, Monistat; clotrimazole, Lotrimin
antiparasitic (an-tye-pair-ah-SIT-tic)	anti- = against -ic = pertaining to	Kill mites or lice.	lindane, Kwell; permethrin, Nix
antipruritic (an-tye-proo-RIGH-tik)	anti- = against -ic = pertaining to	Reduce severe itching.	diphenhydramine, Benadryl; camphor/pramoxine/zinc, Caladryl
antiseptic (an-tye-SEP-tic)	anti- = against -tic = pertaining to	Used to kill bacteria in skin cuts and wounds or at a surgical site.	isopropyl alcohol; hydrogen peroxide
corticosteroid cream		Specific type of powerful anti-inflammatory cream.	hydrocortisone, Cortaid; triamcinolone, Kenalog

Abbreviations

BCC	basal cell carcinoma
BX, bx	biopsy
C&S	culture and sensitivity
decub	decubitus ulcer
Derm, derm	dermatology
FS	frozen section
I&D	incision and drainage
ID	intradermal
MM	malignant melanoma
SCC	squamous cell carcinoma
SG	skin graft
SLE	systemic lupus erythematosus
STSG	split-thickness skin graft
Subc, SubQ	subcutaneous
UV	ultraviolet

MED TERM TIP

Word Watch: Be careful when using the abbreviation *ID* meaning "intradermal" and *I&D* meaning "incision and drainage."

Chapter Review

Real-World Applications

Medical Record Analysis

This Dermatology Consultation Report contains 11 medical terms. Underline each term and write it in the list below the report. Then define each term.

Dermatology Consultation Report

Reason for Consultation:	Possible recurrence of basal cell carcinoma, left cheek.
History of Present Illness:	Patient is a 74-year-old male first seen by his regular physician 5 years ago for persistent facial lesions. Biopsies revealed basal cell carcinoma in two lesions, one on the nasal tip and the other on the left cheek. These were successfully excised. The patient noted that the left cheek lesion returned approximately one year ago. Patient reports pruritus and states the lesion is growing larger.
Results of Physical Exam:	Examination revealed a 10 × 14 mm lesion on left cheek 20 mm anterior to the ear. The lesion displays marked erythema and poorly defined borders. The area immediately around the lesion shows depigmentation with vesicles.
Assessment:	Recurrence of basal cell carcinoma.
Recommendations:	Due to the lesion's size, shape, and reoccurrence, deep excision of the carcinoma through the epidermis and dermis layers followed by dermatoplasty is recommended.

	Term	Definition
1		
2		
3		
4		
5		
6		
7		
8		
9		
10		
11		

Chart Note Transcription

The chart note below contains 10 phrases that can be reworded with a medical term that you learned in this chapter. Each phrase is identified with an underline. Determine the medical term and write your answers in the spaces provided.

Current Complaint: A 64-year-old female with an open sore (1) on her right leg is seen by the specialist in treating diseases of the skin. (2)

Past History: Patient states she first noticed an area of pain, severe itching, (3) and redness of the skin (4) just below her right knee about 6 weeks ago. One week later raised spots containing pus (5) appeared. Patient states the raised spots containing pus ruptured and the open sore appeared.

Signs and Symptoms: Patient has a deep open sore 5 × 3 cm: It is 4 cm distal to the knee on the lateral aspect of the right leg. It appears to extend into the middle skin layer, (6) and the edges show signs of tissue death. (7) The open sore has a small amount of drainage but there is no odor. A sample of the drainage that was grown in the lab to identify the microorganism and determine the best antibiotic (8) of the drainage revealed *Staphylococcus* bacteria in the open sore.

Diagnosis: Inflammation of connective tissue in the skin. (9)

Treatment: Removal of damaged tissue (10) of the open sore followed by application of an antibiotic cream. Patient was instructed to return to the skin disease specialist's office in 2 weeks, or sooner if the open sore does not heal, or if it begins draining pus.

(1) ______________________________

(2) ______________________________

(3) ______________________________

(4) ______________________________

(5) ______________________________

(6) ______________________________

(7) ______________________________

(8) ______________________________

(9) ______________________________

(10) ______________________________

Case Study

Below is a case study presentation of a patient with a condition discussed in this chapter. Read the case study and answer the questions below. Some questions will ask for information not included within this chapter. Use your text, a medical dictionary, journals, technical materials, multimedia resources, electronic media, or any other reference material you choose to answer these questions.

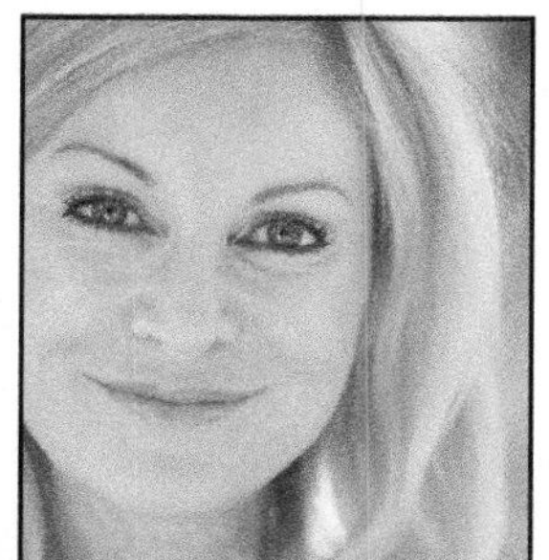
(Monkey Business Images/Shutterstock)

A 40-year-old female is seen in the dermatologist's office, upon the recommendation of her internist, for a workup for suspected SLE. Her presenting symptoms include erythema rash across her cheeks and nose, photosensitivity resulting in raised rash in sun-exposed areas, patches of alopecia, and pain and stiffness in her joints. The dermatologist examines the patient and orders exfoliative cytology and fungal scrapings to rule out other sources of the rash. Her internist had already placed the patient on oral anti-inflammatory medication for joint pain. The dermatologist orders corticosteroid cream for the rash. The patient is advised to use a sunscreen and make a follow-up appointment for results of the biopsy.

1. What pathological condition does the internist think this patient might have? Look this condition up in a reference source, and include a short description of it. SLE is an autoimmune disease. Use a reference source to look up the name of another autoimmune disease.

   ____

   ____

2. List and define each of the patient's presenting symptoms in your own words.

   ____

   ____

3. What diagnostic tests did the dermatologist perform? Describe it in your own words. Why were they important in helping the dermatologist make a diagnosis?

   ____

   ____

4. Each physician initiated a treatment. Describe them in your own words.

   ____

   ____

5. What do you think the term "workup" means?

   ____

   ____

Practice Exercises

A. Complete the Statement

1. The three layers of skin in order starting with the most superficial layer are ______________________, ______________________, and ______________________.

2. The ______________________ layer is the only living layer of the epidermis.

3. The subcutaneous layer of skin is composed primarily of ______________________.

4. Sensory receptors are located in the ______________________ layer of skin.

5. Nails and hair are composed of a hard protein called ______________________.

6. ______________________ is the pigment that gives skin its color.

7. Another name for the dermis is ______________________.

8. The nail body is connected to underlying tissue by the ______________________.

9. ______________________ glands release their product directly into hair follicles while ______________________ glands release their product into a duct.

10. ______________________ glands are sweat glands found in the underarm and pubic areas.

B. Define the Combining Form

	Definition	Example from Chapter
1. **cry/o**	______________________	______________________
2. **cutane/o**	______________________	______________________
3. **diaphor/o**	______________________	______________________
4. **py/o**	______________________	______________________
5. **cyan/o**	______________________	______________________
6. **ungu/o**	______________________	______________________
7. **lip/o**	______________________	______________________
8. **hidr/o**	______________________	______________________
9. **rhytid/o**	______________________	______________________
10. **seb/o**	______________________	______________________
11. **trich/o**	______________________	______________________
12. **necr/o**	______________________	______________________

C. Describe the Type of Burn

1. first degree ______________________________

2. second degree ______________________________

3. third degree ______________________________

D. Terminology Matching

Match each term to its definition.

1.	_______ eczema	a.	decubitus ulcer
2.	_______ nevus	b.	lack of skin pigment
3.	_______ lipoma	c.	acne commonly seen in adults
4.	_______ urticaria	d.	hardened skin
5.	_______ bedsore	e.	redness, vesicles, itching, crusts
6.	_______ acne rosacea	f.	birthmark
7.	_______ acne vulgaris	g.	excessive hair growth
8.	_______ hirsutism	h.	caused by deficient blood supply
9.	_______ alopecia	i.	fatty tumor
10.	_______ gangrene	j.	hives
11.	_______ scleroderma	k.	baldness
12.	_______ albinism	l.	acne of adolescence

E. Define the Term

1. macule ______________________________

2. papule ______________________________

3. cyst ______________________________

4. fissure ______________________________

5. pustule ______________________________

6. wheal ______________________________

7. vesicle ______________________________

8. ulcer ______________________________

9. nodule ______________________________

10. laceration ______________________________

F. Combining Form Practice

The combining form **dermat/o** refers to the skin. Use it to write a term that means:

1. inflammation of the skin ____________________
2. any abnormal skin condition ____________________
3. an instrument for cutting the skin ____________________
4. specialist in skin ____________________
5. surgical repair of the skin ____________________
6. study of the skin ____________________

The combining form **melan/o** means black. Use it to write a term that means a:

7. black tumor ____________________
8. black cell ____________________

The suffix **-derma** means skin. Use it to write a term that means:

9. scaly skin ____________________
10. white skin ____________________
11. red skin ____________________

The combining form **onych/o** refers to the nail. Use it to write a term that means:

12. softening of the nails ____________________
13. infection around the nail ____________________
14. nail eating (biting) ____________________
15. removal of the nail ____________________

G. Procedure Matching

Match each procedure to its definition.

1. ______	debridement	a. surgical removal of wrinkled skin
2. ______	cauterization	b. instrument to cut thin slices of skin
3. ______	chemabrasion	c. removal of fat with suction
4. ______	dermatoplasty	d. use of extreme cold to destroy tissue
5. ______	liposuction	e. skin grafting
6. ______	rhytidectomy	f. removal of lesions with scraper
7. ______	curettage	g. removal of skin with brushes
8. ______	dermabrasion	h. removal of damaged skin
9. ______	dermatome	i. destruction of tissue with electric current
10. ______	cryosurgery	j. chemical peel

H. What's the Abbreviation?

1. frozen section ____________________
2. incision and drainage ____________________
3. intradermal ____________________
4. subcutaneous ____________________
5. ultraviolet ____________________
6. biopsy ____________________

I. What Does it Stand For?

1. C&S ____________________
2. BCC ____________________
3. derm ____________________
4. SG ____________________
5. decub ____________________
6. MM ____________________

J. Fill in the Blank

impetigo	tinea	keloid	exfoliative cytology	xeroderma
petechiae	frozen section	paronychia	scabies	Kaposi's sarcoma

1. The winter climates can cause dry skin. The medical term for this is ____________________.
2. Kim has experienced small pinpoint purplish spots caused by bleeding under the skin. This is called ____________________.
3. Janet has a fungal skin disease. This is called ____________________.
4. A contagious skin disease caused by a mite is ____________________.
5. An infection around the entire nail is called ____________________.
6. A form of skin cancer affecting AIDS patients is called ____________________.
7. Latrivia has a bacterial skin infection that results in pustules crusting and rupturing. It is called ____________________.
8. James's burn scar became a hypertrophic ____________________.
9. For a(n) ____________________ test, cells scraped off the skin are examined under a microscope.
10. During surgery a ____________________ was ordered for a rapid exam of tissue cut from a tumor.

K. Pharmacology Challenge

Fill in the classification for each drug description, then match the brand name.

	Drug Description	Classification	Brand Name
1.	_______ kills fungi	____________________	a. Kwell
2.	_______ reduces severe itching	____________________	b. Cortaid
3.	_______ kills mites and lice	____________________	c. Benadryl
4.	_______ powerful anti-inflammatory	____________________	d. Neosporin
5.	_______ deadens pain	____________________	e. Monistat
6.	_______ kills bacteria	____________________	f. Xylocaine

L. Scenario

Using the Rule of Nines and the descriptions, interpret and rate the degree of burn for each family member in order to communicate the information to health care colleagues.

The Ferris family has just returned from shopping. Mrs. Ferris is holding the baby while heating water on the stove to begin cooking dinner. Derric, who is four, is sitting on the floor playing with some toys while dinner is being prepared. Mr. Ferris is handing a bottle to Mrs. Ferris to quiet the baby while he puts the groceries away. As he turns to walk away his sleeve catches on the handle of the pan and the boiling water flies across the room, burning a large rectangular area on the outside of Mrs. Ferris' lower arm. Blisters immediately begin to show and she also sustains a small oval shaped burn on the side of her face. The water causes a large cone shaped burn on the baby's thigh that is also showing blisters and a small round burn on the back of her hand that has turned red. Derric is hit on his back with the water, leaving a large octagonal shaped burn covering more than 50 percent of his back and a small triangle shaped burn on the top of his neck at the base of his hairline that is intensely red and splotchy. Mr. Ferris tried to reach for the pan and suffers a large burn that covers the entire back of his hand from the stove element. The burn has a charred black appearance and Mr. Ferris is experiencing no pain.

Note: Additional medical resources may be needed to interpret and transcribe the Rule of Nines,

Mrs. Ferris ____________________

Mr. Ferris____________________

Derric____________________

Baby Ferris____________________

Labeling Exercise

Image A

Write the labels for this figure on the numbered lines provided.

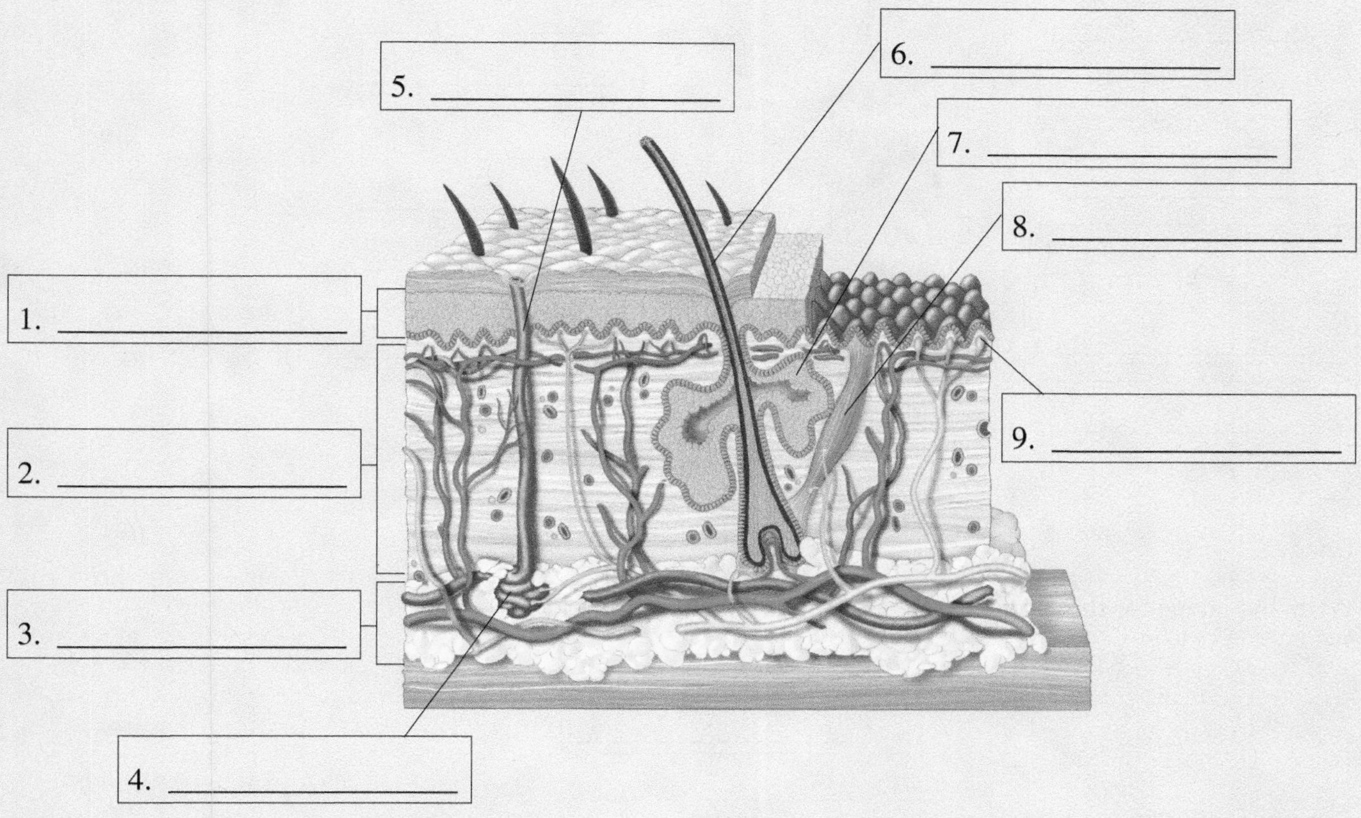

Image B

Write the labels for this figure on the numbered lines provided.

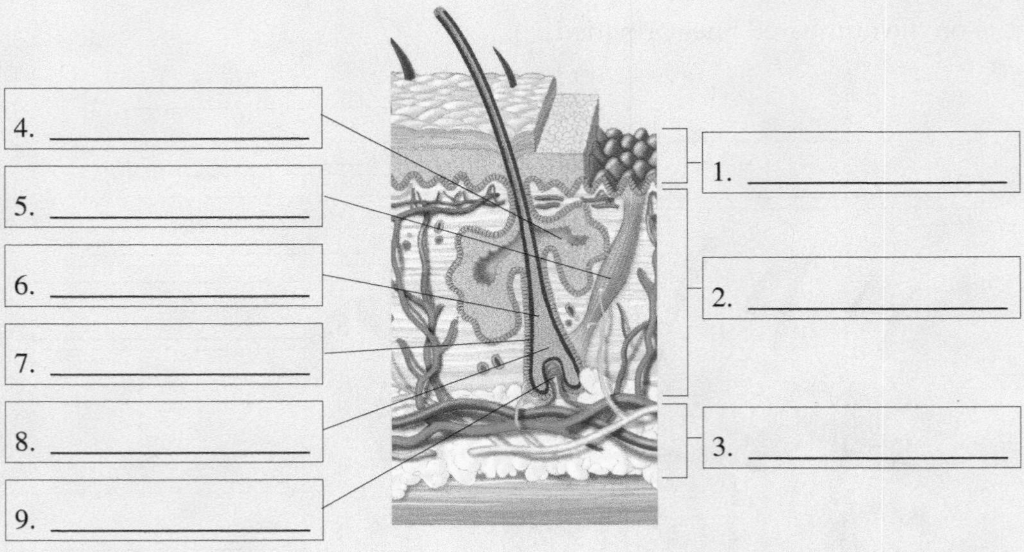

Image C

Write the labels for this figure on the numbered lines provided.

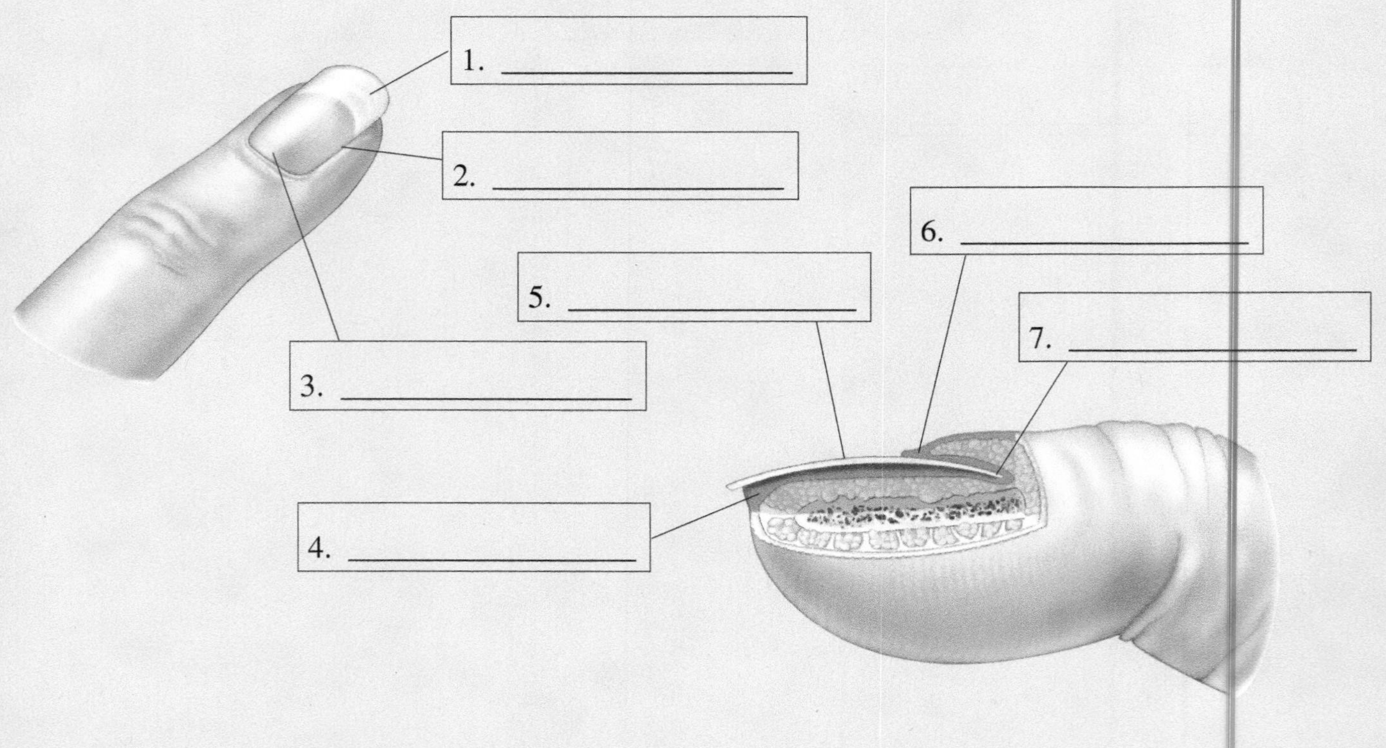

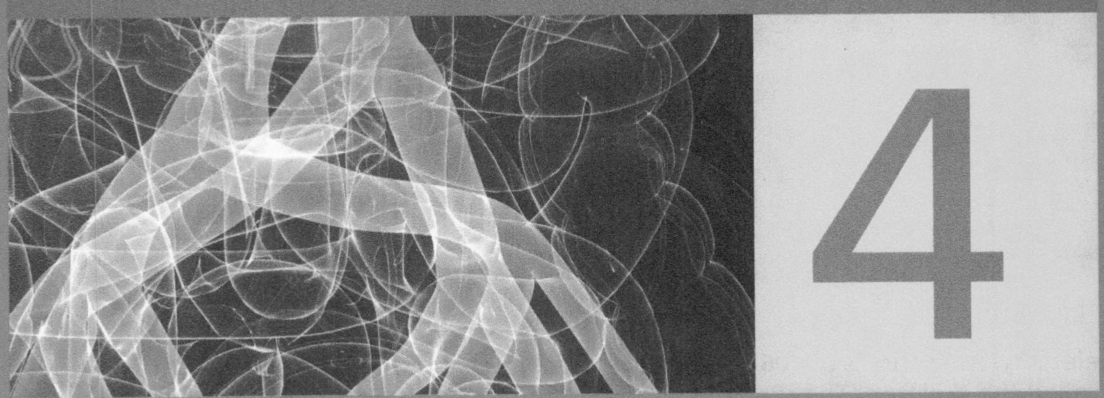

4

MUSCULOSKELETAL SYSTEM

Learning Objectives

Upon completion of this chapter, you will be able to

- Identify and define the combining forms, prefixes, and suffixes introduced in this chapter.
- Correctly spell and pronounce medical terms and major anatomical structures relating to the musculoskeletal system.
- Locate and describe the major organs of the musculoskeletal system and their functions.
- Correctly place bones in either the axial or the appendicular skeleton.
- List and describe the components of a long bone.
- Identify bony projections and depressions.
- Identify the parts of a synovial joint.
- Describe the characteristics of the three types of muscle tissue.
- Use movement terminology correctly.
- Identify and define musculoskeletal system anatomical terms.
- Identify and define selected musculoskeletal system pathology terms.
- Identify and define selected musculoskeletal system diagnostic procedures.
- Identify and define selected musculoskeletal system therapeutic procedures.
- Identify and define selected medications relating to the musculoskeletal system.
- Define selected abbreviations associated with the musculoskeletal system.

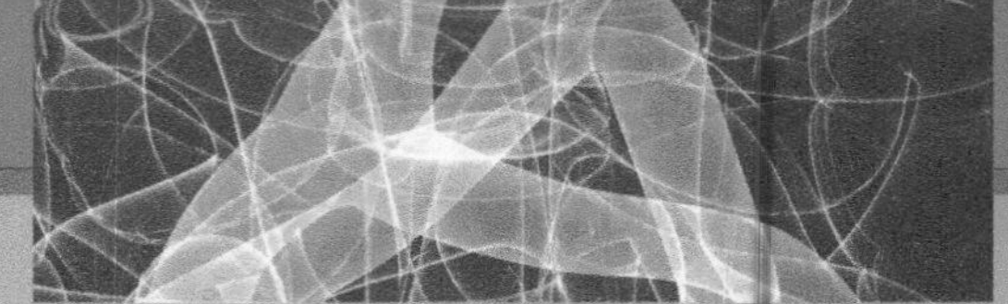

Section I: Skeletal System at a Glance

Function

The skeletal system consists of 206 bones that make up the internal framework of the body, called the skeleton. The skeleton supports the body, protects internal organs, serves as a point of attachment for skeletal muscles for body movement, produces blood cells, and stores minerals.

Structures

Here are the primary structures that comprise the skeletal system.

bones **joints**

Word Parts

Here are the most common word parts (with their meanings) used to build skeletal system terms. For a more comprehensive list, refer to the Terminology section of this chapter.

Combining Forms

ankyl/o	stiff joint
arthr/o	joint
articul/o	joint
burs/o	sac
carp/o	wrist
cervic/o	neck
chondr/o	cartilage
clavicul/o	clavicle
coccyg/o	coccyx
cortic/o	outer portion
cost/o	rib
crani/o	skull
femor/o	femur
fibul/o	fibula
humer/o	humerus
ili/o	ilium
ischi/o	ischium
kyph/o	hump
lamin/o	lamina, part of vertebra
lord/o	bent backwards
lumb/o	low back, loin
mandibul/o	mandible
maxill/o	maxilla
medull/o	inner portion
metacarp/o	metacarpals
metatars/o	metatarsals
myel/o	bone marrow, spinal cord
orth/o	straight
oste/o	bone
patell/o	patella
ped/o	child, foot
pelv/o	pelvis
phalang/o	phalanges
pod/o	foot
prosthet/o	addition
pub/o	pubis
radi/o	radius, ray (X-ray)
sacr/o	sacrum
sarc/o	flesh (muscular substance)
scapul/o	scapula
scoli/o	crooked, bent
spin/o	spine
spondyl/o	vertebrae
stern/o	sternum
synovi/o	synovial membrane
synov/o	synovial membrane
tars/o	ankle
thorac/o	chest
tibi/o	tibia
uln/o	ulna
vertebr/o	vertebra

Suffixes

-blast	immature, embryonic
-clasia	to surgically break
-desis	stabilize, fuse
-listhesis	slipping
-porosis	porous

Skeletal System Illustrated

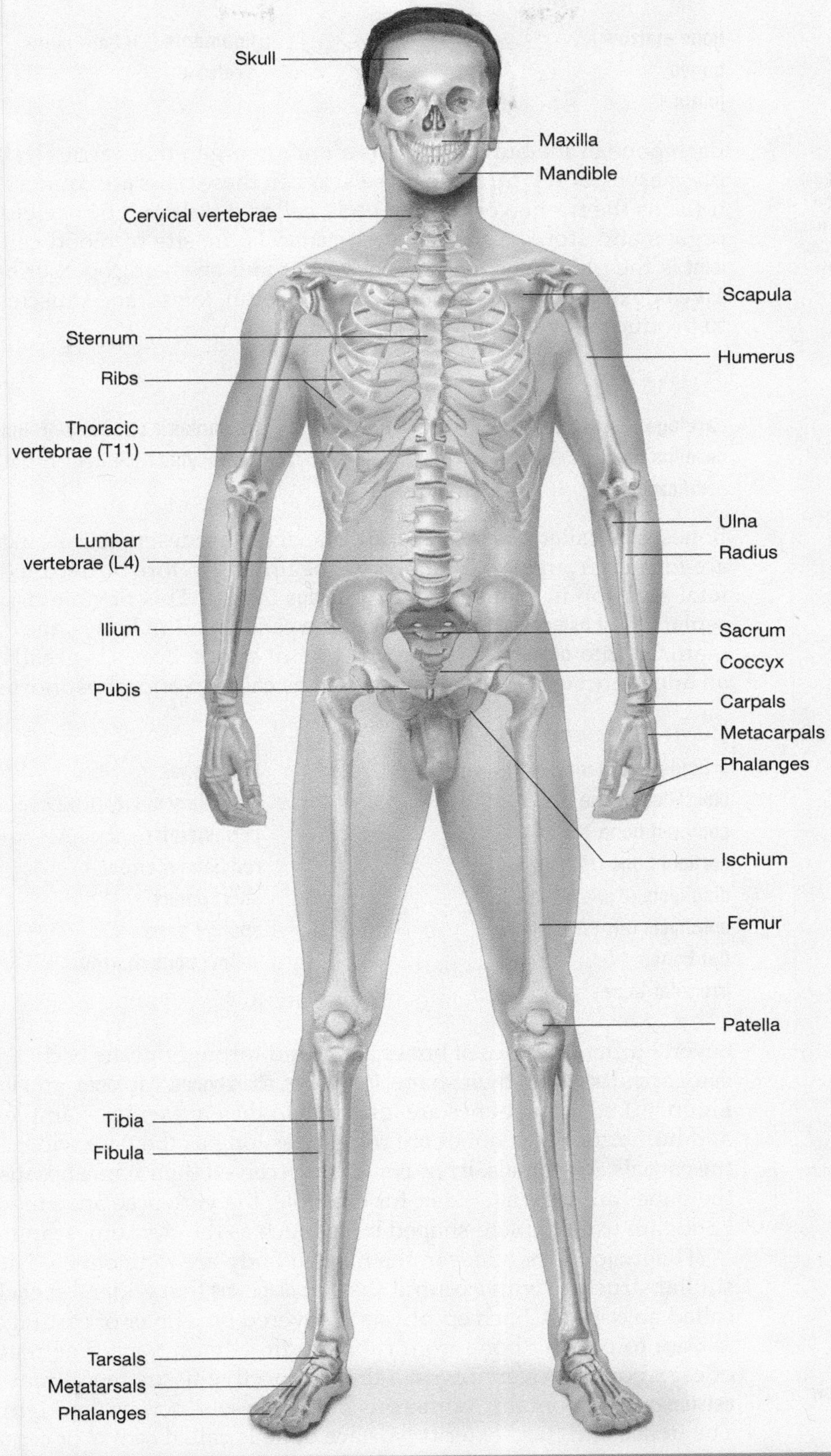

Anatomy and Physiology of the Skeletal System

bone marrow
bones
joints
ligaments (LIG-ah-ments)
skeleton

MED TERM TIP

The term *skeleton*, from the Greek word *skeltos* meaning "dried up," was originally used in reference to a dried-up mummified body, but over time came to be used for bones.

Each bone in the human body is a unique organ that carries its own blood supply, nerves, and lymphatic vessels. When these **bones** are connected to each other it forms the framework of the body called a **skeleton.** The skeleton protects vital organs and stores minerals. **Bone marrow** is the site of blood cell production. A **joint** is the place where two bones meet and are held together by **ligaments.** This gives flexibility to the skeleton. The skeleton, joints, and muscles work together to produce movement.

Bones

cartilage (CAR-tih-lij)
osseous tissue (OSS-ee-us)
ossification (oss-sih-fih-KAY-shun)
osteoblasts (OSS-tee-oh-blasts)
osteocytes (OSS-tee-oh-sights)

Bones, also called **osseous tissue,** are one of the hardest materials in the body. Bones are formed from a gradual process beginning before birth called **ossification.** The fetal skeleton is formed from a **cartilage** model. This flexible tissue is gradually replaced by **osteoblasts,** immature bone cells. In adult bones, the osteoblasts have matured into **osteocytes.** The formation of strong bones is greatly dependent on an adequate supply of minerals such as calcium and phosphorus.

Bone Structure

articular cartilage (ar-TIK-yoo-lar)
cancellous bone (CAN-sell-us)
compact bone
cortical bone (KOR-ti-kal)
diaphysis (dye-AFF-ih-sis)
epiphysis (eh-PIFF-ih-sis)
flat bones
irregular bones
long bones
medullary cavity (MED-you-lair-ee)
periosteum (pair-ee-AH-stee-um)
red bone marrow
short bones
spongy bone
yellow bone marrow

MED TERM TIP

Do not confuse a long bone with a large bone. A long bone is not necessarily a large bone. The bones of your fingers are short in length, but since they are longer than they are wide, they are classified as long bones.

MED TERM TIP

The term *diaphysis* comes from the Greek term meaning "to grow between."

Several different types of bones are found throughout the body and fall into four categories based on their shape: **long bones, short bones, flat bones,** and **irregular bones** (see Figure 4.1 ■). Long bones are longer than they are wide; examples are the femur and humerus. Short bones are roughly as long as they are wide; examples being the carpals and tarsals. Irregular bones received their name because the shapes of the bones are very irregular; for example, the vertebrae are irregular bones. Flat bones are usually plate-shaped bones such as the sternum, scapulae, and pelvis.

The majority of bones in the human body are long bones. These bones have similar structure with a central shaft or **diaphysis** that widens at each end, which is called an **epiphysis.** Each epiphysis is covered by a layer of cartilage called **articular cartilage** to prevent bone from rubbing directly on bone. The remaining surface of each bone is covered with a thin connective tissue membrane called the **periosteum,** which contains numerous blood vessels, nerves, and lymphatic vessels. The dense and hard exterior surface bone is called **cortical** or **compact bone. Cancellous** or **spongy bone** is found inside the bone. As its name indicates, spongy bone

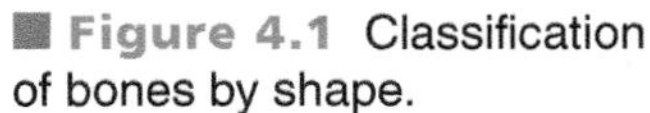

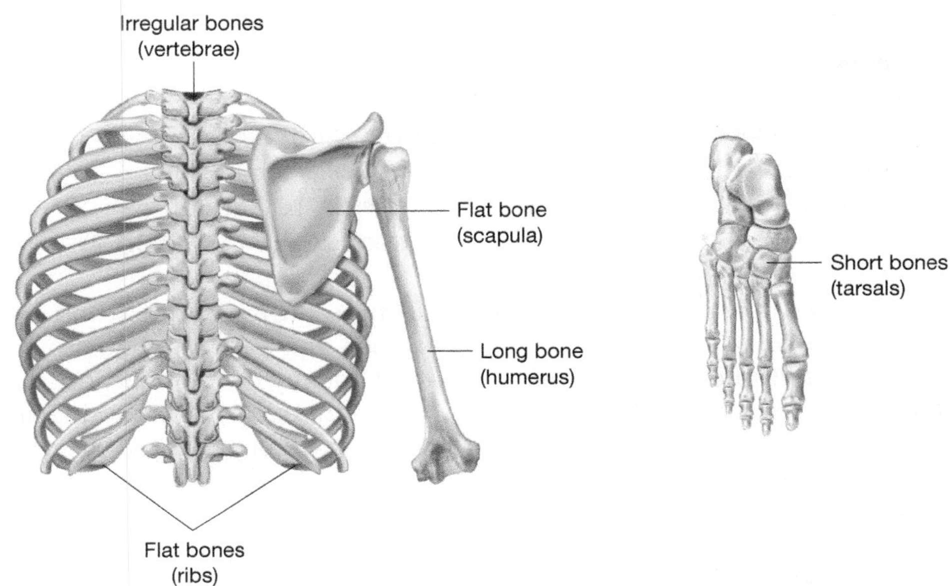

■ **Figure 4.1** Classification of bones by shape.

has spaces in it, giving it a spongelike appearance. These spaces contain **red bone marrow,** which manufactures most of the blood cells and is found in some parts of all bones.

The center of the diaphysis contains an open canal called the **medullary cavity.** Early in life this cavity also contains red bone marrow, but as we age the red bone marrow of the medullary cavity gradually converts to **yellow bone marrow,** which consists primarily of fat cells. Figure 4.2 ■ contains an illustration of the structure of long bones.

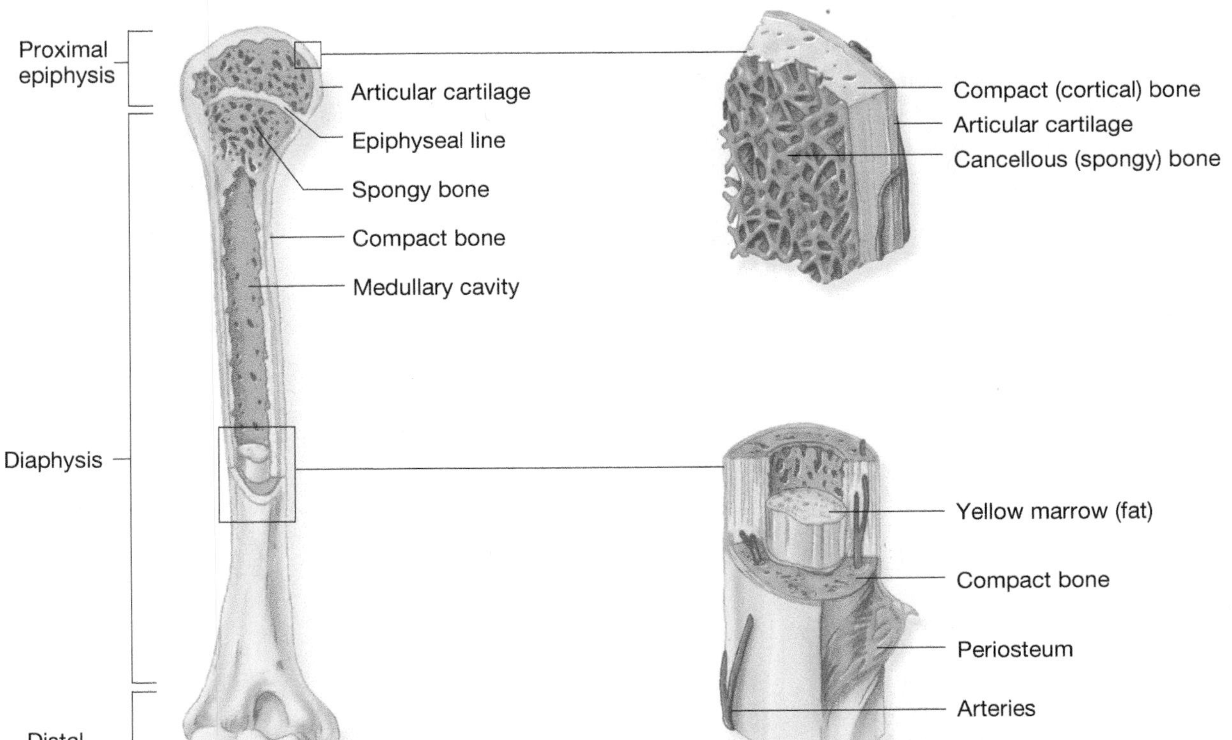

■ **Figure 4.2** Components of a long bone. The entire long bone is on the left side accompanied by a blowup of the proximal epiphysis and a section of the diaphysis.

Bone Projections and Depressions

condyle (KON-dile)
epicondyle (ep-ih-KON-dile)
fissure (FISH-er)
foramen (for-AY-men)
fossa (FOSS-ah)
head
neck
process
sinus (SIGH-nus)
trochanter (tro-KAN-ter)
tubercle (TOO-ber-kl)
tuberosity (too-ber-OSS-ih-tee)

MED TERM TIP

The elbow, commonly referred to as the *funny bone,* is actually a projection of the ulna called the olecranon process.

Bones have many projections and depressions; some are rounded and smooth in order to articulate with another bone in a joint. Others are rough to provide muscles with attachment points. The general term for any bony projection is a **process.** Then there are specific terms to describe the different shapes and locations of various processes. These terms are commonly used on operative reports and in physicians' records for clear identification of areas on the individual bones. Some of the common bony processes include the following:

1. The **head** is a large, smooth, ball-shaped end on a long bone. It may be separated from the body or shaft of the bone by a narrow area called the **neck.**
2. A **condyle** refers to a smooth, rounded portion at the end of a bone.
3. The **epicondyle** is a projection located above or on a condyle.
4. The **trochanter** refers to a large rough process for the attachment of a muscle.
5. A **tubercle** is a small, rough process that provides the attachment for tendons and muscles.
6. The **tuberosity** is a large, rough process that provides the attachment of tendons and muscles.

See Figure 4.3 ■ for an illustration of the processes found on the femur.

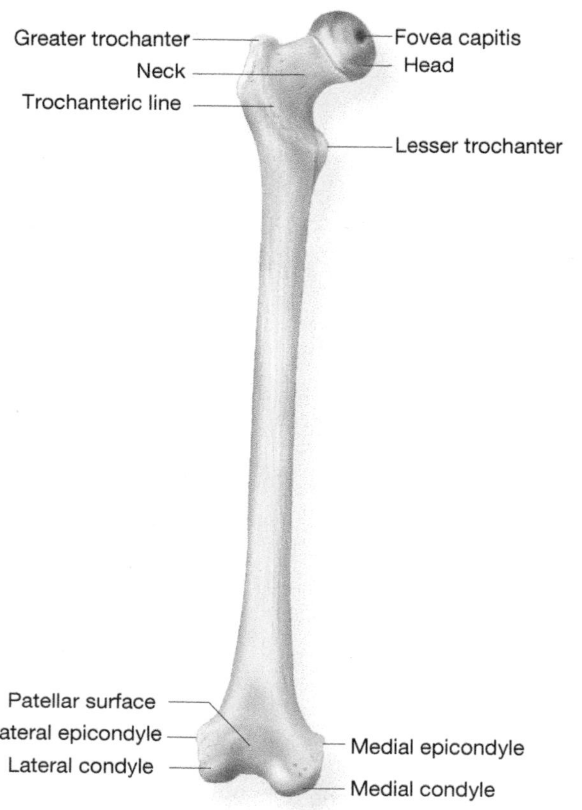

■ **Figure 4.3** Bony processes found on the femur.

Additionally, bones have hollow regions or depressions. The most common are the:

1. **Sinus** is a hollow cavity within a bone.
2. **Foramen** is a smooth, round opening for nerves and blood vessels.
3. **Fossa** consists of a shallow cavity or depression on the surface of a bone.
4. **Fissure** is a slit-type opening.

Skeleton

appendicular skeleton (app-en-DIK-yoo-lar)
axial skeleton (AK-see-al)

The human skeleton has two divisions: the **axial skeleton** and the **appendicular skeleton.** Figures 4.4 and 4.8 illustrate the axial and appendicular skeletons.

MED TERM TIP

Newborn infants have about 300 bones at birth that will fuse into 206 bones as an adult.

Axial Skeleton

cervical vertebrae
coccyx (COCK-six)
cranium (KRAY-nee-um)
ethmoid bone (ETH-moyd)
facial bones
frontal bone
hyoid bone (HIGH-oyd)
intervertebral disc (in-ter-VER-teh-bral)
lacrimal bone (LACK-rim-al)
lumbar vertebrae
mandible (MAN-dih-bl)
maxilla (mack-SIH-lah)
nasal bone
occipital bone (ock-SIP-eh-tal)
palatine bone (PAL-ah-tine)
parietal bone (pah-RYE-eh-tal)
rib cage
sacrum (SAY-crum)
sphenoid bone (SFEE-noyd)
sternum (STER-num)
temporal bone (TEM-por-al)
thoracic vertebrae
vertebral column (VER-teh-bral)
vomer bone (VOH-mer)
zygomatic bone (zeye-go-MAT-ik)

The axial skeleton includes the bones of the head, neck, spine, chest, and trunk of the body (see Figure 4.4 ■). These bones form the central axis for the whole body and protect many of the internal organs such as the brain, lungs, and heart.

The head or skull is divided into two parts consisting of the **cranium** and **facial bones.** These bones surround and protect the brain, eyes, ears, nasal cavity, and oral cavity from injury. The muscles for chewing and moving the head are attached to the cranial bones. The cranium encases the brain and consists of the **frontal, parietal, temporal, ethmoid, sphenoid,** and **occipital bones.** The facial bones surround the mouth, nose, and eyes and include the **mandible, maxilla, zygomatic, vomer, palatine, nasal,** and **lacrimal bones.** The cranial and facial bones are illustrated in Figure 4.5 ■ and described in Table 4.1 ■.

The **hyoid bone** is a single U-shaped bone suspended in the neck between the mandible and larynx. It is a point of attachment for swallowing and speech muscles.

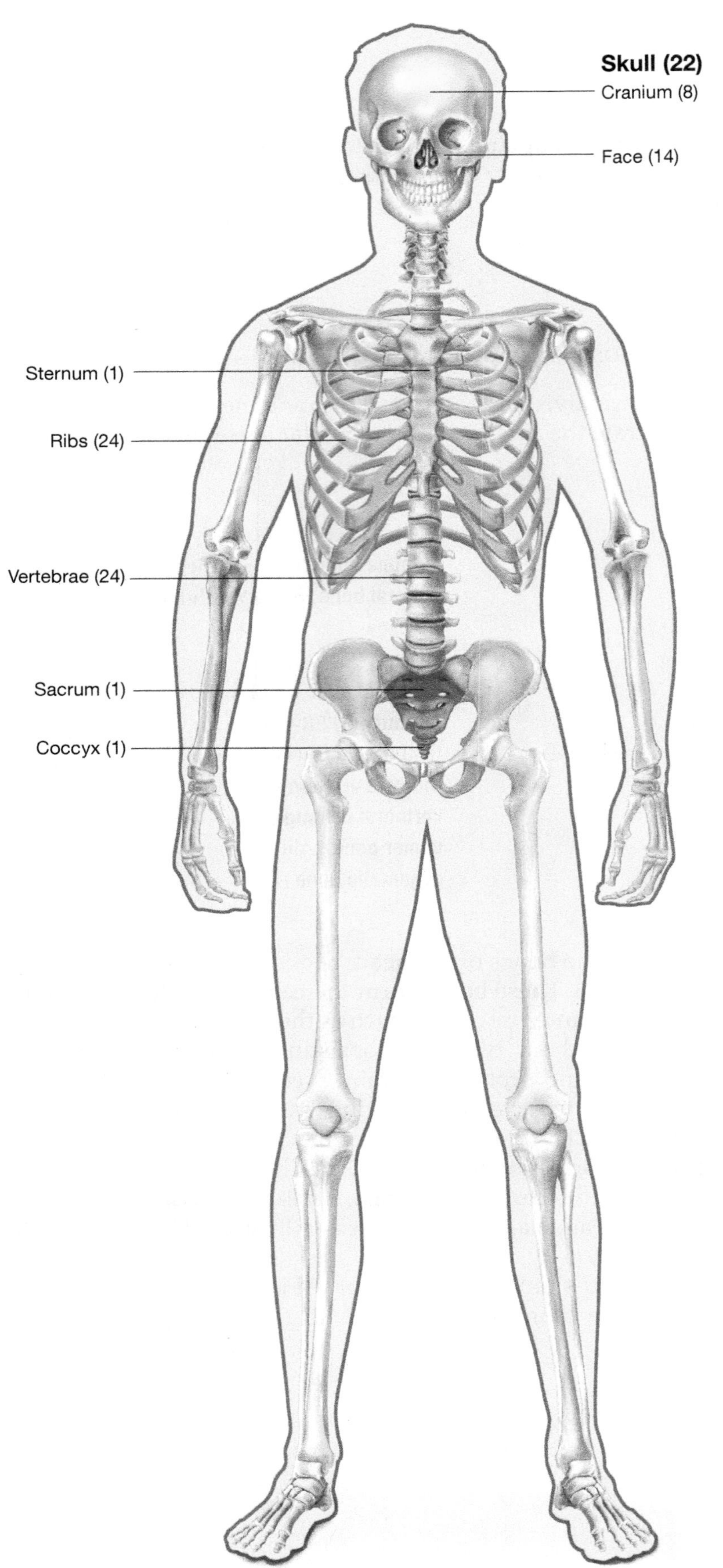

■ **Figure 4.4** Bones of the axial skeleton.

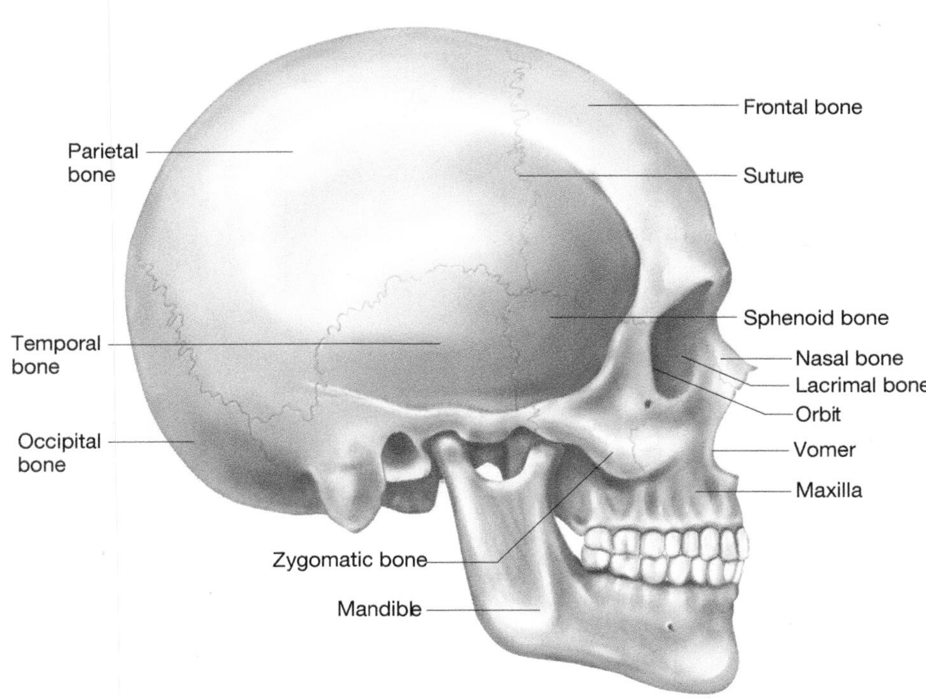

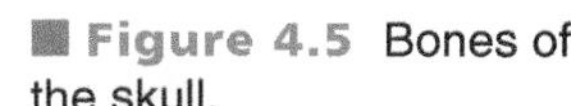
■ **Figure 4.5** Bones of the skull.

Table 4.1 Bones of the Skull

NAME	NUMBER	DESCRIPTION
Cranial Bones		
Frontal bone	1	Forehead
Parietal bone	2	Upper sides of cranium and roof of skull
Occipital bone	1	Back and base of skull
Temporal bone	2	Sides and base of cranium
Sphenoid bone	1	Bat-shaped bone that forms part of the base of the skull, floor, and sides of eye orbit
Ethmoid bone	1	Forms part of eye orbit, nose, and floor of cranium
Facial Bones		
Lacrimal bone	2	Inner corner of each eye
Nasal bone	2	Form part of nasal septum and support bridge of nose
Maxilla	1	Upper jaw
Mandible	1	Lower jawbone; only movable bone of the skull
Zygomatic bone	2	Cheekbones
Vomer bone	1	Base of nasal septum
Palatine bone	1	Hard palate (PAH lat) roof of oral cavity and floor of nasal cavity

The trunk of the body consists of the **vertebral column, sternum,** and **rib cage.** The vertebral or spinal column is divided into five sections: **cervical vertebrae, thoracic vertebrae, lumbar vertebrae, sacrum,** and **coccyx** (see Figure 4.6 ■ and Table 4.2 ■). Located between each pair of vertebrae, from the cervical through the lumbar regions, is an **intervertebral disc.** Each disc is composed of fibrocartilage to provide a cushion between the vertebrae. The rib cage has twelve pairs of ribs attached at the back to the vertebral column. Ten of the pairs are also attached to the sternum in the front (see Figure 4.7 ■). The lowest two pairs are called *floating ribs* and are attached only to the vertebral column. The rib cage serves to provide support for organs, such as the heart and lungs.

MED TERM TIP

The term *coccyx* comes from the Greek word for the cuckoo because the shape of these small bones extending off the sacrum resembles this bird's bill.

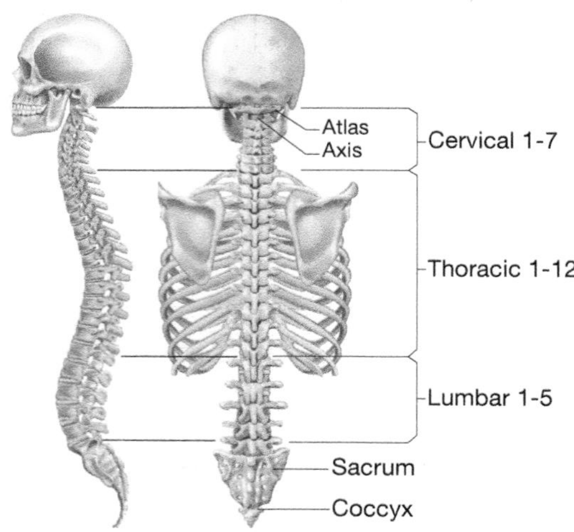

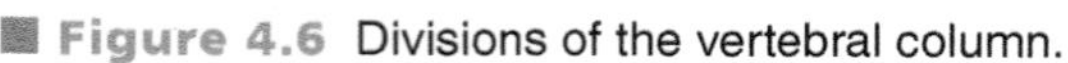

■ Figure 4.6 Divisions of the vertebral column.

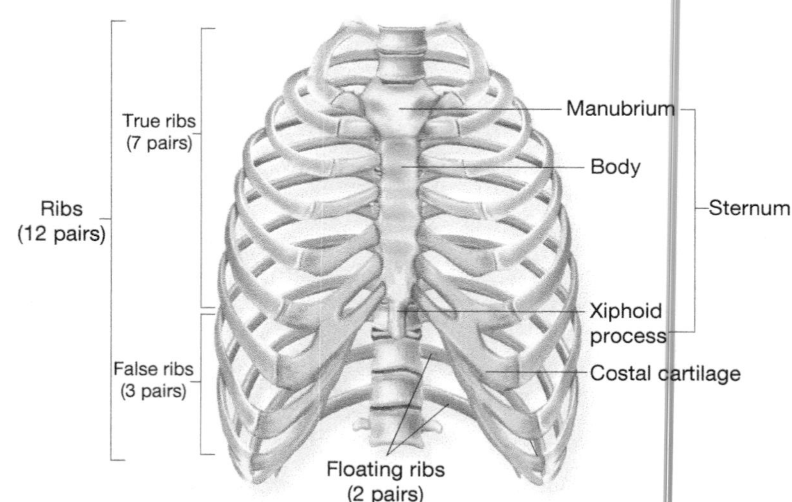

■ Figure 4.7 The structure of the rib cage.

Table 4.2 Bones of the Vertebral/Spinal Column

NAME	NUMBER	DESCRIPTION
Cervical vertebra	7	Vertebrae in the neck region
Thoracic vertebra	12	Vertebrae in the chest region with ribs attached
Lumbar vertebra	5	Vertebrae in the small of the back, about waist level
Sacrum	1	Five vertebrae that become fused into one triangular-shaped flat bone at the base of the vertebral column
Coccyx	1	Three to five very small vertebrae attached to the sacrum, often become fused

Appendicular Skeleton

carpals (CAR-pals)
clavicle (CLAV-ih-kl)
femur (FEE-mer)
fibula (FIB-yoo-lah)
humerus (HYOO-mer-us)
ilium (ILL-ee-um)
innominate bone (ih-NOM-ih-nayt)
ischium (ISS-kee-um)
lower extremities
metacarpals (met-ah-CAR-pals)
metatarsals (met-ah-TAHR-sals)
os coxae (OSS / KOK-sigh)
patella (pah-TELL-ah)
pectoral girdle
pelvic girdle
phalanges (fah-LAN-jeez)
pubis (PYOO-bis)
radius (RAY-dee-us)
scapula (SKAP-yoo-lah)
tarsals (TAHR-sals)
tibia (TIB-ee-ah)
ulna (UHL-nah)
upper extremities

MED TERM TIP

The term *girdle*, meaning something that encircles or confines, refers to the entire bony structure of the shoulder and the pelvis. If just one bone from these areas is being discussed, like the ilium of the pelvis, it would be named as such. If, however, the entire pelvis is being discussed, it would be called the pelvic girdle.

The appendicular skeleton consists of the **pectoral girdle, upper extremities, pelvic girdle,** and **lower extremities** (see Figure 4.8 ■). These are the bones for our appendages or limbs and along with the muscles attached to them, they are responsible for body movement.

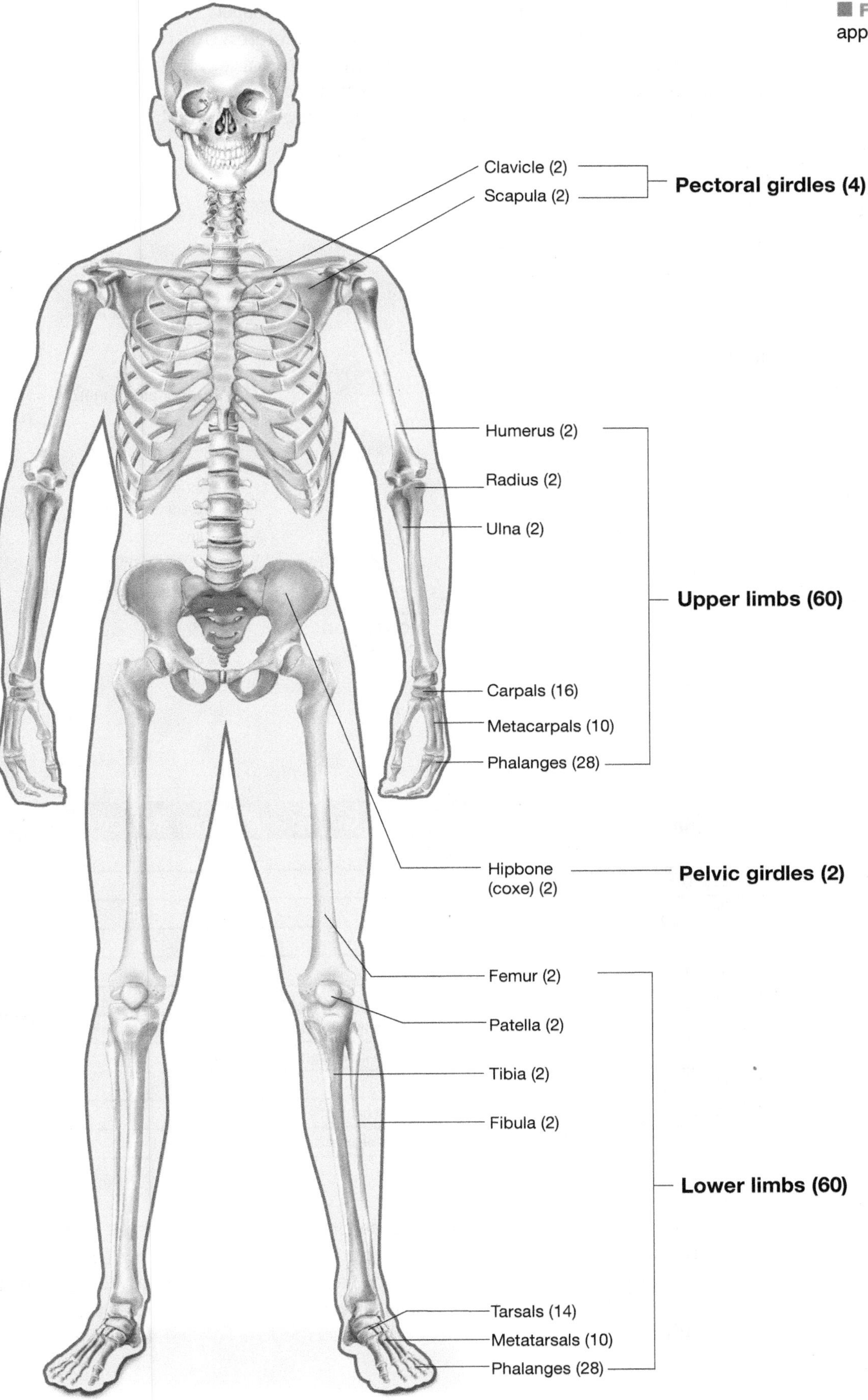

Figure 4.8 Bones of the appendicular skeleton.

The pectoral girdle consists of the **clavicle** and **scapula** bones. It functions to attach the upper extremity, or arm, to the axial skeleton by articulating with the sternum anteriorly and the vertebral column posteriorly. The bones of the upper extremity include the **humerus, ulna, radius, carpals, metacarpals,** and **phalanges.** These bones are illustrated in Figure 4.9 ■ and described in Table 4.3 ■.

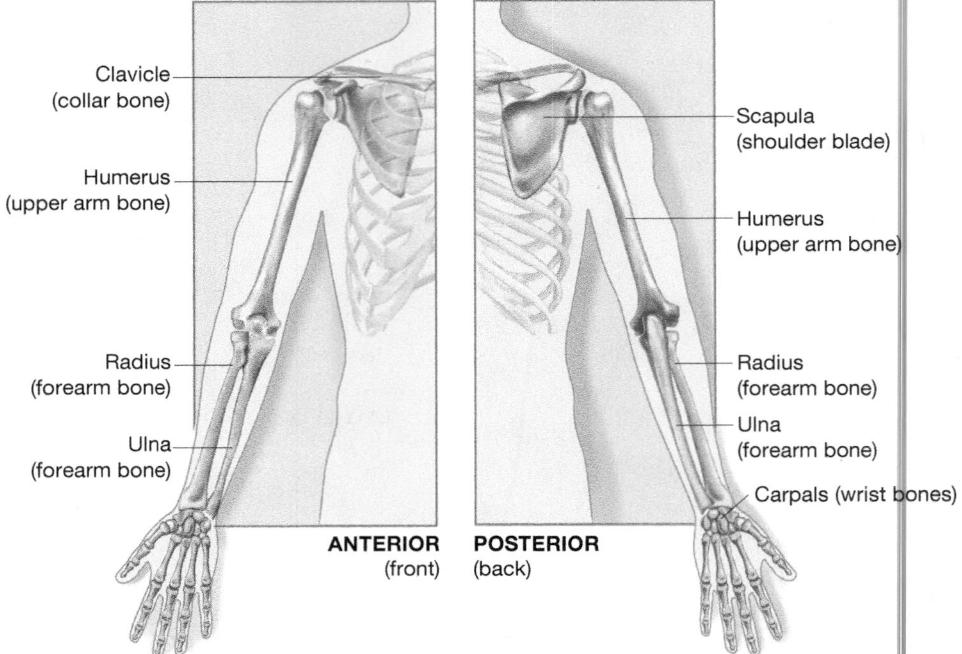

■ **Figure 4.9** Anatomical and common names for the pectoral girdle and upper extremity.

Table 4.3 Bones of the Pectoral Girdle and Upper Extremity

NAME	NUMBER	DESCRIPTION
Pectoral Girdle		
Clavicle	2	Collar bone
Scapula	2	Shoulder blade
Upper Extremity		
Humerus	2	Upper arm bone
Radius	2	Forearm bone on thumb side of lower arm
Ulna	2	Forearm bone on little finger side of lower arm
Carpals	16	Bones of wrist
Metacarpals	10	Bones in palm of hand
Phalanges	28	Finger bones; three in each finger and two in each thumb

The pelvic girdle is called the **os coxae** or the **innominate bone** or hipbone. It contains the **ilium, ischium,** and **pubis.** It articulates with the sacrum posteriorly to attach the lower extremity, or leg, to the axial skeleton. The lower extremity bones include the **femur, patella, tibia, fibula, tarsals, metatarsals,** and phalanges. These bones are illustrated in Figure 4.10 ■ and described in Table 4.4 ■.

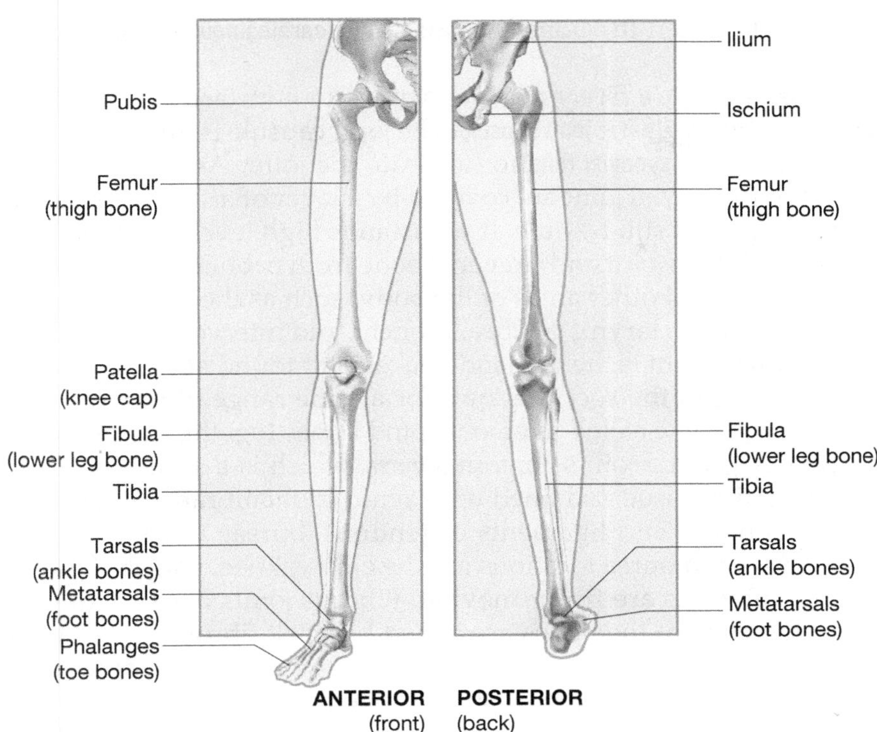

Figure 4.10 Anatomical and common names for the pelvic girdle and lower extremity.

Table 4.4 Bones of the Pelvic Girdle and Lower Extremity

NAME	NUMBER	DESCRIPTION
Pelvic Girdle/Os Coxae		
Ilium	2	Part of the hipbone
Ischium	2	Part of the hipbone
Pubis	2	Part of the hipbone
Lower Extremity		
Femur	2	Upper leg bone; thigh bone
Patella	2	Knee cap
Tibia	2	Shin bone; thicker lower leg bone
Fibula	2	Thinner, long bone in lateral side of lower leg
Tarsals	14	Ankle and heel bones
Metatarsals	10	Forefoot bones
Phalanges	28	Toe bones; three in each toe and two in each great toe

Joints

articulation (ar-tik-yoo-LAY-shun)
bursa (BER-sah)
cartilaginous joints (car-tih-LAJ-ih-nus)
fibrous joints (FYE-bruss)
joint capsule
synovial fluid
synovial joint (sin-OH-vee-al)
synovial membrane

Joints are formed when two or more bones meet. This is also referred to as an **articulation.** There are three types of joints based on the amount of movement allowed between the bones: **synovial joints, cartilaginous joints,** and **fibrous joints** (see Figure 4.11 ■).

Most joints are freely moving synovial joints (see Figure 4.12 ■), which are enclosed by an elastic **joint capsule.** The joint capsule is lined with **synovial membrane,** which secretes **synovial fluid** to lubricate the joint. As noted earlier, the ends of bones in a synovial joint are covered by a layer of articular cartilage. Cartilage is very tough, but still flexible. It withstands high levels of stress to act as a shock absorber for the joint and prevents bone from rubbing against bone. Cartilage is found in several other areas of the body, such as the nasal septum, external ear, eustachian tube, larynx, trachea, bronchi, and intervertebral disks. One example of a synovial joint is the ball-and-socket joint found at the shoulder and hip. The ball rotating in the socket allows for a wide range of motion. Bands of strong connective tissue called ligaments bind bones together at the joint.

Some synovial joints contain a **bursa,** which is a saclike structure composed of connective tissue and lined with synovial membrane. Most commonly found between bones and ligaments or tendons, bursas function to reduce friction. Some common bursa locations are the elbow, knee, and shoulder joints.

Not all joints are freely moving. Fibrous joints allow almost no movement since the ends of the bones are joined by thick fibrous tissue, which may even fuse into solid bone. The sutures of the skull are an example of a fibrous joint. Cartilaginous joints allow for slight movement but hold bones firmly in place by a solid piece of cartilage. An example of this type of joint is the pubic symphysis, the point at which the left and right pubic bones meet in the front of the lower abdomen.

MED TERM TIP

Bursitis is an inflammation of the bursa located between bony prominences such as at the shoulder. Housemaid's knee, a term thought to have originated from the damage to the knees that occurred when maids knelt to scrub floors, is a form of bursitis and carries the medical name *prepatellar bursitis.*

Skull

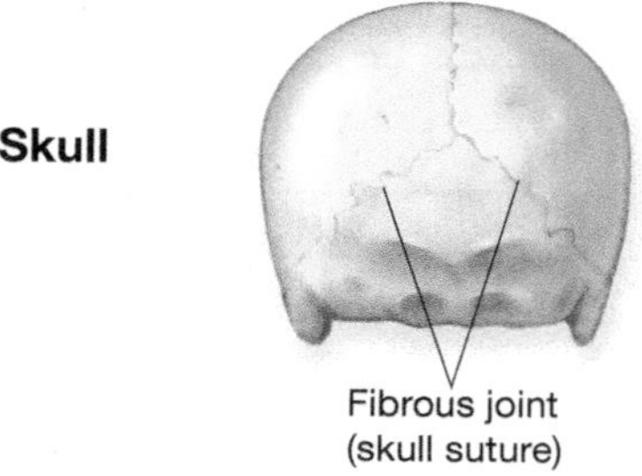

Pelvis

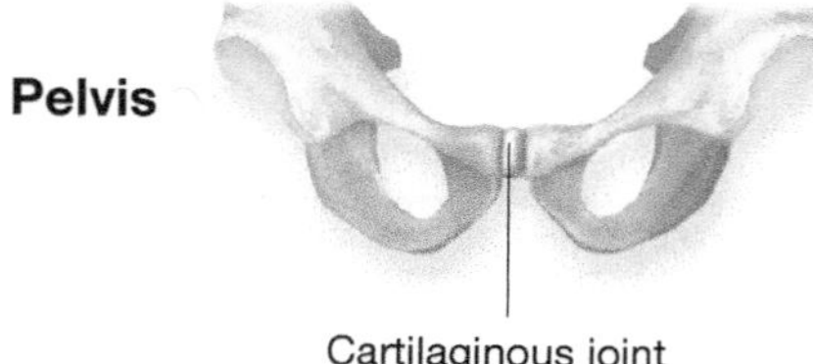

Hand

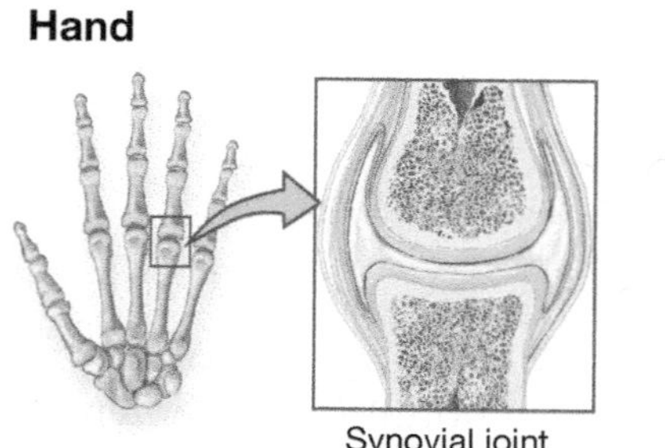

■ **Figure 4.11** Examples of three types of joints found in the body.

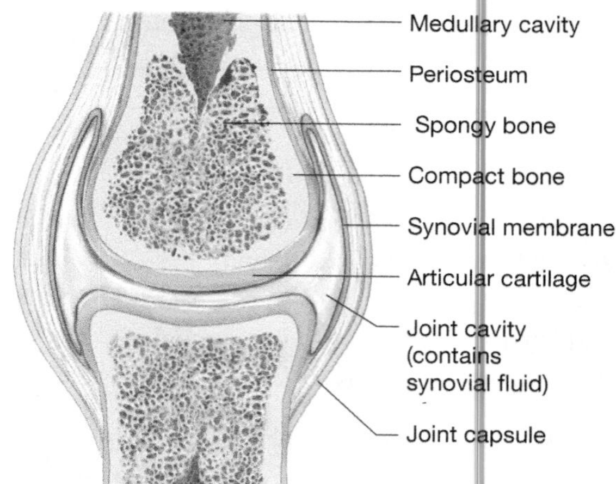

■ **Figure 4.12** Structure of a generalized synovial joint.

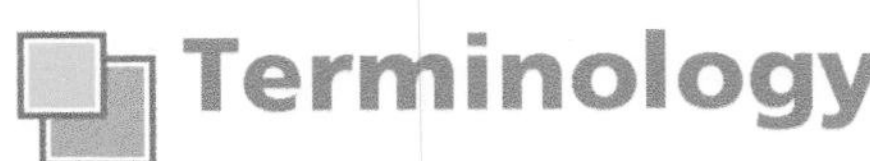

Terminology

Word Parts Used to Build Skeletal System Terms

The following lists contain the combining forms, suffixes, and prefixes used to build terms in the remaining sections of this chapter.

Combining Forms

ankyl/o	stiff joint
arthr/o	joint
articul/o	joint
burs/o	bursa
carp/o	carpus
cervic/o	neck
chondr/o	cartilage
clavicul/o	clavicle
coccyg/o	coccyx
cortic/o	outer portion
cost/o	rib
crani/o	skull
cutane/o	skin
erythr/o	red
femor/o	femur
fibul/o	fibula
humer/o	humerus
ili/o	ilium
ischi/o	ischium

kyph/o	hump
lamin/o	lamina, part of vertebra
lord/o	bent backwards
lumb/o	low back
mandibul/o	mandible
maxill/o	maxilla
medull/o	inner portion
metacarp/o	metacarpus
metatars/o	metatarsus
myel/o	bone marrow
orth/o	straight
oste/o	bone
patell/o	patella
path/o	disease
ped/o	child, foot
pelv/o	pelvis
phalang/o	phalanges
pod/o	foot

prosthet/o	addition
pub/o	pubis
radi/o	radius, ray (X-ray)
sacr/o	sacrum
sarc/o	flesh
scapul/o	scapula
scoli/o	crooked, bent
spin/o	spine
spondyl/o	vertebra
stern/o	sternum
synovi/o	synovial membrane
synov/o	synovial membrane
system/o	system
tars/o	tarsus
thorac/o	thorax
tibi/o	tibia
uln/o	ulna
vertebr/o	vertebra

Suffixes

-ac	pertaining to
-al	pertaining to
-algia	pain
-ar	pertaining to
-ary	pertaining to
-centesis	puncture to withdraw fluid
-clasia	surgically break
-desis	fuse
-eal	pertaining to
-ectomy	surgical removal
-genic	producing

-gram	record
-graphy	process of recording
-iatry	medical treatment
-ic	pertaining to
-itis	inflammation
-listhesis	slipping
-logy	study
-malacia	softening
-metry	process of measuring
-oma	tumor
-ory	pertaining to
-osis	abnormal condition

-otomy	cutting into
-ous	pertaining to
-pathy	disease
-plasty	surgical repair
-porosis	porous
-scope	instrument for viewing
-scopy	process of visually examining
-stenosis	narrowing
-tic	pertaining to
-tome	instrument used to cut

Prefixes

anti-	against
bi-	two
ex-	external, outward
inter-	between
intra-	inside
per-	through
sub-	below, under

Anatomical Terms

TERM	WORD PARTS	DEFINITION
articular (ar-TIK-yoo-lar)	articul/o = joint -ar = pertaining to	pertaining to a joint
carpal (CAR-pal)	carp/o = carpus -al = pertaining to	pertaining to the carpus
cervical (CER-vih-kal)	cervic/o = neck -al = pertaining to	pertaining to the neck
clavicular (cla-VIK-yoo-lar)	clavicul/o = clavicle -ar = pertaining to	pertaining to the clavicle
coccygeal (cock-eh-JEE-all)	coccyg/o = coccyx -eal = pertaining to	pertaining to the coccyx
cortical (KOR-ti-kal)	cortic/o = outer portion -al = petaining to	pertaining to the outer portion
costal (COAST-all)	cost/o = rib -al = pertaining to	pertaining to the rib
cranial (KRAY-nee-all)	crani/o = skull -al = pertaining to	pertaining to the skull
femoral (FEM-or-all)	femor/o = femur -al = pertaining to	pertaining to the femur
fibular (FIB-yoo-lar)	fibul/o = fibula -ar = pertaining to	pertaining to the fibula
humeral (HYOO-mer-all)	humer/o = humerus -al = pertaining to	pertaining to the humerus
iliac (ILL-ee-ack)	ili/o = ilium -ac = pertaining to	pertaining to the ilium
intervertebral (in-ter-VER-teh-bral)	inter- = between vertebr/o = vertebra -al = pertaining to	pertaining to between vertebrae
intracranial (in-trah-KRAY-nee-al)	intra- = inside crani/o = skull -al = pertaining to	pertaining to inside the skull
ischial (ISH-ee-all)	ischi/o = ischium -al = pertaining to	pertaining to the ischium
lumbar (LUM-bar)	lumb/o = low back -ar = pertaining to	pertaining to the low back
mandibular (man-DIB-yoo-lar)	mandibul/o = mandible -ar = pertaining to	pertaining to the mandible
maxillary (mack-sih-LAIR-ree)	maxill/o = maxilla -ary = pertaining to	pertaining to the maxilla

Anatomical Terms *(continued)*

TERM	WORD PARTS	DEFINITION
medullary (MED-you-lair-ee)	medull/o = inner portion -ary = pertaining to	pertaining to the inner portion
metacarpal (met-ah-CAR-pal)	metacarp/o = metacarpus -al = pertaining to	pertaining to the metacarpus
metatarsal (met-ah-TAHR-sal)	metatars/o = metatarsus -al = pertaining to	pertaining to the metatarsus
patellar (pa-TELL-ar)	patell/o = patella -ar = pertaining to	pertaining to the patella
pelvic (PEL-vik)	pelv/o = pelvis -ic = pertaining to	pertaining to the pelvis
phalangeal (fay-lan-JEE-all)	phalang/o = phalanges -eal = pertaining to	pertaining to the phalanges
pubic (PYOO-bik)	pub/o = pubis -ic = pertaining to	pertaining to the pubis
radial (RAY-dee-all)	radi/o = radius -al = pertaining to	pertaining to the radius
sacral (SAY-kral)	sacr/o = sacrum -al = pertaining to	pertaining to the sacrum
scapular (SKAP-yoo-lar)	scapul/o = scapula -ar = pertaining to	pertaining to the scapula
sternal (STER-nal)	stern/o = sternum -al = pertaining to	pertaining to the sternum
synovial (sin-OH-vee-al)	synovi/o = synovial membrane -al = pertaining to	pertaining to the synovial membrane
tarsal (TAHR-sal)	tars/o = tarsus -al = pertaining to	pertaining to the tarsus
thoracic (tho-RASS-ik)	thorac/o = thorax -ic = pertaining to	pertaining to the thorax
tibial (TIB-ee-all)	tibi/o = tibia -al = pertaining to	pertaining to the tibia
ulnar (UHL-nar)	uln/o = ulna -ar = pertaining to	pertaining to the ulna

Pathology

TERM	WORD PARTS	DEFINITION
Medical Specialties		
chiropractic (ki-roh-PRAK-tik)	-tic = pertaining to	Healthcare profession concerned with diagnosis and treatment of malalignment conditions of the spine and musculoskeletal system with the intention of affecting the nervous system and improving health. Healthcare professional is a *chiropractor.*

Pathology *(continued)*

TERM	WORD PARTS	DEFINITION
orthopedics (or-thoh-PEE-diks)	orth/o = straight ped/o = child, foot -ic = pertaining to	Branch of medicine specializing in the diagnosis and treatment of conditions of the musculoskeletal system; also called *orthopedic surgery.* Physician is an *orthopedist* or *orthopedic surgeon.* Name derived from straightening (*orth/o*) deformities in children (*ped/o*).
orthotics (or-THOT-iks)	orth/o = straight -tic = pertaining to	Healthcare profession specializing in making orthopedic appliances such as braces and splints. Person skilled in making and adjusting these appliances is an *orthotist.*
podiatry (po-DYE-ah-tree)	pod/o = foot -iatry = medical treatment	Healthcare profession specializing in diagnosis and treatment of disorders of the feet and lower legs. Healthcare professional is a *podiatrist.*
prosthetics (pross-THET-iks)	prosthet/o = addition -ic = pertaining to	Healthcare profession specializing in making artificial body parts. Person skilled in making and adjusting prostheses is a *prosthetist.*
Signs and Symptoms		
arthralgia (ar-THRAL-jee-ah)	arthr/o = joint -algia = pain	joint pain
bursitis (ber-SIGH-tis)	burs/o = bursa -itis = inflammation	inflammation of a bursa
callus (KAL-us)		The mass of bone tissue that forms at a fracture site during its healing.
chondromalacia (kon-droh-mah-LAY-she-ah)	chondr/o = cartilage -malacia = softening	softening of the cartilage
crepitation (krep-ih-TAY-shun)		The noise produced by bones or cartilage rubbing together in conditions such as arthritis. Also called *crepitus.*
ostealgia (oss-tee-AL-jee-ah)	oste/o = bone -algia = pain	bone pain
osteomyelitis (oss-tee-oh-mi-ell-EYE-tis)	oste/o = bone myel/o = bone marrow -itis = inflammation	inflammation of bone and bone marrow
synovitis (sih-no-VI-tis)	synov/o = synovial membrane -itis = inflammation	inflammation of synovial membrane
Fractures		
closed fracture		Fracture in which there is no open skin wound. Also called a *simple fracture.*

Pathology *(continued)*

TERM	WORD PARTS	DEFINITION
■ **Figure 4.13** (A) Closed (or simple) fracture and (B) open (or compound) fracture.	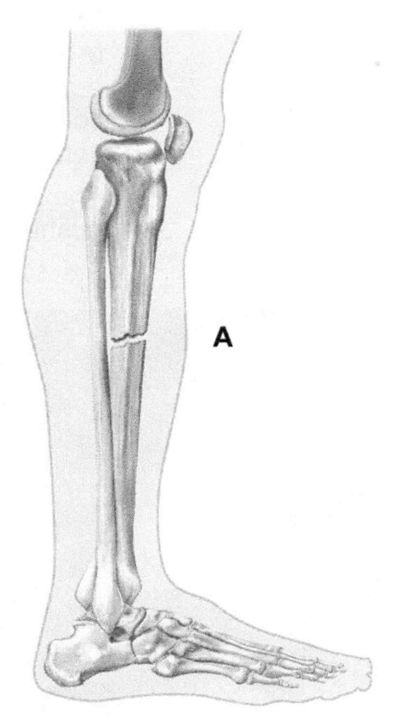	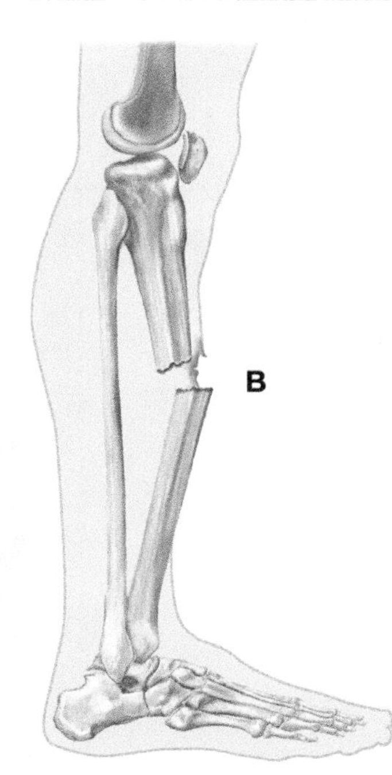
Colles' (COL-eez) **fracture** ■ **Figure 4.14** Colles' fracture. *(Charles Stewart MD FACEP, FAAEM)*	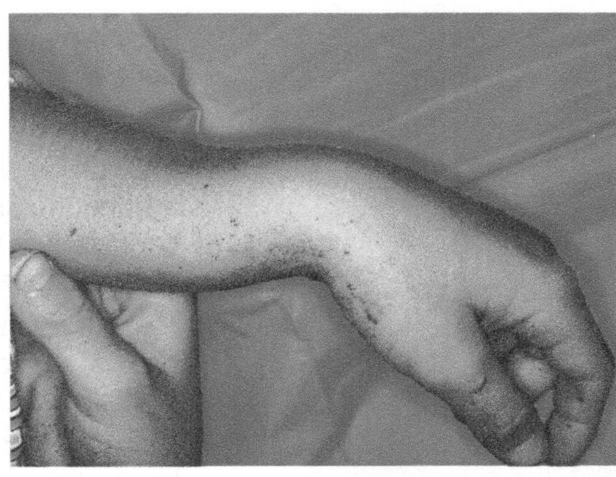	A common type of wrist fracture.
comminuted fracture (kom-ih-NYOOT-ed)		Fracture in which the bone is shattered, splintered, or crushed into many small pieces or fragments.
compound fracture		Fracture in which the skin has been broken through to the fracture. Also called an *open fracture* (see Figure 4.13B ■).
compression fracture		Fracture involving loss of height of a vertebral body. It may be the result of trauma, but in older people, especially women, it may be caused by conditions like osteoporosis.
fracture (FX, Fx)		A broken bone.

Pathology *(continued)*

TERM	WORD PARTS	DEFINITION
greenstick fracture		Fracture in which there is an incomplete break; one side of bone is broken and the other side is bent. This type of fracture is commonly found in children due to their softer and more pliable bone structure.
impacted fracture		Fracture in which bone fragments are pushed into each other.
oblique (oh-BLEEK) fracture 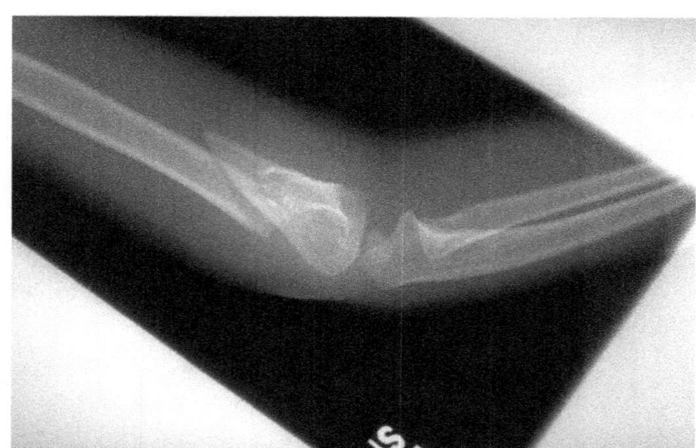 ■ **Figure 4.15** X-ray showing oblique fracture of the humerus. *(Charles Stewart MD)*		Fracture at an angle to the bone.
pathologic (path-a-LOJ-ik) fracture	path/o = disease -logy = study -ic = pertaining to	Fracture caused by diseased or weakened bone.
spiral fracture		Fracture in which the fracture line spirals around the shaft of the bone. Can be caused by a twisting injury and is often slower to heal than other types of fractures.
stress fracture		A slight fracture caused by repetitive low-impact forces, like running, rather than a single forceful impact.
transverse fracture 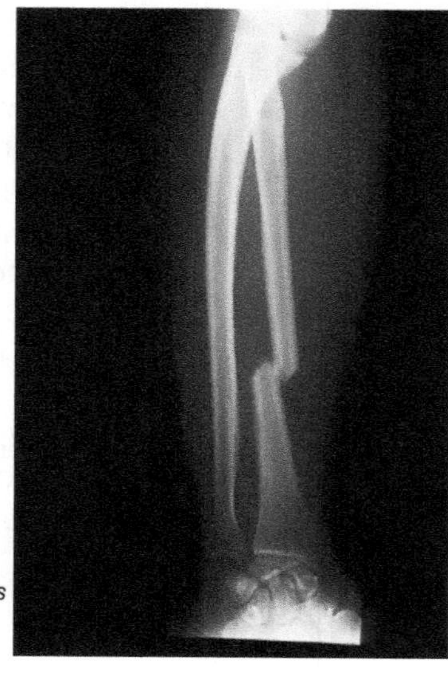 ■ **Figure 4.16** X-ray showing transverse fracture of radius. *(James Stevenson/Science Photo Library/Photo Researchers, Inc.)*		Complete fracture that is straight across the bone at right angles to the long axis of the bone.

Pathology *(continued)*

TERM	WORD PARTS	DEFINITION
Bones		
chondroma (kon-DROH-mah)	chondr/o = cartilage -oma = tumor	A tumor, usually benign, that forms in cartilage.
Ewing's sarcoma (YOO-wings / sar-KOH-mah)	sarc/o = flesh -oma = tumor	Malignant growth found in the shaft of long bones that spreads through the periosteum. Removal is the treatment of choice because this tumor will metastasize or spread to other organs.
exostosis (eck-sos-TOH-sis)	ex- = external, outward oste/o = bone -osis = abnormal condition	A bone spur.
myeloma (my-ah-LOH-mah)	myel/o = bone marrow -oma = tumor	A tumor that forms in bone marrow tissue.
osteochondroma (oss-tee-oh-kon-DROH-mah)	oste/o = bone chondr/o = cartilage -oma = tumor	A tumor, usually benign, that consists of both bone and cartilage tissue.
osteogenic sarcoma (oss-tee-oh-GIN-ik / sark-OH-mah)	oste/o = bone -genic = producing sarc/o = flesh -oma = tumor	The most common type of bone cancer. Usually begins in osteocytes found at the ends of long bones.
osteomalacia (oss-tee-oh-mah-LAY-she-ah)	oste/o = bone -malacia = softening	Softening of the bones caused by a deficiency of calcium. It is thought to be caused by insufficient sunlight and vitamin D in children.
osteopathy (oss-tee-OPP-ah-thee)	oste/o = bone -pathy = disease	A general term for bone disease.
osteoporosis (oss-tee-oh-por-ROH-sis)	oste/o = bone -porosis = porous	Decrease in bone mass producing a thinning and weakening of the bone with resulting fractures. The bone becomes more porous, especially in the spine and pelvis.
Paget's disease (PAH-jets)		A fairly common metabolic disease of the bone from unknown causes. It usually attacks middle-aged and older adults and is characterized by bone destruction and deformity. Named for Sir James Paget, a British surgeon.
rickets (RIK-ets)		Deficiency in calcium and vitamin D found in early childhood that results in bone deformities, especially bowed legs.
Spinal Column		
ankylosing spondylitis (ang-kih-LOH-sing / spon-dih-LYE-tis)	ankyl/o = stiff joint spondyl/o = vertebra -itis = inflammation	Inflammatory spinal condition resembling rheumatoid arthritis and results in gradual stiffening and fusion of the vertebrae. More common in men than women.

Pathology *(continued)*

TERM	WORD PARTS	DEFINITION
herniated nucleus pulposus (HNP) (HER-nee-ated / NOO-klee-us / pull-POH-sus)		Herniation or protrusion of an intervertebral disk; also called *herniated disk* or *ruptured disk.* May require surgery.

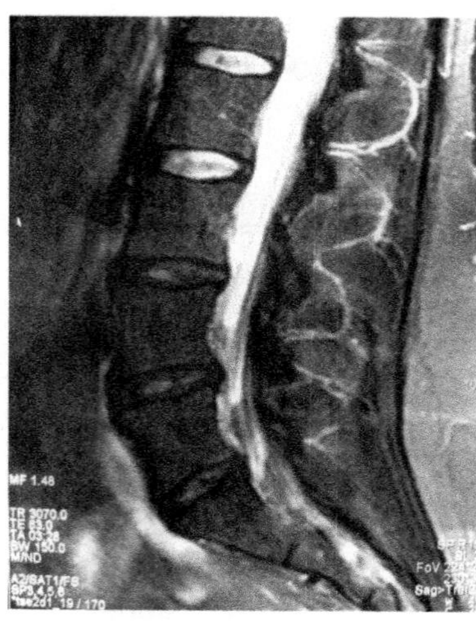

■ **Figure 4.17** Magnetic resonance imaging (MRI) image demonstrating a back herniated disk. *(Michelle Milano/Shutterstock)*

TERM	WORD PARTS	DEFINITION
kyphosis (ki-FOH-sis)	kyph/o = hump -osis = abnormal condition	Abnormal increase in the outward curvature of the thoracic spine. Also known as *hunchback* or *humpback.* See Figure 4.18 ■ for an illustration of abnormal spine curvatures.

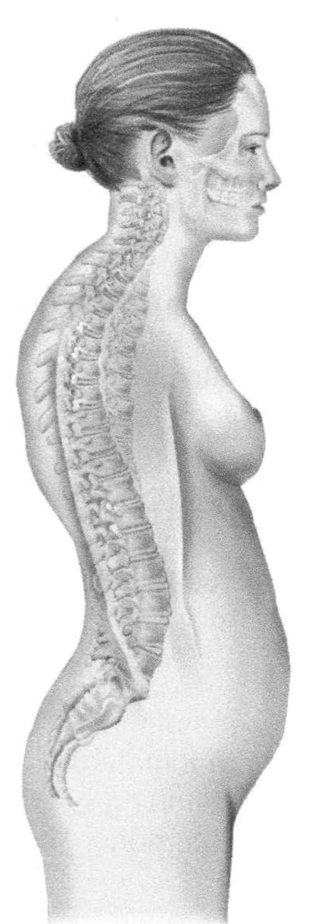

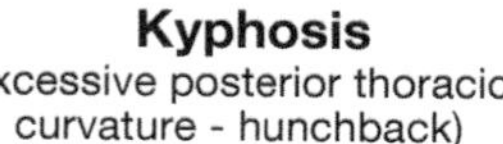

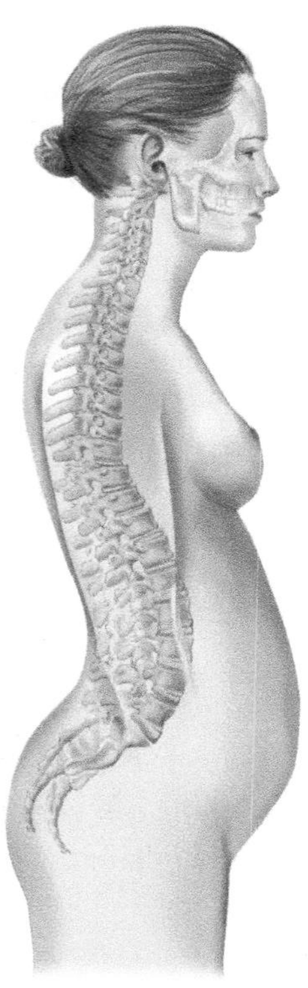

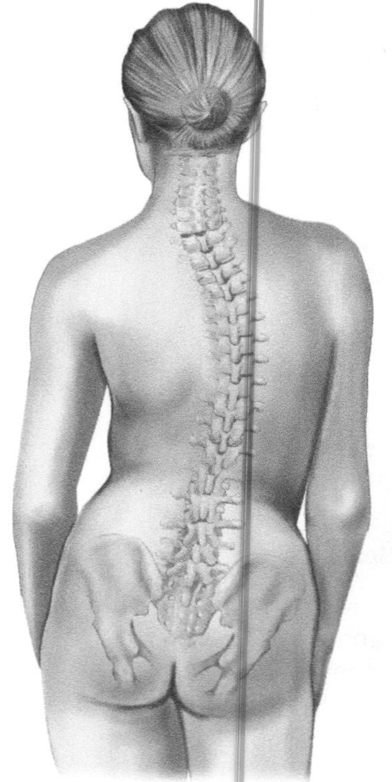

■ **Figure 4.18** Abnormal spinal curvatures: kyphosis, lordosis, and scoliosis.

Pathology *(continued)*

TERM	WORD PARTS	DEFINITION
lordosis (lor-DOH-sis)	lord/o = bent backwards -osis = abnormal condition	Abnormal increase in the forward curvature of the lumbar spine. Also known as *swayback*. See again Figure 4.18 for an illustration of abnormal spine curvatures.
scoliosis (skoh-lee-OH-sis)	scoli/o = crooked, bent -osis = abnormal condition	Abnormal lateral curvature of the spine. See again Figure 4.18 for an illustration of abnormal spine curvatures.
spina bifida (SPY-nah / BIF-ih-dah)	spin/o = spine bi- = two	Congenital anomaly occurring when a vertebra fails to fully form around the spinal cord.
spinal stenosis (ste-NOH-sis)	spin/o = spine -al = pertaining to	Narrowing of the spinal canal causing pressure on the cord and nerves.
spondylolisthesis (spon-dih-loh-liss-THEE-sis)	spondyl/o = vertebra -listhesis = slipping	The forward sliding of a lumbar vertebra over the vertebra below it.
spondylosis (spon-dih-LOH-sis)	spondyl/o = vertebra -osis = abnormal condition	Specifically refers to ankylosing of the spine, but commonly used in reference to any degenerative condition of the vertebral column.
whiplash		Cervical muscle and ligament sprain or strain as a result of a sudden movement forward and backward of the head and neck. Can occur as a result of a rear-end auto collision.
Joints		
bunion (BUN-yun)		Inflammation of the bursa of the first metatarsophalangeal joint (base of the big toe).
dislocation		Occurs when the bones in a joint are displaced from their normal alignment and the ends of the bones are no longer in contact.
osteoarthritis (OA) (oss-tee-oh-ar-THRY-tis)	oste/o = bone arthr/o = joint -itis = inflammation	Arthritis resulting in degeneration of the bones and joints, especially those bearing weight. Results in bone rubbing against bone.
rheumatoid arthritis (RA) (ROO-mah-toyd / ar-THRY-tis)	arthr/o = joint -itis = inflammation	Chronic form of arthritis with inflammation of the joints, swelling, stiffness, pain, and changes in the cartilage that can result in crippling deformities; considered to be an autoimmune disease.

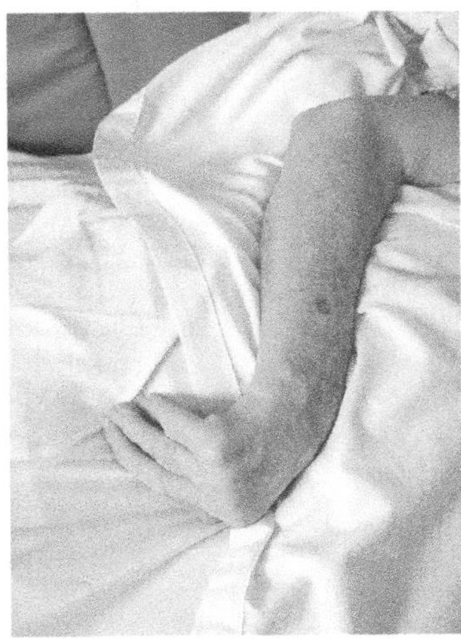

■ **Figure 4.19** Patient with typical rheumatoid arthritis contractures.

Pathology *(continued)*

TERM	WORD PARTS	DEFINITION
sprain		Damage to the ligaments surrounding a joint due to overstretching, but no dislocation of the joint or fracture of the bone.
subluxation (sub-LUCKS-a-shun)	sub- = below, under	An incomplete dislocation, the joint alignment is disrupted, but the ends of the bones remain in contact.
systemic lupus erythematosus (SLE) (sis-TEM-ik / LOOP-us / air-ih-them-ah-TOH-sis)	system/o = system -ic = pertaining to erythr/o = red	Chronic inflammatory autoimmune disease of connective tissue affecting many systems that may include joint pain and arthritis. May be mistaken for rheumatoid arthritis.
talipes (TAL-ih-peez)		Congenital deformity causing misalignment of the ankle joint and foot. Also referred to as a *clubfoot.*

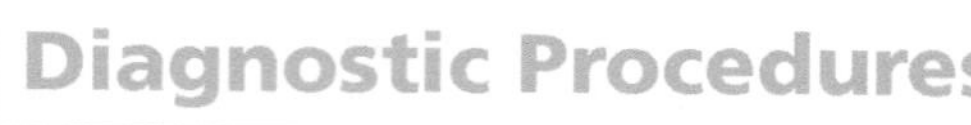

Diagnostic Procedures

TERM	WORD PART	DEFINITION
Diagnostic Imaging		
arthrogram (AR-throh-gram)	arthr/o = joint -gram = record	X-ray record of a joint; usually taken after the joint has been injected by a contrast medium.
arthrography (ar-THROG-rah-fee)	arthr/o = joint -graphy = process of recording	Process of X-raying a joint; usually after injection of a contrast medium into the joint space.
bone scan		Nuclear medicine procedure in which the patient is given a radioactive dye and then scanning equipment is used to visualize bones. It is especially useful in identifying stress fractures, observing progress of treatment for osteomyelitis, and locating cancer metastases to the bone.
dual-energy absorptiometry (DXA) (ab-sorp-she-AHM-eh-tree)	-metry = process of measuring	Measurement of bone density using low-dose X-ray for the purpose of detecting osteoporosis.
myelography (my-eh-LOG-rah-fee)	myel/o = bone marrow -graphy = process of recording	Study of the spinal column after injecting opaque contrast material; particularly useful in identifying herniated nucleus pulposus pinching a spinal nerve.
radiography	radi/o = ray (X-ray) -graphy = process of recording	Diagnostic imaging procedure using X-rays to study the internal structure of the body; especially useful for visualizing bones and joints.
Endoscopic Procedures		
arthroscope (AR-throw-skop)	arthr/o = joint -scope = instrument for viewing	Instrument used to view inside a joint.

Diagnostic Procedures *(continued)*

TERM	WORD PART	DEFINITION
arthroscopy (ar-THROS-koh-pee)	arthr/o = joint -scopy = process of visually examining	Examination of the interior of a joint by entering the joint with an *arthroscope.* The arthroscope contains a small television camera that allows the physician to view the interior of the joint on a monitor during the procedure. Some joint conditions can be repaired during arthroscopy.

Therapeutic Procedures

TERM	WORD PART	DEFINITION
Medical Treatments		
arthrocentesis (ar-thro-sen-TEE-sis)	arthr/o = joint -centesis = puncture to withdraw fluid	Involves the insertion of a needle into the joint cavity in order to remove or aspirate fluid. May be done to remove excess fluid from a joint or to obtain fluid for examination.
orthotic (or-THOT-ik)	orth/o = straight -tic = pertaining to	Orthopedic appliance, such as a brace or splint, used to prevent or correct deformities.
prosthesis (pross-THEE-sis)	prosthet/o = addition	Artificial device used as a substitute for a body part that is either congenitally missing or absent as a result of accident or disease. An example would be an artificial leg.
Surgical Procedures		
amputation (am-pew-TAY-shun)		Partial or complete removal of a limb for a variety of reasons, including tumors, gangrene, intractable pain, crushing injury, or uncontrollable infection.
arthroclasia (ar-throh-KLAY-see-ah)	arthr/o = joint -clasia = surgically break	To forcibly break loose a fused joint while the patient is under anesthetic. Fusion is usually caused by the buildup of scar tissue or adhesions.
arthrodesis (ar-throh-DEE-sis)	arthr/o = joint -desis = fuse	Procedure to stabilize a joint by fusing the bones together.
arthroscopic surgery (ar-throh-SKOP-ic)	arthr/o = joint -scopy = process of visually examining -ic = pertaining to	Performing a surgical procedure while using an arthroscope to view the internal structure, such as a joint.
arthrotomy (ar-THROT-oh-mee)	arthr/o = joint -otomy = cutting into	Surgical procedure that cuts into a joint capsule.
bone graft		Piece of bone taken from the patient used to take the place of a removed bone or a bony defect at another site.
bunionectomy (bun-yun-ECK-toh-mee)	-ectomy = surgical removal	Removal of the bursa at the joint of the great toe.

Therapeutic Procedures *(continued)*

TERM	WORD PART	DEFINITION
bursectomy (ber-SEK-toh-mee)	burs/o = bursa -ectomy = surgical removal	Surgical removal of a bursa.
chondrectomy (kon-DREK-toh-mee)	chondr/o = cartilage -ectomy = surgical removal	Surgical removal of cartilage.
chondroplasty (KON-droh-plas-tee)	chondr/o = cartilage -plasty = surgical repair	Surgical repair of cartilage.
craniotomy (kray-nee-OTT-oh-mee)	chondr/o = cartilage -otomy = cutting into	Surgical procedure that cuts into the skull.
laminectomy (lam-ih-NEK-toh-mee)	lamin/o = lamina, part of vertebra -ectomy = surgical removal	Removal of the vertebral posterior arch to correct severe back problems and pain caused by compression of a spinal nerve.
osteoclasia (oss-tee-oh-KLAY-see-ah)	oste/o = bone -clasia = surgically break	Surgical procedure involving the intentional breaking of a bone to correct a deformity.
osteotome (OSS-tee-oh-tohm)	oste/o = bone -tome = instrument used to cut	Instrument used to cut bone.
osteotomy (oss-tee-OTT-ah-me)	oste/o = bone -otomy = cutting into	Surgical procedure that cuts into a bone.
percutaneous diskectomy (per-kyou-TAY-nee-us / disk-EK-toh-mee)	per- = through cutane/o = skin -ous = pertaining to -ectomy = surgical removal	A thin catheter tube is inserted into the intervertebral disk through the skin and the herniated or ruptured disk material is sucked out or a laser is used to vaporize it.
spinal fusion	spin/o = spine -al = pertaining to	Surgical immobilization of adjacent vertebrae. This may be done for several reasons, including correction for a herniated disk.
synovectomy (sih-no-VEK-toh-mee)	synov/o = synovial membrane -ectomy = surgical removal	Surgical removal of the synovial membrane.
total hip arthroplasty (THA) (ar-thro-PLAS-tee)	arthr/o = joint -plasty = surgical repair	Surgical reconstruction of a hip by implanting a prosthetic or artificial hip joint. Also called *total hip replacement (THR).*
total knee arthroplasty (TKA) (ar-thro-PLAS-tee)	arthr/o = joint -plasty = surgical repair	Surgical reconstruction of a knee joint by implanting a prosthetic knee joint. Also called *total knee replacement (TKR).*

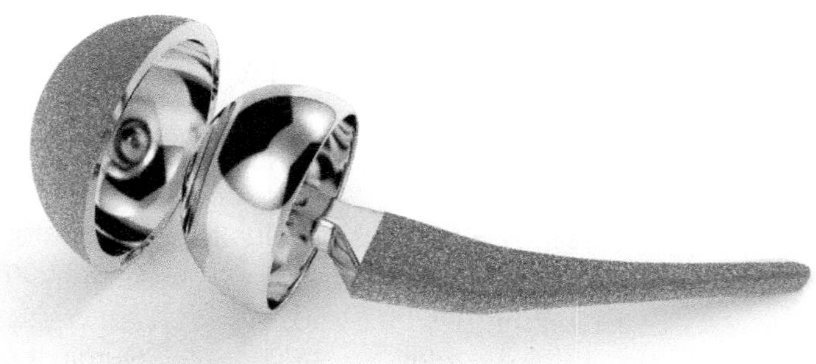

■ **Figure 4.20** Prosthetic hip joint.

Therapeutic Procedures *(continued)*

TERM	WORD PART	DEFINITION
Fracture Care		
cast		Application of a solid material to immobilize an extremity or portion of the body as a result of a fracture, dislocation, or severe injury. It may be made of plaster of Paris or fiberglass.
fixation		Procedure to stabilize a fractured bone while it heals. *External fixation* includes casts, splints, and pins inserted through the skin. *Internal fixation* includes pins, plates, rods, screws, and wires that are applied during an *open reduction.*
reduction		Correcting a fracture by realigning the bone fragments. *Closed reduction* is doing this manipulation without entering the body. *Open reduction* is the process of making a surgical incision at the site of the fracture to do the reduction. This is necessary when bony fragments need to be removed or *internal fixation* such as plates or pins are required.
traction		Applying a pulling force on a fractured or dislocated limb or the vertebral column in order to restore normal alignment.

Pharmacology

CLASSIFICATION	WORD PARTS	ACTION	EXAMPLES
bone reabsorption inhibitors		Conditions that result in weak and fragile bones, such as osteoporosis and Paget's disease, are improved by medications that reduce the reabsorption of bones.	alendronate, Fosamax; ibandronate, Boniva
calcium supplements and vitamin D therapy		Maintaining high blood levels of calcium in association with vitamin D helps maintain bone density; used to treat osteomalacia, osteoporosis, and rickets.	calcium carbonate, Oystercal, Tums; calcium citrate, Cal-Citrate, Citracal
corticosteroids	cortic/o = outer portion	A hormone produced by the adrenal cortex that has very strong anti-inflammatory properties. It is particularly useful in treating rheumatoid arthritis.	prednisone; methylprednisolone, Medrol; dexamethasone, Decadron
nonsteroidal anti-inflammatory drugs (NSAIDs)	-al = pertaining to anti- = against -ory = pertaining to	A large group of drugs that provide mild pain relief and anti-inflammatory benefits for conditions such as arthritis.	ibuprofen, Advil, Motrin; naproxen, Aleve, Naprosyn; salicylates, Aspirin

Abbreviations

AE	above elbow
AK	above knee
BDT	bone density testing
BE	below elbow
BK	below knee
BMD	bone mineral density
C1, C2, etc.	first cervical vertebra, second cervical vertebra, etc.
Ca	calcium
DJD	degenerative joint disease
DXA	dual-energy absorptiometry
FX, Fx	fracture
HNP	herniated nucleus pulposus
JRA	juvenile rheumatoid arthritis
L1, L2, etc.	first lumbar vertebra, second lumbar vertebra, etc.
LE	lower extremity
LLE	left lower extremity
LUE	left upper extremity
NSAID	nonsteroidal anti-inflammatory drug
OA	osteoarthritis
ORIF	open reduction–internal fixation
Orth, ortho	orthopedics
RA	rheumatoid arthritis
RLE	right lower extremity
RUE	right upper extremity
SLE	systemic lupus erythematosus
T1, T2, etc.	first thoracic vertebra, second thoracic vertebra, etc.
THA	total hip arthroplasty
THR	total hip replacement
TKA	total knee arthroplasty
TKR	total knee replacement
UE	upper extremity

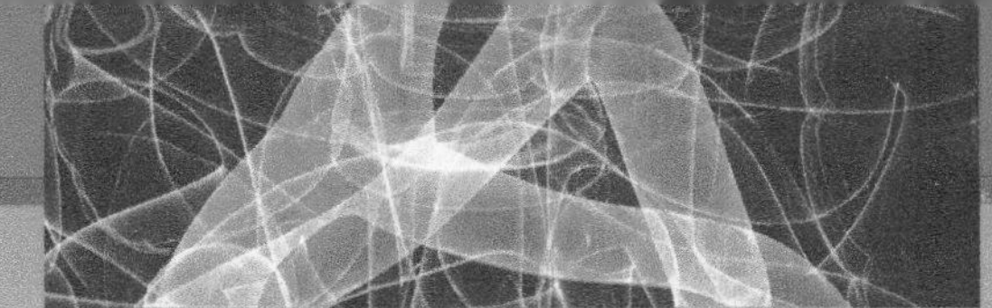

Section II: Muscular System at a Glance

Function

Muscles are bundles, sheets, or rings of tissue that produce movement by contracting and pulling on the structures to which they are attached.

Structures

Here is the primary structure that comprises the muscular system.
muscles

Word Parts

Here are the most common word parts (with their meanings) used to build muscular system terms. For a more comprehensive list, refer to the Terminology section of this chapter.

Combining Forms

duct/o	to bring
extens/o	to stretch out
fasci/o	fibrous band
fibr/o	fibers
flex/o	to bend
kinesi/o	movement
muscul/o	muscle
my/o	muscle
myocardi/o	heart muscle
myos/o	muscle
plant/o	sole of foot
rotat/o	to revolve
ten/o	tendon
tend/o	tendon
tendin/o	tendon
vers/o	to turn

Suffixes

-asthenia	weakness
-ion	action, condition
-kinesia	movement
-tonia	tone

Prefixes

ab-	away from
ad-	toward
circum-	around
e-	outward, without
in-	inward, without

Muscular System Illustrated

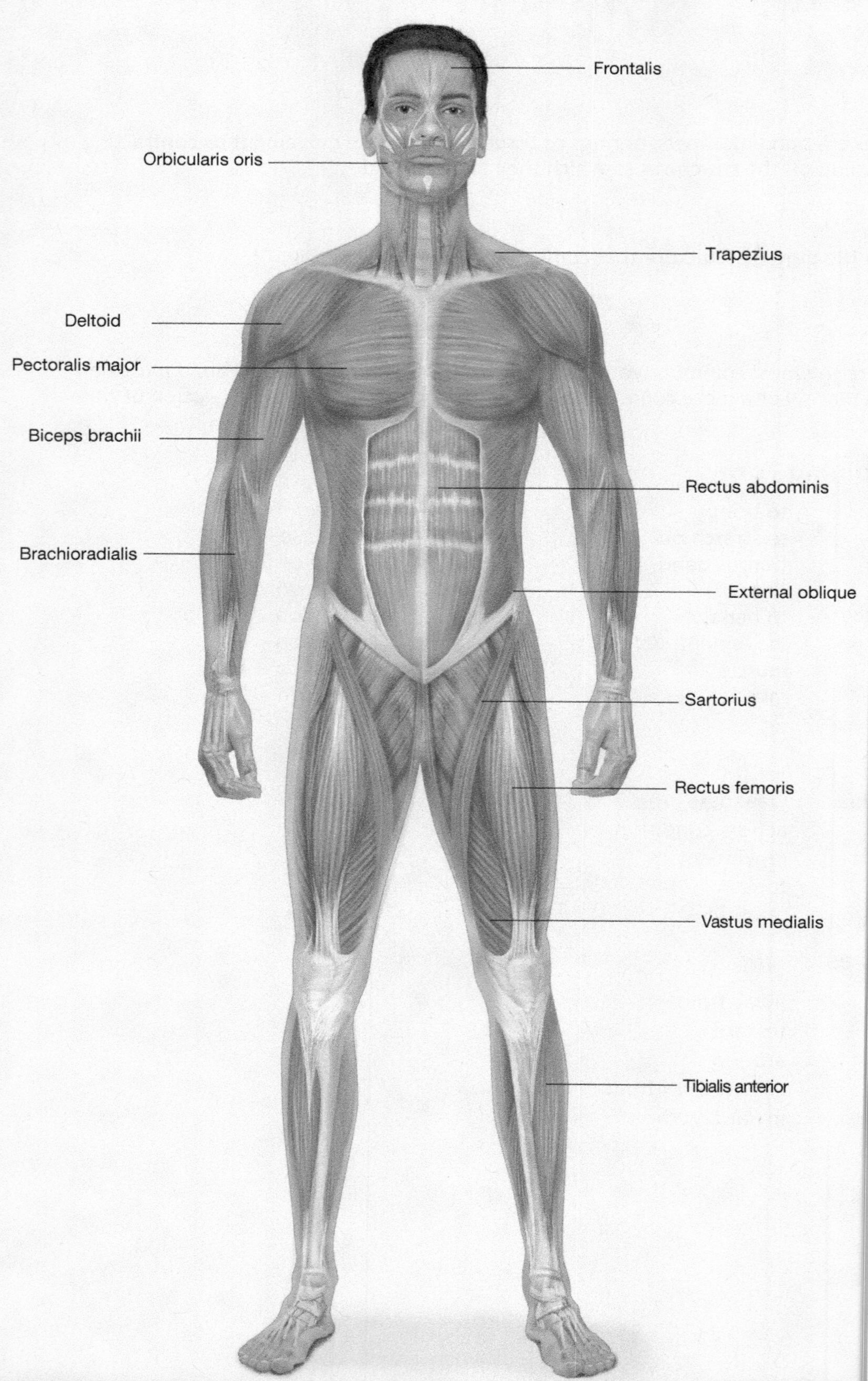

Anatomy and Physiology of the Muscular System

muscle tissue fibers **muscles**

Muscles are bundles of parallel **muscle tissue fibers.** As these fibers contract (shorten in length) they produce movement of or within the body. The movement may take the form of bringing two bones closer together, pushing food through the digestive system, or pumping blood through blood vessels. In addition to producing movement, muscles also hold the body erect and generate heat.

MED TERM TIP

The term *muscle* is the diminutive form of the Latin word *mus* or "little mouse." This is thought to describe how the skin ripples when a muscle contracts, like a little mouse running.

Types of Muscles

cardiac muscle
involuntary muscles
skeletal muscle
smooth muscle
voluntary muscles

The three types of muscle tissue are **skeletal muscle, smooth muscle,** and **cardiac muscle** (see Figure 4.21 ■). Muscle tissue may be either voluntary or involuntary. **Voluntary muscles** are those muscles for which a person consciously chooses to contract and for how long and how hard to contract them. The skeletal muscles of the arm and leg are examples of this type of muscle. **Involuntary muscles** are the muscles under the control of the subconscious regions of the brain. The smooth muscles found in internal organs and cardiac muscles are examples of involuntary muscle tissue.

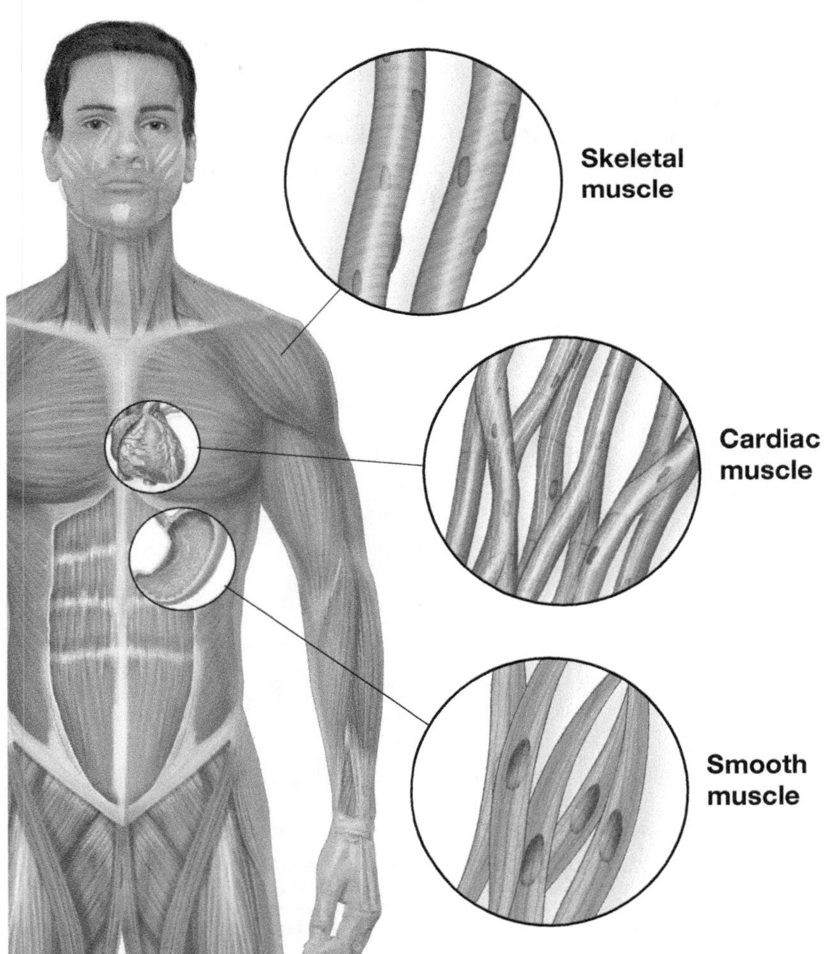

■ **Figure 4.21** The three types of muscles: skeletal, smooth, and cardiac.

Skeletal Muscle

fascia (FASH-ee-ah)
motor neurons
myoneural junction (MY-oh-NOO-rall)
striated muscles (stry-a-ted)
tendon (TEN-dun)

MED TERM TIP

The human body has more than 400 skeletal muscles, which account for almost 50% of the body weight.

A skeletal muscle is directly or indirectly attached to a bone and produces voluntary movement of the skeleton. It is also referred to as a **striated muscle** because of its striped appearance under the microscope (see Figure 4.22 ■). Each muscle is wrapped in layers of fibrous connective tissue called **fascia.** The fascia tapers at each end of a skeletal muscle to form a very strong **tendon.** The tendon then inserts into the periosteum covering a bone to anchor the muscle to the bone. Skeletal muscles are stimulated by **motor neurons** of the nervous system. The point at which the motor nerve contacts a muscle fiber is called the **myoneural junction.**

Smooth Muscle

visceral muscle (vis-she-ral)

Smooth muscle tissue is found in association with internal organs. For this reason, it is also referred to as **visceral muscle.** The name smooth muscle refers to the muscle's microscopic appearance; it lacks the striations of skeletal muscle (see again Figure 4.22). Smooth muscle is found in the walls of the hollow organs, such as the stomach, tube-shaped organs, such as the respiratory airways, and blood vessels. It is responsible for the involuntary muscle action associated with movement of the internal organs, such as churning food, constricting a blood vessel, and uterine contractions.

Cardiac Muscle

myocardium (my-oh-CAR-dee-um)

Cardiac muscle, or **myocardium,** makes up the wall of the heart (see again Figure 4.22). With each involuntary contraction the heart squeezes to pump blood out of its chambers and through the blood vessels.

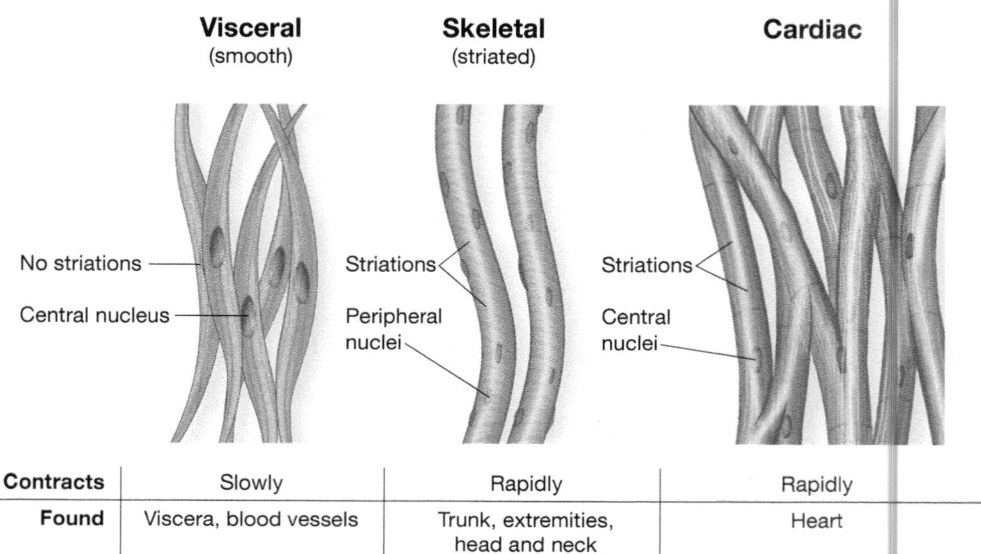

	Visceral (smooth)	Skeletal (striated)	Cardiac
Contracts	Slowly	Rapidly	Rapidly
Found	Viscera, blood vessels	Trunk, extremities, head and neck	Heart
Control	Involuntary	Voluntary	Involuntary

■ **Figure 4.22** Characteristics of the three types of muscles.

Naming Skeletal Muscles

biceps (BYE-seps)
extensor carpi
external oblique
flexor carpi
gluteus maximus (GLOO-tee-us / MACKS-ih-mus)
rectus abdominis (REK-tus / ab-DOM-ih-nis)
sternocleidomastoid (STER-noh-KLY-doh-MASS-toid)

The name of a muscle often reflects its location, origin and insertion, size, action, fiber direction, or number of attachment points, as illustrated by the following examples:

- **Location:** the term **rectus abdominis** means straight (rectus) abdominal muscle.
- **Origin and insertion:** the **sternocleidomastoid** is named for its two origins (stern/o for sternum and cleid/o for clavicle) and single insertion (mastoid process).
- **Size:** when gluteus, meaning rump area, is combined with maximus, meaning large, we have the term **gluteus maximus.**
- **Action:** the **flexor carpi** and **extensor carpi** muscles are named as such because they produce flexion and extension at the wrist.
- **Fiber direction:** the **external oblique** muscle is an abdominal muscle whose fibers run at an oblique angle.
- **Number of attachment points:** the term *bi,* meaning two, can form the medical term **biceps,** which refers to the muscle in the upper arm that has two heads or connecting points.

Skeletal Muscle Actions

action
antagonistic pairs
insertion
origin

Skeletal muscles are attached to two different bones and overlap a joint. When a muscle contracts, the two bones move, but not usually equally. The less movable of the two bones is considered to be the starting point of the muscle and is called the **origin.** The more movable bone is considered to be where the muscle ends and is called the **insertion.** The type of movement a muscle produces is called its **action.** Muscles are often arranged around joints in **antagonistic pairs,** meaning that they produce opposite actions. For example, one muscle will bend a joint while its antagonist is responsible for straightening the joint. Some common terminology for muscle actions are described in Table 4.5 ■.

Table 4.5 Muscle Actions Grouped by Antagonistic Pairs

ACTION	WORD PARTS	DESCRIPTION
abduction (ab-DUCK-shun)	ab- = away from duct/o = to bring -ion = action, condition	Movement away from midline of the body (see Figure 4.23 ■)
adduction (ah-DUCK-shun)	ad- = toward duct/o = to bring -ion = action, condition	Movement toward midline of the body (see again Figure 4.23)
flexion (FLEK-shun)	flex/o = to bend -ion = action, condition	Act of bending or being bent (see Figure 4.24 ■)
extension (eks-TEN-shun)	extens/o = to stretch out -ion = action, condition	Movement that brings limb into or toward a straight condition (see again Figure 4.24)
dorsiflexion (dor-see-FLEK-shun)	dors/o = back of body flex/o = to bend -ion = action, condition	Backward bending, as of hand or foot (see Figure 4.25A ■)
plantar flexion (PLAN-tar / FLEK-shun)	plant/o = sole of foot -ar = pertaining to flex/o = to bend -ion = action, condition	Bending sole of foot; pointing toes downward (see Figure 4.25B ■)

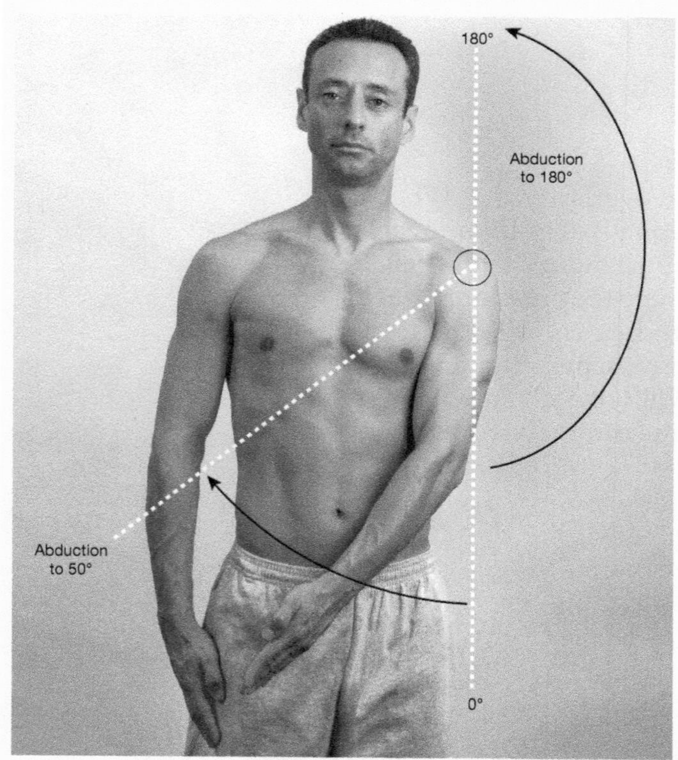

■ **Figure 4.23** Abduction and adduction of the shoulder joint.

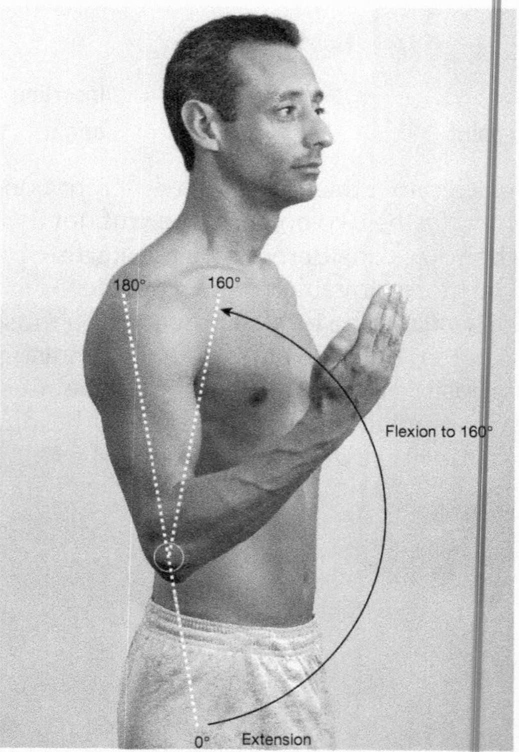

■ **Figure 4.24** Flexion and extension of the elbow joint.

Table 4.5 Muscle Actions Grouped by Antagonistic Pairs (continued)

ACTION	WORD PARTS	DESCRIPTION
eversion (ee-VER-zhun)	e- = outward, without vers/o = to turn -ion = action, condition	Turning outward (see Figure 4.26 ■)
inversion (in-VER-zhun)	in- = inward, without vers/o = to turn -ion = action, condition	Turning inward (see again Figure 4.26)

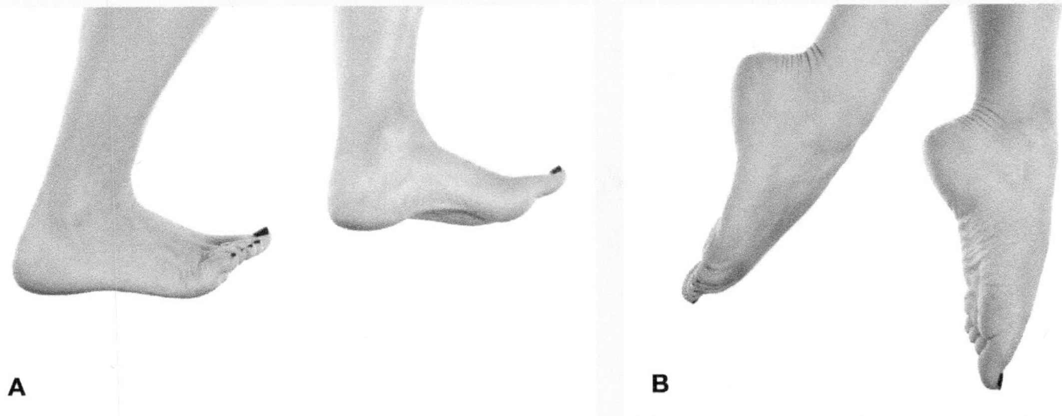

■ **Figure 4.25** Dorsiflexion (A) and plantar flexion (B) of the ankle joint. *(Poulsons Photography/Shutterstock)*

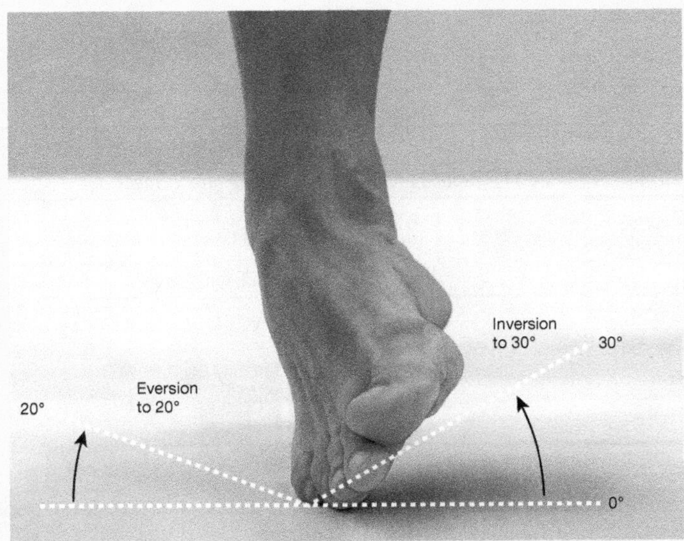

■ **Figure 4.26** Eversion and inversion of the foot.

Table 4.5 Muscle Actions Grouped by Antagonistic Pairs (continued)

ACTION	WORD PARTS	DESCRIPTION
pronation (proh-NAY-shun)		To turn downward or backward as with the hand or foot (see Figure 4.27 ■)
supination (soo-pin-NAY-shun)		Turning the palm or foot upward (see again Figure 4.27)
elevation		To raise a body part, as in shrugging the shoulders
depression		A downward movement, as in dropping the shoulders
The circular actions described below are an exception to the antagonistic pair arrangement.		
circumduction (sir-kum-DUCK-shun)	circum- = around duct/o = to bring -ion = action, condition	Movement in a circular direction from a central point as if drawing a large, imaginary circle in the air
opposition	MED TERM TIP Primates are the only animals with opposable thumbs.	Moving thumb away from palm; the ability to move the thumb into contact with the other fingers
rotation	rotat/o = to revolve -ion = action, condition	Moving around a central axis

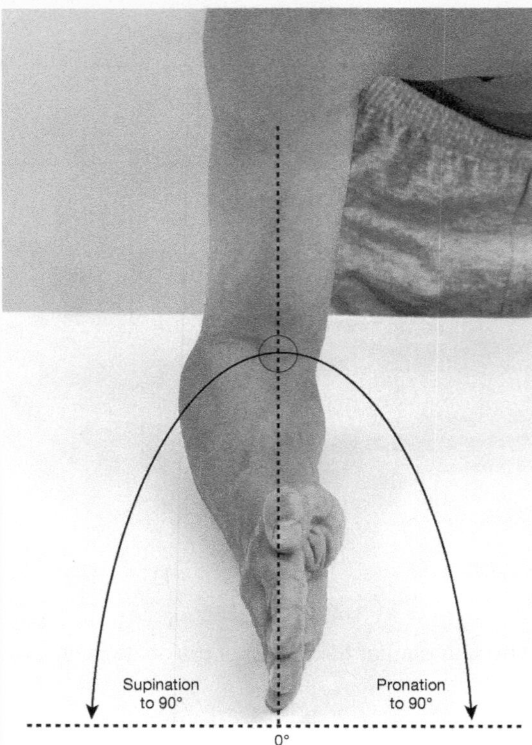

■ **Figure 4.27** Pronation and supination of the forearm.

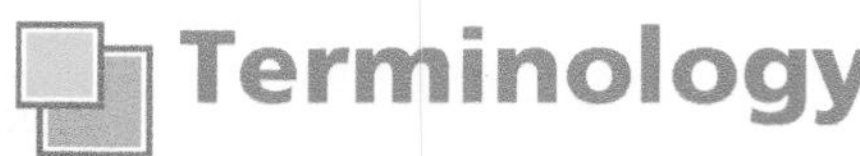

Terminology

Word Parts Used to Build Muscular System Terms

The following lists contain the combining forms, suffixes, and prefixes used to build terms in the remaining sections of this chapter.

Combining Forms

bi/o	life
carp/o	wrist
electr/o	electricity
fasci/o	fibrous band
fibr/o	fibers

kinesi/o	movement
later/o	side
muscul/o	muscle
my/o	muscle
myocardi/o	heart muscle

myos/o	muscle
ten/o	tendon
tend/o	tendon
tendin/o	tendon

Suffixes

-al	pertaining to
-algia	pain
-ar	pertaining to
-asthenia	weakness
-desis	fuse
-dynia	pain
-gram	record

-graphy	process of recording
-itis	inflammation
-kinesia	movement
-logy	study of
-opsy	view of
-otomy	cutting into
-ous	pertaining to

-pathy	disease
-plasty	surgical repair
-rrhaphy	suture
-rrhexis	rupture
-tonia	tone
-trophy	development

Prefixes

a-	without
brady-	slow
dys-	abnormal, difficult, painful

epi-	over
hyper-	excessive
hypo-	insufficient

poly-	many
pseudo-	false

Anatomical Terms

TERM	WORD PARTS	DEFINITION
fascial (FAS-ee-all)	fasci/o = fibrous band -al = pertaining to	pertaining to fascia
muscular (MUSS-kew-lar)	muscul/o = muscle -ar = pertaining to	pertaining to muscles
myocardial (my-oh-CAR-dee-al)	myocardi/o = heart muscle -al = pertaining to	pertaining to heart muscle
skeletal (SKEL-eh-tal)	-al = pertaining to	pertaining to the skeleton
tendinous (TEN-din-us)	tendin/o = tendon -ous = pertaining to	pertaining to tendons

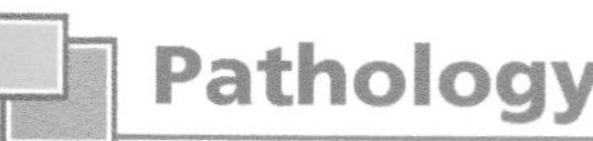

Pathology

TERM	WORD PARTS	DEFINITION
Medical Specialties		
kinesiology (kih-NEE-see-oh-loh-jee)	kinesi/o = movement -logy = study of	The science that studies movement, how it is produced, and the muscles involved.
Signs and Symptoms		
adhesion		Scar tissue forming in the fascia surrounding a muscle, making it difficult to stretch the muscle.
atonia	a- = without -tonia = tone	The lack of muscle tone.
atrophy (AT-rah-fee)	a- = without -trophy = development	Poor muscle development as a result of muscle disease, nervous system disease, or lack of use; commonly referred to as *muscle wasting*.
bradykinesia (brad-ee-kih-NEE-see-ah)	brady- = slow -kinesia = movement	Having slow movements.
contracture (kon-TRACK-chur)		Abnormal shortening of muscle fibers, tendons, or fascia, making it difficult to stretch the muscle.
dyskinesia (dis-kih-NEE-see-ah)	dys- = difficult, painful -kinesia = movement	Having difficult or painful movement.
dystonia	dys- = abnormal -tonia = tone	Having abnormal muscle tone.
hyperkinesia (high-per-kih-NEE-see-ah)	hyper- = excessive -kinesia = movement	Having an excessive amount of movement.
hypertonia	hyper- = excessive -tonia = tone	Having excessive muscle tone.
hypertrophy (high-PER-troh-fee)	hyper- = excessive -trophy = development	Increase in muscle bulk as a result of use, as with lifting weights.
hypokinesia (HI-poh-kih-NEE-see-ah)	hypo- = insufficient -kinesia = movement	Having an insufficient amount of movement.
hypotonia	hypo- = insufficient -tonia = tone	Having insufficient muscle tone.
intermittent claudication (klaw-dih-KAY-shun)		Attacks of severe pain and lameness caused by ischemia of the muscles, typically the calf muscles; brought on by walking even very short distances.
myalgia (my-AL-jee-ah)	my/o = muscle -algia = pain	Muscle pain.
myasthenia (my-ass-THEE-nee-ah)	my/o = muscle -asthenia = weakness	Muscle weakness.
myotonia	my/o = muscle -tonia = tone	Muscle tone.
spasm		Sudden, involuntary, strong muscle contraction.

Pathology *(continued)*

TERM	WORD PARTS	DEFINITION
tenodynia (ten-oh-DIN-ee-ah)	ten/o = tendon -dynia = pain	Tendon pain.
Muscles		
fasciitis (fas-ee-EYE-tis)	fasci/o = fibrous band -itis = inflammation	Inflammation of fascia.
fibromyalgia (figh-broh-my-AL-jee-ah)	fibr/o = fibers my/o = muscle -algia = pain	Condition with widespread aching and pain in the muscles and soft tissue.
lateral epicondylitis (ep-ih-kon-dih-LYE-tis)	later/o = side -al = pertaining to epi- = over -itis = inflammation	Inflammation of the muscle attachment to the lateral epicondyle of the elbow. Often caused by strongly gripping. Commonly called *tennis elbow.*
muscular dystrophy (MD) (MUSS-kew-ler / DIS-troh-fee)	muscul/o = muscle -ar = pertaining to dys- = abnormal -trophy = development	Inherited disease causing a progressive muscle degeneration, weakness, and atrophy.
myopathy (my-OPP-ah-thee)	my/o = muscle -pathy = disease	A general term for muscle disease.
myorrhexis (my-oh-REK-sis)	my/o = muscle -rrhexis = rupture	Tearing a muscle.
polymyositis (pol-ee-my-oh-SIGH-tis)	poly- = many myos/o = muscle -itis = inflammation	The simultaneous inflammation of two or more muscles.
pseudohypertrophic muscular dystrophy (soo-doh-HIGH-per-troh-fic)	pseudo- = false hyper- = excessive -trophy = development muscul/o = muscle -ar = pertaining to dys- = abnormal -trophy = development	A type of inherited muscular dystrophy in which the muscle tissue is gradually replaced by fatty tissue, making the muscle look strong. Also called *Duchenne's muscular dystrophy.*
torticollis (tore-tih-KOLL-iss)		Severe neck spasms pulling the head to one side. Commonly called *wryneck* or a *crick in the neck.*
Tendons, Muscles, and/or Ligaments		
carpal tunnel syndrome (CTS)	carp/o = wrist -al = pertaining to	Repetitive motion disorder with pain caused by compression of the finger flexor tendons and median nerve as they pass through the carpal tunnel of the wrist.
ganglion cyst (GANG-lee-on)		Cyst that forms on tendon sheath, usually on hand, wrist, or ankle.
repetitive motion disorder		Group of chronic disorders involving the tendon, muscle, joint, and nerve damage, resulting from the tissue being subjected to pressure, vibration, or repetitive movements for prolonged periods.

Pathology *(continued)*

TERM	WORD PARTS	DEFINITION
rotator cuff injury		The rotator cuff consists of the joint capsule of the shoulder joint reinforced by the tendons from several shoulder muscles. The high degree of flexibility at the shoulder joint puts the rotator cuff at risk for strain and tearing.
strain		Damage to the muscle, tendons, or ligaments due to overuse or overstretching.
tendinitis (ten-dih-NIGH-tis)	tendin/o = tendon -itis = inflammation	Inflammation of a tendon.

Diagnostic Procedures

TERM	WORD PARTS	DEFINITION
Clinical Laboratory Test		
creatine phosphokinase (CPK) (KREE-ah-teen / foss-foe-KYE-nase)		Muscle enzyme found in skeletal muscle and cardiac muscle. Blood levels become elevated in disorders such as heart attack, muscular dystrophy, and other skeletal muscle pathologies.
Additional Diagnostic Procedures		
deep tendon reflexes (DTR)		Muscle contraction in response to a stretch caused by striking the muscle tendon with a reflex hammer. Test used to determine if muscles are responding properly.
electromyogram (EMG) (ee-lek-troh-MY-oh-gram)	electr/o = electricity my/o = muscle -gram = record	The hardcopy record produced by electromyography.
electromyography (EMG) (ee-lek-troh-my-OG-rah-fee)	electr/o = electricity my/o = muscle -graphy = process of recording	Study and record of the strength and quality of muscle contractions as a result of electrical stimulation.
muscle biopsy (BYE-op-see)	bi/o = life -opsy = view of	Removal of muscle tissue for pathological examination.

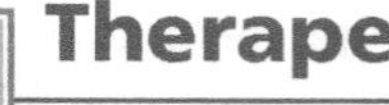

Therapeutic Procedures

TERM	WORD PARTS	DEFINITION
Surgical Procedures		
carpal tunnel release	carp/o = wrist -al = pertaining to	Surgical cutting of the ligament in the wrist to relieve nerve pressure caused by carpal tunnel syndrome, which can result from repetitive motion such as typing.
fasciotomy (fas-ee-OT-oh-mee)	fasci/o = fibrous band -otomy = cutting into	A surgical procedure that cuts into fascia.

Therapeutic Procedures *(continued)*

TERM	WORD PARTS	DEFINITION
myoplasty (MY-oh-plas-tee)	my/o = muscle -plasty = surgical repair	A surgical procedure to repair a muscle.
myorrhaphy (MY-or-ah-fee)	my/o = muscle -rrhaphy = suture	To suture a muscle.
tendoplasty (TEN-doh-plas-tee)	tend/o = tendon -plasty = surgical repair	A surgical procedure to repair a tendon.
tendotomy (tend-OT-oh-mee)	tend/o = tendon -otomy = cutting into	A surgical procedure that cuts into a tendon.
tenodesis (ten-oh-DEE-sis)	ten/o = tendon -desis = fuse	Surgical procedure to stabilize a joint by anchoring down the tendons of the muscles that move the joint.
tenoplasty (TEN-oh-plas-tee)	ten/o = tendon -plasty = surgical repair	A surgical procedure to repair a tendon.
tenorrhaphy (tah-NOR-ah-fee)	ten/o = tendon -rrhaphy = suture	To suture a tendon.

Pharmacology

CLASSIFICATION	WORD PARTS	ACTION	EXAMPLES
skeletal muscle relaxants	-al = pertaining to	Medication to relax skeletal muscles in order to reduce muscle spasms. Also called *antispasmodics*.	cyclobenzaprine, Flexeril; carisoprodol, Soma

Abbreviations

CTS	carpal tunnel syndrome	**EMG**	electromyogram
CPK	creatine phosphokinase	**IM**	intramuscular
DTR	deep tendon reflex	**MD**	muscular dystrophy

Chapter Review

Real-World Applications

Medical Record Analysis

This Discharge Summary contains 10 medical terms. Underline each term and write it in the list below the report. Then define each term.

Discharge Summary

Admitting Diagnosis:	Osteoarthritis bilateral knees.
Final Diagnosis:	Osteoarthritis bilateral knees with right TKA
History of Present Illness:	Patient is a 68-year-old male. He reports he has experienced occasional knee pain and swelling since he injured his knees playing football in high school. These symptoms became worse while he was in his 50s and working on a concrete surface. The right knee has always been more painful than the left. He saw his orthopedic surgeon six months ago because of constant knee pain and swelling severe enough to interfere with sleep and all activities. He required a cane to walk. CT scan indicated severe bilateral osteoarthritis. He is admitted to the hospital at this time for TKR right knee.
Summary of Hospital Course:	Patient tolerated the surgical procedure well. He began intensive physical therapy for lower extremity ROM and strengthening exercises and gait training with a walker. He received occupational therapy instruction in ADLs, especially dressing and personal care. He was able to transfer himself out of bed by the third post-op day and was able to ambulate 150 ft with a walker and dress himself on the fifth post-op day.
Discharge Plans:	Patient was discharged home with his wife one week post-op. He will continue rehabilitation as an outpatient. Return to office for post-op checkup in one week.

	Term	Definition
1	______________	______________________________
2	______________	______________________________
3	______________	______________________________
4	______________	______________________________
5	______________	______________________________
6	______________	______________________________
7	______________	______________________________
8	______________	______________________________
9	______________	______________________________
10	______________	______________________________

Chart Note Transcription

The chart note below contains 11 phrases that can be reworded with a medical term that you learned in this chapter. Each phrase is identified with an underline. Determine the medical term and write your answers in the space provided.

Current Complaint: An 82-year-old female was transported to the Emergency Room via ambulance with severe left hip pain following a fall on the ice.

Past History: Patient suffered a wrist broken bone (1) 2 years earlier that required immobilization by solid material. (2) Following this broken bone, (3) her physician who specializes in treatment of bone conditions (4) diagnosed her with moderate porous bones (5) on the basis of a computer-assisted X-ray. (6)

Signs and Symptoms: Patient reported severe left hip pain, rating it as 8 on a scale of 1 to 10. She held her hip in a bent position (7) and could not tolerate movement toward a straight position. (8) X-rays of the left hip and leg were taken.

Diagnosis: Shattered broken bone (9) in the neck of the left thigh bone. (10)

Treatment: Implantation of an artificial hip joint (11) on the left.

(1) ______________________________

(2) ______________________________

(3) ______________________________

(4) ______________________________

(5) ______________________________

(6) ______________________________

(7) ______________________________

(8) ______________________________

(9) ______________________________

(10) ______________________________

(11) ______________________________

Case Study

Below is a case study presentation of a patient with a condition covered by this chapter. Read the case study and answer the questions below. Some questions will ask for information not included within this chapter. Use your text, a medical dictionary, journals, technical materials, multimedia resources, electronic media, or any other reference material you choose to answer these questions.

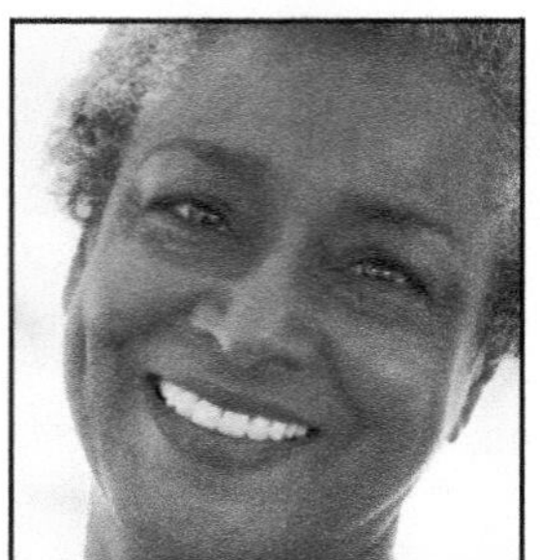

(Monkey Business Images/Shutterstock)

Mary Pearl, age 60, has come into the physician's office complaining of swelling, stiffness, and arthralgia, especially in her elbows, wrists, and hands. A bone scan revealed acute inflammation in multiple joints with damaged articular cartilage and an erythrocyte sedimentation rate blood test indicated a significant level of acute inflammation in the body. A diagnosis of acute episode of rheumatoid arthritis was made. The physician ordered nonsteroidal anti-inflammatory medication and physical therapy. The therapist initiated a treatment program of hydrotherapy and AROM exercises.

1. What pathological condition does this patient have? Look this condition up in a reference source and include a short description of it.

____

____

2. What type of long-term damage may occur in a patient with rheumatoid arthritis?

____

____

3. Describe the other major type of arthritis mentioned in your textbook.

____

____

4. What two diagnostic procedures did the physician order? Describe them in your own words. What were the results?

____

____

5. What treatments were ordered? Explain what the physical therapy procedures involve.

____

____

6. This patient is experiencing an acute episode. Explain what this phrase means and contrast it with chronic.

____

____

Practice Exercises

A. Complete the Statement

1. The two divisions of the human skeleton are the ________________ and ________________.
2. Another name for visceral muscle is ________________ muscle.
3. The five functions of the skeletal system are to ________________, ________________, ________________, ________________, and ________________.
4. Nerves contact skeletal muscle fibers at the ________________ junction.
5. ________________ bones are roughly as long as they are wide.
6. The membrane covering bones is called the ________________.
7. A Colles' fracture occurs in the ________________.
8. Another name for spongy bone is ________________ bone.
9. ________________ joints are the most common joints in the body.
10. The three types of muscle are ________________, ________________, and ________________.
11. A ________________ is a smooth, round opening in bones.
12. The ________________ is the shaft of a long bone.

B. Adjective Form Practice

Give the adjective form for the following bones.

1. femur ________________
2. sternum ________________
3. clavicle ________________
4. coccyx ________________
5. maxilla ________________
6. tibia ________________
7. patella ________________
8. phalanges ________________
9. humerus ________________
10. pubis ________________

C. Combining Form Practice

The combining form **oste/o** refers to bone. Use it to write a term that means:

1. bone cell ____________________
2. embryonic bone cell ____________________
3. porous bone ____________________
4. disease of the bone ____________________
5. cutting into a bone ____________________
6. instrument to cut bone ____________________
7. inflammation of the bone and bone marrow ____________________
8. softening of the bones ____________________
9. tumor composed of both bone and cartilage ____________________

The combining form **my/o** refers to muscle. Use it to write a term that means:

10. muscle disease ____________________
11. surgical repair of muscle ____________________
12. suture of muscle ____________________
13. record of muscle electricity ____________________
14. muscle weakness ____________________

The combining form **ten/o** refers to tendons. Use it to write a term that means:

15. tendon pain ____________________
16. tendon suture ____________________

The combining form **arthr/o** refers to the joints. Use it to write a term that means:

17. surgical fusion of a joint ____________________
18. surgical repair of a joint ____________________
19. cutting into a joint ____________________
20. inflammation of a joint ____________________
21. puncture to withdraw fluid from a joint ____________________
22. pain in the joints ____________________

The combining form **chondr/o** refers to cartilage. Use it to write a term that means:

23. cartilage removal ______________________________

24. cartilage tumor ______________________________

25. cartilage softening ______________________________

D. Name That Suffix

	Suffix	Example from Chapter
1. fuse	______________	__________
2. weakness	______________	__________
3. slipping	______________	__________
4. to surgically break	______________	__________
5. movement	______________	__________
6. porous	______________	__________

E. Spinal Column Practice

Name the five regions of the spinal column and indicate the number of bones in each area.

	Name	Number of Bones
1.	______________	__________
2.	______________	__________
3.	______________	__________
4.	______________	__________
5.	______________	__________

F. Prefix and Suffix Practice

Circle the prefix and/or suffix. Place a *P* for prefix or an *S* for suffix over these word parts then, define the term.

1. arthroscopy ______________________________

2. intervertebral ______________________________

3. chondromalacia ______________________________

4. diskectomy ______________________________

5. intracranial ______________________________

6. subscapular ______________________________

G. Define the Combining Form

	Definition	Example from Chapter
1. lamin/o	______	______
2. ankyl/o	______	______
3. chondr/o	______	______
4. spondyl/o	______	______
5. my/o	______	______
6. orth/o	______	______
7. kyph/o	______	______
8. tend/o	______	______
9. myel/o	______	______
10. articul/o	______	______

H. What's the Abbreviation?

1. intramuscular ______
2. total knee replacement ______
3. herniated nucleus pulposus ______
4. deep tendon reflex ______
5. upper extremity ______
6. fifth lumbar vertebra ______
7. bone density testing ______
8. above the knee ______
9. fracture ______
10. nonsteroidal anti-inflammatory drug ______

I. Define the Term

1. orthopedics ______
2. chiropractic ______
3. podiatry ______
4. orthotics ______
5. prosthetics ______

J. Terminology Matching

Match each term to its definition.

1. _______ abduction
2. _______ rotation
3. _______ plantar flexion
4. _______ extension
5. _______ dorsiflexion
6. _______ flexion
7. _______ adduction
8. _______ opposition

a. backward bending of the foot
b. bending the foot to point toes toward the ground
c. straightening motion
d. motion around a central axis
e. motion away from the body
f. moving the thumb away from the palm
g. motion toward the body
h. bending motion

K. Fill in the Blank

carpal tunnel syndrome	rickets	lateral epicondylitis	systemic lupus erythematosus
scoliosis	osteogenic sarcoma	pseudohypertrophic muscular dystrophy	
herniated nucleus pulposus	osteoporosis		
	spondylolisthesis		

1. Mrs. Lewis, age 84, broke her hip. Her physician will be running tests for what potential ailment? ____________________
2. Jamie, age 6 months, is being given orange juice and vitamin supplements to avoid what condition? ____________________
3. George has severe elbow pain after playing tennis four days in a row. He may have ____________________.
4. Marshall's doctor told him that he had a ruptured disk. The medical term for this is ____________________.
5. Mr. Jefferson's physician has discovered a tumor at the end of his femur. He has been admitted to the hospital for a biopsy to rule out what type of bone cancer? ____________________
6. The school nurse has asked Janelle to bend over so that she may examine her back to see if she is developing a lateral curve. What is the nurse looking for? ____________________
7. Gerald has experienced a gradual loss of muscle strength over the past 5 years even though his muscles look large and healthy. The doctors believe he has an inherited muscle disease. What is that disease? ____________________
8. Roberta has suddenly developed arthritis in her hands and knees. Rheumatoid arthritis had been ruled out, but what other auto-immune disease might Roberta have? ____________________
9. Mark's X-ray demonstrated forward sliding of a lumbar vertebra; the radiologist diagnosed ____________________.
10. The orthopedist determined that Marcia's repetitive wrist movements at work caused her to develop ____________________.

L. Fracture Type Matching

Match each fracture type to its definition.

1.	_______ comminuted	a.	fracture line is at an angle
2.	_______ greenstick	b.	fracture line curves around the bone
3.	_______ compound	c.	bone is splintered or crushed
4.	_______ simple	d.	bone is pressed into itself
5.	_______ impacted	e.	fracture line is straight across bone
6.	_______ transverse	f.	skin has been broken
7.	_______ oblique	g.	no open wound
8.	_______ spiral	h.	bone only partially broken

M. Name That Anatomical Name

1. knee cap ____________________
2. ankle bones ____________________
3. collar bone ____________________
4. thigh bone ____________________
5. toe bones ____________________
6. wrist bones ____________________
7. shin bone ____________________
8. shoulder blade ____________________
9. finger bones ____________________

N. What Does it Stand For?

1. DJD ____________________
2. EMG ____________________
3. C1 ____________________
4. T6 ____________________
5. IM ____________________
6. DTR ____________________
7. JRA ____________________

8. LLE ________________

9. ortho ________________

10. CTS ________________

O. Define the Term

1. chondroplasty ________________
2. bradykinesia ________________
3. osteoporosis ________________
4. lordosis ________________
5. atrophy ________________
6. myeloma ________________
7. prosthesis ________________
8. craniotomy ________________
9. arthrocentesis ________________
10. bursitis ________________

P. Pharmacology Challenge

Fill in the classification for each drug description, then match the brand name.

	Drug Description	Classification	Brand Name
1.	_______ Treats mild pain and anti-inflammatory	________________	a. Flexeril
2.	_______ Hormone with anti-inflammatory properties	________________	b. Aleve
3.	_______ Reduces muscle spasms	________________	c. Fosamax
4.	_______ Treats conditions of weakened bones	________________	d. Oystercal
5.	_______ Maintains blood calcium levels	________________	e. Medrol

Labeling Exercise

Image A

Write the labels for this figure on the numbered lines provided.

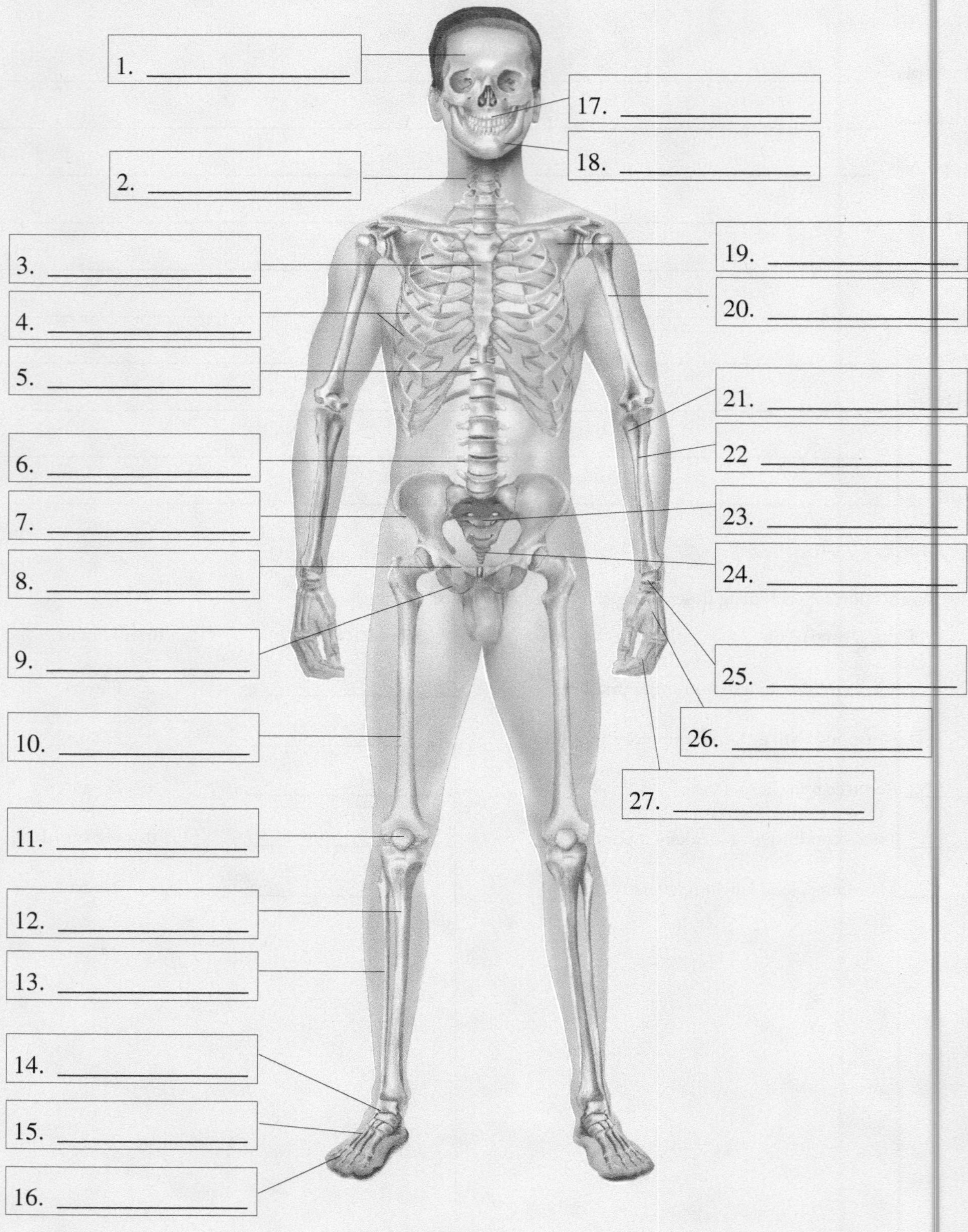

Image B

Write the labels for this figure on the numbered lines provided.

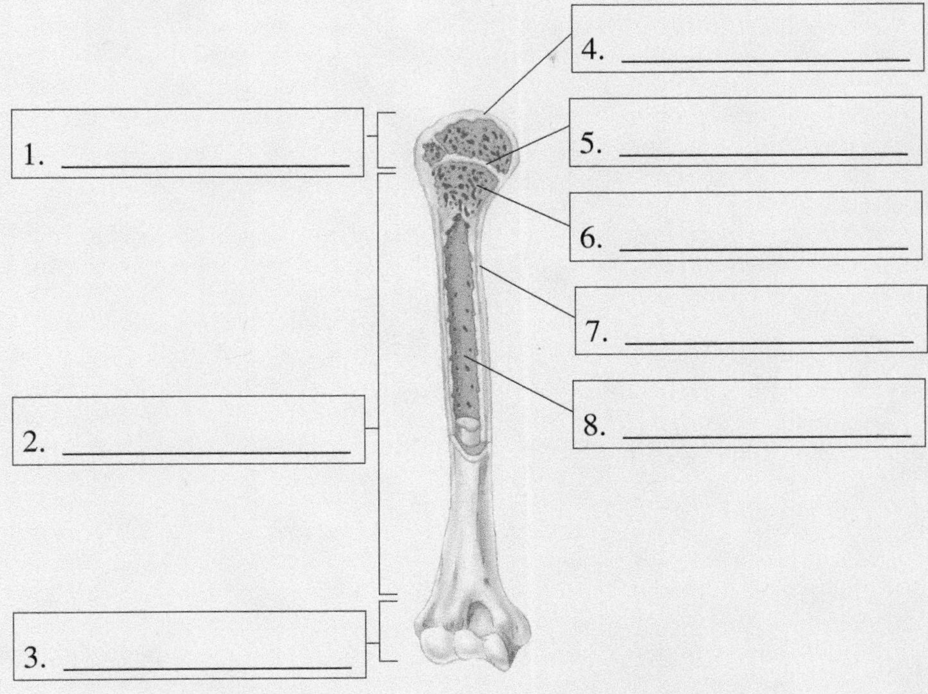

Image C

Write the labels for this figure on the numbered lines provided.

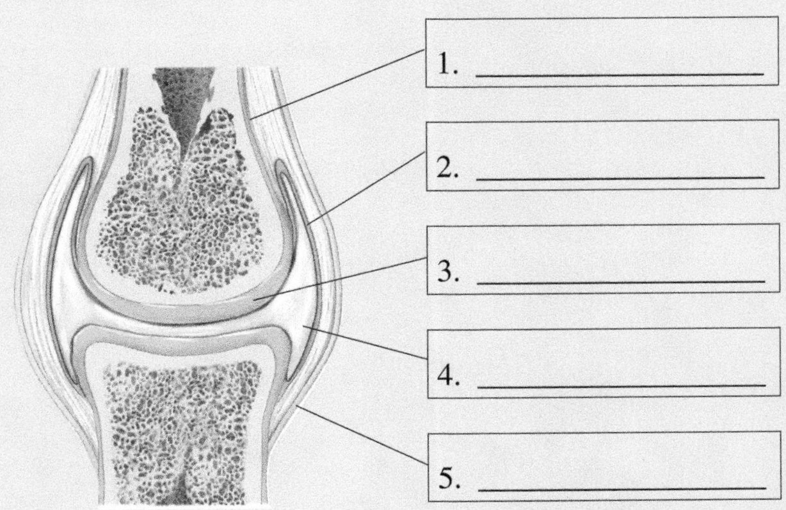

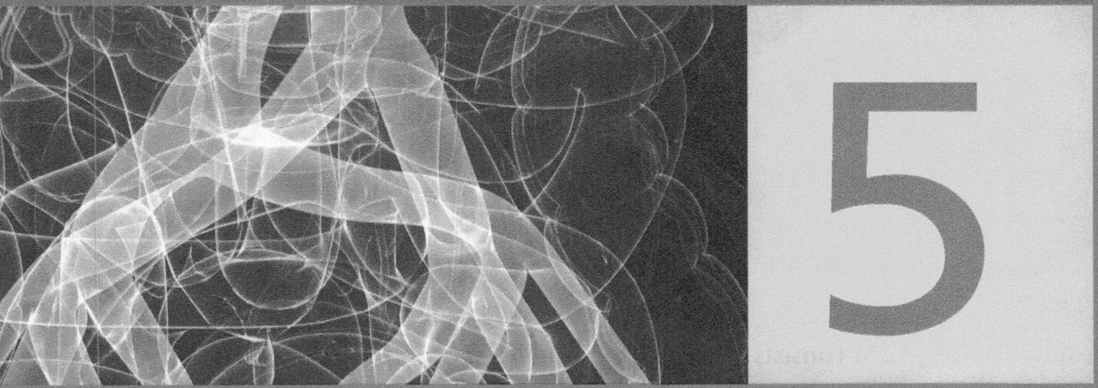

5

CARDIOVASCULAR SYSTEM

Learning Objectives

Upon completion of this chapter, you will be able to

- Identify and define the combining forms and suffixes introduced in this chapter.
- Correctly spell and pronounce medical terms and major anatomical structures relating to the cardiovascular system.
- Describe the major organs of the cardiovascular system and their functions.
- Describe the anatomy of the heart.
- Describe the flow of blood through the heart.
- Explain how the electrical conduction system controls the heartbeat.
- List and describe the characteristics of the three types of blood vessels.
- Define pulse and blood pressure.
- Identify and define cardiovascular system anatomical terms.
- Identify and define selected cardiovascular system pathology terms.
- Identify and define selected cardiovascular system diagnostic procedures.
- Identify and define selected cardiovascular system therapeutic procedures.
- Identify and define selected medications relating to the cardiovascular system.
- Define selected abbreviations associated with the cardiovascular system.

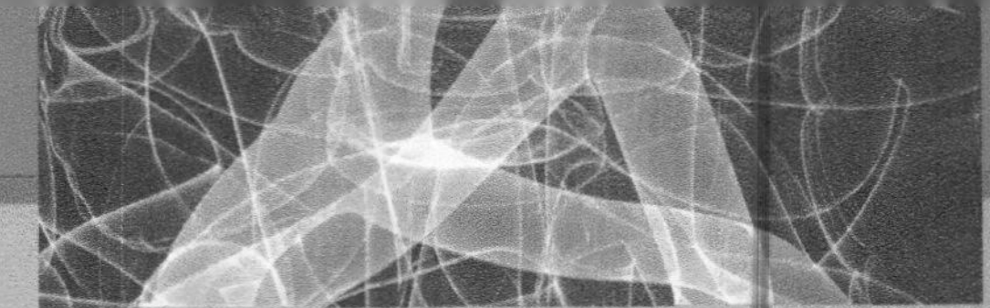

Cardiovascular System at a Glance

Function

The cardiovascular system consists of the pump and vessels that distribute blood to all areas of the body. This system allows for the delivery of needed substances to the cells of the body as well as for the removal of wastes.

Structures

Here are the primary structures that comprise the cardiovascular system.

blood vessels
- **arteries**
- **capillaries**
- **veins**

heart

Word Parts

Here are the most common word parts (with their meanings) used to build cardiovascular system terms. For a more comprehensive list, refer to the Terminology section of this chapter.

Combining Forms

angi/o	vessel
aort/o	aorta
arteri/o	artery
ather/o	fatty substance
atri/o	atrium
cardi/o	heart
coron/o	heart
corpor/o	body
embol/o	plug
isch/o	to hold back
myocardi/o	heart muscle
pect/o	chest
phleb/o	vein
sphygm/o	pulse
steth/o	chest
thromb/o	clot
valv/o	valve
valvul/o	valve
varic/o	dilated vein
vascul/o	blood vessel
vas/o	vessel, duct
ven/o	vein
ventricul/o	ventricle

Suffixes

-manometer	instrument to measure pressure
-ole	small
-tension	pressure
-tonic	pertaining to tone
-ule	small

Cardiovascular System Illustrated

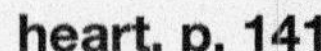

heart, p. 141

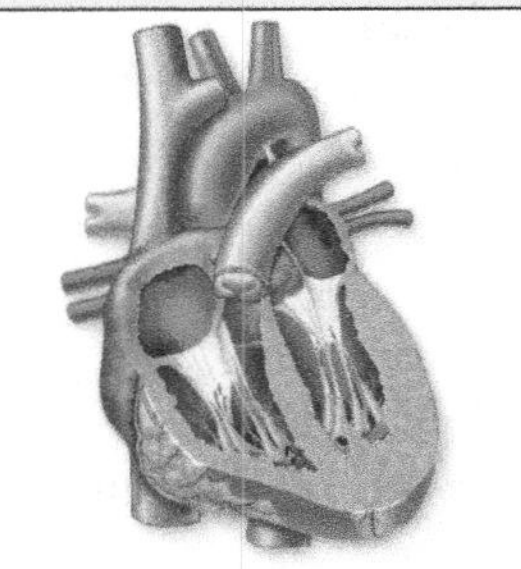

Pumps blood through blood vessels

vein, p. 149

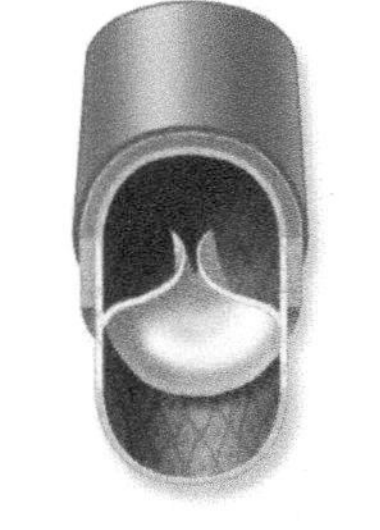

Carries blood towards the heart

artery, p. 147

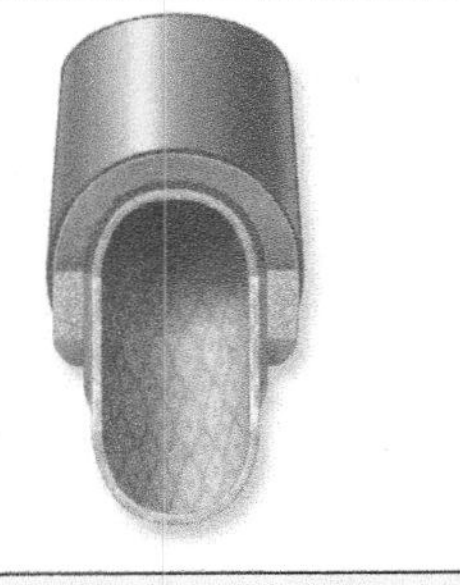

Carries blood away from the heart

capillary, p. 149

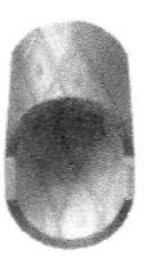

Exchange site between blood and tissues

Anatomy and Physiology of the Cardiovascular System

arteries
blood vessels
capillaries
carbon dioxide
circulatory system
deoxygenated (dee-OK-sih-jen-ay-ted)
heart
oxygen
oxygenated (OK-sih-jen-ay-ted)
pulmonary circulation (PULL-mon-air-ee / ser-kew-LAY-shun)
systemic circulation (sis-TEM-ik / ser-kew-LAY-shun)
veins

The cardiovascular (CV) system, also called the **circulatory system,** maintains the distribution of blood throughout the body and is composed of the **heart** and the **blood vessels—arteries, capillaries,** and **veins.**

The circulatory system is composed of two parts: the **pulmonary circulation** and the **systemic circulation.** The pulmonary circulation, between the heart and lungs, transports **deoxygenated** blood to the lungs to get oxygen, and then back to the heart. The systemic circulation carries **oxygenated** blood away from the heart to the tissues and cells, and then back to the heart (see Figure 5.1 ■). In this way all the body's cells receive blood and oxygen.

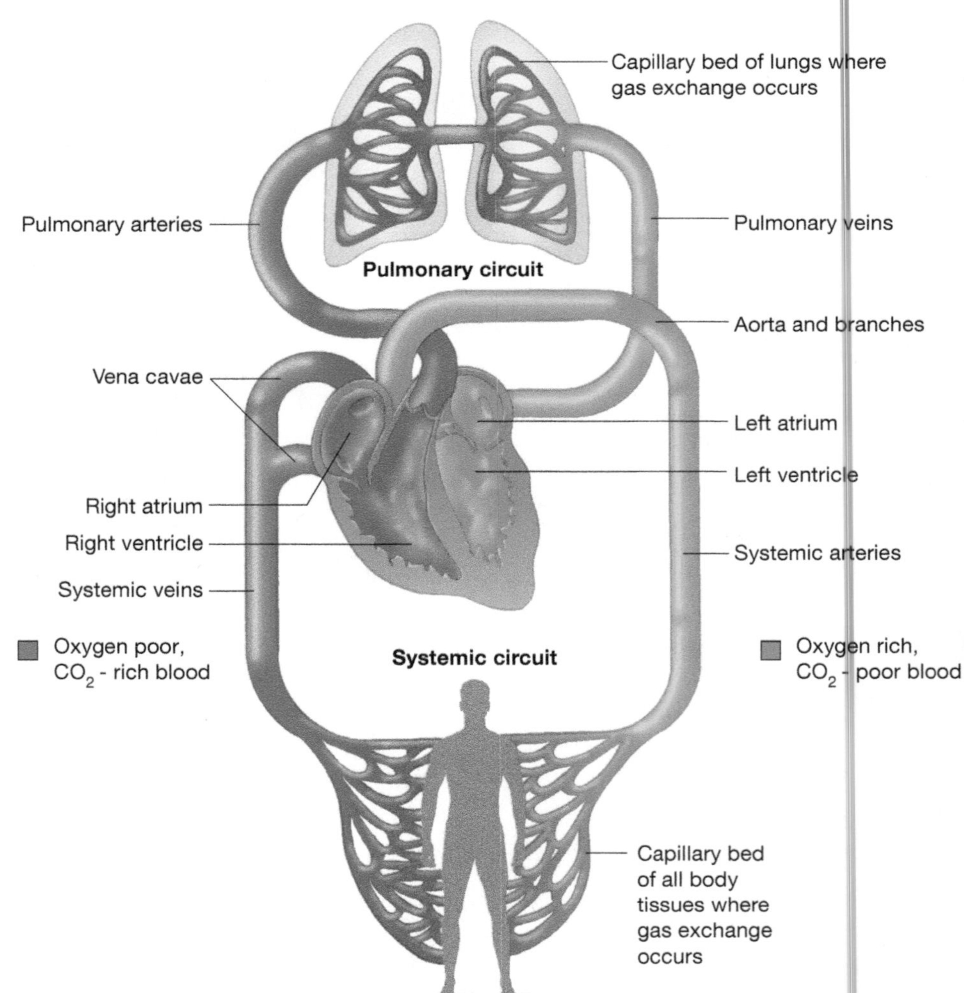

■ **Figure 5.1** A schematic of the circulatory system illustrating the pulmonary circulation picking up oxygen from the lungs and the systemic circulation delivering oxygen to the body.

In addition to distributing **oxygen** and other nutrients, such as glucose and amino acids, the cardiovascular system also collects the waste products from the body's cells. **Carbon dioxide** and other waste products produced by metabolic reaction are transported by the cardiovascular system to the lungs, liver, and kidneys where they are eliminated from the body.

Heart

apex (AY-peks)

cardiac muscle (CAR-dee-ak)

The heart is a muscular pump made up of **cardiac muscle** fibers that could be considered a muscle rather than an organ. It has four chambers, or cavities, and beats an average of 60–100 beats per minute (bpm) or about 100,000 times in one day. Each time the cardiac muscle contracts, blood is ejected from the heart and pushed throughout the body within the blood vessels.

The heart is located in the mediastinum in the center of the chest cavity; however, it is not exactly centered; more of the heart is on the left side of the mediastinum than the right (see Figure 5.2 ■). At about the size of a fist and shaped like an upside-down pear, the heart lies directly behind the sternum. The tip of the heart at the lower edge is called the **apex**.

MED TERM TIP

Your heart is approximately the size of your clenched fist and pumps 4,000 gallons of blood each day. It will beat at least three billion times during your lifetime.

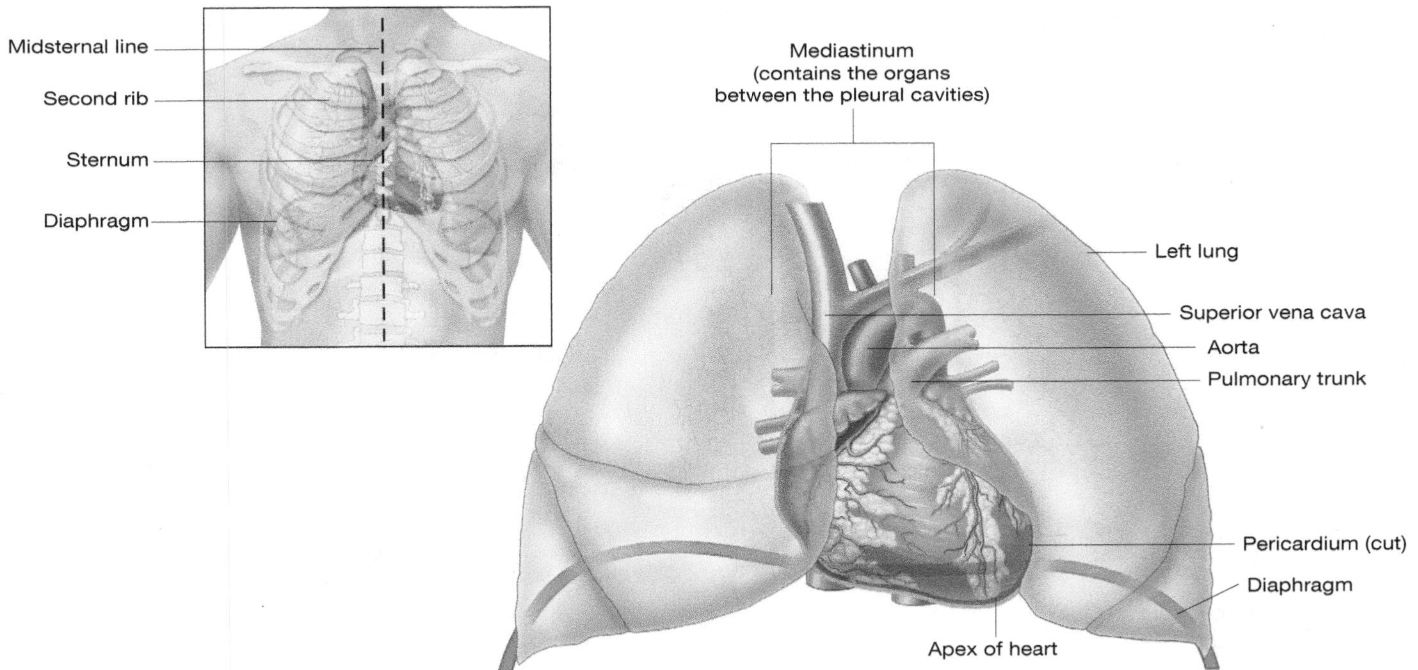

■ **Figure 5.2** Location of the heart within the mediastinum of the thoracic cavity.

Heart Layers

endocardium (en-doh-CAR-dee-um)
epicardium (ep-ih-CAR-dee-um)
myocardium (my-oh-CAR-dee-um)
parietal pericardium (pah-RYE-eh-tal / pair-ih-CAR-dee-um)
pericardium (pair-ih-CAR-dee-um)
visceral pericardium (VISS-er-al / pair-ih-CAR-dee-um)

The wall of the heart is quite thick and composed of three layers (see Figure 5.3 ■):

1. The **endocardium** is the inner layer of the heart lining the heart chambers. It is a very smooth, thin layer that serves to reduce friction as the blood passes through the heart chambers.
2. The **myocardium** is the thick, muscular middle layer of the heart. Contraction of this muscle layer develops the pressure required to pump blood through the blood vessels.
3. The **epicardium** is the outer layer of the heart. The heart is enclosed within a double-layered pleural sac, called the **pericardium.** The epicardium is the **visceral pericardium,** or inner layer of the sac. The outer layer of the sac is the **parietal pericardium.** Fluid between the two layers of the sac reduces friction as the heart beats.

MED TERM TIP

These layers become important when studying the disease conditions affecting the heart. For instance, when the prefix *endo-* is added to *carditis,* forming *endocarditis,* we know that the inflammation is within the "inner layer of the heart." In discussing the muscular action of the heart, the prefix *myo-,* meaning "muscle," is added to *cardium* to form the word *myocardium.* The diagnosis *myocardial infarction* (MI), or heart attack, means that the patient has an infarct or "dead tissue in the muscle of the heart." The prefix *peri-,* meaning "around," when added to the word *cardium* refers to the sac "surrounding the heart." Therefore, *pericarditis* is an "inflammation of the outer sac of the heart."

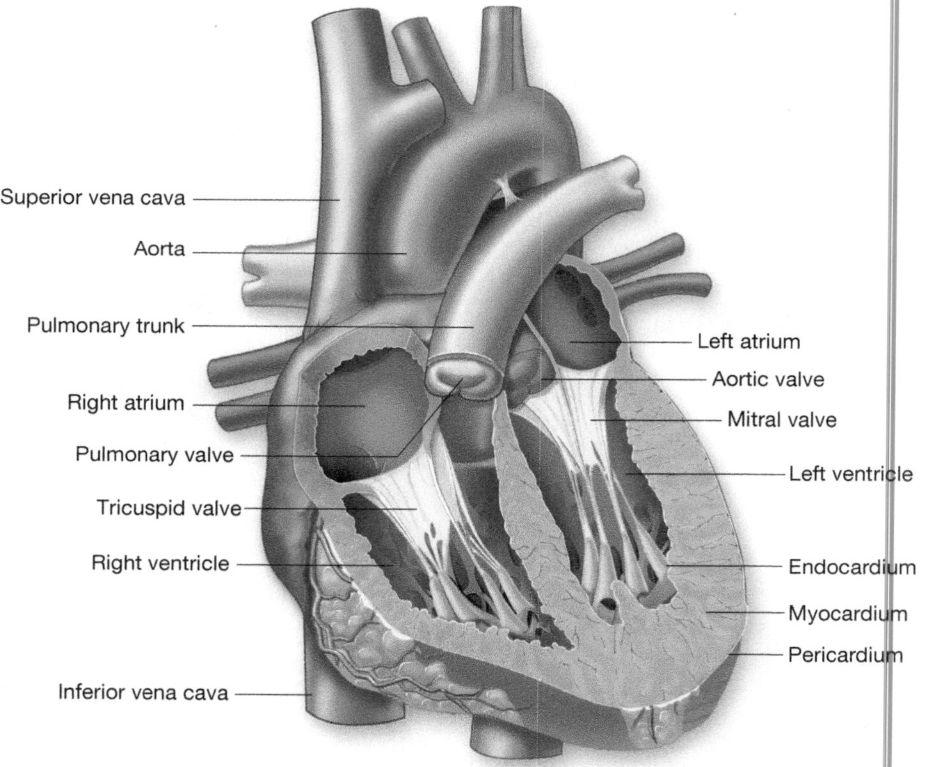

■ **Figure 5.3** Internal view of the heart illustrating the heart chambers, heart layers, and major blood vessels associated with the heart.

Heart Chambers

atria (AY-tree-ah)
interatrial septum (in-ter-AY-tree-al / SEP-tum)
interventricular septum (in-ter-ven-TRIK-yoo-lar / SEP-tum)
ventricles (VEN-trik-lz)

The heart is divided into four chambers or cavities (see Figures 5.3 and 5.4). There are two **atria,** or upper chambers, and two **ventricles,** or lower chambers. These chambers are divided into right and left sides by walls called the **interatrial septum** and the **interventricular septum.** The atria are the receiving chambers of the heart. Blood returning to the heart via veins first collects in the atria. The ventricles are the pumping chambers. They have a much thicker myocardium and their contraction ejects blood out of the heart and into the great arteries.

MED TERM TIP

The term *ventricle* comes from the Latin term *venter,* which means "little belly." Although it originally referred to the abdomen and then the stomach, it came to stand for any hollow region inside an organ.

Heart Valves

aortic valve (ay-OR-tik)
atrioventricular valve (ay-tree-oh-ven-TRIK-yoo-lar)
bicuspid valve (bye-CUSS-pid)
cusps
mitral valve (MY-tral)
pulmonary valve (PULL-mon-air-ee)
semilunar valve (sem-ih-LOO-nar)
tricuspid valve (try-CUSS-pid)

Four valves act as restraining gates to control the direction of blood flow. They are situated at the entrances and exits to the ventricles (see Figure 5.4 ■). Properly functioning valves allow blood to flow only in the forward direction by blocking it from returning to the previous chamber.

The four valves are as follows:

1. **Tricuspid valve:** an **atrioventricular valve** (AV), meaning that it controls the opening between the right atrium and the right ventricle. Once the blood enters the right ventricle, it cannot go back up into the atrium again. The prefix *tri-,* meaning three, indicates that this valve has three leaflets or **cusps.**
2. **Pulmonary valve:** a **semilunar valve.** The prefix *semi-,* meaning half, and the term **lunar,** meaning moon, indicate that this valve looks like a half moon. Located between the right ventricle and the pulmonary artery, this valve prevents blood that has been ejected into the pulmonary artery from returning to the right ventricle as it relaxes.
3. **Mitral valve:** also called the **bicuspid valve,** indicating that it has two cusps. Blood flows through this atrioventricular valve to the left ventricle and cannot go back up into the left atrium.
4. **Aortic valve:** a semilunar valve located between the left ventricle and the aorta. Blood leaves the left ventricle through this valve and cannot return to the left ventricle.

MED TERM TIP

The heart makes two distinct sounds referred to as "lub-dupp." These sounds are produced by the forceful snapping shut of the heart valves. *Lub* is the closing of the atrioventricular valves. *Dupp* is the closing of the semilunar valves.

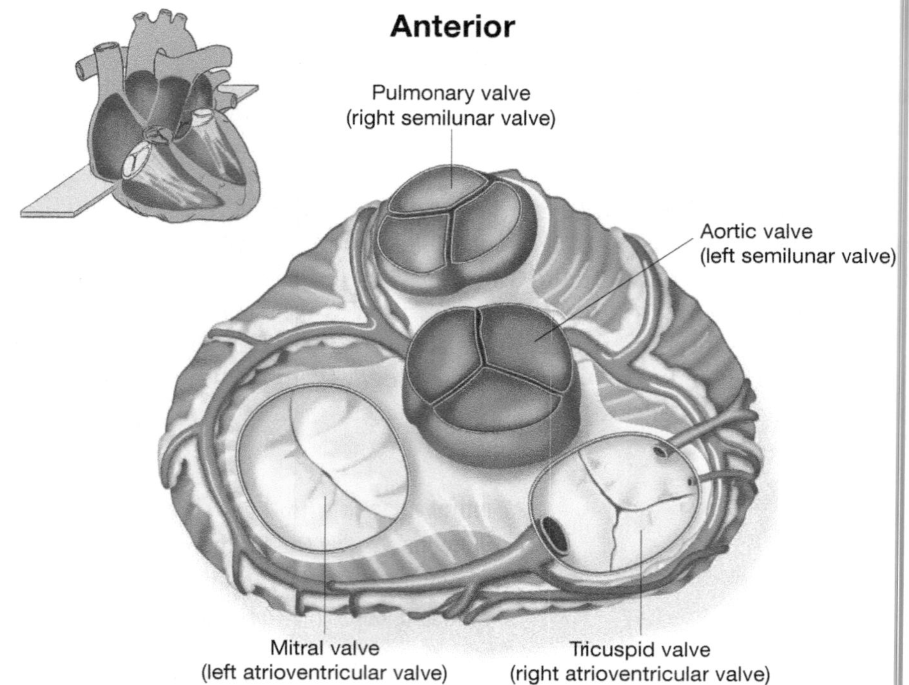

■ **Figure 5.4** Superior view of heart valves illustrating position, size, and shape of each valve.

Blood Flow Through the Heart

aorta (ay-OR-tah)
diastole (dye-ASS-toe-lee)
inferior vena cava (VEE-nah / KAY-vah)
pulmonary artery (PULL-mon-air-ee)
pulmonary veins
superior vena cava
systole (SIS-toe-lee)

The flow of blood through the heart is very orderly (see Figure 5.5 ■). It progresses through the heart to the lungs, where it receives oxygen; then goes back to the heart; and then out to the body tissues and parts. The normal process of blood flow is:

1. Deoxygenated blood from all the tissues in the body enters a relaxed right atrium via two large veins called the **superior vena cava** and **inferior vena cava.**
2. The right atrium contracts and blood flows through the tricuspid valve into the relaxed right ventricle.
3. The right ventricle then contracts and blood is pumped through the pulmonary valve into the **pulmonary artery,** which carries it to the lungs for oxygenation.
4. The left atrium receives blood returning to the heart after being oxygenated by the lungs. This blood enters the relaxed left atrium from the four **pulmonary veins.**
5. The left atrium contracts and blood flows through the mitral valve into the relaxed left ventricle.
6. When the left ventricle contracts, the blood is pumped through the aortic valve and into the **aorta,** the largest artery in the body. The aorta carries blood to all parts of the body.

It can be seen that the heart chambers alternate between relaxing in order to fill and contracting to push blood forward. The period of time a chamber is relaxed is **diastole.** The contraction phase is **systole.**

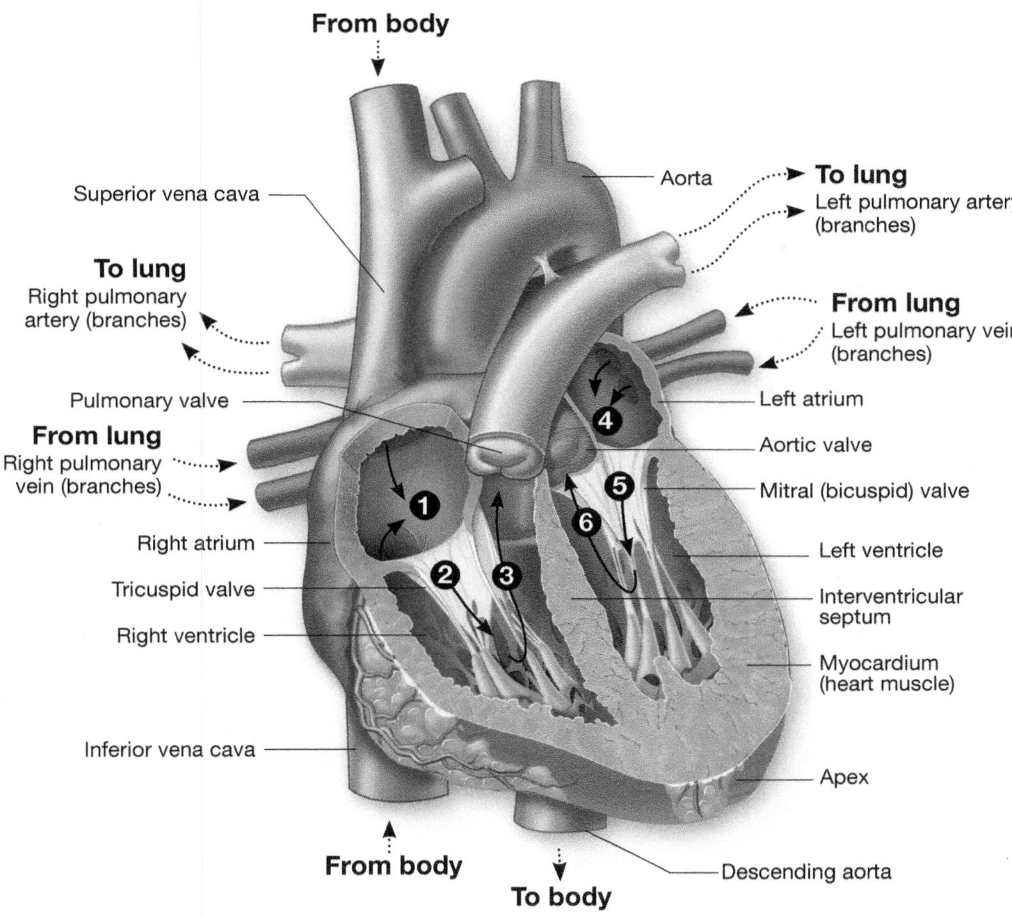

■ **Figure 5.5** The path of blood flow through the chambers of the left and right side of the heart, including the veins delivering blood to the heart and arteries receiving blood ejected from the heart.

Conduction System of the Heart

atrioventricular bundle
atrioventricular node
autonomic nervous system (aw-toh-NOM-ik / NER-vus / SIS-tem)
bundle branches
bundle of His
pacemaker
Purkinje fibers (per-KIN-gee)
sinoatrial node (sigh-noh-AY-tree-al)

The heart rate is regulated by the **autonomic nervous system;** therefore, we have no voluntary control over the beating of our heart. Special tissue within the heart is responsible for conducting an electrical impulse stimulating the different chambers to contract in the correct order.

The path that the impulses travel is as follows (see Figure 5.6 ■):

1. The **sinoatrial (SA) node,** or **pacemaker,** is where the electrical impulses begin. From the sinoatrial node a wave of electricity travels through the atria, causing them to contract, or go into systole.
2. The **atrioventricular node** is stimulated.
3. This node transfers the stimulation wave to the **atrioventricular bundle** (formerly called **bundle of His**).
4. The electrical signal next travels down the **bundle branches** within the interventricular septum.
5. The **Purkinje fibers** out in the ventricular myocardium are stimulated, resulting in ventricular systole.

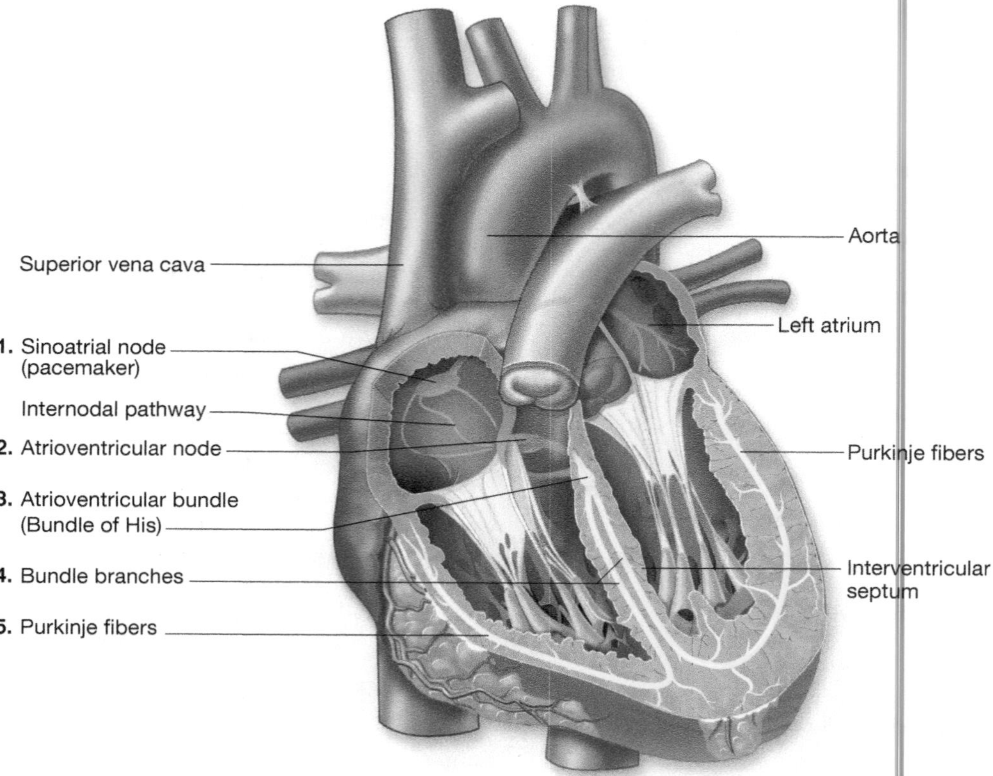

■ **Figure 5.6** The conduction system of the heart; traces the path of the electrical impulse that stimulates the heart chambers to contract in the correct sequence.

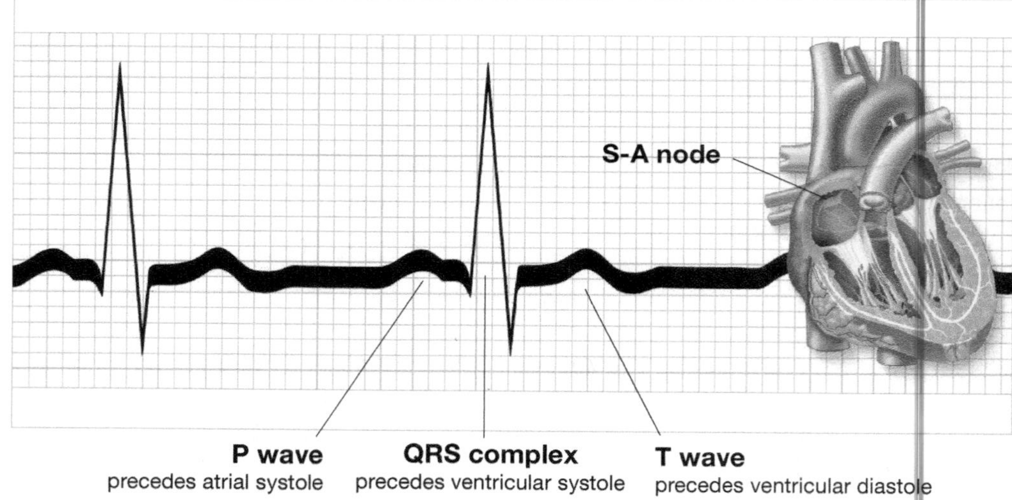

■ **Figure 5.7** An electrocardiogram (EKG) wave, a record of the electrical signal as it moves through the conduction system of the heart. This signal stimulates the chambers of the heart to contract and relax in the proper sequence.

MED TERM TIP

The electrocardiogram, referred to as an EKG or ECG, is a measurement of the electrical activity of the heart (see Figure 5.7 ■). This can give the physician information about the health of the heart, especially the myocardium.

Blood Vessels

lumen (LOO-men)

There are three types of blood vessels: arteries, capillaries, and veins (see Figure 5.8 ■). These are the pipes that circulate blood throughout the body. The **lumen** is the channel within these vessels through which blood flows.

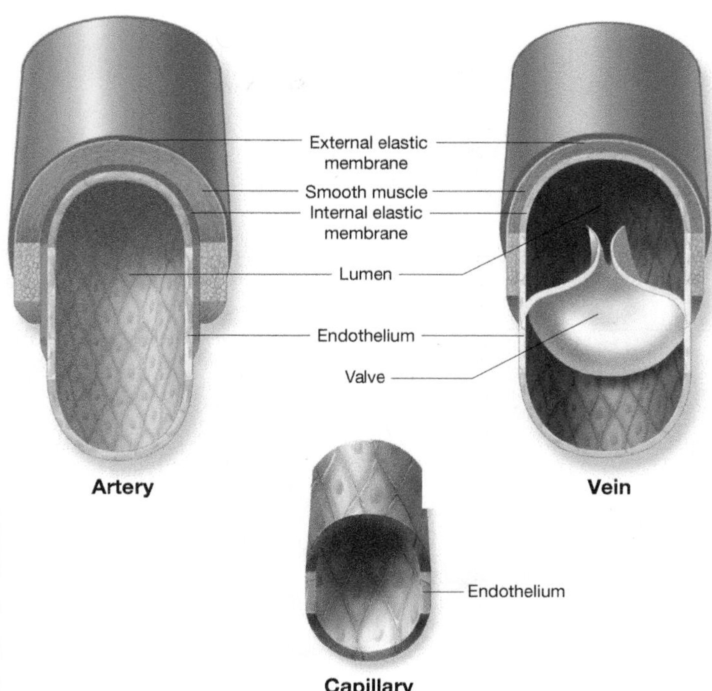

■ **Figure 5.8** Comparative structure of arteries, capillaries, and veins.

Arteries

arterioles (ar-TEE-ree-ohlz)

coronary arteries (KOR-ah-nair-ee / AR-te-reez)

The arteries are the large, thick-walled vessels that carry the blood away from the heart. The walls of arteries contain a thick layer of smooth muscle that can contract or relax to change the size of the arterial lumen. The pulmonary artery carries deoxygenated blood from the right ventricle to the lungs. The largest artery, the aorta, begins from the left ventricle of the heart and carries oxygenated blood to all the body systems. The **coronary arteries** then branch from the aorta and provide blood to the myocardium (see Figure 5.9 ■). As they travel through the body, the arteries branch into progressively smaller sized arteries. The smallest of the arteries, called **arterioles,** deliver blood to the capillaries. Figure 5.10 ■ illustrates the major systemic arteries.

MED TERM TIP

The term *coronary,* from the Latin word for crown, describes how the great vessels encircle the heart as they emerge from the top of the heart.

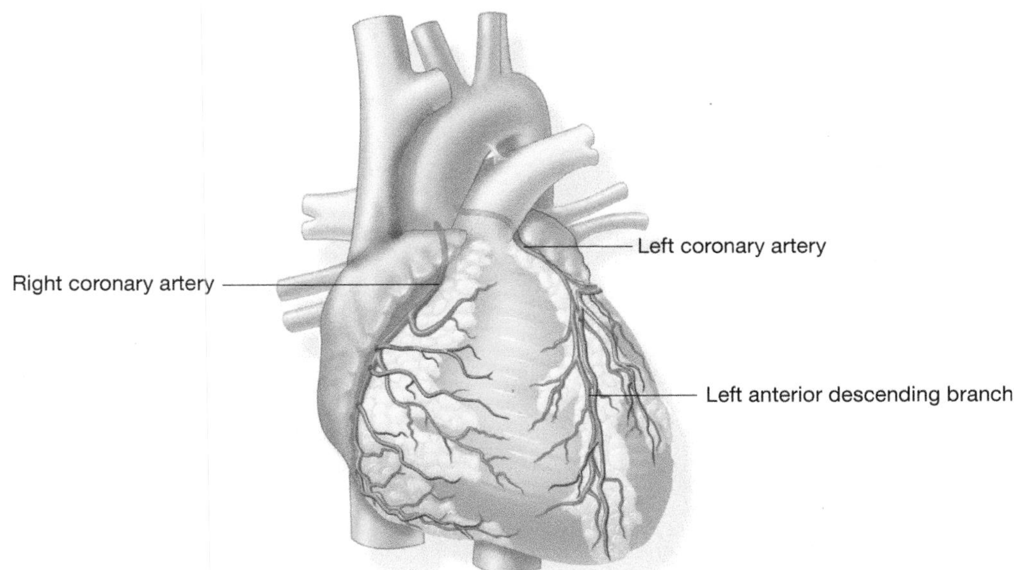

■ **Figure 5.9** The coronary arteries.

Right common carotid artery
Left common carotid artery
Right subclavian artery
Left subclavian artery
Ascending aorta
Aortic arch
Brachial artery
Renal artery
Abdominal aorta
Common iliac artery
Radial artery
Internal iliac artery
Ulnar artery
External iliac artery
Femoral artery
Popliteal artery
Peroneal artery
Anterior tibial artery
Posterior tibial artery

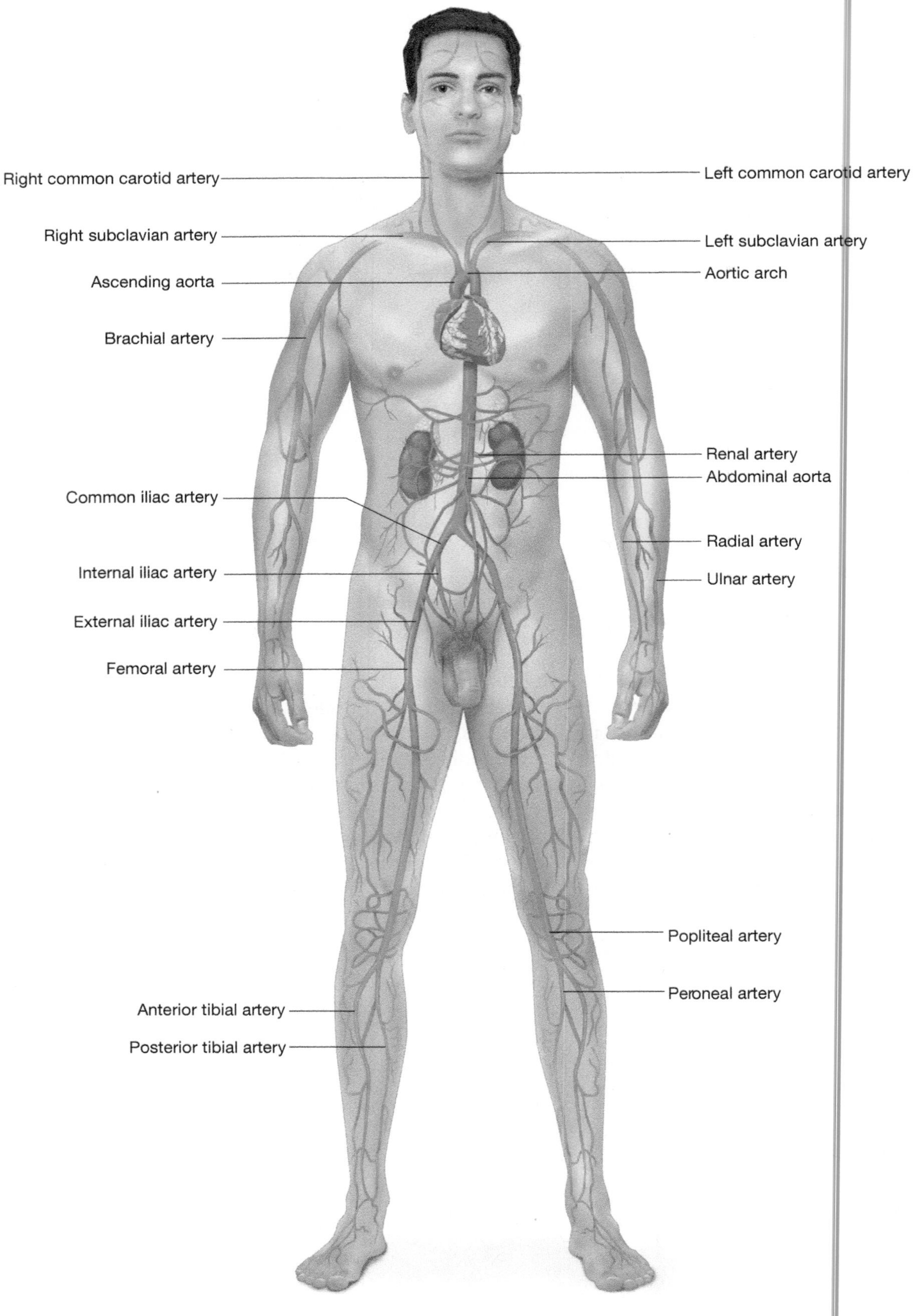

■ **Figure 5.10** The major arteries of the body.

Capillaries

capillary bed

Capillaries are a network of tiny blood vessels referred to as a **capillary bed.** Arterial blood flows into a capillary bed, and venous blood flows back out. Capillaries are very thin walled, allowing for the diffusion of the oxygen and nutrients from the blood into the body tissues (see Figure 5.8). Likewise, carbon dioxide and waste products are able to diffuse out of the body tissues and into the bloodstream to be carried away. Since the capillaries are so small in diameter, the blood will not flow as quickly through them as it does through the arteries and veins. This means that the blood has time for an exchange of nutrients, oxygen, and waste material to take place. As blood exits a capillary bed, it returns to the heart through a vein.

Veins

venules (VEN-yools)

The veins carry blood back to the heart (see Figure 5.8). Blood leaving capillaries first enters small **venules,** which then merge into larger veins. Veins have much thinner walls than arteries, causing them to collapse easily. The veins also have valves that allow the blood to move only toward the heart. These valves prevent blood from backflowing, ensuring that blood always flows toward the heart. The two large veins that enter the heart are the superior vena cava, which carries blood from the upper body, and the inferior vena cava, which carries blood from the lower body. Blood pressure in the veins is much lower than in the arteries. Muscular action against the veins and skeletal muscle contractions help in the movement of blood. Figure 5.11 ■ illustrates the major systemic veins.

Pulse and Blood Pressure

blood pressure (BP)
diastolic pressure (dye-ah-STOL-ik)
pulse
systolic pressure (sis-TOL-ik)

Blood pressure (BP) is a measurement of the force exerted by blood against the wall of a blood vessel. During ventricular systole, blood is under a lot of pressure from the ventricular contraction, giving the highest blood pressure reading—the **systolic pressure.** The **pulse** felt at the wrist or throat is the surge of blood caused by the heart contraction. This is why pulse rate is normally equal to heart rate. During ventricular diastole, blood is not being pushed by the heart at all and the blood pressure reading drops to its lowest point—the **diastolic pressure.** Therefore, to see the full range of what is occurring with blood pressure, both numbers are required. Blood pressure is also affected by several other characteristics of the blood and the blood vessels. These include the elasticity of the arteries, the diameter of the blood vessels, the viscosity of the blood, the volume of blood flowing through the vessels, and the amount of resistance to blood flow.

MED TERM TIP

The instrument used to measure blood pressure is called a *sphygmomanometer.* The combining form *sphygm/o* means "pulse" and the suffix *-manometer* means "instrument to measure pressure." A blood pressure reading is reported as two numbers, for example, 120/80. The 120 is the systolic pressure and the 80 is the diastolic pressure. There is no one "normal" blood pressure number. The normal blood pressure for an adult is a systolic pressure less than 120 and diastolic pressure less than 80.

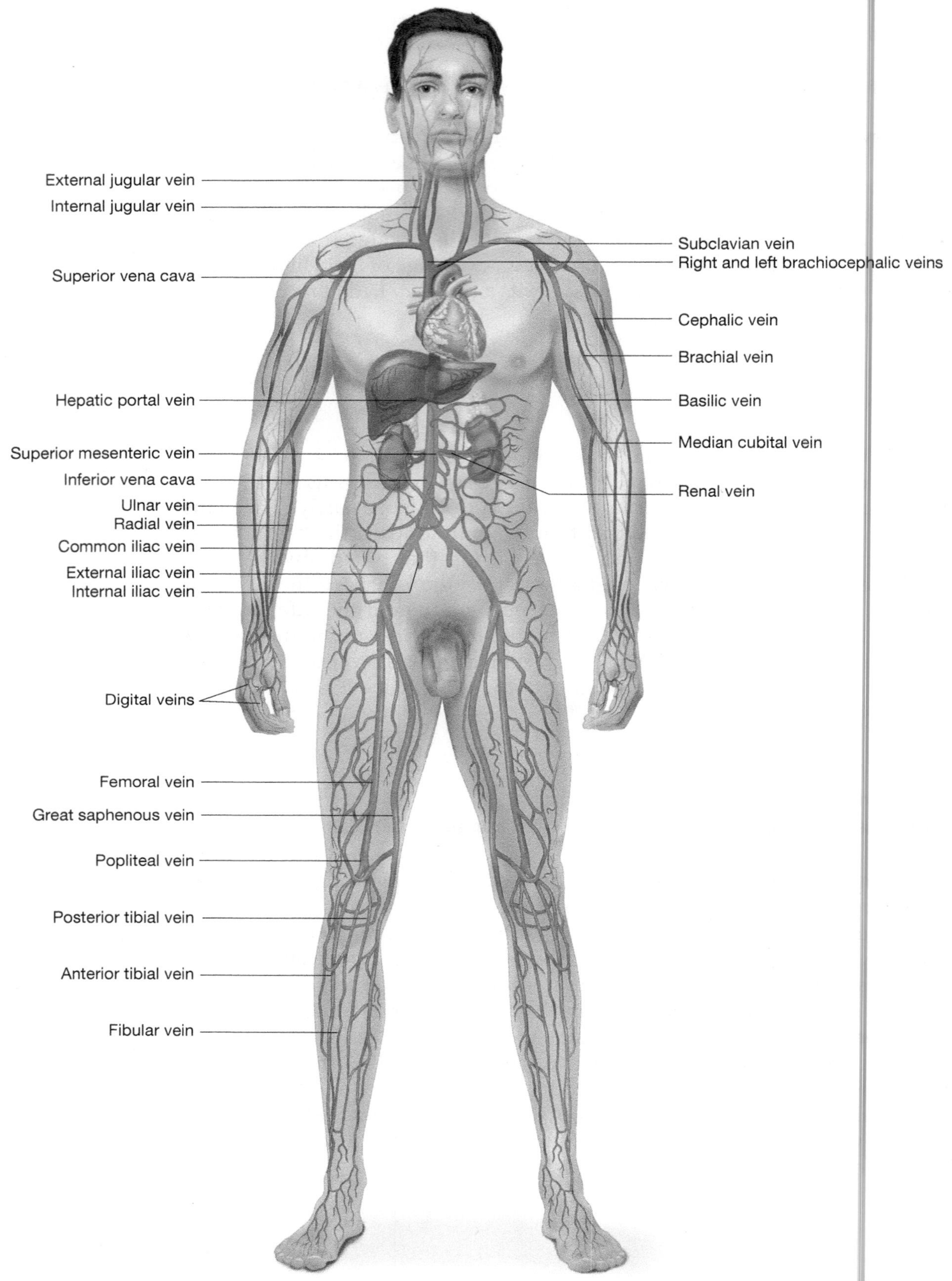
External jugular vein
Internal jugular vein
Superior vena cava
Hepatic portal vein
Superior mesenteric vein
Inferior vena cava
Ulnar vein
Radial vein
Common iliac vein
External iliac vein
Internal iliac vein
Digital veins
Femoral vein
Great saphenous vein
Popliteal vein
Posterior tibial vein
Anterior tibial vein
Fibular vein
Subclavian vein
Right and left brachiocephalic veins
Cephalic vein
Brachial vein
Basilic vein
Median cubital vein
Renal vein

Figure 5.11 The major veins of the body.

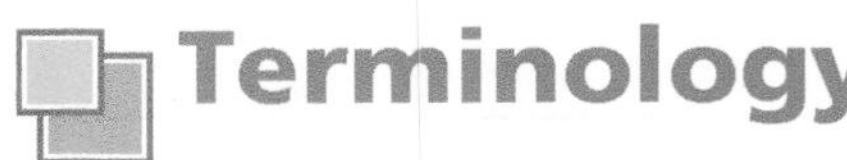

Terminology

Word Parts Used to Build Cardiovascular System Terms

The following lists contain the combining forms, suffixes, and prefixes used to build terms in the remaining sections of this chapter.

Combining Forms

aort/o	aorta
angi/o	vessel
arteri/o	artery
ather/o	fatty substance
atri/o	atrium
cardi/o	heart
coron/o	heart
corpor/o	body
cutane/o	skin
duct/o	to bring
electr/o	electricity

embol/o	plug
hem/o	blood
isch/o	to hold back
lip/o	fat
my/o	muscle
myocardi/o	heart muscle
orth/o	straight
pector/o	chest
phleb/o	vein
pulmon/o	lung
sept/o	a wall

son/o	sound
sphygm/o	pulse
steth/o	chest
thromb/o	clot
valv/o	valve
valvul/o	valve
varic/o	dilated vein
vas/o	vessel
vascul/o	blood vessel
ven/o	vein
ventricul/o	ventricle

Suffixes

-ac	pertaining to
-al	pertaining to
-ar	pertaining to
-ary	pertaining to
-eal	pertaining to
-ectomy	surgical removal
-gram	record
-graphy	process of recording
-ia	condition
-ic	pertaining to
-itis	inflammation

-logy	study of
-lytic	destruction
-manometer	instrument to measure pressure
-megaly	enlarged
-ole	small
-oma	growth
-ose	pertaining to
-ous	pertaining to
-pathy	disease
-plasty	surgical repair

-rrhexis	rupture
-sclerosis	hardening
-scope	instrument for viewing
-spasm	involuntary muscle contraction
-stenosis	narrowing
-tension	pressure
-tic	pertaining to
-tonic	pertaining to tone
-ule	small

Prefixes

a-	without
anti-	against
brady-	slow
de-	without
endo-	inner
extra-	outside of

hyper-	excessive
hypo-	insufficient
inter-	between
intra-	within
per-	through
peri-	around

poly-	many
tachy-	fast
tetra-	four
trans-	across
ultra-	beyond

Anatomical Terms

TERM	WORD PARTS	DEFINITION
aortic (ay-OR-tik)	aort/o = aorta -ic = pertaining to	Pertaining to the aorta
arterial (ar-TEE-ree-al)	arteri/o = artery -al = pertaining to	Pertaining to an artery
arteriole (ar-TEE-ree-ohl)	arteri/o = artery -ole = small	A small (narrow in diameter) artery
atrial (AY-tree-al)	atri/o = atrium -al = pertaining to	Pertaining to the atrium
cardiac (CAR-dee-ak)	cardi/o = heart -ac = pertaining to	Pertaining to the heart
coronary (KOR-ah-nair-ee)	coron/o = heart -ary = pertaining to	Pertaining to the heart
interatrial (in-ter-AY-tree-al)	inter- = between atri/o = atrium -al = pertaining to	Pertaining to between the atria
interventricular (in-ter-ven-TRIK-yoo-lar)	inter- = between ventricul/o = ventricle -ar = pertaining to	Pertaining to between the ventricles
myocardial (my-oh-CAR-dee-al)	myocardi/o = heart muscle -al = pertaining to	Pertaining to heart muscle
valvular (VAL-view-lar)	valvul/o = valve -ar = pertaining to	Pertaining to a valve
vascular (VAS-kwee-lar)	vascul/o = blood vessel -ar = pertaining to	Pertaining to a blood vessel
venous (VEE-nus)	ven/o = vein -ous = pertaining to	Pertaining to a vein
ventricular (ven-TRIK-yoo-lar)	ventricul/o = ventricle -ar = pertaining to	Pertaining to a ventricle
venule (VEN-yool)	ven/o = vein -ule = small	A small (narrow in diameter) vein

Pathology

TERM	WORD PARTS	DEFINITION
Medical Specialties		
cardiology (car-dee-ALL-oh-jee)	cardi/o = heart -logy = study of	The branch of medicine involving diagnosis and treatment of conditions and diseases of the cardiovascular system. Physician is a *cardiologist.*
cardiovascular technician	cardi/o = heart vascul/o = blood vessel -ar = pertaining to	Healthcare professional trained to perform a variety of diagnostic and therapeutic procedures including electrocardiography, echocardiography, and exercise stress tests.

Pathology (continued)

TERM	WORD PARTS	DEFINITION
Signs and Symptoms		
angiitis (an-jee-EYE-tis)	angi/o = vessel -itis = inflammation	Inflammation of a vessel.
angiospasm (AN-jee-oh-spazm)	angi/o = vessel -spasm = involuntary muscle contraction	An involuntary muscle contraction of the smooth muscle in the wall of a vessel; narrows the vessel.
angiostenosis (an-jee-oh-sten-OH-sis)	angi/o = vessel -stenosis = narrowing	The narrowing of a vessel.
bradycardia (brad-ee-CAR-dee-ah)	brady- = slow cardi/o = heart -ia = condition	The condition of having a slow heart rate; typically less than 60 beats/minute; highly trained aerobic persons may normally have a slow heart rate.
embolus (EM-boh-lus)	embol/o = plug	The obstruction of a blood vessel by a blood clot that has broken off from a thrombus somewhere else in the body and traveled to the point of obstruction. If it occurs in a coronary artery, it may result in a myocardial infarction.

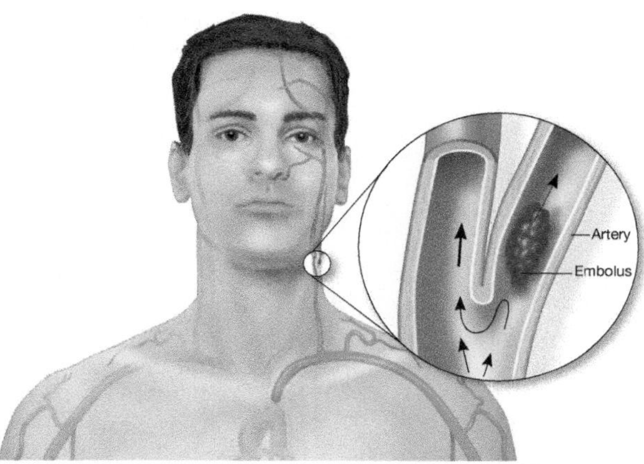

■ **Figure 5.12** Illustration of an embolus floating in an artery. The embolus will become lodged in a blood vessel that is smaller than it is, resulting in occlusion of that artery.

TERM	WORD PARTS	DEFINITION
infarct (IN-farkt)		An area of tissue within an organ or part that undergoes necrosis (death) following the loss of its blood supply.
ischemia (is-KEYH-mee-ah)	isch/o = to hold back hem/o = blood -ia = condition	The localized and temporary deficiency of blood supply due to an obstruction to the circulation.
murmur (MUR-mur)		A sound, in addition to the normal heart sounds, arising from blood flowing through the heart. This extra sound may or may not indicate a heart abnormality.
orthostatic hypotension (or-thoh-STAT-ik)	orth/o = straight hypo- = insufficient -tension = pressure	The sudden drop in blood pressure a person experiences when standing straight up suddenly.
palpitations (pal-pih-TAY-shunz)		Pounding, racing heartbeats.

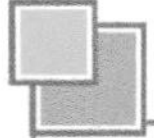

Pathology *(continued)*

TERM	WORD PARTS	DEFINITION
plaque (plak)		A yellow, fatty deposit of lipids in an artery that is the hallmark of atherosclerosis. Also called an *atheroma.*
regurgitation (re-ger-gih-TAY-shun)		To flow backwards. In the cardiovascular system this refers to the backflow of blood through a valve.
tachycardia (tak-ee-CAR-dee-ah)	tachy- = fast cardi/o = heart -ia = condition	The condition of having a fast heart rate; typically more than 100 beats/minute while at rest.
thrombus (THROM-bus)	thromb/o = clot	A blood clot forming within a blood vessel. May partially or completely occlude the blood vessel.

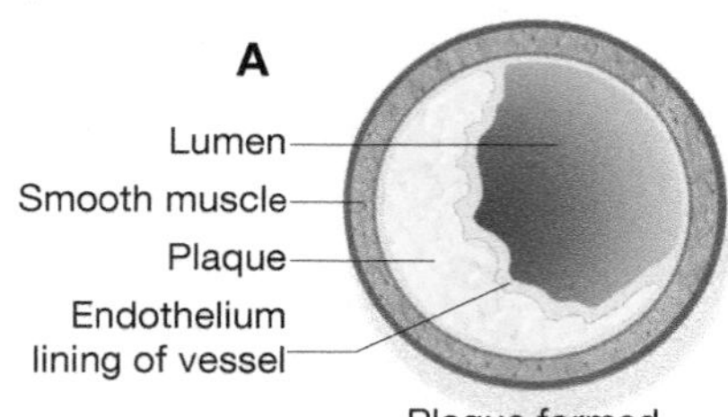

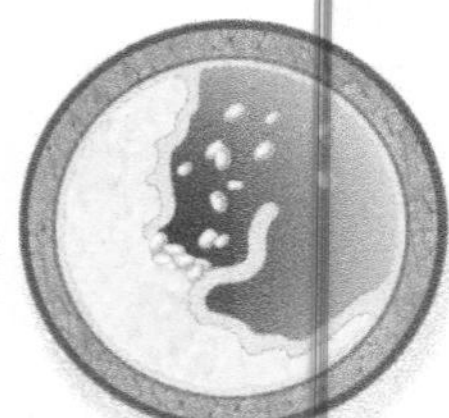

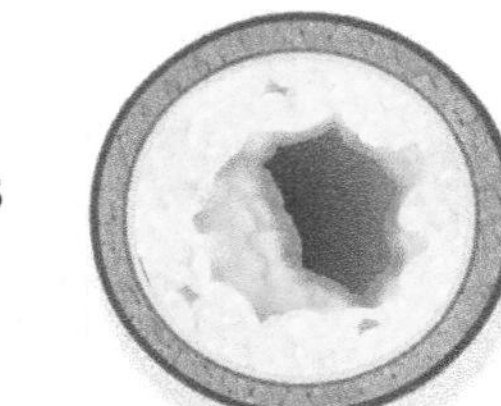

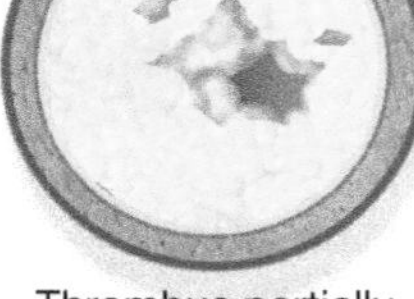

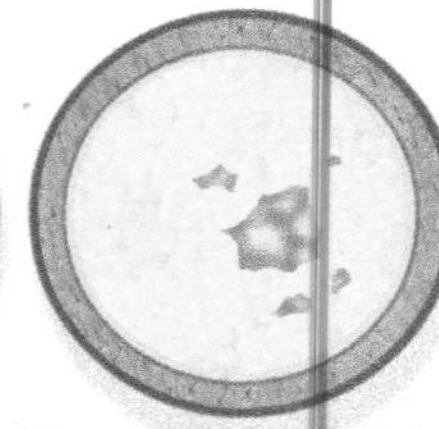

■ **Figure 5.13** Development of an atherosclerotic plaque that progressively narrows the lumen of an artery to the point that a thrombus fully occludes the lumen.

Heart		
angina pectoris (an-JYE-nah / PECK-tor-is)	pector/o = chest	Condition in which there is severe pain with a sensation of constriction around the heart. Caused by a deficiency of oxygen to the heart muscle.
arrhythmia (ah-RITH-mee-ah)	a- = without -ia = condition	Irregularity in the heartbeat or action. Comes in many different forms; some are not serious, while others are life-threatening.
bundle branch block (BBB)		Occurs when the electrical impulse is blocked from traveling down the bundle of His or bundle branches. Results in the ventricles beating at a different rate than the atria. Also called a *heart block.*
cardiac arrest	cardi/o = heart -ac = pertaining to	Complete stopping of heart activity.
cardiomegaly (car-dee-oh-MEG-ah-lee)	cardi/o = heart -megaly = enlarged	An enlarged heart.

Pathology *(continued)*

TERM	WORD PARTS	DEFINITION
cardiomyopathy (car-dee-oh-my-OP-ah-thee)	cardi/o = heart my/o = muscle -pathy = disease	General term for a disease of the myocardium. Can be caused by alcohol abuse, parasites, viral infection, and congestive heart failure. One of the most common reasons a patient may require a heart transplant.
congenital septal defect (CSD)	sept/o = a wall -al = pertaining to	A hole, present at birth, in the septum between two heart chambers; results in a mixture of oxygenated and deoxygenated blood. There can be an *atrial septal defect* (ASD) and a *ventricular septal defect* (VSD).
congestive heart failure (CHF) (kon-JESS-tiv)		Pathological condition of the heart in which there is a reduced outflow of blood from the left side of the heart because the left ventricle myocardium has become too weak to efficiently pump blood. Results in weakness, breathlessness, and edema.
coronary artery disease (CAD) (KOR-ah-nair-ee)	coron/o = heart -ary = pertaining to	Insufficient blood supply to the heart muscle due to an obstruction of one or more coronary arteries. May be caused by atherosclerosis and may cause angina pectoris and myocardial infarction.

MED TERM TIP

All types of cardiovascular disease have been the number one killer of Americans since the 19th century. This disease kills more people annually than the next six causes of death combined.

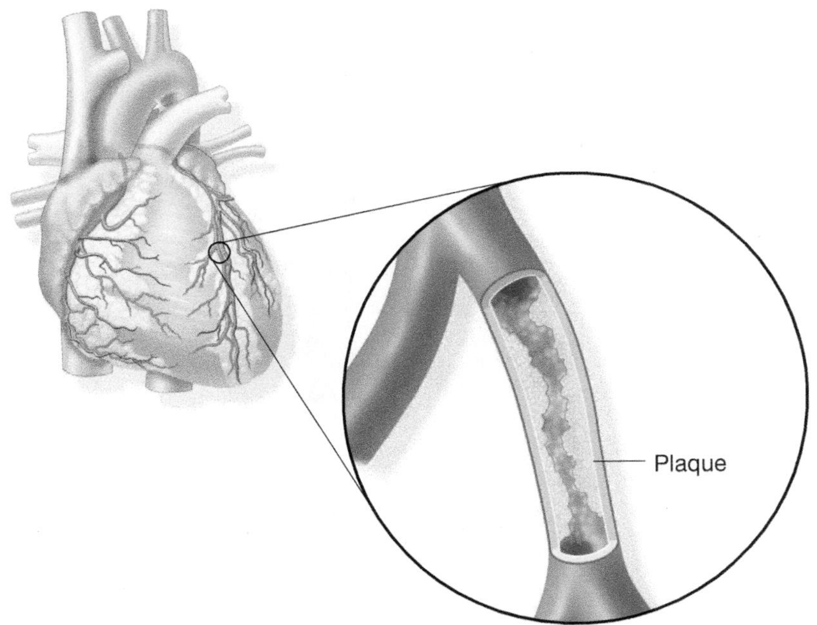

■ **Figure 5.14** Formation of an atherosclerotic plaque within a coronary artery; may lead to coronary artery disease, angina pectoris, and myocardial infarction.

TERM	WORD PARTS	DEFINITION
endocarditis (en-doh-car-DYE-tis)	endo- = inner cardi/o = heart -itis = inflammation	Inflammation of the lining membranes of the heart. May be due to bacteria or to an abnormal immunological response. In bacterial endocarditis, the mass of bacteria that forms is referred to as *vegetation.*

Pathology *(continued)*

TERM	WORD PARTS	DEFINITION
fibrillation (fih-brill-AY-shun)		An extremely serious arrhythmia characterized by an abnormal quivering or contraction of heart fibers. When this occurs in the ventricles, cardiac arrest and death can occur. Emergency equipment to defibrillate, or convert the heart to a normal beat, is necessary.
flutter		An arrhythmia in which the atria beat too rapidly, but in a regular pattern.
heart valve prolapse (PROH-laps)		Condition in which the cusps or flaps of the heart valve are too loose and fail to shut tightly, allowing blood to flow backward through the valve when the heart chamber contracts. Most commonly occurs in the mitral valve, but may affect any of the heart valves.
heart valve stenosis (steh-NOH-sis)	-stenosis = narrowing	The cusps or flaps of the heart valve are too stiff. Therefore, they are unable to open fully, making it difficult for blood to flow through, or shut tightly, allowing blood to flow backward. This condition may affect any of the heart valves.
myocardial infarction (MI) (my-oh-CAR-dee-al / in-FARC-shun)	myocardi/o = heart muscle -al = pertaining to	Condition caused by the partial or complete occlusion or closing of one or more of the coronary arteries. Symptoms include a squeezing pain or heavy pressure in the middle of the chest (angina pectoris). A delay in treatment could result in death. Also referred to as a *heart attack*.

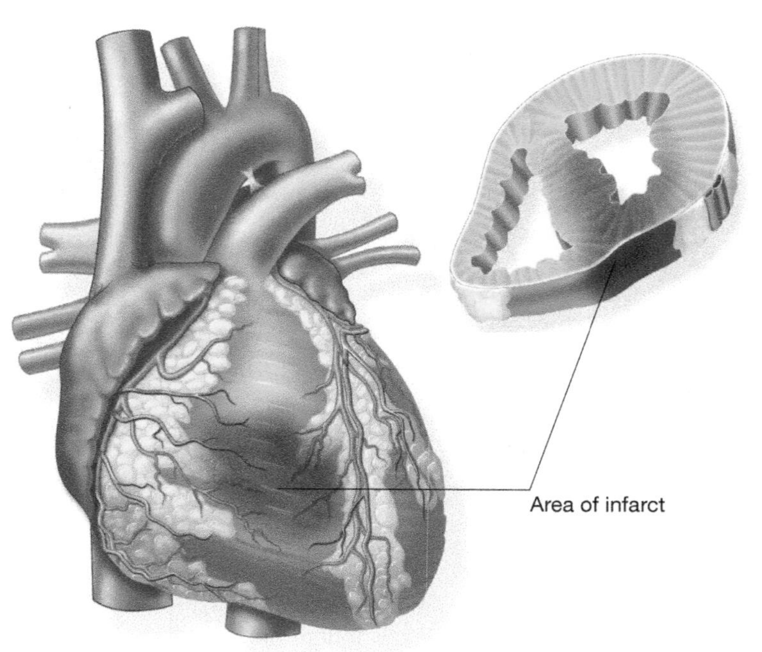

Figure 5.15 External and cross-sectional view of an infarct caused by a myocardial infarction.

Pathology *(continued)*

TERM	WORD PARTS	DEFINITION
myocarditis (my-oh-car-DYE-tis)	myocardi/o = heart muscle -itis = inflammation	Inflammation of the muscle layer of the heart wall.
pericarditis (pair-ih-car-DYE-tis)	peri- = around cardi/o = heart -itis = inflammation	Inflammation of the pericardial sac around the heart.
tetralogy of Fallot (teh-TRALL-oh-jee / fal-LOH)	tetra- = four -logy = study of	Combination of four congenital anomalies: pulmonary stenosis, an interventricular septal defect, improper placement of the aorta, and hypertrophy of the right ventricle. Needs immediate surgery to correct.
valvulitis (val-view-LYE-tis)	valvul/o = valve -itis = inflammation	The inflammation of a heart valve.
Blood Vessels		
aneurysm (AN-yoo-rizm)		Weakness in the wall of an artery resulting in localized widening of the artery. Although an aneurysm may develop in any artery, common sites include the aorta in the abdomen and the cerebral arteries in the brain.

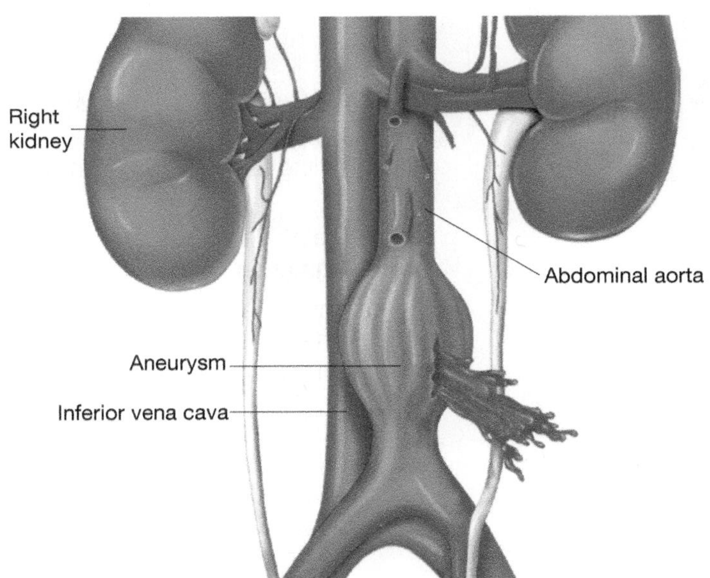

■ **Figure 5.16** Illustration of a large aneurysm in the abdominal aorta that has ruptured.

TERM	WORD PARTS	DEFINITION
arteriorrhexis (ar-tee-ree-oh-REK-sis)	arteri/o = artery -rrhexis = rupture	A ruptured artery; may occur if an aneurysm ruptures an arterial wall.
arteriosclerosis (ar-tee-ree-oh-skleh-ROH-sis)	arteri/o = artery -sclerosis = hardening	Thickening, hardening, and loss of elasticity of the walls of the arteries. Most often due to atherosclerosis.
atheroma (ath-er-OH-mah)	ather/o = fatty substance -oma = growth	A deposit of fatty substance in the wall of an artery that bulges into and narrows the lumen of the artery; a characteristic of atherosclerosis. Also called a *plaque.*

Pathology *(continued)*

TERM	WORD PARTS	DEFINITION
atherosclerosis (ath-er-oh-skleh-ROH-sis)	ather/o = fatty substance -sclerosis = hardening	The most common form of arteriosclerosis. Caused by the formation of yellowish plaques of cholesterol on the inner walls of arteries (see again Figures 5.13 & 5.14).
coarctation of the aorta (CoA) (koh-ark-TAY-shun)		Severe congenital narrowing of the aorta.
hemorrhoid (HIM-oh-royd)	hem/o = blood	Varicose veins in the anal region.
hypertension (HTN) (high-per-TEN-shun)	hyper- = excessive -tension = pressure	Blood pressure above the normal range. *Essential* or *primary hypertension* occurs directly from cardiovascular disease. *Secondary hypertension* refers to high blood pressure resulting from another disease such as kidney disease.
hypotension (high-poh-TEN-shun)	hypo- = insufficient -tension = pressure	Decrease in blood pressure. Can occur in shock, infection, cancer, anemia, or as death approaches.
patent ductus arteriosus (PDA) (PAY-tent / DUCK-tus / ar-tee-ree-OH-sis)	duct/o = to bring arteri/o = artery	Congenital heart anomaly in which the fetal connection between the pulmonary artery and the aorta fails to close at birth. This condition may be treated with medication and resolve with time. However, in some cases surgery is required.
peripheral vascular disease (PVD)	-al = pertaining to vascul/o = blood vessel -ar = pertaining to	Any abnormal condition affecting blood vessels outside the heart. Symptoms may include pain, pallor, numbness, and loss of circulation and pulses.
phlebitis (fleh-BYE-tis)	phleb/o = vein -itis = inflammation	The inflammation of a vein.
polyarteritis (pol-ee-ar-ter-EYE-tis)	poly- = many arteri/o = artery -itis = inflammation	Inflammation of several arteries.
Raynaud's phenomenon (ray-NOZ)		Periodic ischemic attacks affecting the extremities of the body, especially the fingers, toes, ears, and nose. The affected extremities become cyanotic and very painful. These attacks are brought on by arterial constriction due to extreme cold or emotional stress.
thrombophlebitis (throm-boh-fleh-BYE-tis)	thromb/o = clot phleb/o = vein -itis = inflammation	Inflammation of a vein resulting in the formation of blood clots within the vein.
varicose veins (VAIR-ih-kohs)	varic/o = dilated vein -ose = pertaining to	Swollen and distended veins, usually in the legs.

Diagnostic Procedures

TERM	WORD PARTS	DEFINITION
Medical Procedures		
auscultation (oss-kul-TAY-shun)		Process of listening to the sounds within the body by using a stethoscope.
sphygmomanometer (sfig-moh-mah-NOM-eh-ter)	sphygm/o = pulse -manometer = instrument to measure pressure	Instrument for measuring blood pressure. Also referred to as a *blood pressure cuff.*
■ Figure 5.17 Using a sphygmomanometer to measure blood pressure.	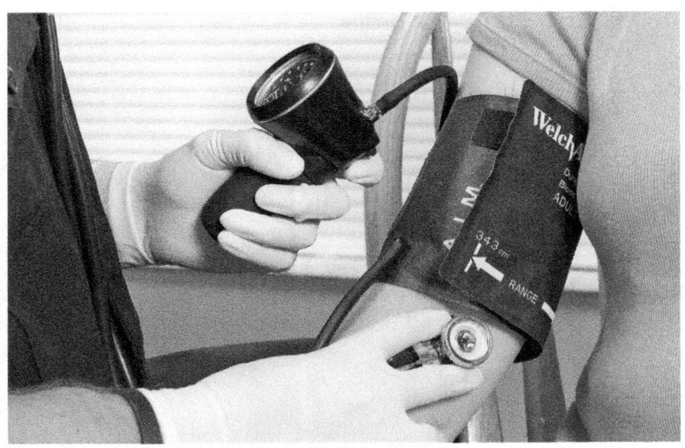	
stethoscope (STETH-oh-scope)	steth/o = chest -scope = instrument for viewing	Instrument for listening to body sounds (auscultation), such as the chest, heart, or intestines.
Clinical Laboratory Tests		
cardiac enzymes (CAR-dee-ak / EN-zyms)	cardi/o = heart -ac = pertaining to	Blood test to determine the level of enzymes specific to heart muscles in the blood. An increase in the enzymes may indicate heart muscle damage such as a myocardial infarction. These enzymes include creatine phosphokinase (CPK), lactate dehydrogenase (LDH), and glutamic oxaloacetic transaminase (GOT).
serum lipoprotein level (SEE-rum / lip-oh-PROH-teen)	lip/o = fat	Blood test to measure the amount of cholesterol and triglycerides in the blood. An indicator of atherosclerosis risk.
Diagnostic Imaging		
angiogram (AN-jee-oh-gram)	angi/o = vessel -gram = record	X-ray record of a vessel taken during angiography.
angiography (an-jee-OG-rah-fee)	angi/o = vessel -graphy = process of recording	X-rays taken after the injection of an opaque material into a blood vessel. Can be performed on the aorta as an aortic angiography, on the heart as angiocardiography, and on the brain as a cerebral angiography.
cardiac scan	cardi/o = heart -ac = pertaining to	Patient is given radioactive thallium intravenously and then scanning equipment is used to visualize the heart. It is especially useful in determining myocardial damage.

Diagnostic Procedures *(continued)*

TERM	WORD PARTS	DEFINITION
Doppler ultrasonography (DOP-ler / ul-trah-son-OG-rah-fee)	ultra- = beyond son/o = sound -graphy = process of recording	Measurement of sound-wave echoes as they bounce off tissues and organs to produce an image. In this system, used to measure velocity of blood moving through blood vessels to look for blood clots or deep vein thromboses.
echocardiography (ek-oh-car-dee-OG-rah-fee)	cardi/o = artery -graphy = process of recording	Noninvasive diagnostic method using ultrasound to visualize internal cardiac structures. Cardiac valve activity can be evaluated using this method.
Cardiac Function Tests		
catheter (KATH-eh-ter)		Flexible tube inserted into the body for the purpose of moving fluids into or out of the body. In the cardiovascular system a catheter is used to place dye into blood vessels so they may be visualized on x-rays.
cardiac catheterization (CAR-dee-ak / cath-eh-ter-ih-ZAY-shun)	cardi/o = heart -ac = pertaining to	Passage of a thin tube catheter through a blood vessel leading to the heart. Done to detect abnormalities, to collect cardiac blood samples, and to determine the blood pressure within the heart.
electrocardiogram (ee-lek-tro-CAR-dee-oh-gram)	electr/o = electricity cardi/o = heart -gram = record	Hard copy record produced by electrocardiography.
electrocardiography (ECG, EKG) (ee-lek-troh-car-dee-OG-rah-fee)	electr/o = electricity cardi/o = heart -graphy = process of recording	Process of recording the electrical activity of the heart. Useful in the diagnosis of abnormal cardiac rhythm and heart muscle (myocardium) damage.
Holter monitor		Portable ECG monitor worn by a patient for a period of a few hours to a few days to assess the heart and pulse activity as the person goes through the activities of daily living. Used to assess a patient who experiences chest pain and unusual heart activity during exercise and normal activities.
stress testing	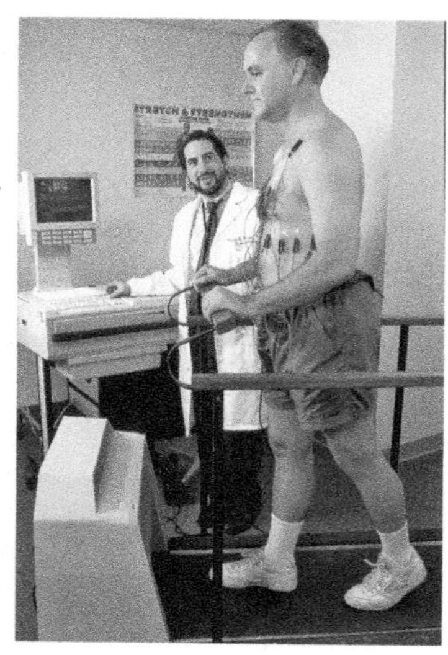	Method for evaluating cardiovascular fitness. The patient is placed on a treadmill or a bicycle and then subjected to steadily increasing levels of work. An EKG and oxygen levels are taken while the patient exercises. The test is stopped if abnormalities occur on the EKG. Also called an *exercise test* or a *treadmill test.*

Figure 5.18 Man undergoing a stress test on a treadmill while physician monitors his condition. *(Jonathan Nourok/PhotoEdit Inc.)*

Therapeutic Procedures

TERM	WORD PARTS	DEFINITION
Medical Procedures		
cardiopulmonary resuscitation (CPR) (car-dee-oh-PULL-mon-air-ee / ree-suss-ih-TAY-shun)	cardi/o = heart pulmon/o = lung -ary = pertaining to	Procedure to restore cardiac output and oxygenated air to the lungs for a person in cardiac arrest. A combination of chest compressions (to push blood out of the heart) and artificial respiration (to blow air into the lungs) performed by one or two CPR-trained rescuers.
defibrillation (dee-fib-rih-LAY-shun)	de- = without	Procedure that converts serious irregular heartbeats, such as fibrillation, by giving electric shocks to the heart using an instrument called a defibrillator. Also called *cardioversion.* Automated external defibrillators (AED) are portable devices that automatically detect life-threatening arrhythmias and deliver the appropriate electrical shock. They are designed to be used by nonmedical personnel and are found in public places such as shopping malls and schools. **Figure 5.19** An emergency medical technician positions defibrillator paddles on the chest of a supine male patient.
extracorporeal circulation (ECC) (EX-tra-core-poor-EE-al)	extra- = outside of corpor/o = body -eal = pertaining to	During open-heart surgery, the routing of blood to a heart-lung machine so it can be oxygenated and pumped to the rest of the body.
implantable cardioverter-defibrillator (ICD) (CAR-dee-oh-ver-ter / de-FIB-rih-lay-tor)	cardi/o = heart de- = without	Device implanted in the heart that delivers an electrical shock to restore a normal heart rhythm. Particularly useful for persons who experience ventricular fibrillation.
pacemaker implantation 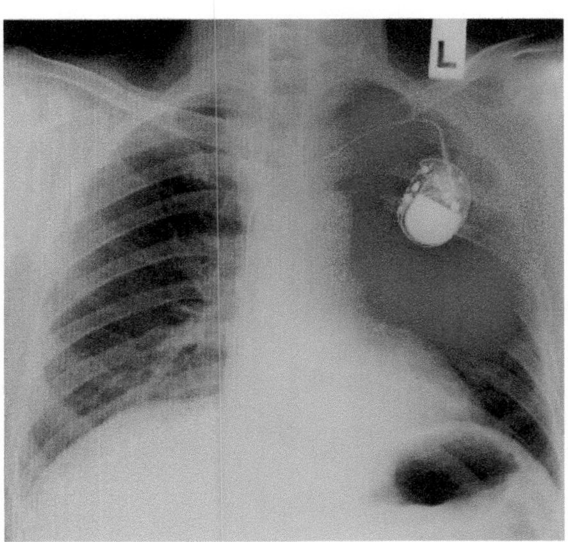		Electrical device that substitutes for the natural pacemaker of the heart. It controls the beating of the heart by a series of rhythmic electrical impulses. An external pacemaker has the electrodes on the outside of the body. An internal pacemaker has the electrodes surgically implanted within the chest wall. **Figure 5.20** Color enhanced X-ray showing a pacemaker implanted in the left side of the chest and the electrode wires running to the heart muscle.

Therapeutic Procedures *(continued)*

TERM	WORD PARTS	DEFINITION
thrombolytic therapy (throm-boh-LIT-ik / THAIR-ah-pee)	thromb/o = clot -lytic = destruction	Process in which drugs, such as streptokinase (SK) or tissue-type plasminogen activator (tPA), are injected into a blood vessel to dissolve clots and restore blood flow.
Surgical Procedures		
aneurysmectomy (an-yoo-riz-MEK-toh-mee)	-ectomy = surgical removal	Surgical removal of the sac of an aneurysm.
arterial anastomosis (ar-TEE-ree-all / ah-nas-toe-MOE-sis)	arteri/o = artery -al = pertaining to	Surgical joining together of two arteries. Performed if an artery is severed or if a damaged section of an artery is removed.
atherectomy (ath-er-EK-toh-mee)	ather/o = fatty substance -ectomy = surgical removal	Surgical procedure to remove a deposit of fatty substance, an atheroma, from an artery.
coronary artery bypass graft (CABG) (KOR-ah-nair-ee)	coron/o = heart -ary = pertaining to	Open-heart surgery in which a blood vessel from another location in the body (often a leg vein) is grafted to route blood around a blocked coronary artery.
embolectomy (em-boh-LEK-toh-mee)	embol/o = plug -ectomy = surgical removal	Removal of an embolus or clot from a blood vessel.
endarterectomy (end-ar-teh-REK-toh-mee)	endo- = inner arteri/o = artery -ectomy = surgical removal	Removal of the diseased or damaged inner lining of an artery. Usually performed to remove atherosclerotic plaques.
heart transplantation		Replacement of a diseased or malfunctioning heart with a donor's heart.
intracoronary artery stent (in-trah-KOR-ah-nair-ee / AR-ter-ee)	intra- = within coron/o = heart -ary = pertaining to	Placement of a stent within a coronary artery to treat coronary ischemia due to atherosclerosis.

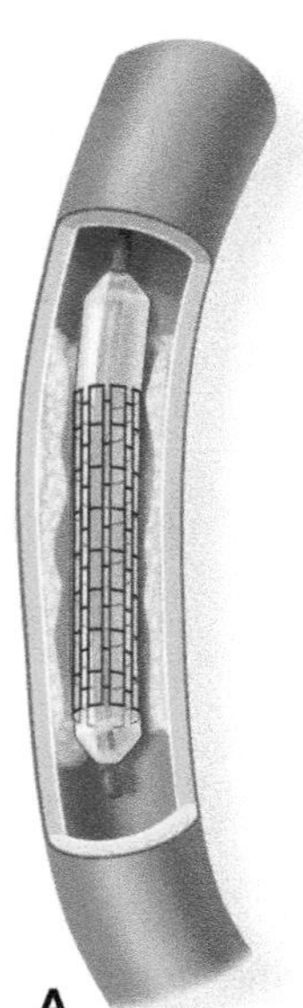

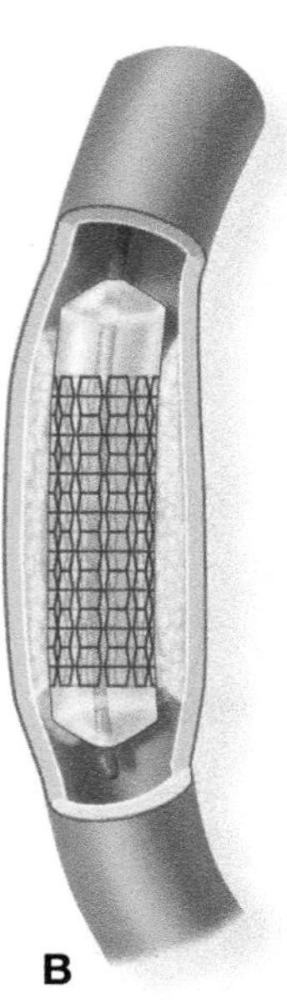

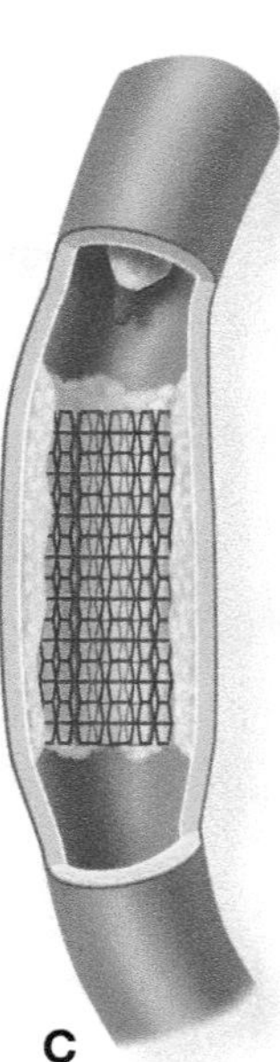

Figure 5.21 The process of placing a stent in a blood vessel. (A) A catheter is used to place a collapsed stent next to an atherosclerotic plaque; (B) stent is expanded; (C) catheter is removed, leaving the expanded stent behind.

Therapeutic Procedures *(continued)*

TERM	WORD PARTS	DEFINITION
ligation and stripping (lye-GAY-shun)		Surgical treatment for varicose veins. The damaged vein is tied off (ligation) and removed (stripping).
percutaneous transluminal coronary angioplasty (PTCA) (per-kyoo-TAY-nee-us / trans-LOO-mih-nal / KOR-ah-nair-ee / AN-jee-oh-plas-tee)	per- = through cutane/o = skin -ous = pertaining to trans- = across -al = pertaining to angi/o = vessel -plasty = surgical repair	Method for treating localized coronary artery narrowing. A balloon catheter is inserted through the skin into the coronary artery and inflated to dilate the narrow blood vessel.

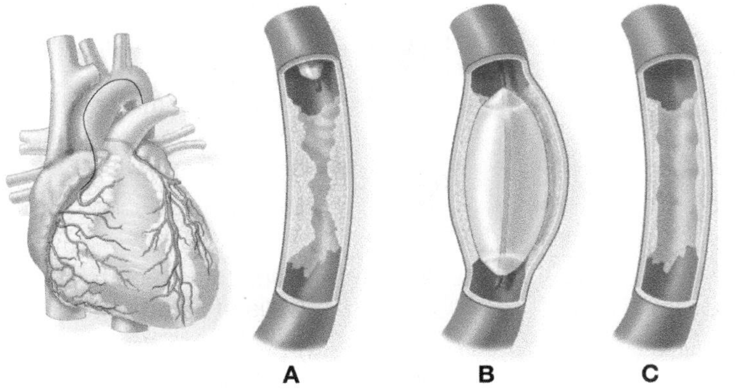

■ **Figure 5.22** Balloon angioplasty: (A) deflated balloon catheter is approaching an atherosclerotic plaque; (B) plaque is compressed by inflated balloon; (C) plaque remains compressed after balloon catheter is removed.

TERM	WORD PARTS	DEFINITION
stent		Stainless steel tube placed within a blood vessel or a duct to widen the lumen (see again Figure 5.21).
valve replacement		Removal of a diseased heart valve and replacement with an artificial valve.
valvoplasty (VAL-voh-plas-tee)	valv/o = valve -plasty = surgical repair	Surgical procedure to repair a heart valve.

Pharmacology

CLASSIFICATION	WORD PARTS	ACTION	EXAMPLES
ACE inhibitor drugs		Produce vasodilation and decrease blood pressure.	benazepril, Lotensin; catopril, Capoten
antiarrhythmic (an-tye-a-RHYTH-mik)	anti- = against a- = without -ic = pertaining to	Reduces or prevents cardiac arrhythmias.	flecainide, Tambocor; ibutilide, Corvert
anticoagulant (an-tye-koh-AG-you-lant)	anti- = against	Prevents blood clot formation.	heparin; warfarin, Coumadin
antilipidemic (an-tye-lip-ih-DEM-ik)	anti- = against lip/o = fat -ic = pertaining to	Reduces amount of cholesterol and lipids in the bloodstream; treats hyperlipidemia.	atorvastatin, Lipitor; simvastatin, Zocor
antiplatelet agents	anti- = against	Inhibits the ability of platelets to clump together as part of a blood clot.	clopidogrel, Plavix; aspirin; ticlopidine, Ticlid

Pharmacology (continued)

CLASSIFICATION	WORD PARTS	ACTION	EXAMPLES
beta-blocker drugs		Treats hypertension and angina pectoris by lowering the heart rate.	metoprolol, Lopressor; propranolol, Inderal
calcium channel blocker drugs		Treats hypertension, angina pectoris, and congestive heart failure by causing the heart to beat less forcefully and less often.	diltiazem, Cardizem; nifedipine, Procardia
cardiotonic (card-ee-oh-TAHN-ik)	cardi/o = heart -tonic = pertaining to tone	Increases the force of cardiac muscle contraction; treats congestive heart failure.	digoxin, Lanoxin
diuretic (dye-you-RET-ik)	-tic = pertaining to	Increases urine production by the kidneys, which works to reduce plasma and therefore blood volume, resulting in lower blood pressure.	furosemide, Lasix
thrombolytic (throm-boh-LIT-ik)	thromb/o = clot -lytic = destruction	Dissolves existing blood clots.	tissue plasminogen activator (tPA); alteplase, Activase
vasoconstrictor (vaz-oh-kon-STRICK-tor)	vas/o = vessel	Contracts smooth muscle in walls of blood vessels; raises blood pressure.	metaraminol, Aramine
vasodilator (vaz-oh-DYE-late-or)	vas/o = vessel	Relaxes the smooth muscle in the walls of arteries, thereby increasing diameter of the blood vessel. Used for two main purposes: increasing circulation to an ischemic area; reducing blood pressure.	nitroglycerine, Nitro-Dur; isoxsuprine, Vasodilan

Abbreviations

AED	automated external defibrillator
AF	atrial fibrillation
AMI	acute myocardial infarction
AS	arteriosclerosis
ASD	atrial septal defect
ASHD	arteriosclerotic heart disease
AV, A-V	atrioventricular
BBB	bundle branch block (L for left; R for right)
BP	blood pressure
bpm	beats per minute
CABG	coronary artery bypass graft
CAD	coronary artery disease
cath	catheterization
CC	cardiac catheterization, chief complaint
CCU	coronary care unit
CHF	congestive heart failure
CoA	coarctation of the aorta
CP	chest pain
CPR	cardiopulmonary resuscitation
CSD	congenital septal defect
CV	cardiovascular
DVT	deep vein thrombosis
ECC	extracorporeal circulation
ECG, EKG	electrocardiogram
ECHO	echocardiogram
GOT	glutamic oxaloacetic transaminase
HTN	hypertension
ICD	implantable cardioverter-defibrillator
ICU	intensive care unit
IV	intravenous

Abbreviations *(continued)*

LVAD	left ventricular assist device
LVH	left ventricular hypertrophy
MI	myocardial infarction, mitral insufficiency
mm Hg	millimeters of mercury
MR	mitral regurgitation
MS	mitral stenosis
MVP	mitral valve prolapse
P	pulse
PAC	premature atrial contraction
PDA	patent ductus arteriosus
PTCA	percutaneous transluminal coronary angioplasty
PVC	premature ventricular contraction
S1	first heart sound
S2	second heart sound
SA, S-A	sinoatrial
SK	streptokinase
tPA	tissue-type plasminogen activator
V fib	ventricular fibrillation
VSD	ventricular septal defect
VT	ventricular tachycardia

MED TERM TIP

Word Watch: Be careful using the abbreviation *MS,* which can mean either "mitral stenosis" or "multiple sclerosis."

Chapter Review

Real-World Applications

Medical Record Analysis

This Discharge Summary contains 12 medical terms. Underline each term and write it in the list below the report. Then define each term.

PGH **PEARSON GENERAL HOSPITAL**

5500 University Avenue, Metropolis, TX
Phone: (211) 594-4000 • Fax: (211) 594-4001

Medical Consultation Osteology
Date 6/1/2013
Patient Jorge Johnson
Patient complaint: Sever pain in the right ankle with any movement of lower limb.

Discharge Summary

Admitting Diagnosis:	Difficulty breathing, hypertension, tachycardia
Final Diagnosis:	CHF secondary to mitral valve prolapse
History of Present Illness:	Patient was brought to the Emergency Room by her family because of difficulty breathing and palpitations. Patient reports that she has experienced these symptoms for the past 6 months, but this episode is more severe than any previous. Upon admission in the ER, heart rate was 120 beats per minute and blood pressure was 180/110. The results of an EKG and cardiac enzyme blood tests were normal. She was admitted for a complete workup for tachycardia and hypertension.
Summary of Hospital Course:	Patient underwent a full battery of diagnostic tests. A prolapsed mitral valve was observed by echocardiography. A stress test had to be stopped early due to onset of severe difficulty in breathing. Angiocardiography failed to demonstrate significant CAD. Blood pressure and tachycardia were controlled with medications. At discharge, HR was 88 beats per minute and blood pressure was 165/98.
Discharge Plans:	There was no evidence of a myocardial infarction or significant CAD. Patient was placed on a low-salt and low-cholesterol diet. She received instructions on beginning a carefully graded exercise program. She is to continue her medications. If symptoms are not controlled by these measures, a mitral valve replacement will be considered.

	Term	Definition
1		
2		
3		
4		
5		
6		
7		
8		
9		
10		
11		
12		

Chart Note Transcription

The chart note below contains 11 phrases that can be reworded with a medical term that you learned in this chapter. Each phrase is identified with an underline. Determine the medical term and write your answers in the space provided.

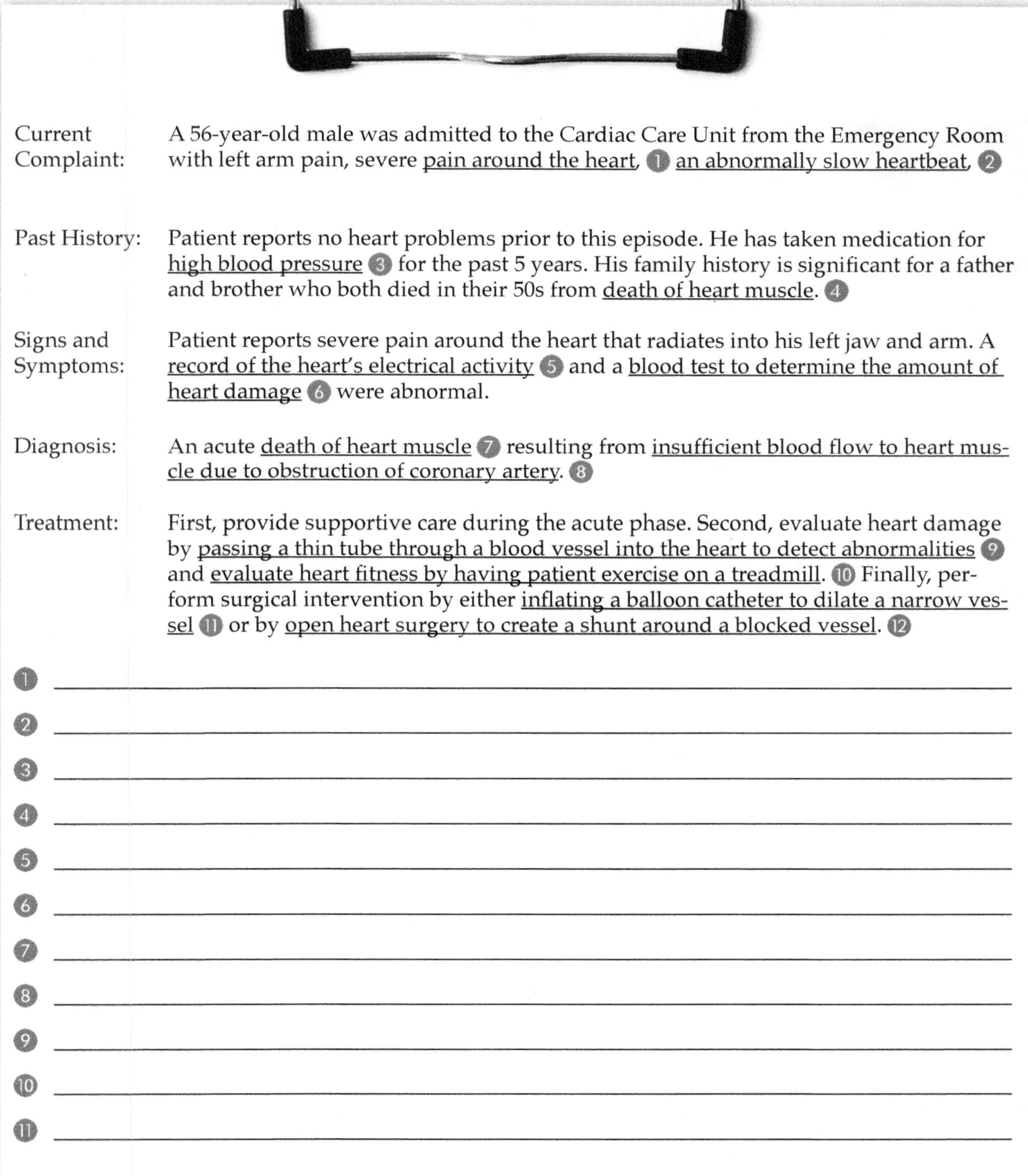

Current Complaint:	A 56-year-old male was admitted to the Cardiac Care Unit from the Emergency Room with left arm pain, severe pain around the heart, (1) an abnormally slow heartbeat, (2)
Past History:	Patient reports no heart problems prior to this episode. He has taken medication for high blood pressure (3) for the past 5 years. His family history is significant for a father and brother who both died in their 50s from death of heart muscle. (4)
Signs and Symptoms:	Patient reports severe pain around the heart that radiates into his left jaw and arm. A record of the heart's electrical activity (5) and a blood test to determine the amount of heart damage (6) were abnormal.
Diagnosis:	An acute death of heart muscle (7) resulting from insufficient blood flow to heart muscle due to obstruction of coronary artery. (8)
Treatment:	First, provide supportive care during the acute phase. Second, evaluate heart damage by passing a thin tube through a blood vessel into the heart to detect abnormalities (9) and evaluate heart fitness by having patient exercise on a treadmill. (10) Finally, perform surgical intervention by either inflating a balloon catheter to dilate a narrow vessel (11) or by open heart surgery to create a shunt around a blocked vessel. (12)

(1) ______________________

(2) ______________________

(3) ______________________

(4) ______________________

(5) ______________________

(6) ______________________

(7) ______________________

(8) ______________________

(9) ______________________

(10) ______________________

(11) ______________________

Case Study

Below is a case study presentation of a patient with a condition covered by this chapter. Read the case study and answer the questions below. Some questions will ask for information not included within this chapter. Use your text, a medical dictionary, journals, technical materials, multimedia resources, electronic media, or any other reference material you choose to answer these questions.

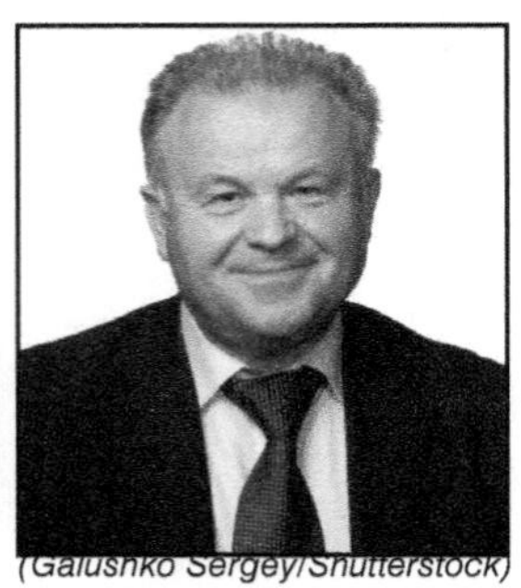
(Galushko Sergey/Shutterstock)

Mr. Thomas is a 62-year-old man who has been diagnosed with an acute myocardial infarction with the following symptoms and history. His chief complaint is a persistent, crushing chest pain that radiates to his left arm, jaw, neck, and shoulder blade. He describes the pain, which he has had for the past 12 hours, as a "squeezing" sensation around his heart. He has also suffered nausea, dyspnea, and diaphoresis. He has a low-grade temperature and his blood pressure is within a normal range at 130/82. He states that he smokes two packs of cigarettes a day, is overweight by 50 pounds, and has a family history of hypertension and coronary artery disease. He leads a relatively sedentary lifestyle.

1. What is the common name for Mr. Thomas's acute condition? Look this condition up in a reference source and include a short description of it.

____

____

2. What do you think the phrase "chief complaint" means?

____

____

3. What is the medical term for this patient's chief complaint? Define this term.

____

____

4. List and define each of the patient's additional symptoms in your own words. (These terms appear in other chapters of the book or use a medical dictionary.)

____

____

5. Using your text as a resource, name and describe three diagnostic tests that may be performed to determine the extent of the patient's heart damage.

____

____

6. What risk factors for developing heart disease does Mr. Thomas have? What changes should he make?

____

____

Practice Exercises

A. Complete the Statement

1. The study of the heart is called ____________________.
2. The three layers of the heart are ____________________, ____________________, and ____________________.
3. The impulse for the heartbeat (the pacemaker) originates in the ____________________.
4. Arteries carry blood ____________________ the heart.
5. The four heart valves are ____________________, ____________________, ____________________, and ____________________.
6. The ____________________ are the receiving chambers of the heart and the ____________________ are the pumping chambers.
7. The ____________________ circulation carries blood to and from the lungs.
8. The pointed tip of the heart is called the ____________________.
9. The ____________________ divides the heart into left and right halves.
10. ____________________ is the contraction phase of the heartbeat and ____________________ is the relaxation phase.

B. Combining Form Practice

The combining form **cardi/o** refers to the heart. Use it to write a term that means:

1. pertaining to the heart ____________________
2. disease of the heart muscle ____________________
3. enlargement of the heart ____________________
4. abnormally fast heart rate ____________________
5. abnormally slow heart rate ____________________
6. record of heart electricity ____________________

The combining form **angi/o** refers to the vessel. Use it to write a term that means:

7. vessel narrowing ____________________
8. vessel inflammation ____________________
9. involuntary muscle contraction of a vessel ____________________

The combining form **arteri/o** refers to the artery. Use it to write a term that means:

10. pertaining to an artery ____________________
11. hardening of an artery ____________________
12. small artery ____________________

C. Prefix Practice

Add the appropriate prefix to **-carditis** to form the term that matches each definition.

1. inflammation of the inner lining of the heart ______________________________
2. inflammation of the outer layer of the heart ______________________________
3. inflammation of the muscle of the heart ______________________________

D. Define the Combining Form

	Definition	Example from Chapter
1. **cardi/o**	______________________	______________
2. **valvul/o**	______________________	______________
3. **steth/o**	______________________	______________
4. **arteri/o**	______________________	______________
5. **phleb/o**	______________________	______________
6. **angi/o**	______________________	______________
7. **ventricul/o**	______________________	______________
8. **thromb/o**	______________________	______________
9. **atri/o**	______________________	______________
10. **ather/o**	______________________	______________

E. Name That Term

1. pertaining to a vein ______________________________
2. study of the heart ______________________________
3. record of a vein ______________________________
4. process of recording electrical activity of the heart ______________________________
5. high blood pressure ______________________________
6. low blood pressure ______________________________
7. surgical repair of valve ______________________________
8. pertaining to between ventricles ______________________________
9. removal of fatty substance ______________________________
10. narrowing of the arteries ______________________________

F. Name That Suffix

	Suffix	Example from Chapter
1. pressure	______________	______________
2. abnormal narrowing	______________	______________
3. instrument to measure pressure	______________	______________
4. small	______________	______________
5. hardening	______________	______________

G. Terminology Matching

Match each term to its definition.

1. _______ arrhythmia	a.	swollen, distended veins
2. _______ thrombus	b.	inflammation of vein
3. _______ bradycardia	c.	serious congenital anomaly
4. _______ murmur	d.	slow heart rate
5. _______ phlebitis	e.	insertion of thin tubing
6. _______ hypotension	f.	irregular heartbeat
7. _______ varicose vein	g.	an abnormal heart sound
8. _______ tetralogy of Fallot	h.	clot in blood vessel
9. _______ catheterization	i.	low blood pressure
10. _______ sphygmomanometer	j.	blood pressure cuff

H. What Does it Stand For?

1. BP ______________________________
2. CHF ______________________________
3. MI ______________________________
4. CCU ______________________________
5. PVC ______________________________
6. CPR ______________________________
7. CAD ______________________________
8. CP ______________________________
9. EKG ______________________________
10. S1 ______________________________

I. What's the Abbreviation?

1. mitral valve prolapse ______________________________
2. ventricular septal defect ______________________________
3. percutaneous transluminal coronary angioplasty ______________________________
4. ventricular fibrillation ______________________________
5. deep vein thrombosis ______________________________
6. lactate dehydrogenase ______________________________
7. coarctation of the aorta ______________________________
8. tissue-type plasminogen activator ______________________________
9. cardiovascular ______________________________
10. extracorporeal circulation ______________________________

J. Procedure Matching

Match each procedure to its definition.

1.	_______ cardiac enzymes	a.	visualizes heart after patient is given radioactive thallium
2.	_______ Doppler ultrasound	b.	uses ultrasound to visualize heart beating
3.	_______ Holter monitor	c.	blood test that indicates heart muscle damage
4.	_______ cardiac scan	d.	uses treadmill to evaluate cardiac fitness
5.	_______ stress testing	e.	removes varicose veins
6.	_______ echocardiography	f.	clot-dissolving drugs
7.	_______ extracorporeal circulation	g.	measures velocity of blood moving through blood vessels
8.	_______ ligation and stripping	h.	balloon angioplasty
9.	_______ thrombolytic therapy	i.	use of a heart-lung machine
10.	_______ PTAC	j.	portable EKG monitor

K. Define the Term

1. catheter ______________________________
2. infarct ______________________________
3. thrombus ______________________________
4. palpitation ______________________________
5. regurgitation ______________________________

6. aneurysm ____

7. cardiac arrest ____

8. fibrillation ____

9. myocardial infarction ____

10. hemorrhoid ____

L. Fill in the Blank

angiography	murmur	varicose veins	echocardiogram
pacemaker	CHF	defibrillation	angina pectoris
Holter monitor	hypertension	MI	CCU

1. Tiffany was born with a congenital condition resulting in an abnormal heart sound called a(n) ____________________.
2. Joseph suffered an arrhythmia resulting in cardiac arrest. The emergency team used an instrument to give electric shocks to the heart to create a normal heart rhythm. This procedure is called ____________________.
3. Marguerite has been placed on a low-sodium diet and medication to bring her blood pressure down to a normal range. She suffers from ____________________.
4. Tony has had an artificial device called a(n) ____________________ inserted to control the beating of his heart by producing rhythmic electrical impulses.
5. Derrick's physician determined that he had ____________________ after examining his legs and finding swollen, tortuous veins.
6. Laura has persistent chest pains that require medication. The term for the pain is ____________________.
7. La Tonya will be admitted to what hospital unit after surgery to correct her heart condition? ____________________
8. Stephen is going to have a coronary artery bypass graft to correct the blockage in his coronary arteries. He recently suffered a heart attack as a result of this occlusion. His attack is called a(n) ____________________.
9. Stephen's physician scheduled a(n) ____________________, an X-ray to determine the extent of his blood vessel damage.
10. A patient scheduled to have a diagnostic procedure that uses ultrasound to produce an image of the heart valves is going to have a(n) ____________________.
11. Eric must wear a device for 24 hours that will keep track of his heart activity as he performs his normal daily routine. This device is called a(n) ____________________.
12. Lydia is 82 years old and is suffering from a heart condition that causes weakness, edema, and breathlessness. Her heart failure is the cause of her lung congestion. This condition is called ____________________.

M. Pharmacology Challenge

Fill in the classification for each drug description, then match the brand name.

	Drug Description	Classification	Brand Name
1.	_______ prevents arrhthymia	______________________	a. tPA
2.	_______ reduces cholesterol	______________________	b. Coumadin
3.	_______ increases force of heart contraction	______________________	c. Cardizem
4.	_______ increases urine production	______________________	d. Nitro-Dur
5.	_______ prevents blood clots	______________________	e. Tambocor
6.	_______ dissolves blood clots	______________________	f. Lanoxin
7.	_______ relaxes smooth muscle in artery wall	______________________	g. Lipitor
8.	_______ cause heart to beat less forcefully	______________________	h. Lasix

Labeling Exercise

Image A

Write the labels for this figure on the numbered lines provided.

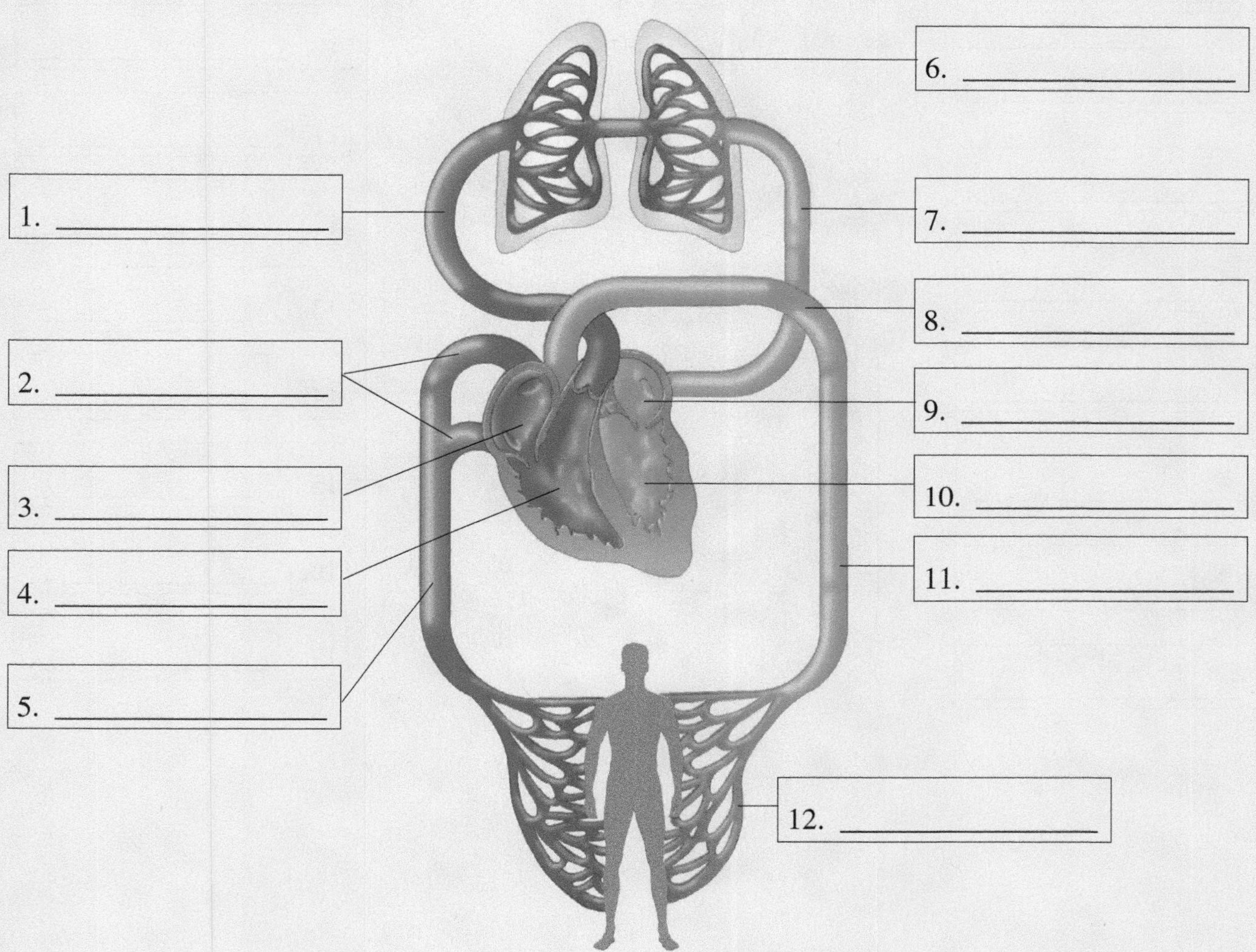

Image B

Write the labels for this figure on the numbered lines provided.

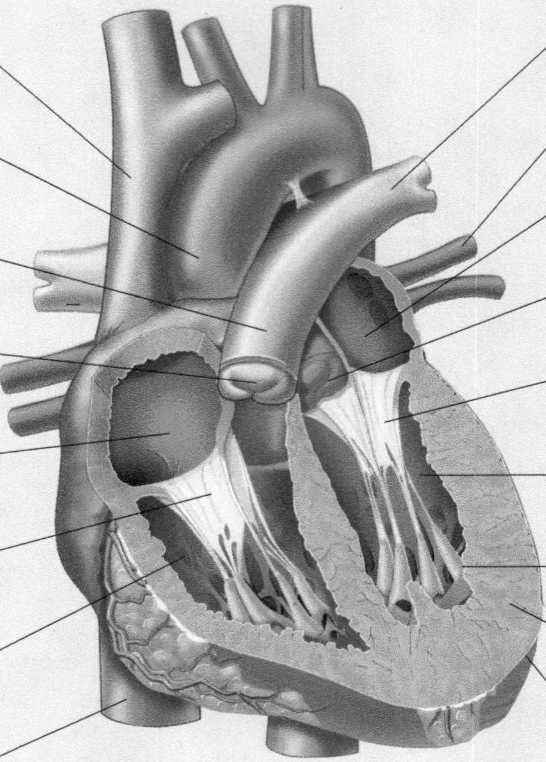

1. ____________________

2. ____________________

3. ____________________

4. ____________________

5. ____________________

6. ____________________

7. ____________________

8. ____________________

9. ____________________

10. ____________________

11. ____________________

12. ____________________

13. ____________________

14. ____________________

15. ____________________

16. ____________________

17. ____________________

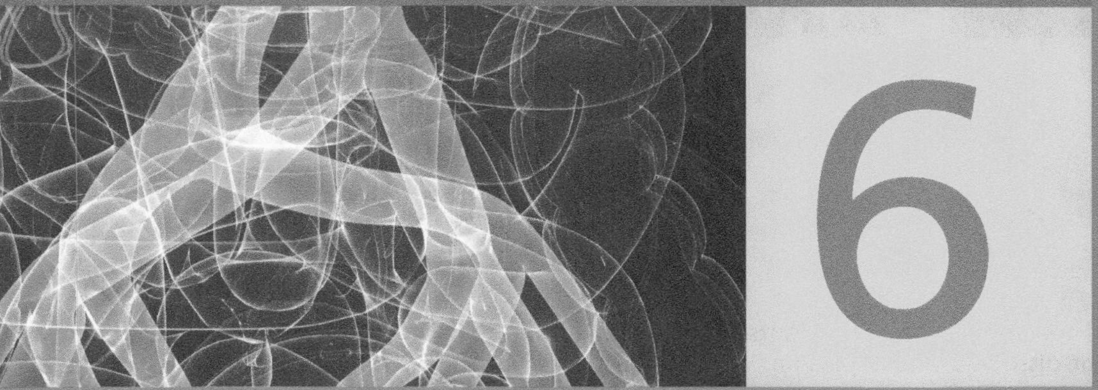

6

BLOOD AND THE LYMPHATIC AND IMMUNE SYSTEMS

Learning Objectives

Upon completion of this chapter, you will be able to

- Recognize the combining forms and suffixes introduced in this chapter.
- Gain the ability to pronounce medical terms and major anatomical structures.
- List the major components, structures, and organs of the blood and lymphatic and immune systems and their functions.
- Describe the blood typing systems.
- Discuss immunity, the immune response, and standard precautions.
- Identify and define blood and lymphatic and immune system anatomical terms.
- Identify and define selected blood and lymphatic and immune system pathology terms.
- Identify and define selected blood and lymphatic and immune system diagnostic procedures.
- Identify and define selected blood and lymphatic and immune system therapeutic procedures.
- Identify and define selected medications associated with blood and the lymphatic and immune systems.
- Define selected abbreviations associated with blood and the lymphatic and immune systems.

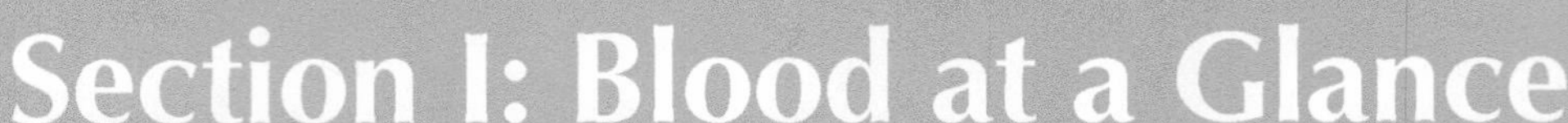

Section I: Blood at a Glance

Function

Blood transports gases, nutrients, and wastes to all areas of the body either attached to red blood cells or dissolved in the plasma. White blood cells fight infection and disease, and platelets initiate the blood clotting process.

Structures

Here are the primary components that comprise blood.

formed elements
- **erythrocytes**
- **leukocytes**
- **platelets**

plasma

Word Parts

Here are the most common word parts (with their meanings) used to build blood terms. For a more comprehensive list, refer to the Terminology section of this chapter.

Combining Forms

agglutin/o	clumping
bas/o	base
chrom/o	color
coagul/o	clotting
cyt/o	cell
eosin/o	rosy red
erythr/o	red
fibrin/o	fibers, fibrous
fus/o	pouring
granul/o	granules
hem/o	blood
hemat/o	blood
leuk/o	white
lymph/o	lymph
morph/o	shape
neutr/o	neutral
phag/o	eat, swallow
sanguin/o	blood
septic/o	infection
thromb/o	clot

Suffixes

-apheresis	removal, carry away
-crit	separation of
-cytosis	more than the normal number of cells
-emia	blood condition
-globin	protein
-penia	abnormal decrease, too few
-phil	attracted to
-poiesis	formation
-stasis	standing still

Staying Current

Many diseases and other disabling conditions are spread through the blood stream. As a member of the health care team it is essential that you remain up to date on the most current practices and procedures used to treat these blood borne conditions. Schedule regular intervals to examine medical and dental dictionaries and other medical resources including electronic media, integrate these resources to interpret technical materials and employ increasingly precise language to communicate your findings with your colleagues.

Cardiovascular System Illustrated

heart, p. 133

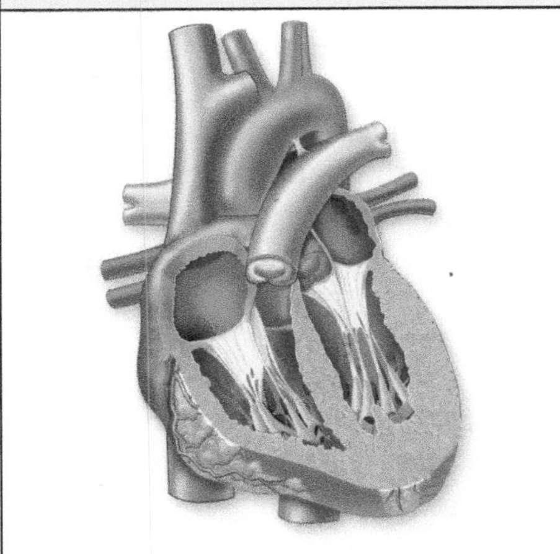

Pumps blood through blood vessels

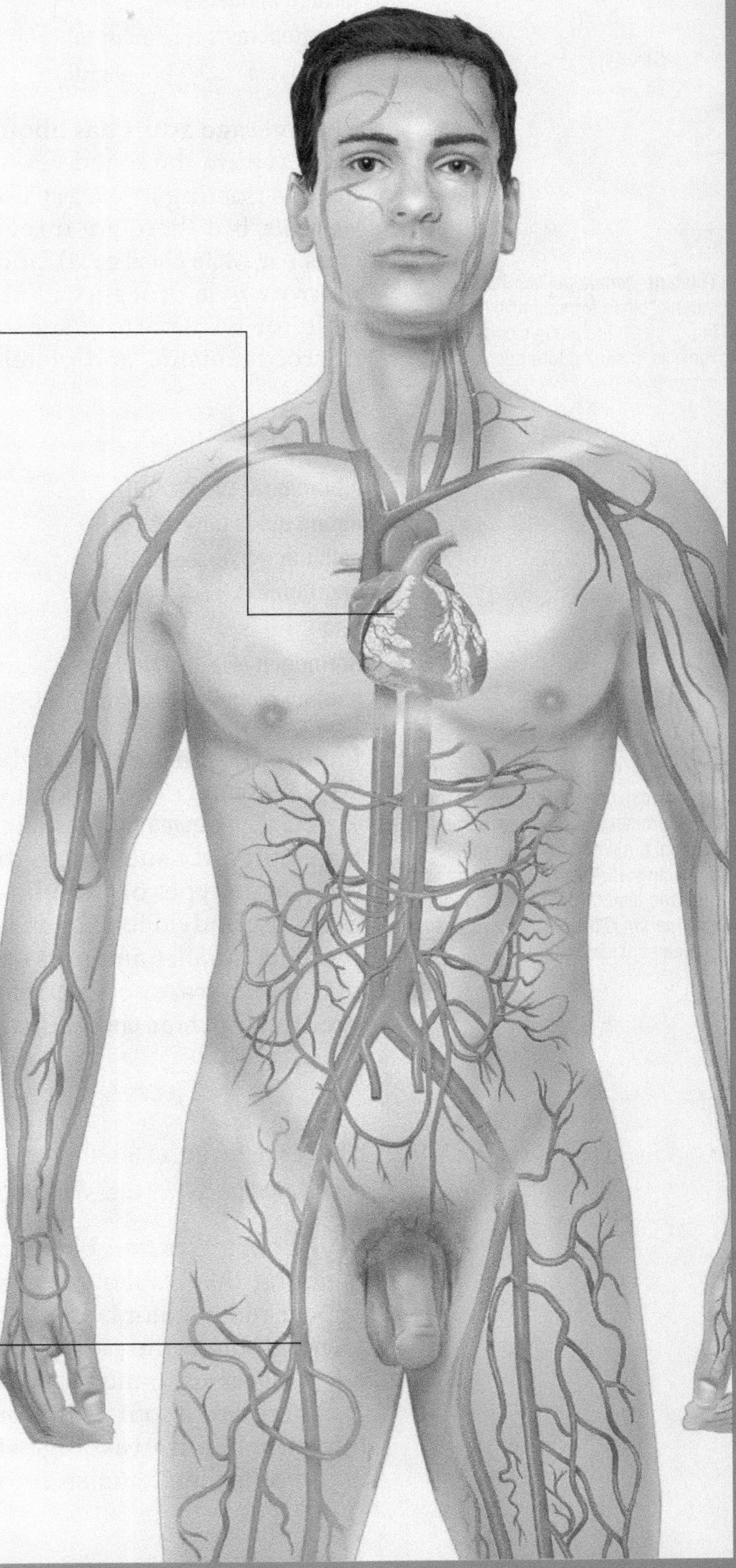

artery, p. 138

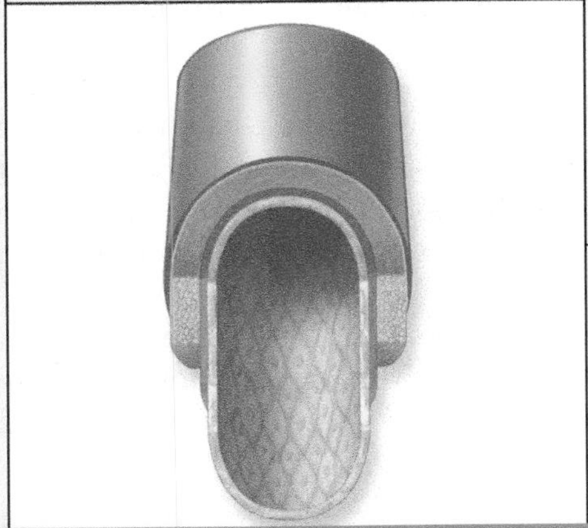

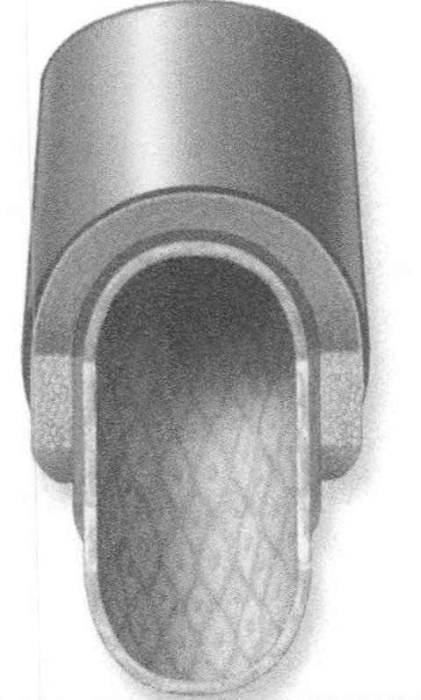

Anatomy and Physiology of Blood

erythrocytes (eh-RITH-roh-sights)
formed elements
hematopoiesis (hee-mah-toh-poy-EE-sis)
leukocytes (LOO-koh-sights)
plasma (PLAZ-mah)
platelets (PLAYT-lets)
red blood cells
white blood cells

MED TERM TIP

The term *hematopoiesis* literally means "blood formation" by combining hemat/o (meaning blood) with -poiesis (meaning formation).

The average adult has about five liters of blood that circulates throughout the body within the blood vessels of the cardiovascular system. Blood is a mixture of cells floating in watery **plasma.** As a group, these cells are referred to as **formed elements,** but there are three different kinds: **erythrocytes** (or **red blood cells**), **leukocytes** (or **white blood cells**), and **platelets.** Blood cells are produced in the red bone marrow by a process called **hematopoiesis.** Plasma and erythrocytes are responsible for transporting substances, leukocytes protect the body from invading microorganisms, and platelets play a role in controlling bleeding.

Plasma

albumin (al-BEW-min)
amino acids (ah-MEE-noh)
calcium (KAL-see-um)
creatinine (kree-AT-in-in)
fats
fibrinogen (fye-BRIN-oh-jen)
gamma globulin (GAM-ah / GLOB-yoo-lin)
globulins (GLOB-yew-lenz)
glucose (GLOO-kohs)
plasma proteins
potassium (poh-TASS-ee-um)
sodium
urea (yoo-REE-ah)

MED TERM TIP

Word Watch: *Plasma* and *serum* are not interchangeable words. Serum is plasma, but with fibrinogen removed or inactivated. This way it can be handled and tested without it clotting. The term *serum* is also sometimes used to mean antiserum or antitoxin.

Liquid plasma composes about 55% of whole blood in the average adult and is 90–92% water. The remaining 8–10% portion of plasma is dissolved substances, especially **plasma proteins** such as **albumin, globulins,** and **fibrinogen.** Albumin helps transport fatty substances that cannot dissolve in the watery plasma. There are three main types of globulins; the most commonly known one, **gamma globulin,** acts as an antibody. Fibrinogen is a blood-clotting protein. In addition to the plasma proteins, smaller amounts of other important substances are also dissolved in the plasma for transport: **calcium, potassium, sodium, glucose, amino acids, fats,** and waste products such as **urea** and **creatinine.**

Erythrocytes

bilirubin (bil-ly-ROO-bin)
enucleated (ee-NEW-klee-ate-ed)
hemoglobin (hee-moh-GLOH-bin)

Erythrocytes, or red blood cells (RBCs), are biconcave disks that are **enucleated,** meaning they no longer contain a nucleus (see Figure 6.1 ■). Red blood cells appear red in color because they contain **hemoglobin,** an iron-containing pigment. Hemoglobin is the part of the red blood cell that picks up oxygen from the lungs and delivers it to the tissues of the body.

There are about 5 million erythrocytes per cubic millimeter of blood. The total number in an average-sized adult is 35 trillion, with males having more red blood cells than females. Erythrocytes have an average lifespan of 120 days, and

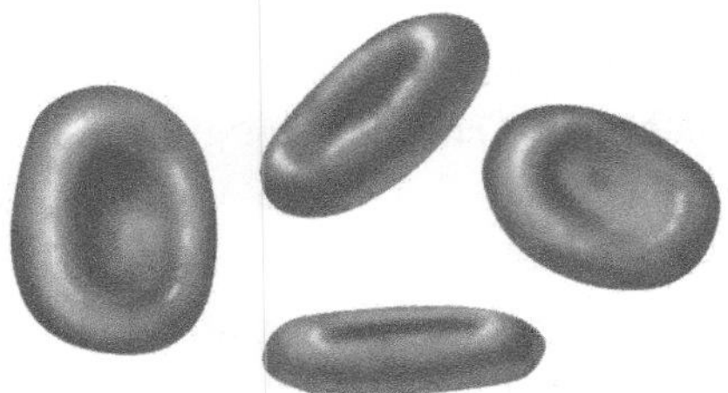

■ **Figure 6.1** The biconcave disk shape of erythrocytes (red blood cells).

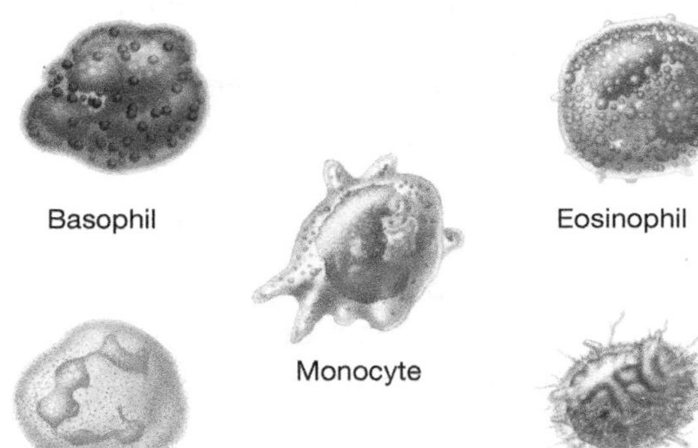

■ **Figure 6.2** The five different types of leukocytes (white blood cells).

then the spleen removes the worn-out and damaged ones from circulation. Much of the red blood cell, such as the iron, can be reused, but one portion, **bilirubin,** is a waste product disposed of by the liver.

> **MED TERM TIP**
>
> Your body makes about 2 million erythrocytes every second. Of course, it must then destroy 2 million every second to maintain a relatively constant 30 trillion red blood cells.

Leukocytes

agranulocytes (ah-GRAN-yew-loh-sights)
granulocytes (GRAN-yew-loh-sights)
pathogens (PATH-oh-ginz)

Leukocytes, also referred to as white blood cells (WBCs), provide protection against the invasion of **pathogens** such as bacteria, viruses, and other foreign material. In general, white blood cells have a spherical shape with a large nucleus, and there are about 8,000 per cubic millimeter of blood (see Figure 6.2 ■). There are five different types of white blood cells, each with its own strategy for protecting the body. The five can be subdivided into two categories: **granulocytes** (with granules in the cytoplasm) and **agranulocytes** (without granules in the cytoplasm). The name and function of each type is presented in Table 6.1 ■.

> **MED TERM TIP**
>
> A *phagocyte* is a cell that has the ability to ingest (phag/o = eat; -cyte = cell) and digest bacteria and other foreign particles. This process, *phagocytosis*, is critical for the control of bacteria within the body.

Table 6.1 Leukocyte Classification

LEUKOCYTE	FUNCTION
Granulocytes	
Basophils (basos) (BAY-soh-fillz)	Release histamine and heparin to damaged tissues
Eosinophils (eosins) (ee-oh-SIN-oh-fillz)	Destroy parasites and increase during allergic reactions
Neutrophils (NOO-troh-fillz)	Engulfs foreign and damaged cells (phagocytosis); most numerous of the leukocytes
Agranulocytes	
Monocytes (monos) (MON-oh-sights)	Engulfs foreign and damaged cells (phagocytosis)
Lymphocytes (lymphs) (LIM-foh-sights)	Plays several different roles in immune response

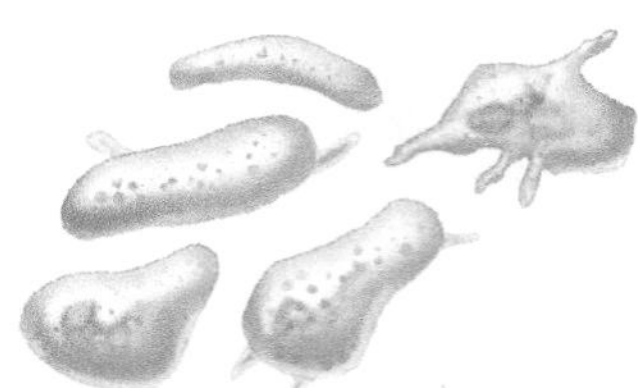

■ Figure 6.3 Platelet structure.

MED TERM TIP

You can find a clue to the meaning of many terms associated with platelets because they contain word parts:

- fibrinogen: fibrin/o = fibers + -gen = that which produces
- hemostasis: hem/o = blood + -stasis = standing still
- agglutinate: agglutin/o = clumping
- prothrombin: pro- = before + thromb/o = clot
- thromboplastin: thromb/o = clot + -plastin = formation

Platelets

agglutinate (ah-GLOO-tih-nayt)
fibrin (FYE-brin)
hemostasis (hee-moh-STAY-sis)
prothrombin (proh-THROM-bin)
thrombin (THROM-bin)
thrombocyte (THROM-boh-sight)
thromboplastin (throm-boh-PLAS-tin)

Platelet, the modern term for **thrombocyte,** refers to the smallest of all the formed blood elements. Platelets are not whole cells, but rather are formed when the cytoplasm of a large precursor cell shatters into small plate-like fragments (see Figure 6.3 ■). There are between 200,000 and 300,000 per cubic millimeter in the body.

Platelets play a critical part in the blood-clotting process or **hemostasis.** They **agglutinate** or clump together into small clusters when a blood vessel is cut or damaged. Platelets also release a substance called **thromboplastin,** which, in the presence of calcium, reacts with **prothrombin** (a clotting protein in the blood) to form **thrombin.** Then thrombin, in turn, works to convert fibrinogen to **fibrin,** which eventually becomes the meshlike blood clot.

Blood Typing

ABO system
blood typing
Rh factor

Each person's blood is different due to the presence of antigens or markers on the surface of erythrocytes. Before a person receives a blood transfusion, it is important to do **blood typing.** This laboratory test determines if the donated blood is compatible with the recipient's blood. There are many different subgroups of blood markers, but the two most important ones are the **ABO system** and **Rh factor.**

ABO System

type A
type AB
type B
type O
universal donor
universal recipient

In the ABO blood system there are two possible red blood cell markers, A and B. A marker is one method by which cells identify themselves. A person with an A marker is said to have **type A** blood. Type A blood produces anti-B antibodies that will attack type B blood. The presence of a B marker gives **type B** blood and anti-A antibodies (that will attack type A blood). If both markers are present, the blood is **type AB** and does not contain any antibodies. Therefore, type AB blood will not attack any other blood type. The absence of either an A or a B marker results in **type O** blood, which contains both anti-A and anti-B antibodies. Type O blood will attack all other blood types (A, B, and AB). For further information on antibodies, refer to the lymphatic section later in this chapter.

Because type O blood does not have either marker A or B, it will not react with anti-A or anti-B antibodies. For this reason, a person with type O blood is referred to as a **universal donor.** In extreme cases, type O blood may be given to a person with any of the other blood types. Similarly, type AB blood is the **universal recipient.** A person with type AB blood has no antibodies against the other blood types and, therefore, in extreme cases, can receive any type of blood.

Rh Factor

Rh-negative **Rh-positive**

Rh factor is not as difficult to understand as the ABO system. A person with the Rh factor on his or her red blood cells is said to be **Rh-positive** (Rh+). Since this person has the factor, he or she will not make anti-Rh antibodies. A person without the Rh factor is **Rh-negative** (Rh–) and will produce anti-Rh antibodies. Therefore, an Rh+ person may receive both an Rh+ and an Rh– transfusion, but an Rh– person can receive only Rh– blood.

Terminology

Word Parts Used to Build Blood Terms

The following lists contain the combining forms, suffixes, and prefixes used to build terms in the remaining sections of this chapter.

Combining Forms

bas/o	base
chrom/o	color
coagul/o	clotting
cyt/o	cell
eosin/o	rosy red
erythr/o	red
fibrin/o	fibers

fus/o	pouring
granul/o	granules
hem/o	blood
hemat/o	blood
leuk/o	white
lip/o	fat
lymph/o	lymph

morph/o	shape
neutr/o	neutral
phleb/o	vein
sanguin/o	blood
septic/o	infection
thromb/o	clot

Suffixes

-apheresis	removal, carry away
-crit	separation of
-cyte	cell
-cytosis	more than the normal number of cells
-emia	blood condition
-globin	protein

-ia	condition
-ic	pertaining to
-ion	action
-logy	study of
-lytic	destruction
-oma	swelling
-otomy	cutting into

-ous	pertaining to
-penia	too few
-phil	attracted to
-plastic	pertaining to development
-rrhage	abnormal flow
-rrhagic	pertaining to abnormal flow

Prefixes

a-	without
an-	without
anti-	against
auto-	self

dys-	abnormal
homo-	same
hyper-	excessive
hypo-	insufficient

mono-	one
pan-	all
poly-	many
trans-	across

Anatomical Terms

TERM	WORD PARTS	DEFINITION
agranulocyte (ah-GRAN-yew-loh-sight)	a- = without granul/o = granules -cyte = cell	A leukocyte without granules in its cytoplasm; monocytes and lymphocytes.
basophil (BAY-soh-fill)	bas/o = base -phil = attracted to	A granulocytic leukocyte that attracts a basic pH stain.
eosinophil (ee-oh-SIN-oh-fill)	eosin/o = rosy red -phil = attracted to	A granulocytic leukocyte that attracts a rosy red stain.
erythrocyte (eh-RITH-roh-sight)	erythr/o = red -cyte = cell	A red blood cell.
fibrinous (fye-brin-us)	fibrin/o = fibers -ous = pertaining to	Pertaining to fibers.
granulocyte (GRAN-yew-loh-sight)	granul/o = granules -cyte = cell	A leukocyte with granules in its cytoplasm; basophils, eosinophils, neutrophils.
hematic (hee-MAT-ik)	hemat/o = blood -ic = pertaining to	Pertaining to blood.
leukocyte (LOO-koh-sight)	leuk/o = white -cyte = cell	A white blood cell.
lymphocyte (LIM-foh-sight)	lymph/o = lymph -cyte = cell	An agranulocytic leukocyte formed in lymphatic tissue.
monocyte (MON-oh-sight)	mono- = one -cyte = cell	An agranulocytic leukocyte with a single, large nucleus.
neutrophil (NOO-troh-fill)	neutr/o = neutral -phil = attracted to	A granulocytic leukocyte that attracts a neutral pH stain.
sanguinous (SANG-gwih-nus)	sanguin/o = blood -ous = pertaining to	Pertaining to blood.
thrombocyte (THROM-boh-sight)	thromb/o = clot -cyte = cell	A clotting cell; a platelet.

Pathology

TERM	WORD PARTS	DEFINITION
Medical Specialties		
hematology (hee-mah-TALL-oh-jee)	hemat/o = blood -logy = study of	The branch of medicine specializing in treatment of diseases and conditions of the blood. Physician is a *hematologist*.
Signs and Symptoms		
blood clot		The hard collection of fibrin, blood cells, and tissue debris that is the end result of hemostasis or the blood-clotting process (see Figure 6.4 ■).

Pathology *(continued)*

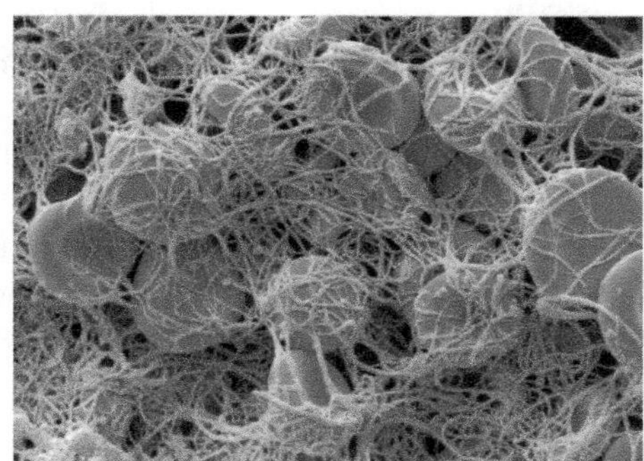

Figure 6.4 Electronmicrograph showing a blood clot composed of fibrin, red blood cells, and tissue debris.

TERM	WORD PARTS	DEFINITION
coagulate (koh-ag-YOO-late)	coagul/o = clotting	To convert from a liquid to a gel or solid, as in blood coagulation.
dyscrasia (dis-CRAZ-ee-ah)	dys- = abnormal -ia = condition	A general term indicating the presence of a disease affecting blood.
hematoma (hee-mah-TOH-mah)	hemat/o = blood -oma = swelling	The collection of blood under the skin as the result of blood escaping into the tissue from damaged blood vessels. Commonly referred to as a *bruise.*
	MED TERM TIP Word Watch: The term *hematoma* is confusing. Its simple translation is "blood tumor." However, it is used to refer to blood that has leaked out of a blood vessel and has pooled in the tissues causing swelling.	
hemorrhage (HEM-er-rij)	hem/o = blood -rrhage = abnormal flow	Rapid flow of blood.
Blood		
hemophilia (hee-moh-FILL-ee-ah)	hem/o = blood -phil = attracted to -ia = condition	Hereditary blood disease in which blood-clotting time is prolonged due to a lack of one vital clotting factor. It is transmitted by a sex-linked trait from females to males, appearing almost exclusively in males.
hyperlipidemia (HYE-per-lip-id-ee-mee-ah)	hyper- = excessive lip/o = fat -emia = blood condition	Condition of having too high a level of lipids such as cholesterol in the bloodstream. A risk factor for developing atherosclerosis and coronary artery disease.
pancytopenia (pan-sigh-toe-PEN-ee-ah)	pan- = all cyt/o = cell -penia = too few	Having too few of all cells.
septicemia (sep-tih-SEE-mee-ah)	septic/o = infection -emia = blood condition	Having bacteria or their toxins in the bloodstream. *Sepsis* is a term that means putrefaction or infection. Commonly referred to as *blood poisoning.*

Pathology *(continued)*

TERM	WORD PARTS	DEFINITION
Erythrocytes		
anemia (an-NEE-mee-ah)	an- = without -emia = blood condition	A large group of conditions characterized by a reduction in the number of red blood cells or the amount of hemoglobin in the blood; results in less oxygen reaching the tissues.
aplastic anemia (a-PLAS-tik / an-NEE-mee-ah)	a- = without -plastic = pertaining to development an- = without -emia = blood condition	Severe form of anemia that develops as a consequence of loss of functioning red bone marrow. Results in a decrease in the number of all the formed elements. Treatment may eventually require a bone marrow transplant.
erythrocytosis (ee-RITH-row-sigh-toe-sis)	erythr/o = red -cytosis = more than normal number of cells	The condition of having too many red blood cells.
erythropenia (ee-RITH-row-pen-ee-ah)	erythr/o = red -penia = too few	The condition of having too few red blood cells.
hemolytic anemia (hee-moh-LIT-ik / an-NEE-mee-ah)	hem/o = blood -lytic = destruction an- = without -emia = blood condition	An anemia that develops as the result of the destruction of erythrocytes.
hemolytic reaction (hee-moh-LIT-ik)	hem/o = blood -lytic = destruction	The destruction of a patient's erythrocytes that occurs when receiving a transfusion of an incompatible blood type. Also called a *transfusion reaction.*
hypochromic anemia (hi-poe-CHROME-ik / an-NEE-mee-ah)	hypo- = insufficient chrom/o = color -ic = pertaining to an- = without -emia = blood condition	Anemia resulting from having insufficient hemoglobin in the erythrocytes. Named because the hemoglobin molecule is responsible for the dark red color of the erythrocytes.
iron-deficiency anemia	an- = without -emia = blood condition	Anemia resulting from not having sufficient iron to manufacture hemoglobin.
pernicious anemia (PA) (per-NISH-us / an-NEE-mee-ah)	an- = without -emia = blood condition	Anemia associated with insufficient absorption of vitamin B_{12} by the digestive system. Vitamin B_{12} is necessary for erythrocyte production.
polycythemia vera (pol-ee-sigh-THEE-mee-ah / VAIR-rah)	poly- = many cyt/o = cell hem/o = blood -ia = condition	Production of too many red blood cells by the bone marrow. Blood becomes too thick to easily flow through the blood vessels.
sickle cell anemia	an- = without -emia = blood condition	A genetic disorder in which erythrocytes take on an abnormal curved or "sickle" shape. These cells are fragile and are easily damaged, leading to a hemolytic anemia (see Figure 6.5 ■).

Pathology *(continued)*

TERM	WORD PARTS	DEFINITION
■ **Figure 6.5** Comparison of normal-shaped erythrocytes and the abnormal sickle shape noted in patients with sickle cell anemia.	**Normal red blood cells**	**Sickled cells**
thalassemia (thal-ah-SEE-mee-ah)	-emia = blood condition	A genetic disorder in which the body is unable to make functioning hemoglobin, resulting in anemia.
Leukocytes		
leukemia (loo-KEE-mee-ah)	leuk/o = white -emia = blood condition	Cancer of the white blood cell–forming red bone marrow resulting in a large number of abnormal and immature white blood cells circulating in the blood.
leukocytosis (LOO-koh-sigh-toh-sis)	leuk/o = white -cytosis = more than normal number of cells	The condition of having too many white blood cells.
leukopenia (LOO-koh-pen-ee-ah)	leuk/o = white -penia = too few	The condition of having too few white blood cells.
Platelets		
thrombocytosis (throm-boh-sigh-TOH-sis)	thromb/o = clot -cytosis = more than normal number of cells	The condition of having too many platelets.
thrombopenia (THROM-boh-pen-ee-ah)	thromb/o = clot -penia = too few	The condition of having too few platelets.

Diagnostic Procedures

TERM	WORD PARTS	DEFINITION
Clinical Laboratory Tests		
blood culture and sensitivity (C&S)		Sample of blood is incubated in the laboratory to check for bacterial growth. If bacteria are present, they are identified and tested to determine which antibiotics they are sensitive to.
complete blood count (CBC)		Combination of blood tests including red blood cell count (RBC), white blood cell count (WBC), hemoglobin (Hgb), hematocrit (Hct), white blood cell differential, and platelet count.

Diagnostic Procedures *(continued)*

TERM	WORD PARTS	DEFINITION
erythrocyte sedimentation rate (ESR, sed rate) (eh-RITH-roh-sight / sed-ih-men-TAY-shun)	erythr/o = red -cyte = cell	Blood test to determine the rate at which mature red blood cells settle out of the blood after the addition of an anticoagulant. This is an indicator of the presence of an inflammatory disease.
hematocrit (HCT, Hct, crit) (hee-MAT-oh-krit)	hemat/o = blood -crit = separation of	Blood test to measure the volume of red blood cells (erythrocytes) within the total volume of blood.
hemoglobin (Hgb, hb, HGB) (hee-moh-GLOH-bin)	hem/o = blood -globin = protein	A blood test to measure the amount of hemoglobin present in a given volume of blood.
platelet count (PLAYT-let)		Blood test to determine the number of platelets in a given volume of blood.
prothrombin time (pro-time, PT) (proh-THROM-bin)	thromb/o = clot	A measure of the blood's coagulation abilities by measuring how long it takes for a clot to form after prothrombin has been activated.
red blood cell count (RBC)		Blood test to determine the number of erythrocytes in a volume of blood. A decrease in red blood cells may indicate anemia; an increase may indicate polycythemia.
red blood cell morphology	morph/o = shape -logy = study of	Examination of a specimen of blood for abnormalities in the shape (morphology) of the erythrocytes. Used to determine diseases like sickle cell anemia.
sequential multiple analyzer computer (SMAC)		Machine for doing multiple blood chemistry tests automatically.
white blood cell count (WBC)		Blood test to measure the number of leukocytes in a volume of blood. An increase may indicate the presence of infection or a disease such as leukemia. A decrease in white blood cells may be caused by radiation therapy or chemotherapy.
white blood cell differential (diff) (diff-er-EN-shal)		Blood test to determine the number of each variety of leukocytes.
Medical Procedures		
bone marrow aspiration (as-pih-RAY-shun)		Sample of bone marrow is removed by aspiration with a needle and examined for diseases such as leukemia or aplastic anemia.
phlebotomy (fleh-BOT-oh-me)	phleb/o = vein -otomy = cutting into	Incision into a vein in order to remove blood for a diagnostic test. Also called *venipuncture.*

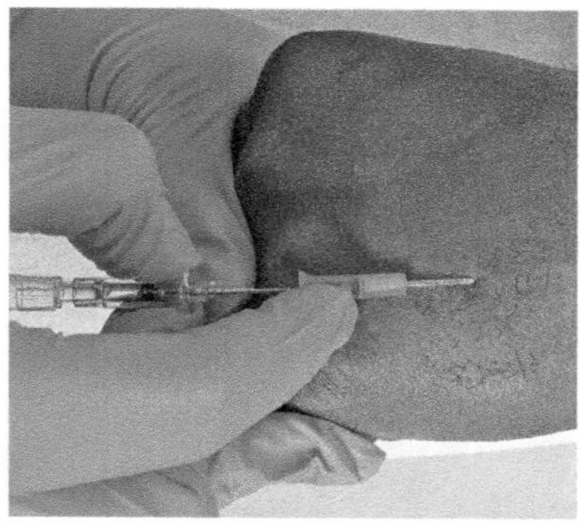

Figure 6.6 Phlebotomist using a needle to withdraw blood.

Therapeutic Procedures

TERM	WORD PARTS	DEFINITION
Medical Procedures		
autologous transfusion (aw-TALL-oh-gus / trans-FYOO-zhun)	auto- = self	Procedure for collecting and storing a patient's own blood several weeks prior to the actual need. It can then be used to replace blood lost during a surgical procedure.
blood transfusion (trans-FYOO-zhun)	trans- = across fus/o = pouring -ion = action	Artificial transfer of blood into the bloodstream.
	MED TERM TIP Before a patient receives a blood transfusion, the laboratory performs a **type and cross-match.** This test first double-checks the blood type of both the donor's and recipient's blood. Then a cross-match is performed. This process mixed together small samples of both bloods and observes the mixture for adverse reactions.	
bone marrow transplant (BMT)		Patient receives red bone marrow from a donor after the patient's own bone marrow has been destroyed by radiation or chemotherapy.
homologous transfusion (hoh-MALL-oh-gus / trans-FYOO-zhun)	homo- = same	Replacement of blood by transfusion of blood received from another person.
packed red cells		A transfusion in which most of the plasma, leukocytes, and platelets have been removed, leaving on erythrocytes.
plasmapheresis (plaz-mah-fah-REE-sis)	-apheresis = removal, carry away	Method of removing plasma from the body without depleting the formed elements. Whole blood is removed and the cells and plasma are separated. The cells are returned to the patient along with a donor plasma transfusion.
whole blood		Refers to the mixture of both plasma and formed elements.

Pharmacology

CLASSIFICATION	WORD PARTS	ACTION	EXAMPLES
anticoagulant (an-tih-koh-AG-yoo-lant)	anti- = against coagul/o = clotting	Substance that prevents blood clot formation. Commonly referred to as *blood thinners.*	heparin, HepLock; warfarin, Coumadin
antihemorrhagic (an-tih-hem-er-RAJ-ik)	anti- = against hem/o = blood -rrhagic = pertaining to abnormal flow	Substance that prevents or stops hemorrhaging; a *hemostatic agent.*	aminocaproic acid, Amicar; vitamin K
antiplatelet agents (an-tih-PLATE-let)	anti- = against	Substance that interferes with the action of platelets. Prolongs bleeding time. Used to prevent heart attacks and strokes.	clopidogrel, Plavix; ticlopidine, Ticlid

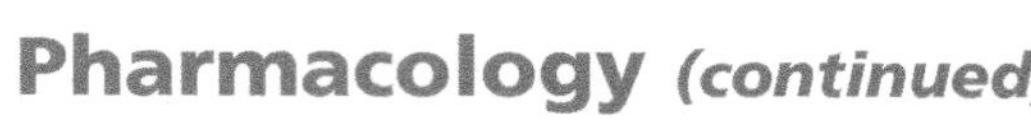

Pharmacology (continued)

CLASSIFICATION	WORD PARTS	ACTION	EXAMPLES
hematinic (hee-mah-TIN-ik)	hemat/o = blood -ic = pertaining to	Substance that increases the number of erythrocytes or the amount of hemoglobin in the blood.	epoetin alfa, Procrit; darbepoetin alfa, Aranesp
thrombolytic (throm-boh-LIT-ik)	thromb/o = clot -lytic = destruction	Term meaning able to dissolve existing blood clots.	alteplase, Activase; streptokinase, Streptase

Abbreviations

ALL	acute lymphocytic leukemia
AML	acute myelogenous leukemia
basos	basophils
BMT	bone marrow transplant
CBC	complete blood count
CLL	chronic lymphocytic leukemia
CML	chronic myelogenous leukemia
diff	differential
eosins, eos	eosinophils
ESR, SR, sed rate	erythrocyte sedimentation rate
HCT, Hct, crit	hematocrit
Hgb, Hb, HGB	hemoglobin
lymphs	lymphocytes
monos	monocytes
PA	pernicious anemia
PCV	packed cell volume
PMN, polys	polymorphonuclear neutrophil
PT, pro-time	prothrombin time
RBC	red blood cell
Rh+	Rh-positive
Rh–	Rh-negative
segs	segmented neutrophils
SMAC	sequential multiple analyzer computer
WBC	white blood cell

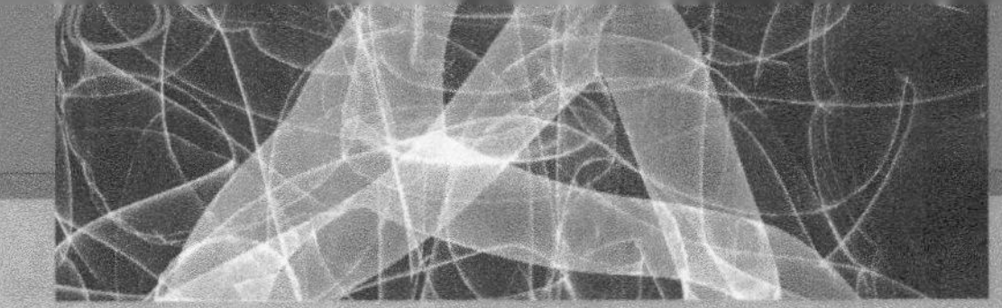

Section II: The Lymphatic and Immune Systems at a Glance

Function

The lymphatic system consists of a network of lymph vessels that pick up excess tissue fluid, cleanse it, and return it to the circulatory system. It also picks up fats that have been absorbed by the digestive system. The immune system fights disease and infections.

Structures

Here are the primary structures that comprise the lymphatic and immune system.

lymph nodes
lymphatic vessels
spleen
thymus gland
tonsils

Word Parts

Here are the most common word parts (with their meanings) used to build lymphatic and immune system terms. For a more comprehensive list, refer to the Terminology section of this chapter.

Combining Forms

adenoid/o	adenoids
axill/o	axilla, underarm
immun/o	protection
inguin/o	groin region
lymph/o	lymph
lymphaden/o	lymph node
lymphangi/o	lymph vessel
nucle/o	nucleus
path/o	disease
splen/o	spleen
thym/o	thymus gland
tonsill/o	tonsils
tox/o	poison

Suffixes

-edema	swelling
-globulin	protein

The Lymphatic and Immune Systems Illustrated

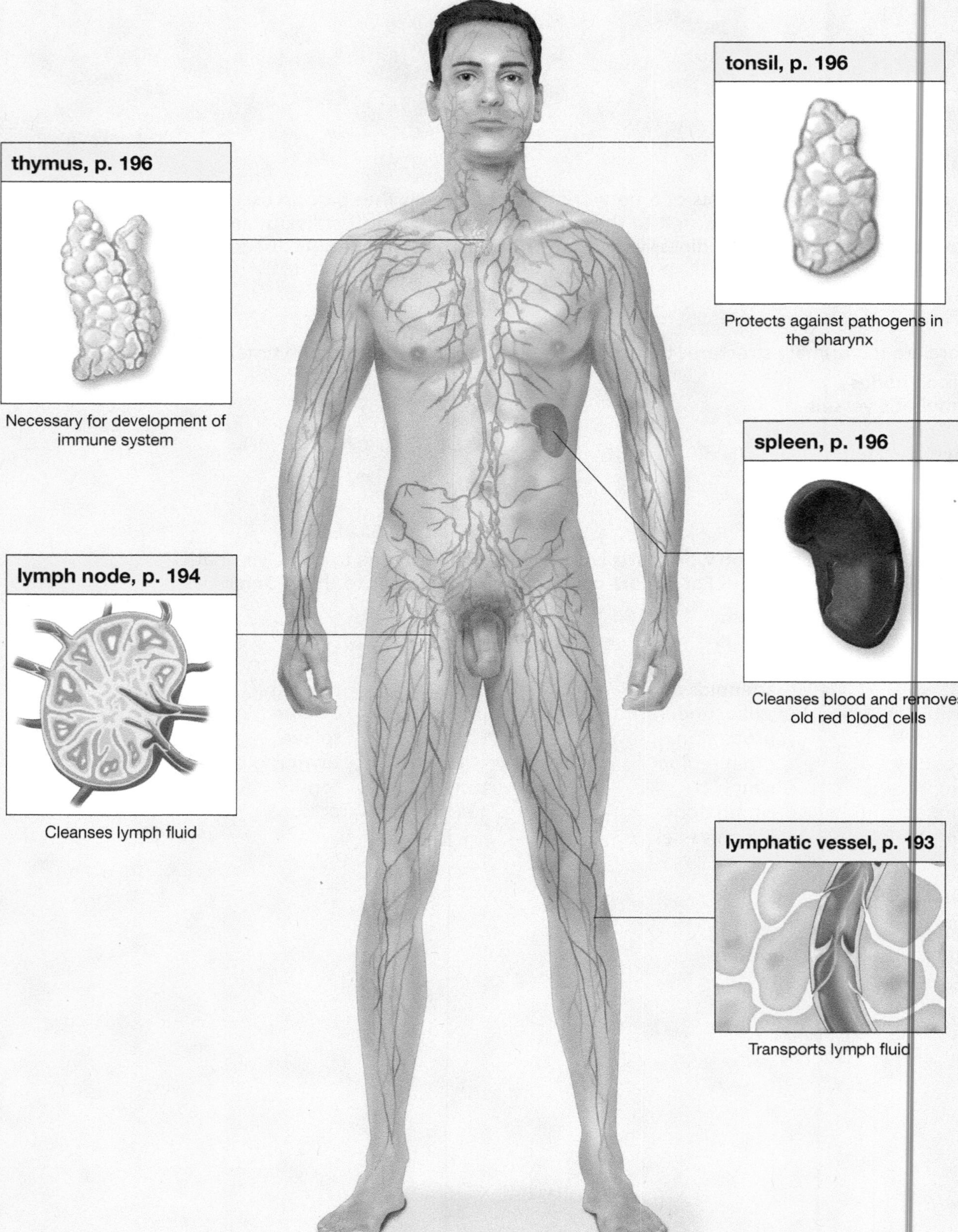

Anatomy and Physiology of the Lymphatic and Immune Systems

lacteals (lack-TEE-als)
lymph (LIMF)
lymph nodes
lymphatic vessels (lim-FAT-ik)
spleen
thymus gland (THIGH-mus)
tonsils (TON-sulls)

The lymphatic system consists of a network of **lymphatic vessels, lymph nodes,** the **spleen,** the **thymus gland,** and the **tonsils.** These organs perform several quite diverse functions for the body. First, they collect excess tissue fluid throughout the body and return it to the circulatory system. The fluid, once inside a lymphatic vessel, is referred to as **lymph.** Lymph vessels located around the small intestines, called **lacteals,** are able to pick up absorbed fats for transport. Additionally, the lymphatic system works with the immune system to form the groups of cells, tissues, organs, and molecules that serve as the body's primary defense against the invasion of pathogens. These systems work together defending the body against foreign invaders and substances, as well as removing our own cells that have become diseased.

Lymphatic Vessels

lymphatic capillaries (CAP-ih-lair-eez)
lymphatic ducts
right lymphatic duct
thoracic duct
valves

The lymphatic vessels form an extensive network of ducts throughout the entire body. However, unlike the circulatory system, these vessels are not in a closed loop. Instead, they serve as one-way pipes conducting lymph from the tissues toward the thoracic cavity (see Figure 6.7 ■). These vessels begin as very small

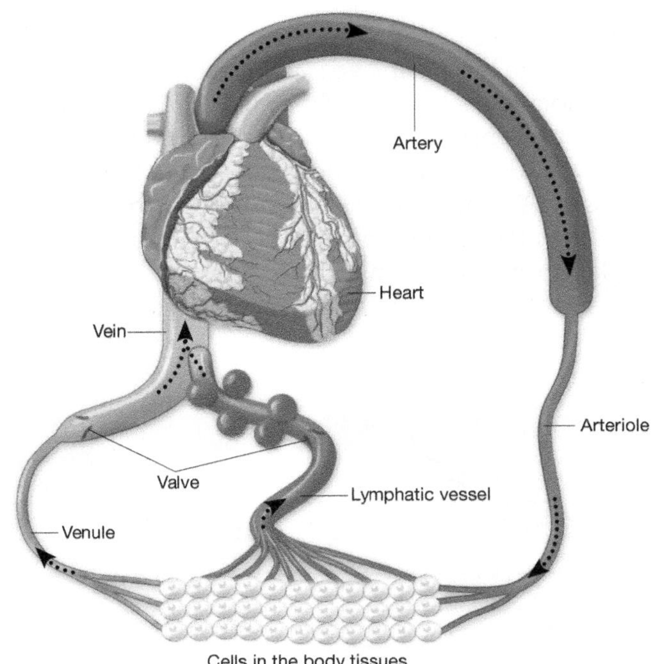

■ **Figure 6.7** Lymphatic vessels (green) pick up excess tissue fluid, purify it in lymph nodes, and return it to the circulatory system.

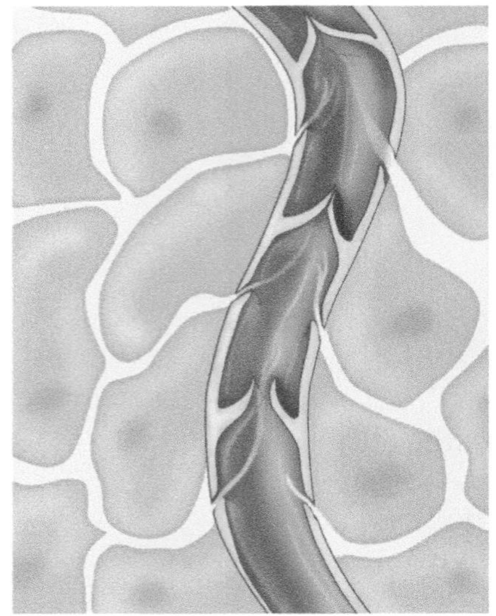

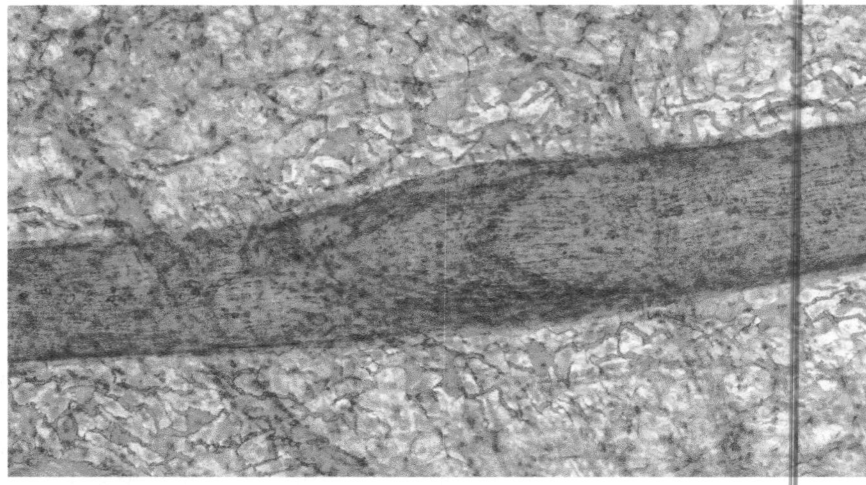

■ **Figure 6.8** (A) Lymphatic vessel with valves within tissue cells; (B) photomicrograph of lymphatic vessel with valve clearly visible. *(Michael Abbey/Photo Researchers, Inc.)*

lymphatic capillaries in the tissues. Excessive tissue fluid enters these capillaries to begin the trip back to the circulatory system. The capillaries merge into larger lymphatic vessels. This is a very low pressure system, so these vessels have **valves** along their length to ensure that lymph can only move forward toward the thoracic cavity (see Figure 6.8 ■). These vessels finally drain into one of two large **lymphatic ducts,** the **right lymphatic duct** or the **thoracic duct.** The smaller right lymphatic duct drains the right arm and the right side of the head, neck, and chest. This duct empties lymph into the right subclavian vein. The larger thoracic duct drains lymph from the rest of the body and empties into the left subclavian vein (see Figure 6.9 ■).

MED TERM TIP

The term *capillary* is also used to describe the minute blood vessels within the circulatory system. This is one of several general medical terms, such as valves, cilia, and hair, that are used in several systems.

Lymph Nodes

lymph glands

Lymph nodes are small organs composed of lymphatic tissue located along the route of the lymphatic vessels. These nodes, also referred to as **lymph glands,** house lymphocytes and antibodies and therefore work to remove pathogens and cell debris as lymph passes through them on its way back to the thoracic cavity (see Figure 6.10 ■). Lymph nodes also serve to trap and destroy cells from cancerous tumors. Although found throughout the body, lymph nodes are particularly concentrated in several regions. For example, lymph nodes concentrated in the neck region drain lymph from the head. See again Figure 6.9 and Table 6.2 ■ for a description of some of the most important sites for lymph nodes.

MED TERM TIP

In surgical procedures to remove a malignancy from an organ, such as a breast, the adjacent lymph nodes are also tested for cancer. If cancerous cells are found in the tested lymph nodes, the disease is said to have spread or *metastasized.* Tumor cells may then spread to other parts of the body by means of the lymphatic system.

Table 6.2 Sites for Lymph Nodes

NAME	LOCATION	FUNCTION
axillary (AK-sih-lair-ee)	armpits	Drain arms and shoulder region; cancer cells from breasts may be present
cervical (SER-vih-kal)	neck	Drain head and neck; may be enlarged during upper respiratory infections
inguinal (ING-gwih-nal)	groin	Drain legs and lower pelvis
mediastinal (mee-dee-ass-TYE-nal)	chest	Drain chest cavity

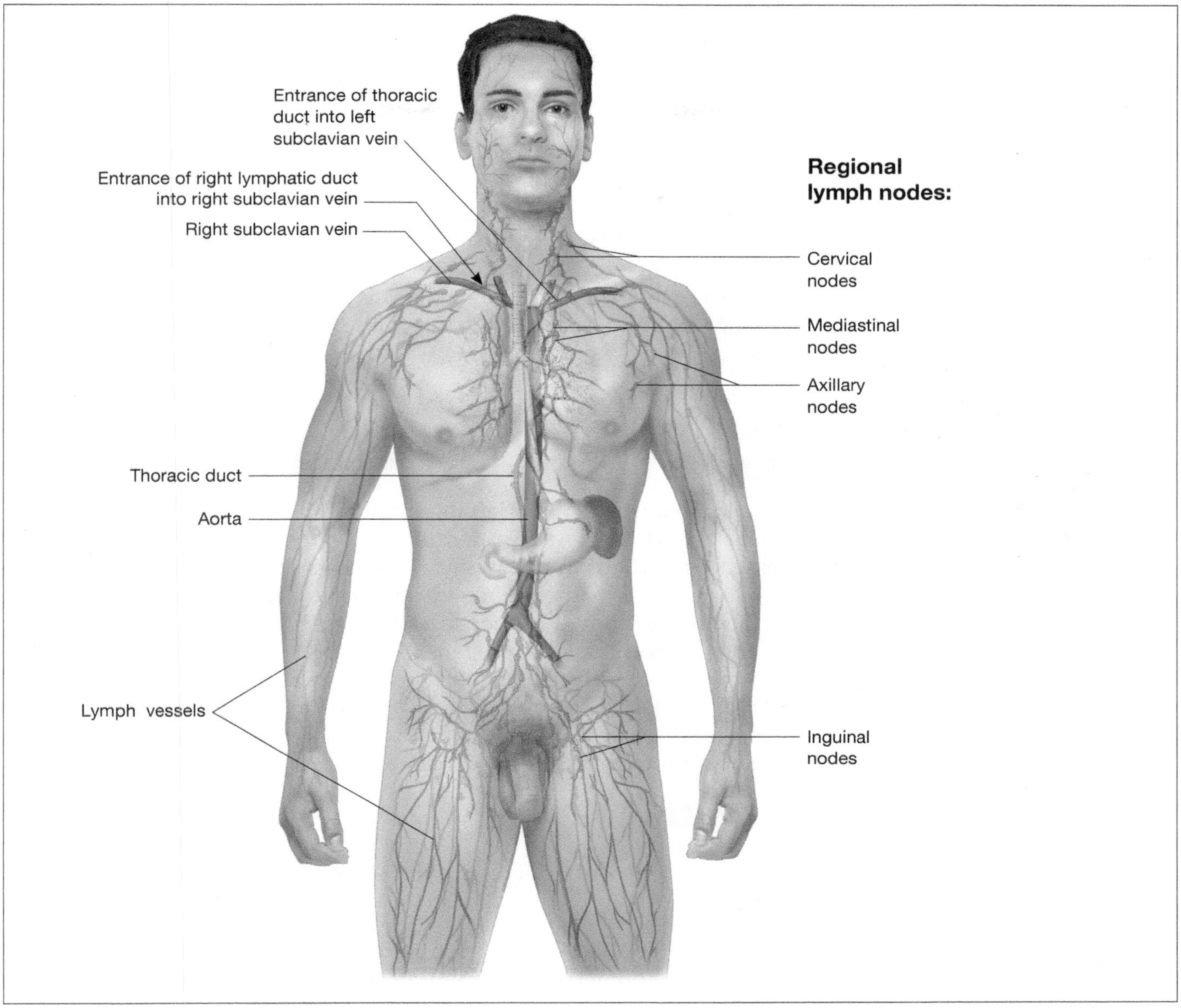

Entrance of thoracic duct into left subclavian vein
Entrance of right lymphatic duct into right subclavian vein
Right subclavian vein
Thoracic duct
Aorta
Lymph vessels
Regional lymph nodes:
Cervical nodes
Mediastinal nodes
Axillary nodes
Inguinal nodes

Figure 6.9 Location of lymph vessels, lymphatic ducts, and areas of lymph node concentrations.

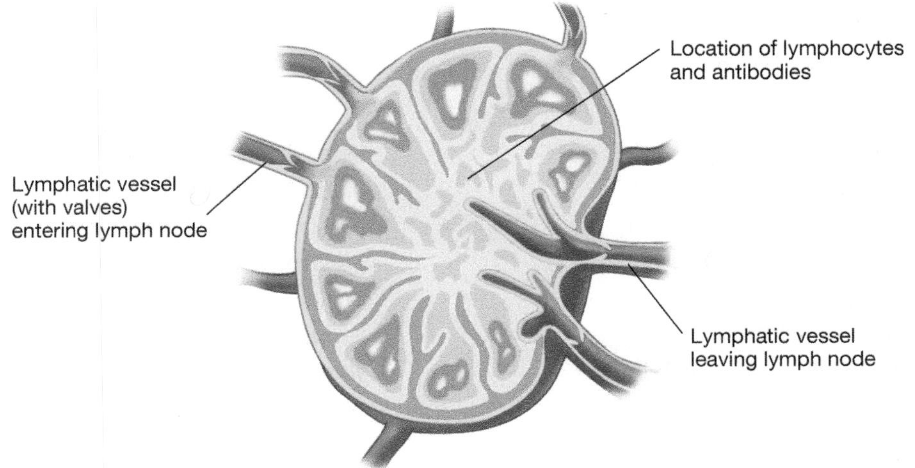

Figure 6.10 Structure of a lymph node.

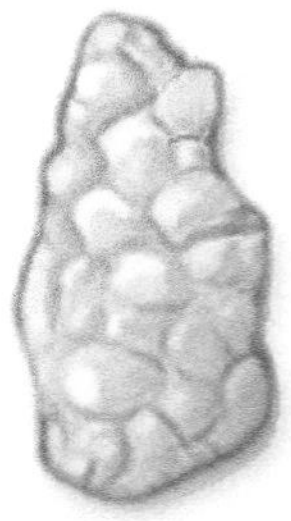

■ Figure 6.11 Shape of a tonsil.

Tonsils

adenoids (ADD-eh-noydz)
lingual tonsils (LING-gwal)
palatine tonsils (PAL-ah-tyne)
pharyngeal tonsils (fair-IN-jee-al)
pharynx (FAIR-inks)

The tonsils are collections of lymphatic tissue located on each side of the throat or **pharynx** (see Figure 6.11 ■). There are three sets of tonsils: **palatine tonsils, pharyngeal tonsils** (commonly referred to as the **adenoids**), and **lingual tonsils.** All tonsils contain a large number of leukocytes and act as filters to protect the body from the invasion of pathogens through the digestive or respiratory systems. Tonsils are not vital organs and can safely be removed if they become a continuous site of infection.

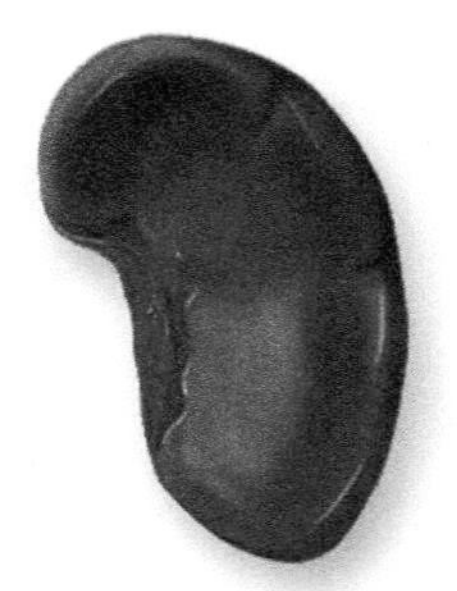

■ Figure 6.12 Shape of the spleen.

Spleen

blood sinuses
macrophages (MACK-roh-fayj-ez)

The spleen, located in the upper left quadrant of the abdomen, consists of lymphatic tissue that is highly infiltrated with blood vessels (see Figure 6.12 ■). These vessels spread out into slow-moving **blood sinuses.** The spleen filters out and destroys old red blood cells, recycles the iron, and also stores some of the blood supply for the body. Phagocytic **macrophages** line the blood sinuses in the spleen to engulf and remove pathogens. Because the blood is moving through the organ slowly, the macrophages have time to carefully identify pathogens and worn-out red blood cells. The spleen is also not a vital organ and can be removed due to injury or disease. However, without the spleen, a person's susceptibility to a bloodstream infection may be increased.

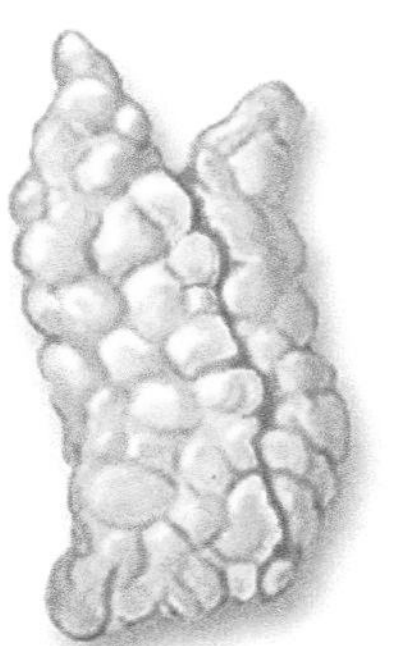

■ Figure 6.13 Shape of the thymus gland.

Thymus Gland

T cells
T lymphocytes
thymosin (thigh-MOH-sin)

The thymus gland, located in the upper portion of the mediastinum, is essential for the proper development of the immune system (see Figure 6.13 ■). It assists the body with the immune function and the development of antibodies. This organ's hormone, **thymosin,** changes lymphocytes to **T lymphocytes** (simply called **T cells**), which play an important role in the immune response. The thymus is active in the unborn child and throughout childhood until adolescence, when it begins to shrink in size.

Immunity

acquired immunity
active acquired immunity
bacteria (bak-TEE-ree-ah)
cancerous tumors
fungi (FUN-jee)
immune response
immunity (im-YOO-nih-tee)
immunizations (im-yoo-nih-ZAY-shuns)
natural immunity
passive acquired immunity
protozoans (proh-toh-ZOH-anz)
toxins
vaccinations (vak-sih-NAY-shuns)
viruses

Immunity is the body's ability to defend itself against pathogens, such as **bacteria, viruses, fungi, protozoans, toxins,** and **cancerous tumors.** Immunity comes in two forms: **natural immunity** and **acquired immunity.** Natural immunity, also called *innate immunity,* is not specific to a particular disease and does not require prior exposure to the pathogenic agent. A good example of natural immunity is the macrophage. These leukocytes are present throughout all the tissues of the body, but are concentrated in areas of high exposure to invading bacteria, like the lungs and digestive system. They are very active phagocytic cells, ingesting and digesting any pathogen they encounter (see Figure 6.14 ■).

Acquired immunity is the body's response to a specific pathogen and may be established either passively or actively. **Passive acquired immunity** results when a person receives protective substances produced by another human or animal. This may take the form of maternal antibodies crossing the placenta to a baby or an antitoxin or gamma globulin injection. **Active acquired immunity** develops following direct exposure to the pathogenic agent. The agent stimulates the body's **immune response,** a series of different mechanisms all geared to neutralize the agent. For example, a person typically can catch chickenpox only once because once the body has successfully fought the virus, it will be able to more quickly recognize and kill it in the future. **Immunizations** or **vaccinations** are special types of active acquired immunity. Instead of actually being exposed to the infectious agent and having the disease, a person is exposed to a modified or weakened pathogen that is still capable of stimulating the immune response but not actually causing the disease.

Immune Response

antibody (AN-tih-bod-ee)
antibody-mediated immunity
antigen–antibody complex
antigens (AN-tih-jens)
B cells
B lymphocytes
cell-mediated immunity
cellular immunity
cytotoxic (sigh-toh-TOK-sik)
humoral immunity (HYOO-mor-al)
natural killer (NK) **cells**

Disease-causing agents are recognized as being foreign because they display proteins that are different from a person's own natural proteins. Those foreign proteins, called **antigens,** stimulate the immune response. The immune response consists of two distinct and different processes: **humoral immunity** (also called **antibody-mediated immunity**) and **cellular immunity** (also called **cell-mediated immunity**).

MED TERM TIP

The term *humoral* comes from the Latin word for "liquid." It is the old-fashioned term to refer to the fluids of the body.

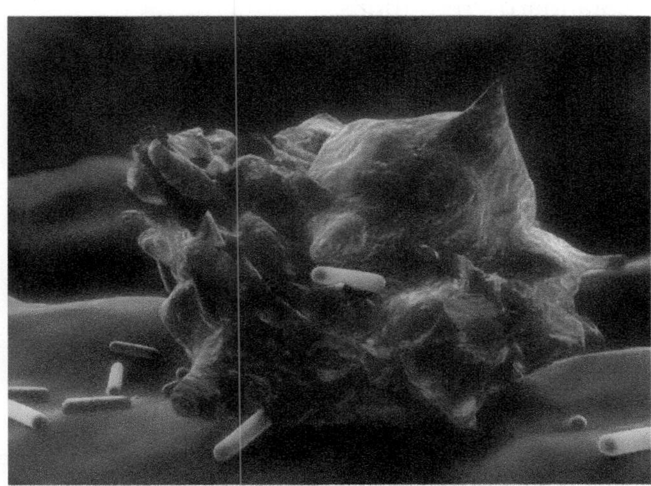

■ **Figure 6.14** Enhanced photomicrograph showing a macrophage (purple) attacking bacillus *Escherichia coli* (green). *(Sebastian Kaulitzki/ Shutterstock)*

Humoral immunity refers to the production of **B lymphocytes,** also called **B cells,** which respond to antigens by producing a protective protein, an **antibody.** Antibodies combine with the antigen to form an **antigen–antibody complex.** This complex either targets the foreign substance for phagocytosis or prevents the infectious agent from damaging healthy cells.

Cellular immunity involves the production of T cells and **natural killer** (NK) **cells.** These defense cells are **cytotoxic,** meaning that they physically attack and destroy pathogenic cells.

MED TERM TIP

Analyzing the word parts that make up the term *cytotoxic* gives you a quick idea of this cell's function.

- cyt/o = cell
- tox/o = poison
- -ic = pertaining to

Standard Precautions

cross-infection
nosocomial infection (no-so-KOH-mee-all)
Occupational Safety and Health Administration (OSHA)
reinfection
self-inoculation

Hospitals and other healthcare settings contain a large number of infective pathogens. Patients and healthcare workers are exposed to each other's pathogens and sometimes become infected. An infection acquired in this manner, as a result of hospital exposure, is referred to as a **nosocomial infection.** Nosocomial infections can spread in several ways. **Cross-infection** occurs when a person, either a patient or healthcare worker, acquires a pathogen from another patient or healthcare worker. **Reinfection** takes place when a patient becomes infected again with the same pathogen that originally brought him or her to the hospital. **Self-inoculation** occurs when a person becomes infected in a different part of the body by a pathogen from another part of his or her own body—such as intestinal bacteria spreading to the urethra.

With the appearance of the hepatitis B virus (HBV) in the mid-1960s and the human immunodeficiency virus (HIV) in the mid-1980s, the fight against spreading infections took on even greater significance. In 1987 the **Occupational Safety and Health Administration** (OSHA) issued mandatory guidelines to ensure that all employees at risk of exposure to body fluids are provided with personal protective equipment. These guidelines state that all human blood, tissue, and body fluids must be treated as if they were infected with HIV, HBV, or other bloodborne pathogens. These guidelines were expanded in 1992 and 1996 to encourage the fight against not just bloodborne pathogens, but all nosocomial infections spread by contact with blood, mucous membranes, nonintact skin, and all body fluids (including amniotic fluid, vaginal secretions, pleural fluid, cerebrospinal fluid, peritoneal fluid, pericardial fluid, and semen). These guidelines are commonly referred to as the Standard Precautions:

MED TERM TIP

The simple act of thoroughly washing your hands is the most effective method of preventing the spread of infectious diseases.

1. Wash hands before putting on and after removing gloves and before and after working with each patient or patient equipment.
2. Wear gloves when in contact with any body fluid, mucous membrane, or nonintact skin or if you have chapped hands, a rash, or open sores.
3. Wear a nonpermeable gown or apron during procedures that are likely to expose you to any body fluid, mucous membrane, or nonintact skin.
4. Wear a mask and protective equipment or a face shield when patients are coughing often or if body fluid droplets or splashes are likely.
5. Wear a facemask and eyewear that seal close to the face during procedures that cause body tissues to be vaporized.
6. Remove for proper cleaning any shared equipment—such as a thermometer, stethoscope, or blood pressure cuff—that has come into contact with body fluids, mucous membrane, or nonintact skin.

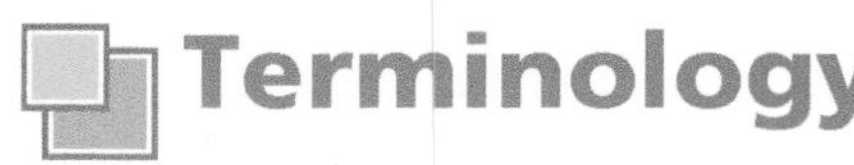

Terminology

Word Parts Used to Build Lymphatic and Immune System Terms

The following lists contain the combining forms, suffixes, and prefixes used to build terms in the remaining sections of this chapter.

Combining Forms

adenoid/o	adenoids	lymph/o	lymph	pneumon/o	lung
axill/o	axilla, underarm	lymphaden/o	lymph node	sarc/o	flesh
cortic/o	outer region, cortex	lymphangi/o	lymph vessel	splen/o	spleen
immun/o	protection	nucle/o	nucleus	thym/o	thymus gland
inguin/o	groin	path/o	disease	tonsill/o	tonsils

Suffixes

-al	pertaining to	-globulin	protein	-logy	study of
-ar	pertaining to	-gram	record	-megaly	enlarged
-ary	pertaining to	-graphy	process of recording	-oma	tumor
-atic	pertaining to	-ia	condition	-osis	abnormal condition
-ectomy	surgical removal	-iasis	abnormal condition	-pathy	disease
-edema	swelling	-ic	pertaining to	-therapy	treatment
-genic	producing	-itis	inflammation		

Prefixes

anti-	against	auto-	self	mono-	one

Anatomical Terms

TERM	WORD PARTS	DEFINITION
axillary (AK-sih-lair-ee)	axill/o = axilla, underarm -ary = pertaining to	Pertaining to the underarm region.
immunoglobulins (im-yoo-noh-GLOB-yoo-linz)	immun/o = protection -globulin = protein	Antibodies secreted by the B cells. All antibodies are immunoglobulins and assist in protecting the body and its surfaces from the invasion of bacteria. For example, the immunoglobulin IgA in colostrum, the first milk from the mother, helps to protect the newborn from infection.
inguinal (ING-gwih-nal)	inguin/o = groin -al = pertaining to	Pertaining to the groin region.
lymphangial (lim-FAN-gee-al)	lymphangi/o = lymph vessel -al = pertaining to	Pertaining to lymph vessels.

Anatomical Terms *(continued)*

TERM	WORD PARTS	DEFINITION
lymphatic (lim-FAT-ik)	lymph/o = lymph -atic = pertaining to	Pertaining to lymph.
splenic (SPLEN-ik)	splen/o = spleen -ic = pertaining to	Pertaining to the spleen.
thymic (THIGH-mik)	thym/o = thymus gland -ic = pertaining to	Pertaining to the thymus gland.
tonsillar (ton-sih-lar)	tonsill/o = tonsils -ar = pertaining to	Pertaining to the tonsils.

Pathology

TERM	WORD PARTS	DEFINITION
Medical Specialties		
allergist (AL-er-jist)		A physician who specializes in testing for and treating allergies.
immunology (im-yoo-NALL-oh-jee)	immun/o = protection -logy = study of	A branch of medicine concerned with diagnosis and treatment of infectious diseases and other disorders of the immune system. Physician is an *immunologist.*
pathology (path-OL-oh-gee)	path/o = disease -logy = study of	A branch of medicine concerned with determining the underlying causes and development of diseases. Physician is an *immunologist.*
Signs and Symptoms		
hives		Appearance of wheals as part of an allergic reaction.
inflammation (in-flah-MA-shun)		The tissues' response to injury from pathogens or physical agents. Characterized by redness, pain, swelling, and feeling hot to touch.

MED TERM TIP

Word Watch: The terms *inflammation* and *inflammatory* are spelled with two *m*'s, while *inflame* and *inflamed* each have only one *m*. These may be the most commonly misspelled terms by medical terminology students.

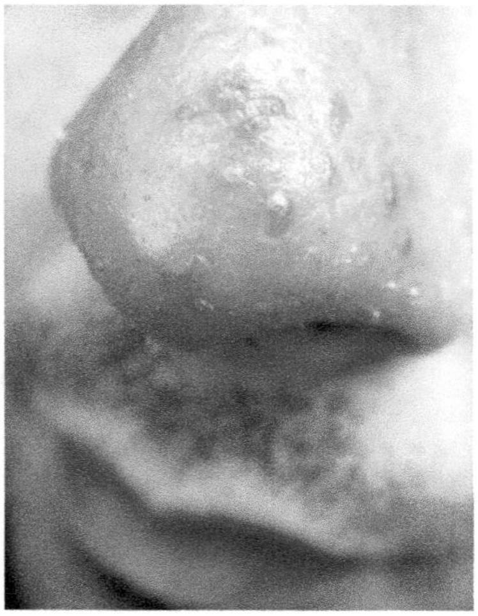

Figure 6.15 Inflammation as illustrated by cellulitis of the nose. Note that the area is red and swollen. It is also painful and hot to touch.

Pathology (continued)

TERM	WORD PARTS	DEFINITION
lymphedema (limf-eh-DEE-mah)	lymph/o = lymph -edema = swelling	Edema appearing in the extremities due to an obstruction of the lymph flow through the lymphatic vessels.
pathogenic (path-oh-JEN-ik)	path/o = disease -genic = producing	An adjective term to describe something—such as bacteria, viruses, or toxins—that produce disease.
splenomegaly (splee-noh-MEG-ah-lee)	splen/o = spleen -megaly = enlarged	An enlarged spleen.
urticaria (er-tih-KAY-ree-ah)		Severe itching associated with hives, usually linked to food allergy, stress, or drug reactions.
Allergic Reactions		
allergy (AL-er-jee)		Hypersensitivity to a common substance in the environment or to a medication. The substance causing the allergic reaction is called an *allergen.*
anaphylactic shock (an-ah-fih-LAK-tik)		Life-threatening condition resulting from a severe allergic reaction. Examples of instances that may trigger this reaction include bee stings, medications, or the ingestion of foods. Circulatory and respiratory problems occur, including respiratory distress, hypotension, edema, tachycardia, and convulsions. Also called **anaphylaxis.**
Lymphatic System		
adenoiditis (add-eh-noyd-EYE-tis)	adenoid/o = adenoids -itis = inflammation	Inflammation of the adenoids.
autoimmune disease	auto- = self	A disease resulting from the body's immune system attacking its own cells as if they were pathogens. Examples include systemic lupus erythematosus, rheumatoid arthritis, and multiple sclerosis.
elephantiasis (el-eh-fan-TYE-ah-sis)	-iasis = abnormal condition	Inflammation, obstruction, and destruction of the lymph vessels resulting in enlarged tissues due to edema.
Hodgkin's disease (HD) (HOJ-kins)		Also called *Hodgkin's lymphoma.* Cancer of the lymphatic cells found in concentration in the lymph nodes. Named after Thomas Hodgkin, a British physician, who first described it.
lymphadenitis (lim-fad-en-EYE-tis)	lymphaden/o = lymph node -itis = inflammation	Inflammation of the lymph nodes. Referred to as *swollen glands.*
lymphadenopathy (lim-fad-eh-NOP-ah-thee)	lymphaden/o = lymph node -pathy = disease	A general term for lymph node diseases.
lymphangioma (lim-fan-jee-OH-mah)	lymphangi/o = lymph vessel -oma = tumor	A tumor in a lymphatic vessel.

Pathology *(continued)*

TERM	WORD PARTS	DEFINITION
lymphoma (lim-FOH-mah)	lymph/o = lymph -oma = tumor	A tumor in lymphatic tissue.
mononucleosis (mono) (mon-oh-nook-lee-OH-sis)	mono- = one nucle/o = nucleus -osis = abnormal condition	Acute infectious disease with a large number of abnormal mononuclear lymphocytes. Caused by the Epstein–Barr virus. Abnormal liver function may occur.
non-Hodgkin's lymphoma (NHL)	lymph/o = lymph -oma = tumor	Cancer of the lymphatic tissues other than Hodgkin's lymphoma.
■ **Figure 6.16** Photo of the neck of a patient with non-Hodgkin's lymphoma showing the swelling associated with enlarged lymph nodes.		
thymoma (thigh-MOH-mah)	thym/o = thymus gland -oma = tumor	A tumor of the thymus gland.
tonsillitis (ton-sil-EYE-tis)	tonsill/o = tonsils -itis = inflammation	Inflammation of the tonsils.
Immune System		
acquired immunodeficiency syndrome (AIDS) (ac-quired / im-you-noh-dee-FIH-shen-see / SIN-drohm)	immun/o = protection	Disease involving a defect in the cell-mediated immunity system. A syndrome of opportunistic infections occurring in the final stages of infection with the human immunodeficiency virus (HIV). This virus attacks T4 lymphocytes and destroys them, reducing the person's ability to fight infection.
AIDS-related complex (ARC)		Early stage of AIDS. There is a positive test for the virus, but only mild symptoms of weight loss, fatigue, skin rash, and anorexia.
graft versus host disease (GVHD)		Serious complication of bone marrow transplant (graft). Immune cells from the donor bone marrow attack the recipient's (host's) tissues.
human immunodeficiency virus (HIV) (im-yoo-noh-dee-FIH-shen-see)	immun/o = protection	Virus that causes AIDS; also known as a **retrovirus**.

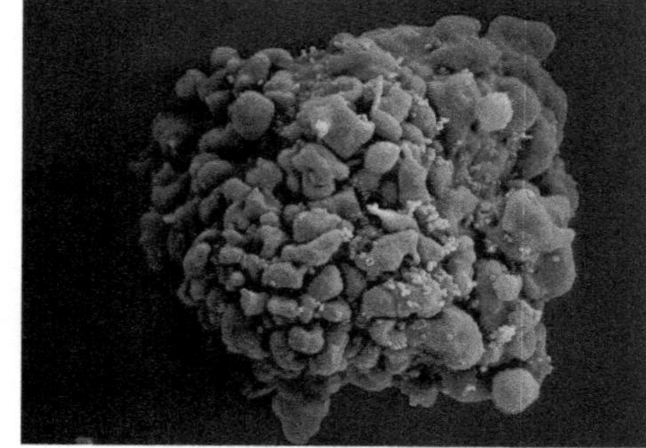

■ **Figure 6.17** Color-enhanced scanning electron micrograph of HIV virus (red) infecting T-helper cells (green).

Pathology *(continued)*

TERM	WORD PARTS	DEFINITION
immunocompromised (im-you-noh-KOM-pro-mized)	immun/o = protection	Having an immune system that is unable to respond properly to pathogens. Also called *immunodeficiency disorder.*
Kaposi's sarcoma (KS) (KAP-oh-seez / sar-KOH-mah)	sarc/o = flesh -oma = tumor	Form of skin cancer frequently seen in patients with AIDS. It consists of brownish-purple papules that spread from the skin and metastasize to internal organs. Named for Moritz Kaposi, an Austrian dermatologist.
opportunistic infections		Infectious diseases associated with patients who have compromised immune systems and therefore a lowered resistance to infections and parasites. May be the result of HIV infection.
pneumocystis pneumonia (PCP) (noo-moh-SIS-tis / new-MOH-nee-ah)	pneumon/o = lung -ia = condition	Pneumonia common in patients with weakened immune systems, such as AIDS patients, caused by the *Pneumocystis jiroveci* fungus.
sarcoidosis (sar-koyd-OH-sis)	-osis = abnormal condition	Disease of unknown cause that forms fibrous lesions commonly appearing in the lymph nodes, liver, skin, lungs, spleen, eyes, and small bones of the hands and feet.
severe combined immunodeficiency syndrome (SCIDS)	immun/o = protection	Disease seen in children born with a non-functioning immune system. Often these children are forced to live in sealed sterile rooms.

Diagnostic Procedures

TERM	WORD PARTS	DEFINITION
Clinical Laboratory Tests		
enzyme-linked immunosorbent assay (ELISA) (EN-zym / LINK'T / im-yoo-noh-sor-bent / ASS-say)	immun/o = protection	Blood test for an antibody to the HIV virus. A positive test means that the person has been exposed to the virus. There may be a false-positive reading, and then the Western blot test would be used to verify the results.
Western blot		Test used as a backup to the ELISA blood test to detect the presence of the antibody to HIV (AIDS virus) in the blood.
Diagnostic Imaging		
lymphangiogram (lim-FAN-jee-oh-gram)	lymphangi/o = lymph vessel -gram = record	X-ray record of the lymphatic vessels produced by lymphangiography.
lymphangiography (lim-FAN-jee-oh-graf-ee)	lymphangi/o = lymph vessel -graphy = process of recording	X-ray taken of the lymph vessels after the injection of dye into the foot. The lymph flow through the chest is traced.

Diagnostic Procedures *(continued)*

TERM	WORD PARTS	DEFINITION
Additional Diagnostic Procedures		
Monospot		Blood test for infectious mononucleosis.
scratch test		Form of allergy testing in which the body is exposed to an allergen through a light scratch on the skin.

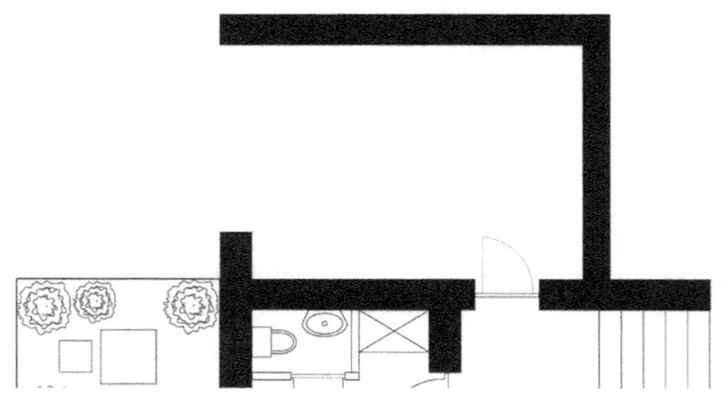

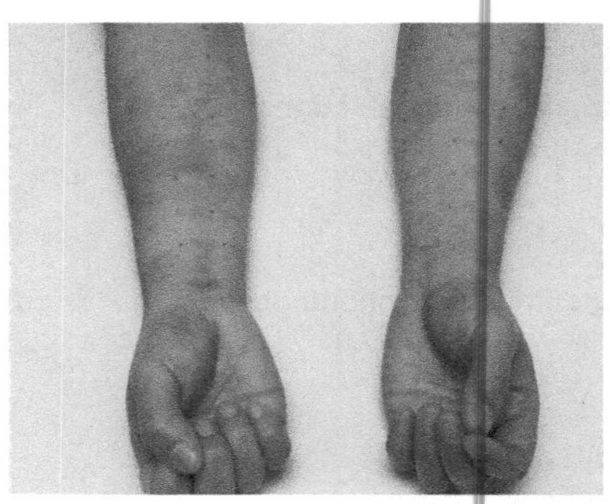

■ **Figure 6.18** (A) Scratch test; patient is exposed to allergens through a light scratch on the skin; (B) Positive scratch test results. Inflammation indicates person is allergic to that substance.

Therapeutic Procedures

TERM	WORD PARTS	DEFINITION
Medical Procedures		
immunotherapy (IM-yoo-noh-thair-ah-pee)	immun/o = protection -therapy = treatment	Giving a patient an injection of immunoglobulins or antibodies in order to treat a disease. The antibodies may be produced by another person or animal, for example, antivenom for snake bites. More recent developments include treatments to boost the activity of the immune system, especially to treat cancer and AIDS.
vaccination (vak-sih-NAY-shun)		Exposure to a weakened pathogen that stimulates the immune response and antibody production in order to confer protection against the full-blown disease. Also called *immunization*.

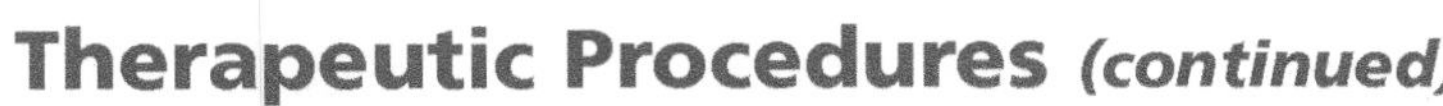

Therapeutic Procedures *(continued)*

TERM	WORD PARTS	DEFINITION
Surgical Procedures		
adenoidectomy (add-eh-noyd-EK-toh-mee)	adenoid/o = adenoids -ectomy = surgical removal	Surgical removal of the adenoids.
lymphadenectomy (lim-fad-eh-NEK-toh-mee)	lymphaden/o = lymph node -ectomy = surgical removal	Removal of a lymph node. This is usually done to test for malignancy.
splenectomy (splee-NEK-toh-mee)	splen/o = spleen -ectomy = surgical removal	Surgical removal of the spleen.
thymectomy (thigh-MEK-toh-mee)	thym/o = thymus gland -ectomy = surgical removal	Surgical removal of the thymus gland.
tonsillectomy (ton-sih-LEK-toh-mee)	tonsill/o = tonsils -ectomy = surgical removal	Surgical removal of the tonsils.

Pharmacology

CLASSIFICATION		ACTION	EXAMPLES
antihistamine (an-tih-HIST-ah-meen)	anti- = against	Blocks the effects of histamine released by the body during an allergic reaction.	cetirizine, Zyrtec; diphenhydramine, Benadryl
corticosteroids (core-tih-koh-STARE-royds)	cortic/o = outer region, cortex	A hormone produced by the adrenal cortex that has very strong anti-inflammatory properties. Particularly useful in treating autoimmune diseases.	prednisone; methylprednisolone, Solu-Medrol
immunosuppressants (im-yoo-noh-sue-PRESS-antz)	immun/o = protection	Blocks certain actions of the immune system. Required to prevent rejection of a transplanted organ.	mycophenolate mofetil, CellCept; cyclosporine, Neoral
protease inhibitor drugs (PROH-tee-ace)		Inhibits protease, an enzyme viruses need to reproduce.	indinavir, Crixivan; saquinavir, Fortovase
reverse transcriptase inhibitor drugs (trans-KRIP-tays)		Inhibits reverse transcriptase, an enzyme needed by viruses to reproduce.	lamivudine, Epivir; zidovudine, Retrovir

Abbreviations

AIDS	acquired immunodeficiency syndrome	**KS**	Kaposi's sarcoma
ARC	AIDS-related complex	**mono**	mononucleosis
ELISA	enzyme-linked immunosorbent assay	**NHL**	non-Hodgkin's lymphoma
GVHD	graft versus host disease	**NK**	natural killer cells
HD	Hodgkin's disease	**PCP**	pneumocystis pneumonia
HIV	human immunodeficiency virus	**SCIDS**	severe combined immunodeficiency syndrome
Ig	immunoglobulins (IgA, IgD, IgE, IgG, IgM)		

Chapter Review

Real-World Applications

Medical Record Analysis

This Discharge Summary contains 11 medical terms. Underline each term and write it in the list below the report. Then define each term. Note: Some terms are defined in other chapters; use your glossary-index to locate and define these terms.

Discharge Summary

Admitting Diagnosis:	Splenomegaly, weight loss, diarrhea, fatigue, chronic cough
Final Diagnosis:	Non-Hodgkin's lymphoma of spleen; splenectomy
History of Present Illness:	Patient is a 36-year-old businessman who was first seen in the office with complaints of feeling generally "run down," intermittent diarrhea, weight loss, and, more recently, a dry cough. He states he has been aware of these symptoms for approximately six months. Monospot and ELISA are both negative. In spite of a 35-pound weight loss, he has abdominal swelling and splenomegaly was detected. He was admitted to the hospital for further evaluation and treatment.
Summary of Hospital Course:	Full-body MRI confirmed splenomegaly and located a 3-cm encapsulated tumor in the spleen. Biopsies taken from the splenic tumor confirmed the diagnosis of non-Hodgkin's lymphoma. The patient underwent splenectomy for removal of the tumor.
Discharge Plans:	Patient was discharged home following recovery from the splenectomy. The abdominal swelling and diarrhea were resolved, but the dry cough persisted. He was referred to an oncologist for evaluation and surveillance for metastases.

	Term	Definition
1	____________	____________
2	____________	____________
3	____________	____________
4	____________	____________
5	____________	____________
6	____________	____________
7	____________	____________
8	____________	____________
9	____________	____________
10	____________	____________
11	____________	____________

Chart Note Transcription

The chart note below contains 10 phrases that can be reworded with a medical term that you learned in this chapter. Each phrase is identified with an underline. Determine the medical term and write your answers in the space provided.

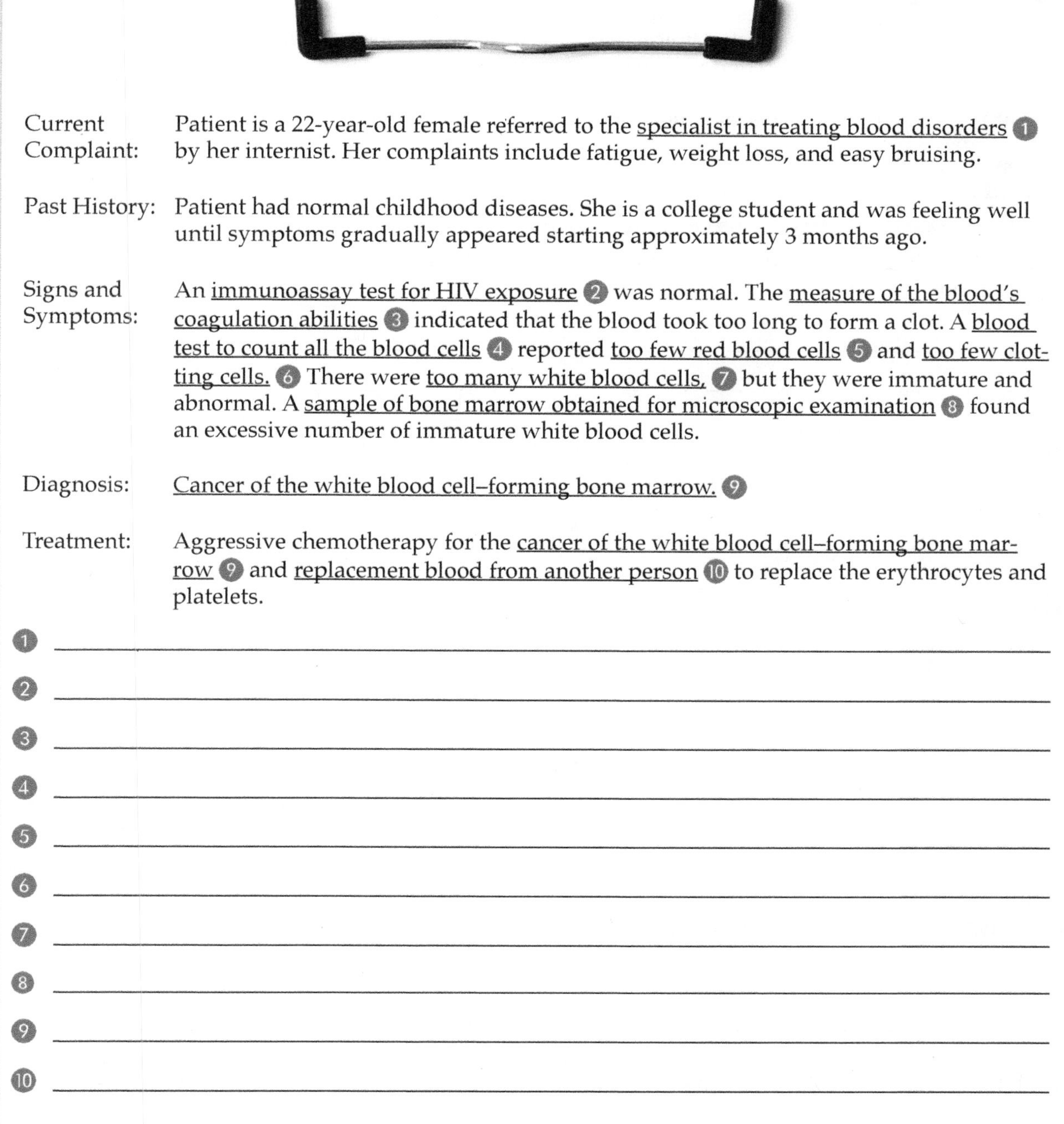

Current Complaint:	Patient is a 22-year-old female referred to the specialist in treating blood disorders ❶ by her internist. Her complaints include fatigue, weight loss, and easy bruising.
Past History:	Patient had normal childhood diseases. She is a college student and was feeling well until symptoms gradually appeared starting approximately 3 months ago.
Signs and Symptoms:	An immunoassay test for HIV exposure ❷ was normal. The measure of the blood's coagulation abilities ❸ indicated that the blood took too long to form a clot. A blood test to count all the blood cells ❹ reported too few red blood cells ❺ and too few clotting cells. ❻ There were too many white blood cells, ❼ but they were immature and abnormal. A sample of bone marrow obtained for microscopic examination ❽ found an excessive number of immature white blood cells.
Diagnosis:	Cancer of the white blood cell–forming bone marrow. ❾
Treatment:	Aggressive chemotherapy for the cancer of the white blood cell–forming bone marrow ❾ and replacement blood from another person ❿ to replace the erythrocytes and platelets.

❶ ______________________________

❷ ______________________________

❸ ______________________________

❹ ______________________________

❺ ______________________________

❻ ______________________________

❼ ______________________________

❽ ______________________________

❾ ______________________________

❿ ______________________________

Case Study

Below is a case study presentation of a patient with a condition covered in this chapter. Read the case study and answer the questions below. Some questions will ask for information not included within this chapter. Use your text, a medical dictionary, journals, technical materials, multimedia resources, electronic media, or any other reference material you choose to answer these questions.

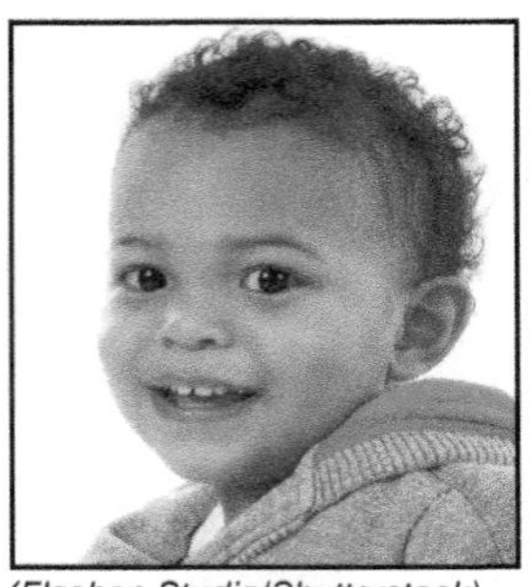

(Flashon Studio/Shutterstock)

A 2-year-old boy is being seen by a hematologist. The child's symptoms include the sudden onset of high fevers, thrombopenia, epistaxis, gingival bleeding, petechiae, and ecchymoses after minor traumas. The physician has ordered a bone marrow aspiration to confirm the clinical diagnosis of acute lymphocytic leukemia. If the diagnosis is positive, the child will be placed immediately on intensive chemotherapy. The physician has informed the parents that treatment produces remission in 90% of children with ALL, especially those between the ages of 2 and 8.

1. What pathological condition does the hematologist suspect? Look this condition up in a reference source and include a short description of it.

___

___

2. List and define each of the patient's presenting symptoms in your own words.

___

___

3. What diagnostic test did the physician perform? Describe it in your own words.

___

___

4. Explain the phrase "clinical diagnosis" in your own words.

___

___

5. If the suspected diagnosis is correct, explain the treatment that will begin.

___

___

6. What do you think the term "remission" means?

___

___

Practice Exercises

A. Complete the Statement

1. The study of the blood is called ____________________.
2. The organs of the lymphatic system other than lymphatic vessels and lymph nodes are the ____________________, ____________________, and ____________________.
3. The two lymph ducts are the ____________________ and ____________________.
4. The primary concentrations of lymph nodes are the ____________________, ____________________, ____________________, and ____________________ regions.
5. The process whereby cells ingest and destroy bacteria within the body is ____________________.
6. The formed elements of blood are the ____________________, ____________________, and ____________________.
7. The fluid portion of blood is called ____________________.
8. ____________________ immunity develops following direct exposure to a pathogen.
9. Humoral immunity is also referred to as ____________________ immunity.
10. The medical term for blood clotting is ____________________.

B. Suffix Practice

Use the following suffixes to create medical terms for the following definitions.

-penia	-globin	-cytosis	-cyte	–globulin

1. too few white (cells) ____________________
2. too few red (cells) ____________________
3. too few clotting (cells) ____________________
4. too few of all cells ____________________
5. increase in white cells ____________________
6. increase in red cells ____________________
7. increase in clotting cells ____________________
8. blood protein ____________________
9. immunity protein ____________________
10. red cell ____________________
11. white cell ____________________
12. lymph cell ____________________

C. Combining Form Practice

The combining form **splen/o** refers to the spleen. Use it to write a term that means:

1. enlargement of the spleen ______
2. surgical removal of the spleen ______
3. cutting into the spleen ______

The combining form **lymph/o** refers to the lymph. Use it to write a term that means:

4. lymph cells ______
5. tumor of the lymph system ______

The combining form **lymphaden/o** refers to the lymph nodes. Use it to write a term that means:

6. disease of a lymph gland ______
7. tumor of a lymph gland ______
8. inflammation of a lymph gland ______

The combining form **immun/o** refers to the immune system. Use it to write a term that means:

9. specialist in the study of the immune system ______
10. immune protein ______
11. study of the immune system ______

The combining form **hemat/o** refers to blood. Use it to write a term that means:

12. relating to the blood ______
13. blood tumor or mass ______
14. blood formation ______

The combining form **hem/o** refers to blood. Use it to write a term that means:

15. blood destruction ______
16. blood protein ______

D. What Does it Stand For?

1. basos ______
2. CBC ______
3. Hgb ______
4. PT ______
5. GVHD ______

6. RBC ______

7. PCV ______

8. ESR ______

9. diff ______

10. lymphs ______

E. Terminology Matching

Match each term to its definition.

1.	______ thalassemia	a.	fluid portion of blood
2.	______ lacteals	b.	disease in which blood does not clot
3.	______ A, B, AB, O	c.	conditions with reduced number of RBCs
4.	______ plasma	d.	mass of blood
5.	______ dyscrasia	e.	blood type
6.	______ hematoma	f.	blood-clotting protein
7.	______ anemia	g.	type of anemia
8.	______ serum	h.	general term for blood disorders
9.	______ hemophilia	i.	lymph vessels around intestine
10.	______ fibrinogen	j.	plasma with inactivated fibrinogen

F. What's the Abbreviation?

1. acquired immunodeficiency syndrome ______
2. AIDS-related complex ______
3. human immunodeficiency virus ______
4. acute lymphocytic leukemia ______
5. bone marrow transplant ______
6. mononucleosis ______
7. Kaposi's sarcoma ______
8. eosinophils ______
9. immunoglobulin ______
10. severe combined immunodeficiency syndrome ______

G. Define the Combining Form

	Combining Form	Example from Chapter
1. lymph node	______	______
2. clot	______	______
3. blood	______	______
4. tonsil	______	______
5. poison	______	______
6. eat/swallow	______	______
7. lymph vessel	______	______
8. disease	______	______
9. spleen	______	______
10. lymph	______	______

H. Fill in the Blank

Kaposi's sarcoma	mononucleosis	Hodgkin's disease	aplastic
polycythemia vera	anaphylactic shock	AIDS	pernicious
pneumocystis	HIV		

1. The condition characterized by the production of too many red blood cells is called ______.
2. The Epstein–Barr virus is thought to be responsible for what infectious disease? ______.
3. A life-threatening allergic reaction is ______.
4. The virus responsible for causing AIDS is ______.
5. A cancer that is seen frequently in AIDS patients is ______.
6. An ELISA is used to test for ______.
7. Malignant tumors concentrate in lymph nodes with this disease: ______.
8. A type of pneumonia seen in AIDS patients is ______ pneumonia.
9. ______ anemia is a severe form of anemia caused by nonfunctioning red bone marrow.
10. ______ anemia is the result of a vitamin B_{12} deficiency.

I. Terminology Matching

Match each term to its definition.

1.	_______ allergy	a.	seen in an allergic reaction
2.	_______ nosocomial	b.	substance that stimulates antibody formation
3.	_______ phagocytosis	c.	a hypersensitivity reaction
4.	_______ hives	d.	engulfing
5.	_______ antibody	e.	protective blood protein
6.	_______ antigen	f.	a type of cancer
7.	_______ Hodgkin's disease	g.	autoimmune disease
8.	_______ sarcoidosis	h.	infection acquired in the hospital
9.	_______ vaccination	i.	blood test for AIDS
10.	_______ ELISA	j.	immunization

J. Pharmacology Challenge

Fill in the classification for each drug description, then match the brand name.

	Drug Description	Classification	Brand Name
1.	_______ inhibits enzyme needed for viral reproduction	_______________	a. HepLock
2.	_______ prevents blood clot formation	_______________	b. Activase
3.	_______ stops bleeding	_______________	c. Solu-Medrol
4.	_______ blocks effects of histamine	_______________	d. Amicar
5.	_______ prevents rejection of a transplanted organ	_______________	e. Epivir
6.	_______ dissolves existing blood clots	_______________	f. CellCept
7.	_______ increases number of erythrocytes	_______________	g. Procrit
8.	_______ strong anti-inflammatory properties	_______________	h. Zyrtec
9.	_______ interferes with action of platelets	_______________	i. Plavix

K. Terminology Matching

Match each term to its definition.

1. _______ culture and sensitivity
2. _______ hematocrit
3. _______ complete blood count
4. _______ erythrocyte sedimentation rate
5. _______ prothrombin time
6. _______ white cell differential
7. _______ red cell morphology

a. measure of blood's clotting ability
b. counts number of each type of blood cell
c. examines cells for abnormal shape
d. checks blood for bacterial growth and best antibiotic to use
e. determines number of each type of white blood cell
f. measures percent of whole blood that is red blood cells
g. an indicator of the presence of an inflammatory condition

L. Scenario

You are preparing to be a Clinical Laboratory Technologist and are currently working in a hospital research laboratory as an intern. A new patient has arrived at the hospital with symptoms that could indicate he may have contracted the Ebola virus. The lab is currently working with the CDC to help find a treatment to manage the virus and even potentially a cure. You have been invited to join the research team. Specifically, you have been asked to study the history of the disease, methods of transmission, symptoms, most current treatment approved by the FDA, locations in the world where it is most prevalent as recorded by the WHO, percentage of patients who survive under current treatment protocols, and the most current research taking place. As a member of the team you will exhibit your ability to cooperate, contribute, and collaborate as you report the results of your research.

Examine medical dictionaries, multimedia resources including electronic media and employ precise medical language to prepare a report of your findings. Cite a specific resource by name for each of the following where additional information was used

1. Medical Journal ____
2. Multimedia Resource____
3. Electronic Media____
4. Medical Dictionary____
5. Technical Materials____
6. Other resource____

Labeling Exercise

Image A

Write the labels for this figure on the numbered lines provided.

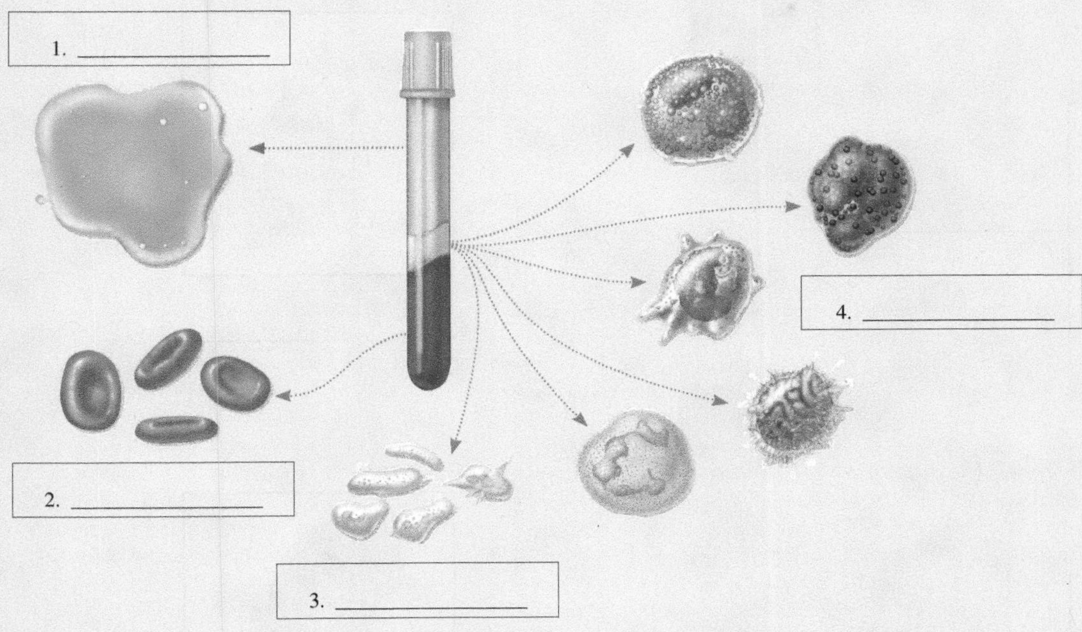

Image B

Write the labels for this figure on the numbered lines provided.

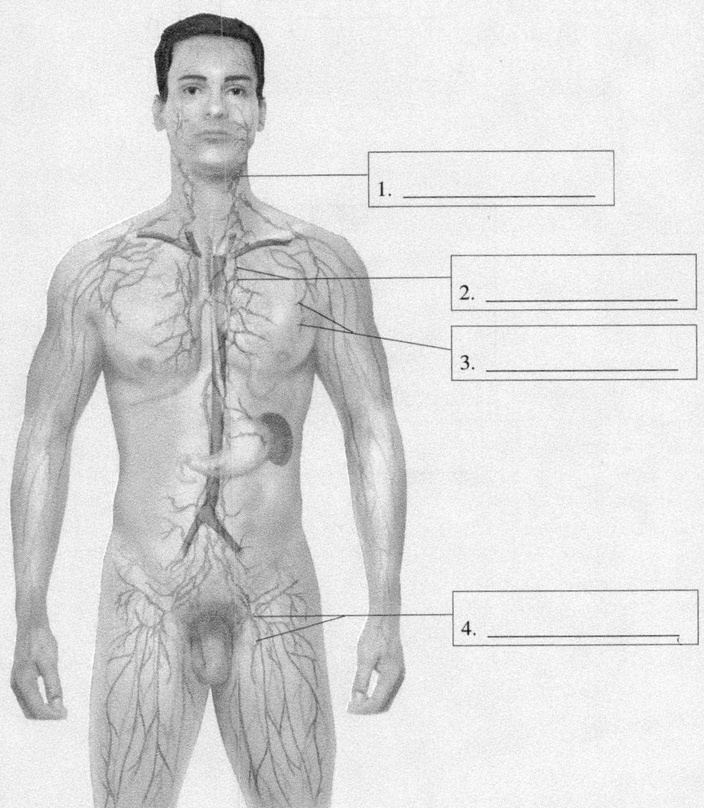

Image C

Write the labels for this figure on the numbered lines provided.

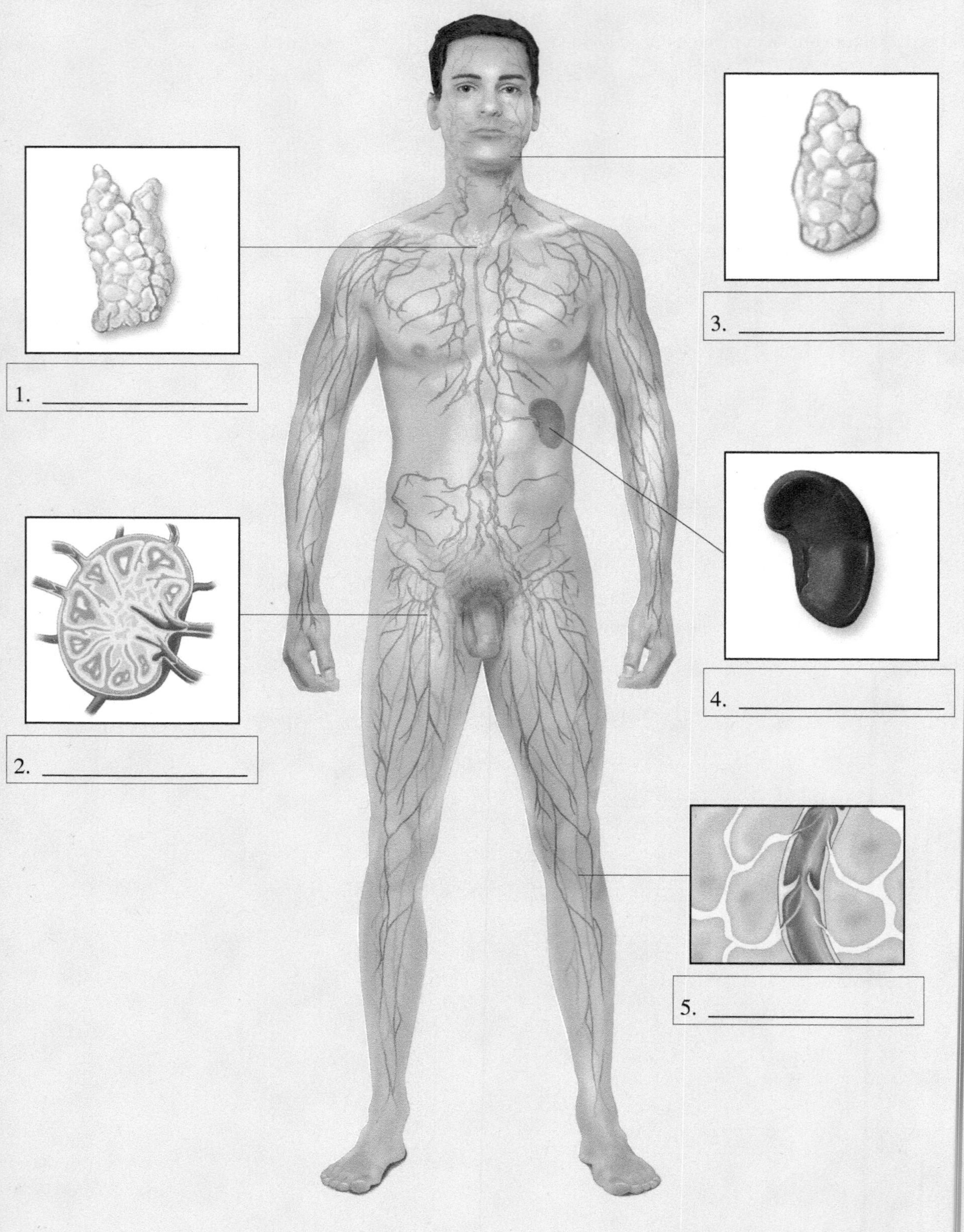

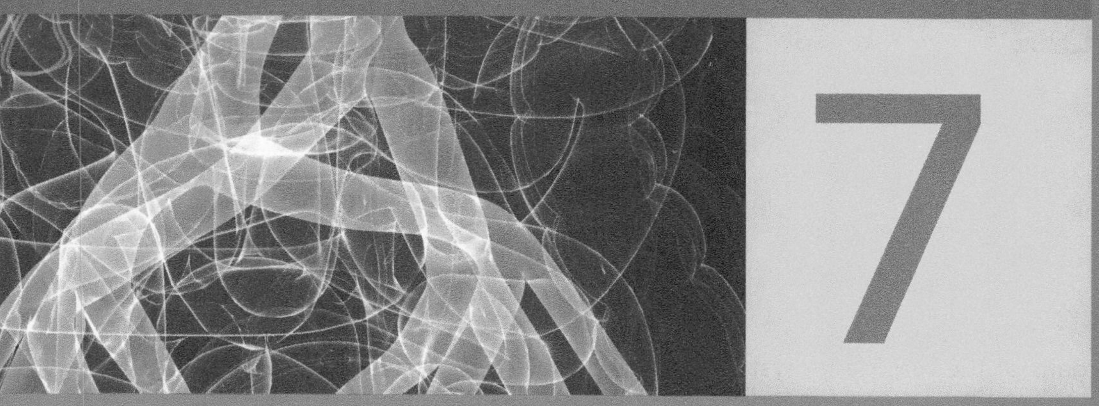

7

RESPIRATORY SYSTEM

Learning Objectives

Upon completion of this chapter, you will be able to

- Identify and define the combining forms and suffixes introduced in this chapter.
- Correctly spell and pronounce medical terms and major anatomical structures relating to the respiratory system.
- Locate and describe the major organs of the respiratory system and their functions.
- List and describe the lung volumes and capacities.
- Describe the process of respiration.
- Identify and define respiratory system anatomical terms.
- Identify and define selected respiratory system pathology terms.
- Identify and define selected respiratory system diagnostic procedures.
- Identify and define selected respiratory system therapeutic procedures.
- Identify and define selected medications relating to the respiratory system.
- Define selected abbreviations associated with the respiratory system.

Respiratory System at a Glance

Function

The organs of the respiratory system are responsible for bringing fresh air into the lungs, exchanging oxygen for carbon dioxide between the air sacs of the lungs and the blood stream, and exhaling the stale air.

Structures

Here are the primary structures that comprise the respiratory system.

nasal cavity	**trachea**
pharynx	**bronchial tubes**
larynx	**lungs**

Word Parts

Here are the most common word parts (with their meanings) used to build respiratory system terms. For a more comprehensive list, refer to the Terminology section of this chapter.

Combining Forms

aer/o	air	orth/o	straight, upright
alveol/o	alveolus; air sac	ox/o, ox/i	oxygen
anthrac/o	coal	pharyng/o	pharynx
atel/o	incomplete	pleur/o	pleura
bronch/o	bronchus	pneum/o	lung, air
bronchi/o	bronchus	pneumon/o	lung, air
bronchiol/o	bronchiole	pulmon/o	lung
coni/o	dust	rhin/o	nose
diaphragmat/o	diaphragm	sept/o	wall
epiglott/o	epiglottis	sinus/o	sinus
laryng/o	larynx	spir/o	breathing
lob/o	lobe	trache/o	trachea, windpipe
nas/o	nose	tuss/o	cough
muc/o	mucus		

Suffixes

-capnia	carbon dioxide	-pnea	breathing
-osmia	smell	-ptysis	spitting
-phonia	voice	-spasm	involuntary muscle contraction
-plegia	paralysis	-thorax	chest

Respiratory System Illustrated

pharynx & larynx, p. 222

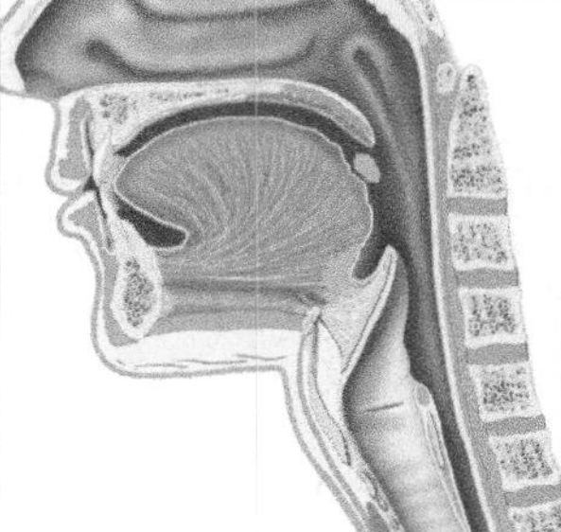

Carries air to the trachea through the voice box

trachea, p. 223

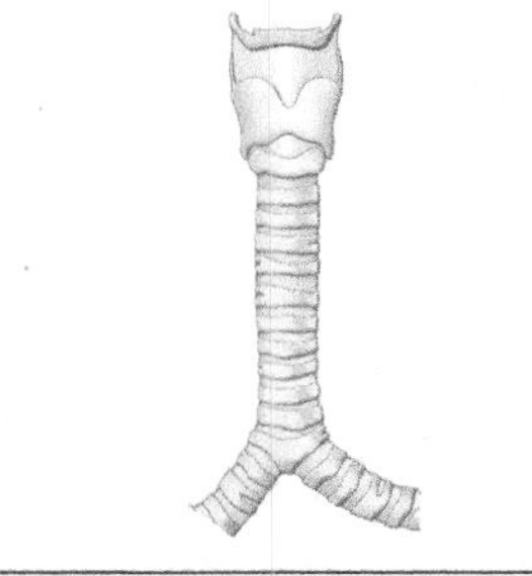

Transports air to and from lungs

nasal cavity, p. 220

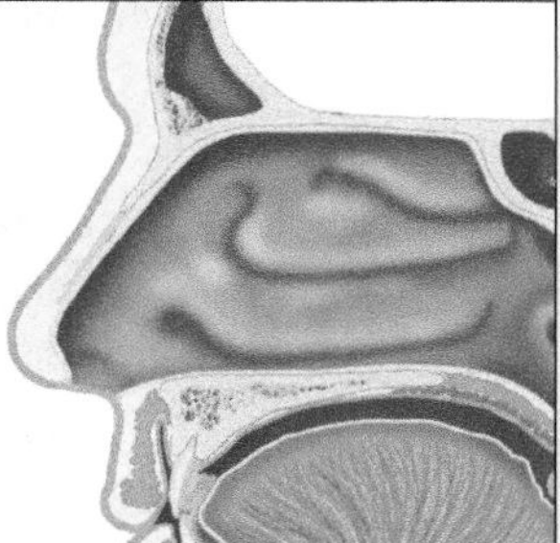

Cleanses, warms, and humidifies inhaled air

bronchial tubes, p. 223

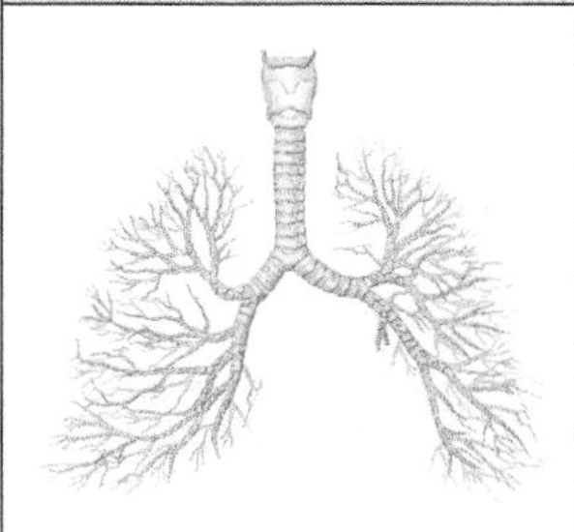

Air passageways inside the lung

lungs, p. 224

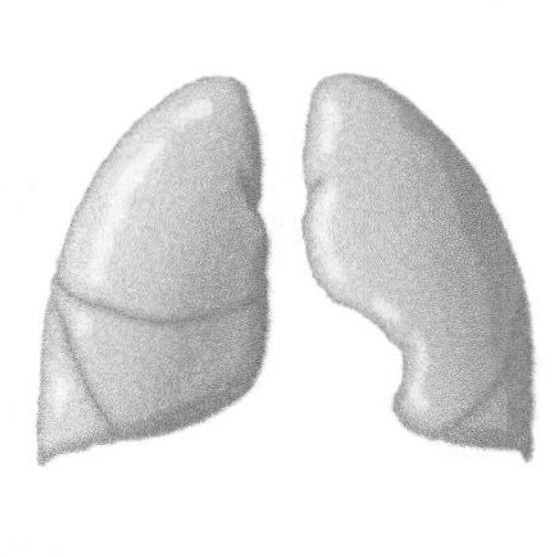

Site of gas exchange between air and blood

Anatomy and Physiology of the Respiratory System

bronchial tubes (BRONG-key-all)
carbon dioxide
exhalation (eks-hah-LAY-shun)
external respiration
inhalation (in-hah-LAY-shun)
internal respiration
larynx (LAIR-inks)
lungs
nasal cavity (NAY-zl)
oxygen (OK-sih-jen)
pharynx (FAIR-inks)
trachea (TRAY-kee-ah)
ventilation

The organs of the respiratory system include the **nasal cavity, pharynx, larynx, trachea, bronchial tubes,** and **lungs.** These organs function together to perform the mechanical and, for the most part, unconscious mechanism of respiration. The cells of the body require the continuous delivery of oxygen and removal of carbon dioxide. The respiratory system works in conjunction with the cardiovascular system to deliver oxygen to all the cells of the body. The process of respiration must be continuous; interruption for even a few minutes can result in brain damage and/or death.

The process of respiration can be subdivided into three distinct parts: **ventilation, external respiration,** and **internal respiration.** Ventilation is the flow of air between the outside environment and the lungs. **Inhalation** is the flow of air into the lungs, and **exhalation** is the flow of air out of the lungs. Inhalation brings fresh **oxygen** (O_2) into the air sacs, while exhalation removes **carbon dioxide** (CO_2) from the body.

> **MED TERM TIP**
> The terms *inhalation* and *inspiration* (in- = inward + spir/o = breathing) can be used interchangeably. Similarly, the terms *exhalation* and *expiration* (ex- = outward + spir/o = breathing) are interchangeable.

External respiration refers to the exchange of oxygen and carbon dioxide that takes place in the lungs. These gases diffuse in opposite directions between the air sacs of the lungs and the bloodstream. Oxygen enters the bloodstream from the air sacs to be delivered throughout the body. Carbon dioxide leaves the bloodstream and enters the air sacs to be exhaled from the body.

Internal respiration is the process of oxygen and carbon dioxide exchange at the cellular level when oxygen leaves the bloodstream and is delivered to the tissues. Oxygen is needed for the body cells' metabolism, all the physical and chemical changes within the body that are necessary for life. The by-product of metabolism is the formation of a waste product, carbon dioxide. The carbon dioxide enters the bloodstream from the tissues and is transported back to the lungs for disposal.

Nasal Cavity

cilia (SIL-ee-ah)
mucus (MYOO-kus)
mucous membrane
nares (NAIR-eez)
nasal septum
palate (PAL-at)
paranasal sinuses (pair-ah-NAY-zl)

> **MED TERM TIP**
> Anyone who has experienced a nosebleed, or *epistaxis*, is aware of the plentiful supply of blood vessels in the nose.

The process of ventilation begins with the nasal cavity. Air enters through two external openings in the nose called the **nares.** The nasal cavity is divided down the middle by the **nasal septum,** a cartilaginous plate. The **palate** in the roof of the mouth separates the nasal cavity above from the mouth below. The walls of the nasal cavity and the nasal septum are made up of flexible cartilage covered with **mucous membrane** (see Figure 7.1 ■). In fact, much of the respiratory tract is

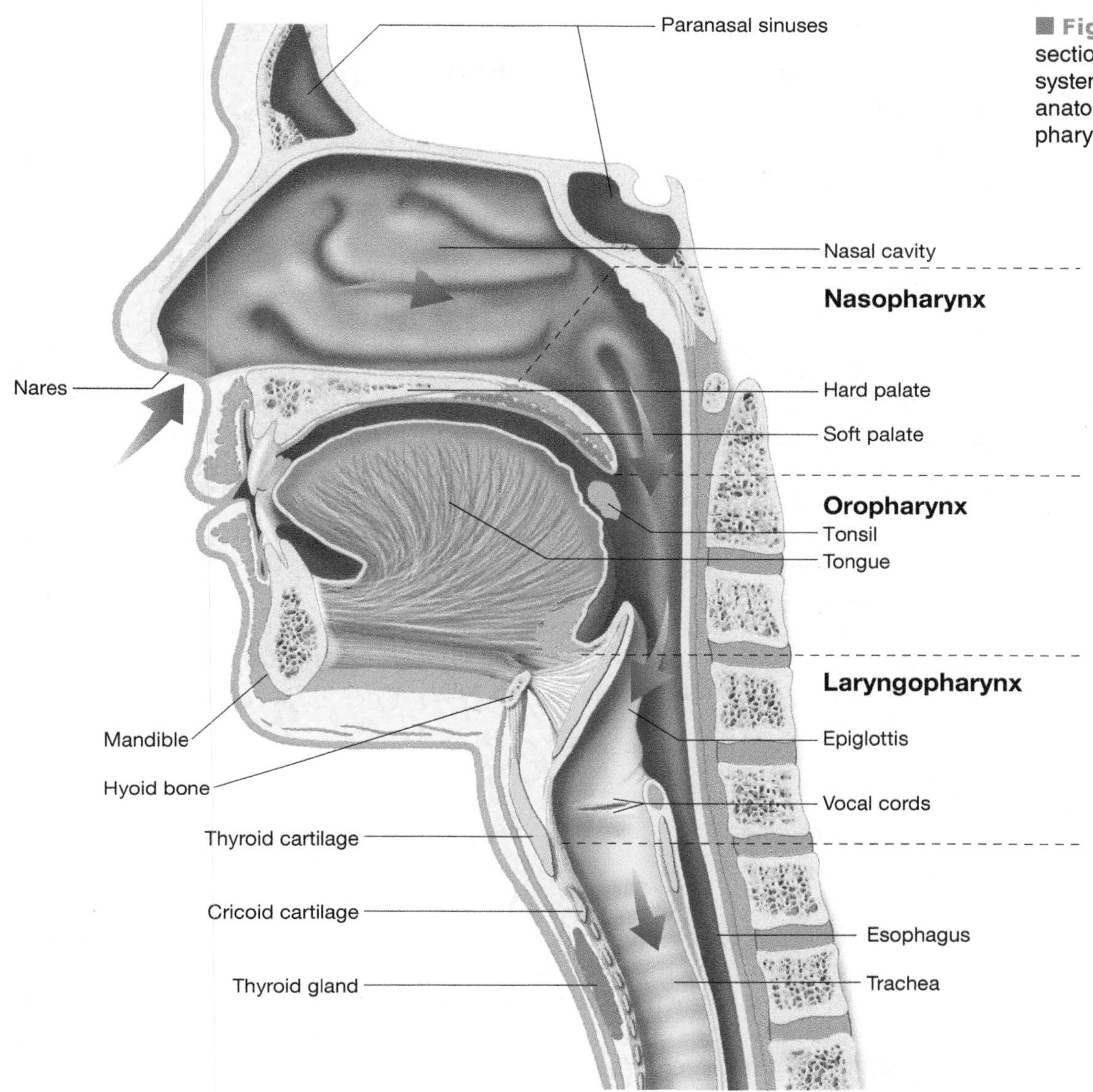

■ **Figure 7.1** Sagittal section of upper respiratory system illustrating the internal anatomy of the nasal cavity, pharynx, larynx, and trachea.

covered with mucous membrane, which secretes a sticky fluid, **mucus,** to help cleanse the air by trapping dust and bacteria. Since this membrane is also wet, it moisturizes inhaled air as it passes by the surface of the cavity. Very small hairs or **cilia** line the opening to the nose (as well as much of the airways), and filter out large dirt particles before they can enter the lungs. Capillaries in the mucous membranes warm inhaled air as it passes through the airways. Additionally, several **paranasal sinuses,** or air-filled cavities, are located within the facial bones. The sinuses act as an echo chamber during sound production and give resonance to the voice.

MED TERM TIP

Word Watch: The term *cilia* means hair, and there are other body systems that have cilia or cilia-like processes. For example, when discussing the eye, *cilia* means eyelashes.

Pharynx

adenoids (ADD-eh-noydz)
auditory tube
eustachian tube (yoo-STAY-she-en)
laryngopharynx (lair-ring-goh-FAIR-inks)
lingual tonsils (LING-gwal)
nasopharynx (nay-zoh-FAIR-inks)
oropharynx (or-oh-FAIR-inks)
palatine tonsils (PAL-ah-tine)
pharyngeal tonsils (fair-IN-jee-al)

Air next enters the pharynx, also called the *throat*, which is used by both the respiratory and digestive systems. At the end of the pharynx, air enters the trachea while food and liquids are shunted into the esophagus.

The pharynx is roughly a 5-inch-long tube consisting of three parts: the upper **nasopharynx,** middle **oropharynx,** and lower **laryngopharynx** (see again Figure 7.1). Three pairs of tonsils (collections of lymphatic tissue) are located in the pharynx. Tonsils are strategically placed to help keep pathogens from entering the body through either the air breathed or food and liquid swallowed. The nasopharynx, behind the nose, contains the **adenoids** or **pharyngeal tonsils.** The oropharynx, behind the mouth, contains the **palatine tonsils** and the **lingual tonsils.** Tonsils are considered a part of the lymphatic system.

The opening of the **eustachian** or **auditory tube** is also found in the nasopharynx. The other end of this tube is in the middle ear. Each time you swallow, this tube opens to equalize air pressure between the middle ear and the outside atmosphere.

MED TERM TIP

In the early 1970s it was common practice to remove the tonsils and adenoids in children suffering from repeated infections. However, it is now understood how important these organs are to remove pathogens from the air we breathe and the food we eat. Antibiotic treatment has also reduced the severity of infections.

Larynx

epiglottis (ep-ih-GLOT-iss)
glottis (GLOT-iss)
thyroid cartilage (THIGH-royd / CAR-tih-lij)
vocal cords

The larynx, or *voice box,* is a muscular structure located between the pharynx and the trachea and contains the **vocal cords** (see again Figure 7.1 and Figure 7.2 ■). The vocal cords are not actually cordlike in structure, but rather they are folds of membranous tissue that produce sound by vibrating as air passes through the **glottis,** the opening between the two vocal cords.

MED TERM TIP

Stuttering may actually result from faulty neuromuscular control of the larynx. Some stutterers can sing or whisper without difficulty. Both singing and whispering involve movements of the larynx that differ from those required for regular speech.

A flap of cartilaginous tissue, the **epiglottis,** sits above the glottis and provides protection against food and liquid being inhaled into the lungs. The epiglottis covers the larynx and trachea during swallowing and shunts food and liquid from the pharynx into the esophagus. The walls of the larynx are composed of several cartilage plates held together with ligaments and muscles. One of these cartilages, the **thyroid cartilage,** forms what is known as the *Adam's apple.* The thyroid cartilage is generally larger in males than in females and helps to produce the deeper male voice.

MED TERM TIP

The term *Adam's apple* is thought to come from a fable that when Adam realized he had sinned in the Garden of Eden, he was unable to swallow the apple in his throat.

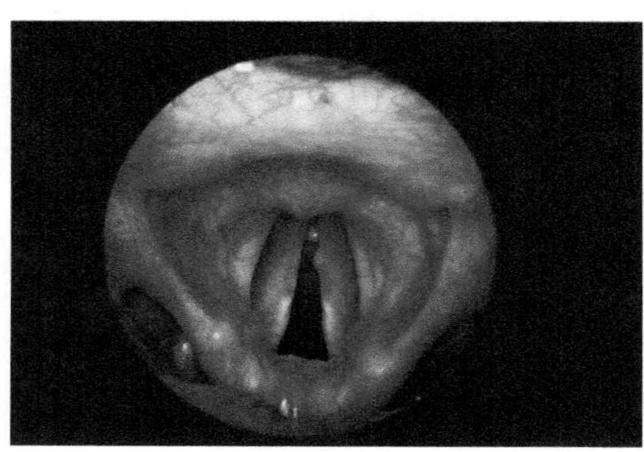

■ **Figure 7.2** The vocal cords within the larynx, superior view from the pharynx. *(CNRI/Photo Researchers, Inc.)*

Trachea

The trachea, also called the *windpipe,* is the passageway for air that extends from the pharynx and larynx down to the main bronchi (see Figure 7.3 ■). Measuring approximately 4 inches in length, it is composed of smooth muscle and cartilage rings and is lined by mucous membrane and cilia. Therefore, it also assists in cleansing, warming, and moisturizing air as it travels to the lungs.

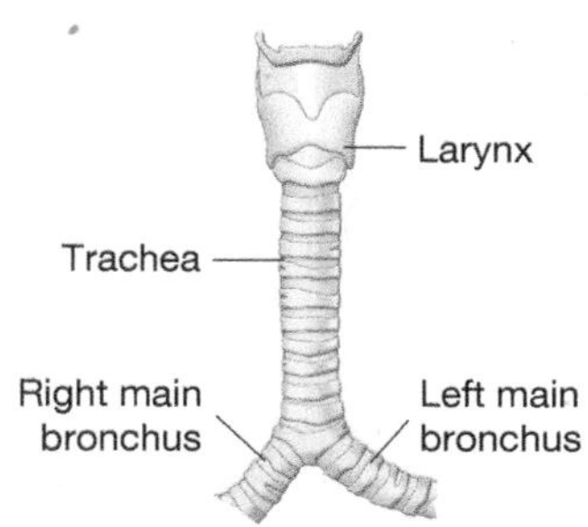

■ **Figure 7.3** Structure of the trachea, which extends from the larynx above to the main bronchi below.

Bronchial Tubes

alveoli (al-VEE-oh-lye)
bronchioles (BRONG-key-ohlz)
bronchus (BRONG-kus)
pulmonary capillaries
respiratory membrane

The distal end of the trachea divides to form the left and right main (primary) bronchi. Each **bronchus** enters one of the lungs and branches repeatedly to form secondary and tertiary bronchi. Each branch becomes narrower until the narrowest branches, the **bronchioles,** are formed (see Figure 7.4 ■). Each bronchiole terminates in a small group of air sacs, called **alveoli.** Each lung has approximately 150 million alveoli. The walls of alveoli are elastic, giving them the ability to expand to hold air and then recoil to their original size. A network of **pulmonary capillaries** from the pulmonary blood vessels tightly encases each alveolus (see Figure 7.5 ■). In fact, the walls of the alveoli and capillaries are so tightly associated with each other they are referred to as a single unit, the **respiratory membrane.** The exchange of oxygen and carbon dioxide between the air within the alveolus and the blood inside the capillaries takes place across the respiratory membrane.

MED TERM TIP

The respiratory system can be thought of as an upside-down tree and its branches. The trunk of the tree consists of the pharynx, larynx, and trachea. The trachea then divides into two branches, the bronchi. Each bronchus divides into smaller and smaller branches. In fact, this branching system of tubes is referred to as the *bronchial tree.*

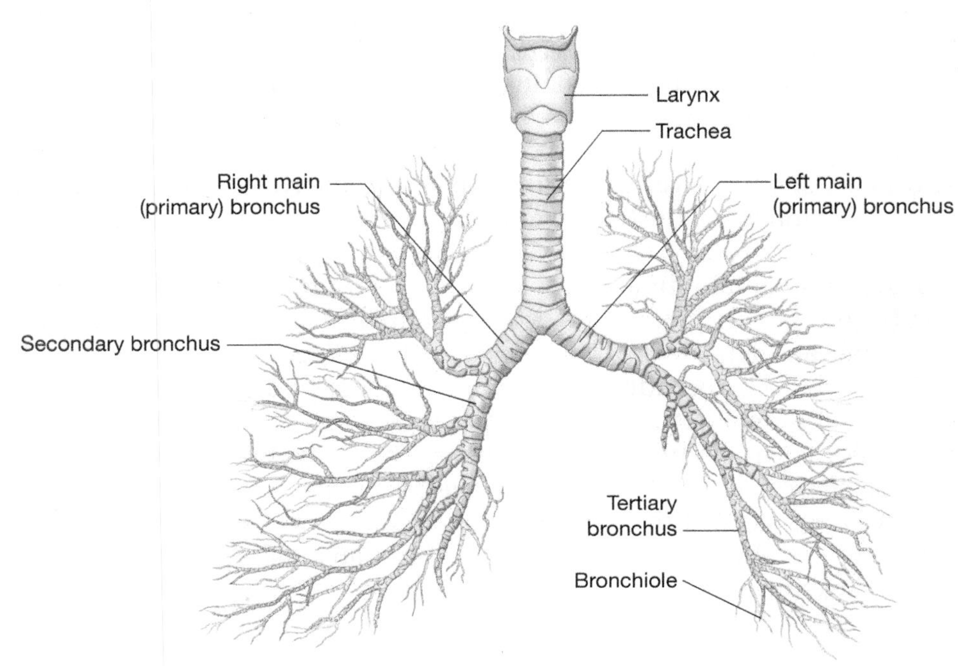

■ **Figure 7.4** The bronchial tree. Note how each main bronchus enters a lung and then branches into smaller and smaller primary bronchi, secondary bronchi, and bronchioles.

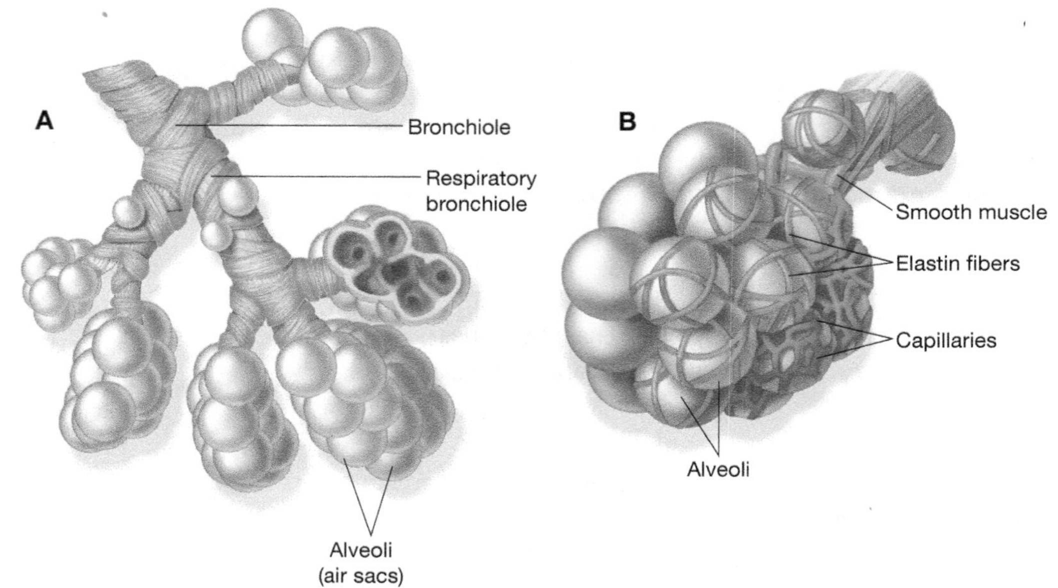

■ **Figure 7.5** (A) Each bronchiole terminates in an alveolar sac, a group of alveoli; (B) alveoli encased by network capillaries, forming the respiratory membrane.

Lungs

apex
base
hilum (HYE-lum)
lobes
mediastinum (mee-dee-ass-TYE-num)
parietal pleura (pah-RYE-eh-tal)
pleura (PLOO-rah)
pleural cavity
serous fluid (SEER-us)
visceral pleura (VISS-er-al)

Each lung is the total collection of the bronchi, bronchioles, and alveoli. They are spongy to the touch because they contain air. The lungs are protected by a double membrane called the **pleura.** The pleura's outer membrane is the **parietal pleura,** which also lines the wall of the chest cavity. The inner membrane, or **visceral pleura,** adheres to the surface of the lungs. The pleural membrane is folded in such a way that it forms a sac around each lung, referred to as the **pleural cavity.** There is normally slippery, watery **serous fluid** between the two layers of the pleura that reduces friction when the two layers rub together as the lungs repeatedly expand and contract.

MED TERM TIP

Some of the abnormal lung sounds heard with a stethoscope, such as crackling and rubbing, are made when the parietal and/or visceral pleura become inflamed and rub against one another.

The lungs contain divisions or **lobes.** There are three lobes in the larger right lung (right upper, right middle, and right lower lobes) and two in the left lung (left upper and left lower lobes). The pointed superior portion of each lung is the **apex,** while the broader lower area is the **base.** Entry of structures like the bronchi, pulmonary blood vessels, and nerves into each lung occurs along its medial border in an area called the **hilum.** The lungs within the thoracic cavity are protected from puncture and damage by the ribs. The area between the right and left lung is called the **mediastinum** and contains the heart, aorta, esophagus, thymus gland, and trachea. See Figure 7.6 ■ for an illustration of the lungs within the chest cavity.

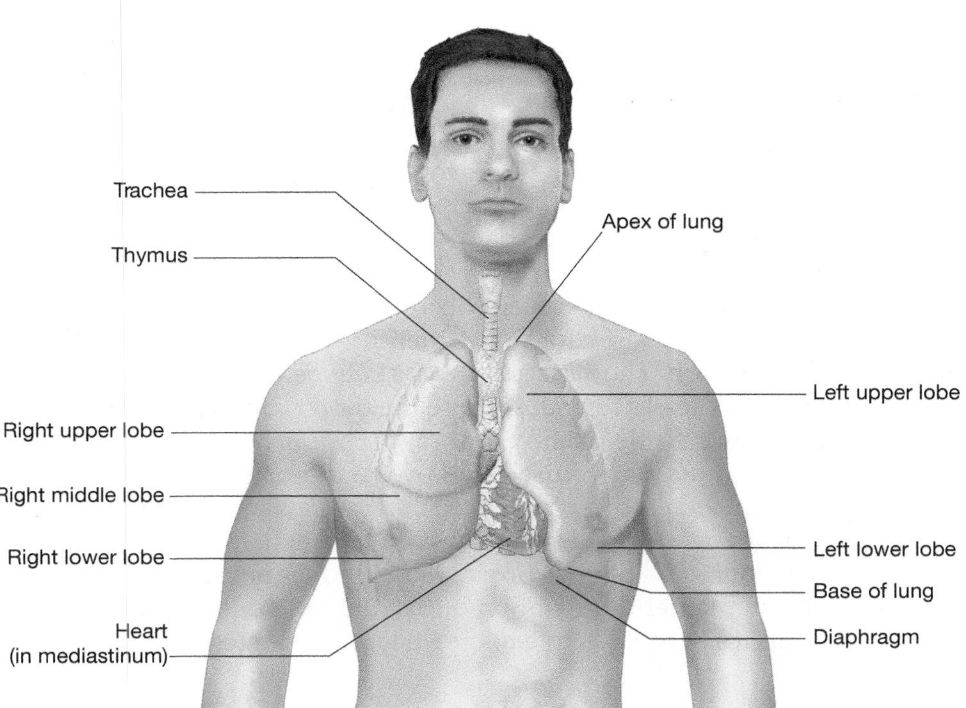

■ **Figure 7.6** Position of the lungs within the thoracic cavity; anterior view illustrating regions of the lungs and their relationship to other thoracic organs.

Lung Volumes and Capacities

pulmonary function test **respiratory therapist**

For some types of medical conditions, like emphysema, it is important to measure the volume of air flowing in and out of the lungs to determine lung capacity. Lung volumes are measured by **respiratory therapists** to aid in determining the functioning level of the respiratory system. Collectively, these measurements are called **pulmonary function tests.** Table 7.1 ■ lists and defines the four lung volumes and four lung capacities.

Table 7.1 Lung Volumes and Capacities

TERM	DEFINITION
Tidal volume (TV)	The amount of air that enters the lungs in a single inhalation or leaves the lungs in a single exhalation of quiet breathing. In an adult this is normally 500 mL.*
Inspiratory reserve volume (IRV)	The amount of air that can be forcibly inhaled after a normal inspiration. Also called *complemental air;* generally measures around 3,000 mL.*
Expiratory reserve volume (ERV)	The amount of air that can be forcibly exhaled after a normal quiet exhalation. This is also called *supplemental air;* approximately 1,000 mL.*
Residual volume (RV)	The air remaining in the lungs after a forced exhalation; about 1,500 mL* in the adult.
Inspiratory capacity (IC)	The volume of air inhaled after a normal exhale.
Functional residual capacity (FRC)	The air that remains in the lungs after a normal exhalation has taken place.
Vital capacity (VC)	The total volume of air that can be exhaled after a maximum inhalation. This amount will be equal to the sum of TV, IRV, and ERV.
Total lung capacity (TLC)	The volume of air in the lungs after a maximal inhalation.

*There is a normal range for measurements of the volume of air exchanged. The numbers given are for the average measurement.

Respiratory Muscles

diaphragm **intercostal muscles** (in-ter-COS-tal)

Air moves in and out of the lungs due to the difference between the atmospheric pressure and the pressure within the chest cavity. The **diaphragm,** the muscle separating the abdomen from the thoracic cavity, produces this difference in pressure. To do this, the diaphragm contracts and moves downward. This increase in thoracic cavity volume causes a decrease in pressure, or negative thoracic pressure, within the chest cavity. Air then flows into the lungs (inhalation) to equalize the pressure. The **intercostal muscles** between the ribs assist in inhalation by raising the rib cage to further enlarge the thoracic cavity. See Figure 7.7 ■ for an illustration of the role of the diaphragm in inhalation. Similarly, when the diaphragm and intercostal muscles relax, the thoracic cavity becomes smaller. This produces an increase in pressure within the cavity, or positive thoracic pressure, and air flows out of the lungs, resulting in exhalation. Therefore, a quiet, unforced exhalation is a passive process since it does not require any muscle contraction. When a forceful inhalation or exhalation is required, additional chest and neck muscles become active to create larger changes in thoracic pressure.

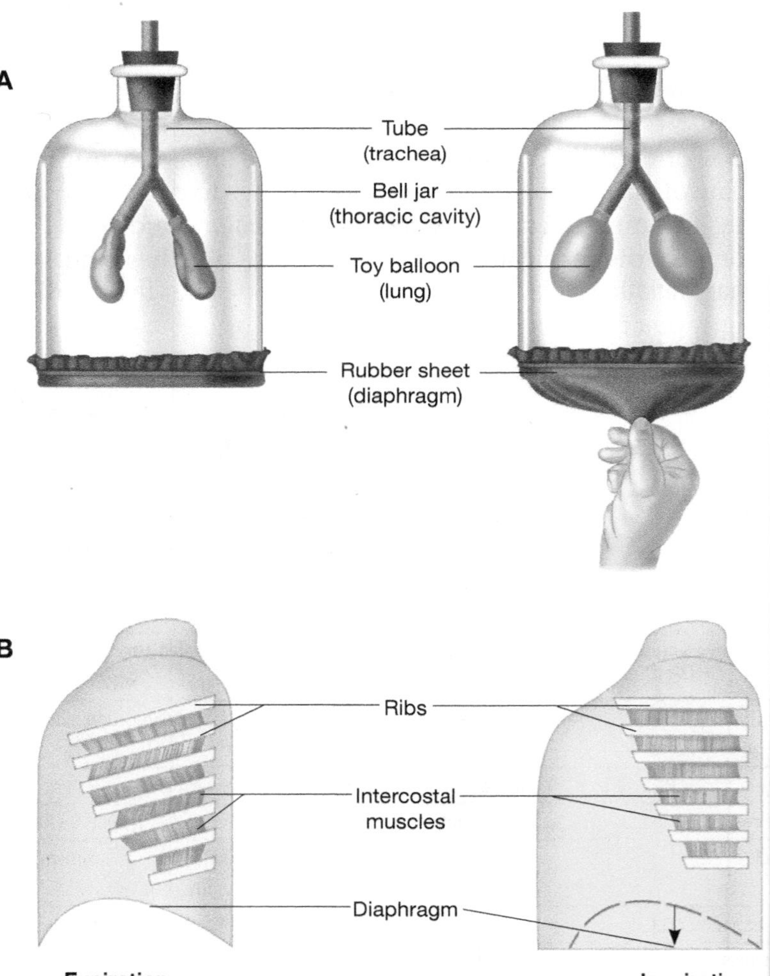

■ **Figure 7.7** (A) Bell jar apparatus demonstrating how downward movement of the diaphragm results in air flowing into the lungs; (B) action of the intercostal muscles lifts the ribs to assist the diaphragm in enlarging the volume of the thoracic cavity.

Respiratory Rate

vital signs

Respiratory rate (measured in breaths per minute) is one of our **vital signs** (VS), along with heart rate, temperature, and blood pressure. The respiratory rate is normally regulated by the level of CO_2 in the blood. When the CO_2 level is high, we breathe more rapidly to expel the excess. Likewise, when CO_2 levels drop, our respiratory rate will also drop.

When the respiratory rate falls outside the range of normal, it may indicate an illness or medical condition. For example, when a patient is running an elevated temperature and has shortness of breath (SOB) due to pneumonia, the respiratory rate may increase dramatically. Or a brain injury or some medications, such as those for pain, can cause a decrease in the respiratory rate. See Table 7.2 ■ for normal respiratory rate ranges for different age groups.

MED TERM TIP

Diaphragmatic breathing is taught to singers and public speakers. You can practice this type of breathing by allowing your abdomen to expand during inhalation and contract during exhalation while your shoulders remain motionless.

MED TERM TIP

When divers wish to hold their breath longer, they first hyperventilate (breath faster and deeper) in order to get rid of as much CO_2 as possible. This will hold off the urge to breathe longer, allowing a diver to stay submerged longer.

Table 7.2 Respiratory Rates for Different Age Groups

AGE	RESPIRATIONS PER MINUTE
Newborn	30–60
1-year-old	18–30
16-year-old	16–20
Adult	12–20

Terminology

Word Parts Used to Build Respiratory System Terms

The following lists contain the combining forms, suffixes, and prefixes used to build terms in the remaining sections of this chapter.

Combining Forms

aer/o	air
alveol/o	alveolus
angi/o	vessel
anthrac/o	coal
arteri/o	artery
atel/o	incomplete
bi/o	life
bronch/o	bronchus
bronchi/o	bronchus
bronchiol/o	bronchiole
carcin/o	cancer
cardi/o	heart
coni/o	dust
cortic/o	outer region, cortex
cyan/o	blue
cyst/o	cyst, bladder

cyt/o	cell
diaphragmat/o	diaphragm
embol/o	plug
epiglott/o	epiglottis
fibr/o	fibers
hem/o	blood
hist/o	tissue
laryng/o	larynx
lob/o	lobe
muc/o	mucus
nas/o	nose
orth/o	straight
ot/o	ear
ox/i	oxygen
ox/o	oxygen

pharyng/o	pharynx
pleur/o	pleura
pneum/o	air
pneumon/o	lung
pulmon/o	lung
py/o	pus
rhin/o	nose
sept/o	wall
sinus/o	sinus
somn/o	sleep
spir/o	breathing
thorac/o	chest
trache/o	trachea
tuss/o	cough

Suffixes

-al	pertaining to
-algia	pain
-ar	pertaining to
-ary	pertaining to
-capnia	carbon dioxide
-centesis	puncture to withdraw fluid
-dynia	pain
-eal	pertaining to
-ectasis	dilation
-ectomy	surgical removal
-emia	blood condition
-genic	produced by
-gram	record
-graphy	process of recording
-ia	condition

-ial	pertaining to
-ic	pertaining to
-ism	state of
-itis	inflammation
-logy	study of
-lytic	destruction
-meter	instrument to measure
-metry	process of measuring
-oma	tumor
-osis	abnormal condition
-osmia	smell
-ostomy	surgically create an opening
-otomy	cutting into
-phonia	voice

-plasm	formation
-plasty	surgical repair
-plegia	paralysis
-pnea	breathing
-ptysis	spitting
-rrhagia	abnormal flow condition
-rrhea	discharge
-scope	instrument for viewing
-scopy	process of visually examining
-spasm	involuntary muscle spasm
-stenosis	narrowing
-thorax	chest
-tic	pertaining to

Prefixes

a-	without
an-	without
anti-	against
brady-	slow
de-	without

dys-	abnormal, difficult
endo-	within
eu-	normal
hyper-	excessive

hypo-	insufficient
pan-	all
poly-	many
tachy-	fast

Anatomical Terms

TERM	WORD PARTS	DEFINITION
alveolar (al-VEE-oh-lar)	alveol/o = alveolus -ar = pertaining to	Pertaining to the alveoli.
bronchial (BRONG-ee-all)	bronch/o = bronchus -ial = pertaining to	Pertaining to a bronchus.
bronchiolar (brong-KEY-oh-lar)	bronchiol/o = bronchiole -ar = pertaining to	Pertaining to a bronchiole.
diaphragmatic (dye-ah-frag-MAT-ik)	diaphragmat/o = diaphragm -ic = pertaining to	Pertaining to the diaphragm.
epiglottic (ep-ih-GLOT-ik)	epiglott/o = epiglottis -ic = pertaining to	Pertaining to the epiglottis.
laryngeal (lair-in-GEE-all)	laryng/o = larynx -eal = pertaining to	Pertaining to the larynx.

Anatomical Terms *(continued)*

TERM	WORD PARTS	DEFINITION
nasal (NAY-zal)	nas/o = nose -al = pertaining to	Pertaining to the nose or nasal cavity.
pharyngeal (fair-in-GEE-all)	pharyng/o = pharynx -eal = pertaining to	Pertaining to the pharynx.
pleural (PLOO-ral)	pleur/o = pleura -al = pertaining to	Pertaining to the pleura.
pulmonary (PULL-mon-air-ee)	pulmon/o = lung -ary = pertaining to	Pertaining to the lung.
septal (SEP-tal)	sept/o = wall -al = pertaining to	Pertaining to the nasal septum.
thoracic (tho-RASS-ik)	thorac/o = chest -ic = pertaining to	Pertaining to the chest.
tracheal (TRAY-key-al)	trache/o = trachea -al = pertaining to	Pertaining to the trachea.

Pathology

TERM	WORD PARTS	DEFINITION
Medical Specialties		
internal medicine		Branch of medicine involving the diagnosis and treatment of diseases and conditions of internal organs such as the respiratory system. The physician is an *internist.*
otorhinolaryngology (ENT) (oh-toh-rye-noh-lair-in-GOL-oh-jee)	ot/o = ear rhin/o = nose laryng/o = larynx -logy = study of	Branch of medicine involving the diagnosis and treatment of conditions and diseases of the ear, nose, and throat region. The physician is an *otorhinolaryngologist.* This medical specialty may also be referred to as *otolaryngology.*
pulmonology (pull-mon-ALL-oh-jee)	pulmon/o = lung -logy = study of	Branch of medicine involved in the diagnosis and treatment of diseases and disorders of the respiratory system. Physician is a *pulmonologist.*
respiratory therapy	spir/o = breathing	Allied health specialty that assists patients with respiratory and cardiopulmonary disorders. Duties of a *respiratory therapist* include conducting pulmonary function tests, monitoring oxygen and carbon dioxide levels in the blood, administering breathing treatments, and ventilator management.
thoracic surgery (tho-RASS-ik)	thorac/o = chest -ic = pertaining to	Branch of medicine involving the diagnosis and treatment of conditions and diseases of the respiratory system by surgical means. Physician is a *thoracic surgeon.*

Pathology *(continued)*

TERM	WORD PARTS	DEFINITION
Signs and Symptoms		
anosmia (ah-NOZ-mee-ah)	an- = without -osmia = smell	Lack of the sense of smell.
anoxia (ah-NOK-see-ah)	an- = without ox/o = oxygen -ia = condition	Condition of receiving almost no oxygen from inhaled air.
aphonia (a-FOH-nee-ah)	a- = without -phonia = voice	Condition of being unable to produce sounds.
apnea (AP-nee-ah)	a- = without -pnea = breathing	Not breathing.
asphyxia (as-FIK-see-ah)	a- = without -ia = condition	Lack of oxygen that can lead to unconsciousness and death if not corrected immediately; also called *asphyxiation* or *suffocation.* Common causes include drowning, foreign body in the respiratory tract, poisoning, and electric shock.
aspiration (as-peer-RAY-shun)	spir/o = breathing	Refers to withdrawing fluid from a body cavity using suction. For example, using a long needle and syringe to withdraw fluid from the pleural cavity, or using a vacuum pump to remove phlegm from a patient's airways. Additionally, it refers to inhaling food, liquid, or a foreign object into the airways, which may lead to the development of pneumonia.
bradypnea (bray-DIP-nee-ah)	brady- = slow -pnea = breathing	Breathing too slowly; a low respiratory rate.
bronchiectasis (brong-key-EK-tah-sis)	bronchi/o = bronchus -ectasis = dilation	Dilated bronchus.
bronchospasm (BRONG-koh-spazm)	bronch/o = bronchus -spasm = involuntary muscle spasm	Involuntary muscle spasm of the smooth muscle in the wall of the bronchus.
Cheyne–Stokes respiration (CHAIN / STOHKS / res-pir-AY-shun)	spir/o = breathing	Abnormal breathing pattern in which there are long periods (10–60 seconds) of apnea followed by deeper, more rapid breathing. Named for John Cheyne, a Scottish physician, and Sir William Stokes, an Irish surgeon.
clubbing		Abnormal widening and thickening of the ends of the fingers and toes associated with chronic oxygen deficiency. Seen in patients with chronic respiratory conditions or circulatory problems.
crackles		Abnormal sound made during inspiration. Usually indicates the presence of fluid or mucus in the small airways. Also called *rales.*

Pathology *(continued)*

TERM	WORD PARTS	DEFINITION
cyanosis (sigh-ah-NO-sis)	cyan/o = blue -osis = abnormal condition	Refers to the bluish tint of skin that is receiving an insufficient amount of oxygen or circulation.
dysphonia (dis-FOH-nee-ah)	dys- = difficult, abnormal -phonia = voice	Condition of having difficulty producing sounds or producing abnormal sounds.
dyspnea (DISP-nee-ah)	dys- = abnormal, difficult -pnea = breathing	Term describing difficult or labored breathing.
epistaxis (ep-ih-STAKS-is)		Nosebleed.
eupnea (yoop-NEE-ah)	eu- = normal -pnea = breathing	Normal breathing and respiratory rate.
hemoptysis (hee-MOP-tih-sis)	hem/o = blood -ptysis = spitting	To cough up blood or blood-stained sputum.
hemothorax (hee-moh-THOH-raks)	hem/o = blood -thorax = chest	Presence of blood in the chest cavity.
hypercapnia (high-per-CAP-nee-ah)	hyper- = excessive -capnia = carbon dioxide	Condition of having excessive carbon dioxide in the body.
hyperpnea (high-per-NEE-ah)	hyper- = excessive -pnea = breathing	Taking deep breaths.
hyperventilation (HYE-per-vent-ill-a-shun)	hyper- = excessive	Breathing both too fast (tachypnea) and too deep (hyperpnea).
hypocapnia (high-poh-CAP-nee-ah)	hypo- = insufficient -capnia = carbon dioxide	An insufficient level of carbon dioxide in the body; a very serious problem because it is the presence of carbon dioxide that stimulates respiration, not the absence of oxygen. Therefore, a person with low carbon dioxide levels would respond with an increased respiratory rate.
hypopnea (high-POP-nee-ah)	hypo- = insufficient -pnea = breathing	Taking shallow breaths.
hypoventilation (HYE-poh-vent-ill-a-shun)	hypo- = insufficient	Breathing both too slow (bradypnea) and too shallow (hypopnea).
hypoxemia (high-pox-EE-mee-ah)	hypo- = insufficient ox/o = oxygen -emia = blood condition	Condition of having an insufficient amount of oxygen in the bloodstream.
hypoxia (high-POX-ee-ah)	hypo- = insufficient ox/o = oxygen -ia = condition	Condition of receiving an insufficient amount of oxygen from inhaled air.
laryngoplegia (lair-RING-goh-plee-gee-ah)	laryng/o = larynx -plegia = paralysis	Paralysis of the muscles controlling the larynx.

Pathology *(continued)*

TERM	WORD PARTS	DEFINITION
orthopnea (or-THOP-nee-ah)	orth/o = straight -pnea = breathing	Term describing dyspnea that is worsened by lying flat. The patient feels able to breath easier while sitting straight up; a common occurrence in those with pulmonary disease.
pansinusitis (pan-sigh-nus-EYE-tis)	pan- = all sinus/o = sinus -itis = inflammation	Inflammation of all the paranasal sinuses.
patent (PAY-tent)		Open or unblocked, such as a patent airway.
phlegm (FLEM)		Thick mucus secreted by the membranes lining the respiratory tract. When phlegm is coughed through the mouth, it is called *sputum.* Phlegm is examined for color, odor, and consistency and tested for the presence of bacteria, viruses, and fungi.
pleural rub (PLOO-ral)	pleur/o = pleura -al = pertaining to	Grating sound made when the two layers of the pleura rub together during respiration. It is caused when one of the surfaces becomes thicker as a result of inflammation or other disease conditions. This rub can be felt through the fingertips when placed on the chest wall or heard through a stethoscope.
pleurodynia (ploor-oh-DIN-ee-ah)	pleur/o = pleura -dynia = pain	Pleural pain.
pyothorax (pye-oh-THOH-raks)	py/o = pus -thorax = chest	Presence of pus in the chest cavity; indicates a bacterial infection.
rhinitis (rye-NYE-tis)	rhin/o = nose -itis = inflammation	Inflammation of the nasal cavity.
rhinorrhagia (rye-noh-RAH-jee-ah)	rhin/o = nose -rrhagia = abnormal flow condition	Rapid flow of blood from the nose.
rhinorrhea (rye-noh-REE-ah)	rhin/o = nose -rrhea = discharge	Discharge from the nose; commonly called a *runny nose.*
rhonchi (RONG-kigh)		Somewhat musical sound during expiration, often found in asthma or infection. Caused by spasms of the bronchial tubes. Also called *wheezing.*
shortness of breath (SOB)		Term used to indicate that a patient is having some difficulty breathing; also called *dyspnea.* The causes can range from mild SOB after exercise to SOB associated with heart disease.
sputum (SPEW-tum)		Mucus or phlegm coughed up from the lining of the respiratory tract.

MED TERM TIP

The term *sputum,* from the Latin word meaning "to spit," now refers to the material coughed up and spit out from the respiratory system.

Pathology *(continued)*

TERM	WORD PARTS	DEFINITION
stridor (STRIGH-dor)		Harsh, high-pitched, noisy breathing sound made when there is an obstruction of the bronchus or larynx. Found in conditions such as croup in children.
tachypnea (tak-ip-NEE-ah)	tachy- = fast -pnea = breathing	Breathing fast; a high respiratory rate.
thoracalgia (thor-ah-KAL-jee-ah)	thorac/o = chest -algia = pain	Chest pain. Does not refer to angina pectoris.
tracheostenosis (tray-kee-oh-steh-w-sis)	trache/o = trachea -stenosis = narrowing	Narrowing of the trachea.
Upper Respiratory System		
croup (KROOP)		Acute respiratory condition found in infants and children characterized by a barking type of cough or stridor.
diphtheria (dif-THEAR-ee-ah)	-ia = condition	Bacterial upper respiratory infection characterized by the formation of a thick membranous film across the throat and a high mortality rate. Rare now due to the DPT (diphtheria, pertussis, tetanus) vaccine.
laryngitis (lair-in-JYE-tis)	laryng/o = larynx -itis = inflammation	Inflammation of the larynx.
nasopharyngitis (nay-zoh-fair-in-JYE-tis)	nas/o = nose pharyng/o = pharynx -itis = inflammation	Inflammation of the nasal cavity and pharynx; commonly called the *common cold.*
pertussis (per-TUH-is)	tuss/o = cough	Commonly called *whooping cough,* due to the whoop sound made when coughing. An infectious bacterial disease of the upper respiratory system that children receive immunization against as part of their DPT shots.
pharyngitis (fair-in-JYE-tis)	pharyng/o = pharynx -itis = inflammation	Inflammation of the pharynx; commonly called a *sore throat.*
rhinomycosis (rye-noh-my-KOH-sis)	rhin/o = nose myc/o = fungus -osis = abnormal condition	Fungal infection of the nasal cavity.
Bronchial Tubes		
asthma (AZ-mah)		Disease caused by various conditions, like allergens, and resulting in constriction of the bronchial airways, dyspnea, coughing, and wheezing. Can cause violent spasms of the bronchi (bronchospasms) but is generally not a life-threatening condition. Medication can be very effective.

MED TERM TIP

The term *asthma,* from the Greek word meaning "panting," describes the breathing pattern of a person having an asthma attack.

Pathology *(continued)*

TERM	WORD PARTS	DEFINITION
bronchiectasis (brong-key-EK-tah-sis)	bronchi/o = bronchus -ectasis = dilation	Abnormal enlargement of bronchi; may be the result of a lung infection. This condition can be irreversible and result in destruction of the bronchial walls. Major symptoms include coughing up a large amount of purulent sputum, crackles, and hemoptysis.
bronchitis (brong-KIGH-tis)	bronch/o = bronchus -itis = inflammation	Inflammation of a bronchus.
bronchogenic carcinoma (brong-koh-JEN-ik / car-sin-OH-mah)	bronch/o = bronchus -genic = produced by carcin/o = cancer -oma = tumor	Malignant tumor originating in the bronchi. Usually associated with a history of cigarette smoking.

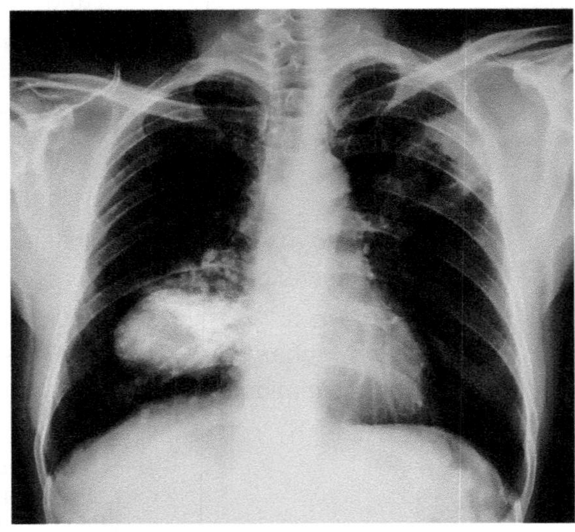

■ **Figure 7.8** Color-enhanced X-ray of large malignant tumor in the right lung.

TERM	WORD PARTS	DEFINITION
Lungs		
adult respiratory distress syndrome (ARDS)	spir/o = breathing -al = pertaining to	Acute respiratory failure in adults characterized by tachypnea, dyspnea, cyanosis, tachycardia, and hypoxemia. May follow trauma, pneumonia, or septic infections. Also called *acute respiratory distress syndrome.*
anthracosis (an-thra-KOH-sis)	anthrac/o = coal -osis = abnormal condition	Type of pneumoconiosis that develops from the collection of coal dust in the lung. Also called *black lung* or *miner's lung.*
asbestosis (az-bes-TOH-sis)	-osis = abnormal condition	Type of pneumoconiosis that develops from collection of asbestos fibers in the lungs. May lead to the development of lung cancer.

Pathology *(continued)*

TERM	WORD PARTS	DEFINITION
atelectasis (at-eh-LEK-tah-sis)	atel/o = incomplete -ectasis = dilation	Condition in which the alveoli in a portion of the lung collapse, preventing the respiratory exchange of oxygen and carbon dioxide. Can be caused by a variety of conditions, including pressure on the lung from a tumor or other object. Term also used to describe the failure of a newborn's lungs to expand.
chronic obstructive pulmonary disease (COPD) (PULL-mon-air-ee)	pulmon/o = lung -ary = pertaining to	Progressive, chronic, and usually irreversible group of conditions, like emphysema, in which the lungs have a diminished capacity for inspiration (inhalation) and expiration (exhalation). The person may have dyspnea upon exertion and a cough.
cystic fibrosis (CF) (SIS-tik / fye-BROH-sis)	cyst/o = cyst, bladder -ic = pertaining to fibr/o = fibers -osis = abnormal condition	Hereditary condition causing the exocrine glands to malfunction. The patient produces very thick mucus that causes severe congestion within the lungs and digestive system. Through more advanced treatment, many children are now living into adulthood with this disease. The term *cystic* in cystic fibrosis refers to cysts that form in the pancreas.
emphysema (em-fih-SEE-mah)		Pulmonary condition characterized by the destruction of the walls of the alveoli, resulting in fewer overexpanded air sacs. Can occur as a result of long-term heavy smoking. Air pollution also worsens this disease. The patient may not be able to breathe except in a sitting or standing position.
histoplasmosis (his-toh-plaz-MOH-sis)	hist/o = tissue -plasm = formation -osis = abnormal condition	Pulmonary infection caused by the fungus *Histoplasma capsulatum,* found in dust and in the droppings of pigeons and chickens. The translation of the name of this condition reflects the microscopic appearance of the fungus.
infant respiratory distress syndrome (IRDS)	spir/o = breathing	Lung condition most commonly found in premature infants that is characterized by tachypnea and respiratory grunting. The condition is caused by a lack of surfactant necessary to keep the lungs inflated. Also called *hyaline membrane disease* (HMD) and *respiratory distress syndrome of the newborn.*
influenza (in-floo-EN-za)		Viral infection of the respiratory system characterized by chills, fever, body aches, and fatigue. Commonly called the *flu.*
Legionnaires' disease (lee-jen-AYRZ)		Severe, often fatal bacterial infection characterized by pneumonia and liver and kidney damage. Named after people who came down with it at an American Legion convention in 1976.

Pathology *(continued)*

TERM	WORD PARTS	DEFINITION
***Mycoplasma* pneumonia** (MY-koh-plaz-ma)	myc/o = fungus -plasm = formation	Less severe but longer lasting form of pneumonia caused by the *Mycoplasma pneumoniae* bacteria. Also called *walking pneumonia.* The translation of the name of this condition reflects the microscopic appearance of the bacteria.
pneumoconiosis (noo-moh-koh-nee-OH-sis)	pneum/o = lung coni/o = dust -osis = abnormal condition	Condition that is the result of inhaling environmental particles that become toxic. Can be the result of inhaling coal dust (anthracosis) or asbestos (asbestosis).
pneumocystis pneumonia (PCP) (noo-moh-SIS-tis / new-MOH-nee-ah)	pneum/o = lung cyst/o = cyst, bladder pneumon/o = lung -ia = condition	Pneumonia with a nonproductive cough, very little fever, and dyspnea caused by the fungus *Pneumocystis jiroveci.* An opportunistic infection often seen in those with weakened immune systems, such as AIDS patients.
pneumonia (new-MOH-nee-ah)	pneumon/o = lung -ia = condition	Inflammatory condition of the lung that can be caused by bacteria, viruses, fungi, and aspirated substances. Results in the filling of the alveoli and air spaces with fluid.
pulmonary edema (PULL-mon-air-ee / eh-DEE-mah)	pulmon/o = lung -ary = pertaining to	Condition in which lung tissue retains an excessive amount of fluid, especially in the alveoli. Results in dyspnea.
pulmonary embolism (PULL-mon-air-ee / EM-boh-lizm)	pulmon/o = lung -ary = pertaining to embol/o = plug -ism = state of	Obstruction of the pulmonary artery or one of its branches by an embolus (often a blood clot broken away from another area of the body). May cause an infarct in the lung tissue.
pulmonary fibrosis (fi-BROH-sis)	pulmon/o = lung -ary = pertaining to fibr/o = fibers -osis = abnormal condition	Formation of fibrous scar tissue in the lungs that leads to decreased ability to expand the lungs. May be caused by infections, pneumoconiosis, autoimmune diseases, and toxin exposure.
severe acute respiratory syndrome (SARS)	spir/o = breathing	Acute viral respiratory infection that begins like the flu but quickly progresses to severe dyspnea; high fatality rate. First appeared in China in 2003.
silicosis (sil-ih-KOH-sis)	-osis = abnormal condition	Type of pneumoconiosis that develops from the inhalation of silica (quartz) dust found in quarrying, glass works, sandblasting, and ceramics.
sleep apnea (AP-nee-ah)	a- = without -pnea = breathing	Condition in which breathing stops repeatedly during sleep long enough to cause a drop in oxygen levels in the blood.
sudden infant death syndrome (SIDS)		Unexpected and unexplained death of an apparently well infant under 1 year of age. The child suddenly stops breathing for unknown reasons.

Pathology *(continued)*

TERM	WORD PARTS	DEFINITION
tuberculosis (TB) (too-ber-kyoo-LOH-sis)	-osis = abnormal condition	Infectious disease caused by the bacteria *Mycobacterium tuberculosis.* Most commonly affects the respiratory system and causes inflammation and calcification in the lungs. Tuberculosis incidence is on the increase and is seen in many patients with weakened immune systems. Multidrug-resistant tuberculosis is a particularly dangerous form of the disease because some bacteria have developed a resistance to the standard drug therapy.
Pleural Cavity		
empyema (em-pye-EE-mah)	py/o = pus	Pus with in the pleural space usually associated with a bacterial infection. Also called *pyothorax.*
pleural effusion (PLOO-ral / eh-FYOO-zhun)	pleur/o = pleura -al = pertaining to	Abnormal accumulation of fluid in the pleural cavity preventing the lungs from fully expanding. Physicians can detect the presence of fluid by tapping the chest (percussion) or listening with a stethoscope (auscultation).
pleurisy (PLOOR-ih-see)	pleur/o = pleura	Inflammation of the pleura characterized by sharp chest pain with each breath. Also called *pleuritis.*
pneumothorax (new-moh-THOH-raks)	pneum/o = air -thorax = chest	Collection of air or gas in the pleural cavity, which may result in collapse of the lung.

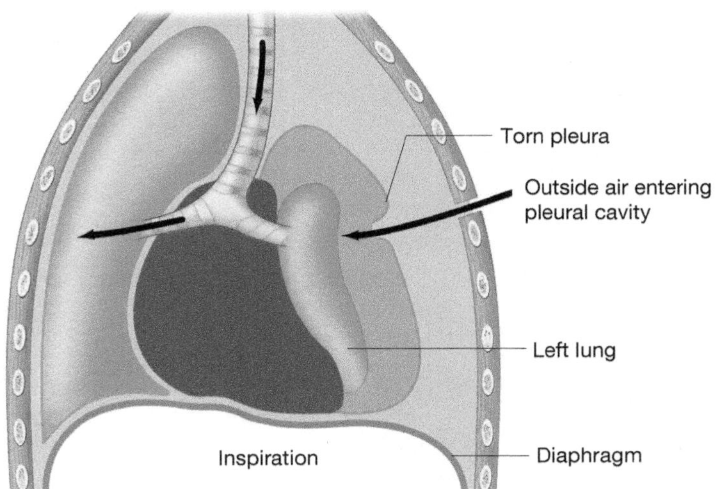

■ **Figure 7.9** Pneumothorax. Figure illustrates how puncture of thoracic wall and tearing of pleural membrane allows air into lung and results in collapsed lung.

Diagnostic Procedures

TERM	WORD PARTS	DEFINITION
Clinical Laboratory Tests		
arterial blood gases (ABGs) (ar-TEE-ree-al)	arteri/o = artery -al = pertaining to	Testing for the gases present in the blood. Generally used to assist in determining the levels of oxygen (O_2) and carbon dioxide (CO_2) in the blood.
sputum culture and sensitivity (C&S) (SPEW-tum)		Testing sputum by placing it on a culture medium and observing any bacterial growth. The specimen is then tested to determine antibiotic effectiveness.
sputum cytology (SPEW-tum / sigh-TALL-oh-jee)	cyt/o = cell -logy = study of	Examining sputum for malignant cells.
Diagnostic Imaging		
bronchogram (BRONG-koh-gram)	bronch/o = bronchus -gram = record	X-ray record of the bronchus produced by bronchography.
bronchography (brong-KOG-rah-fee)	bronch/o = bronchus -graphy = process of recording	X-ray of the lung after a radiopaque substance has been inserted into the trachea or bronchial tube. Resulting X-ray is called a *bronchogram.*
chest X-ray (CXR)		Taking a radiographic picture of the lungs and heart from the back and sides.
pulmonary angiography (PULL-mon-air-ee / an-jee-OG-rah-fee)	pulmon/o = lung -ary = pertaining to angi/o = vessel -graphy = process of recording	Injecting dye into a blood vessel for the purpose of taking an X-ray of the arteries and veins of the lungs.
ventilation-perfusion scan (per-FUSE-shun)		Nuclear medicine diagnostic test that is especially useful in identifying pulmonary emboli. Radioactive air is inhaled for the ventilation portion to determine if air is filling the entire lung. Radioactive intravenous injection shows if blood is flowing to all parts of the lung.
Endoscopic Procedures		
bronchoscope (BRONG-koh-scope)	bronch/o = bronchus -scope = instrument for viewing	Instrument used to view inside a bronchus during a *bronchoscopy.*
bronchoscopy (Bronch) (brong-KOSS-koh-pee)	bronch/o = bronchus -scopy = process of visually examining	Visual examination of the inside of the bronchi; uses an instrument called a *bronchoscope* (see Figure 7.10 ■).
laryngoscope (lair-RING-go-scope)	laryng/o = larynx -scope = instrument for viewing	Instrument used to view inside the larynx during a *laryngoscopy.*
laryngoscopy (lair-in-GOSS-koh-pee)	laryng/o = larynx -scopy = process of visually examining	Examination of the interior of the larynx with a lighted instrument called a *laryngoscope.*

Diagnostic Procedures *(continued)*

TERM	WORD PARTS	DEFINITION
■ **Figure 7.10** Bronchoscopy. Figure illustrates physician using a bronchoscope to inspect the patient's bronchial tubes. Advances in technology include using a videoscope, which projects the internal view of the bronchus onto a video screen.	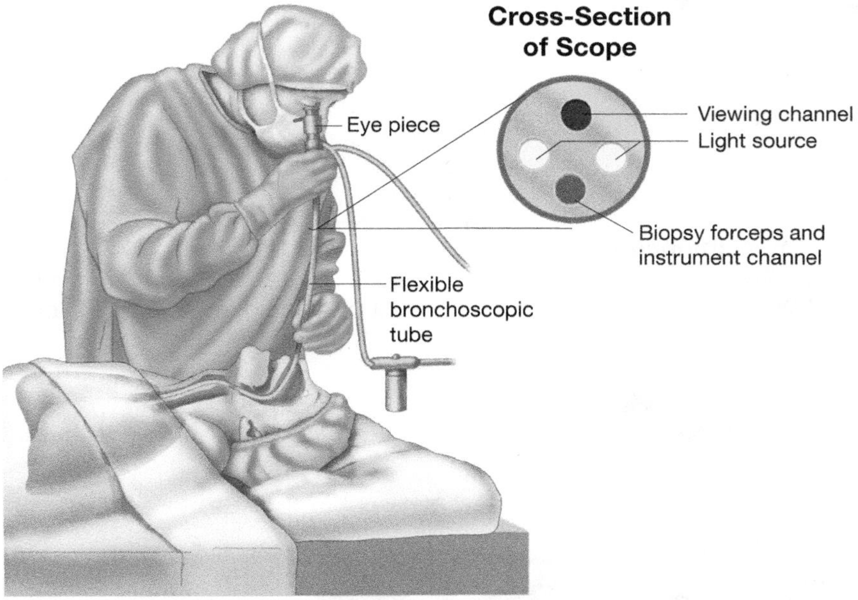	
Pulmonary Function Tests		
oximeter (ox-IM-eh-ter)	ox/i = oxygen -meter = instrument to measure	Instrument that measures the amount of oxygen in the bloodstream.
oximetry (ox-IM-eh-tree)	ox/i = oxygen -metry = process of measuring	Measures the oxygen level in the blood using a device, an *oximeter,* placed on the patient's fingertip or earlobe.
pulmonary function test (PFT) (PULL-mon-air-ee)	pulmon/o = lung -ary = pertaining to	Group of diagnostic tests that give information regarding air flow in and out of the lungs, lung volumes, and gas exchange between the lungs and bloodstream.
spirometer (spy-ROM-eh-ter)	spir/o = breathing -meter = instrument to measure	Instrument to measure lung capacity used for *spirometry.*
spirometry (spy-ROM-eh-tree)	spir/o = breathing -metry = process of measuring	Procedure to measure lung capacity using a *spirometer.*
Additional Diagnostic Procedures		
polysomnography (polly-som-NOG-rah-fee)	poly- = many somn/o = sleep -graphy = process of recording	Monitoring a patient while sleeping to identify sleep apnea. Also called *sleep apnea study.*
sweat test		Test for cystic fibrosis. Patients with this disease have an abnormally large amount of salt in their sweat.
tuberculin skin tests (TB test) (too-BER-kyoo-lin)		Applying the tuberculin purified protein derivative (PPD) under the surface of the skin to determine if the patient has been exposed to tuberculosis. Also called a *Mantoux test.*

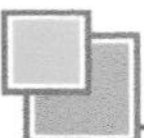

Therapeutic Procedures

TERM	WORD PARTS	DEFINITION
Respiratory Therapy		
aerosol therapy (AIR-oh-sol)	aer/o = air	Medication suspended in a mist intended for inhalation. Delivered by a *nebulizer,* which provides the mist for a period of time while the patient breathes, or a *metered-dose inhaler* (MDI), which delivers a single puff of mist.
endotracheal intubation (en-doh-TRAY-kee-al / in-too-BAY-shun)	endo- = within trache/o = trachea -al = pertaining to	Placing of a tube through the mouth, through the glottis, and into the trachea to create a patent airway.

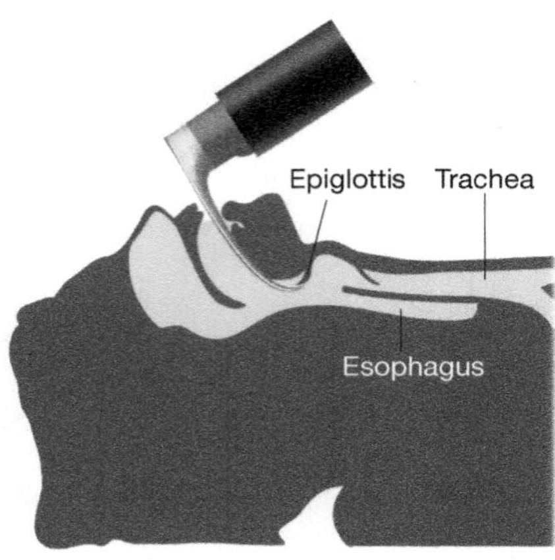

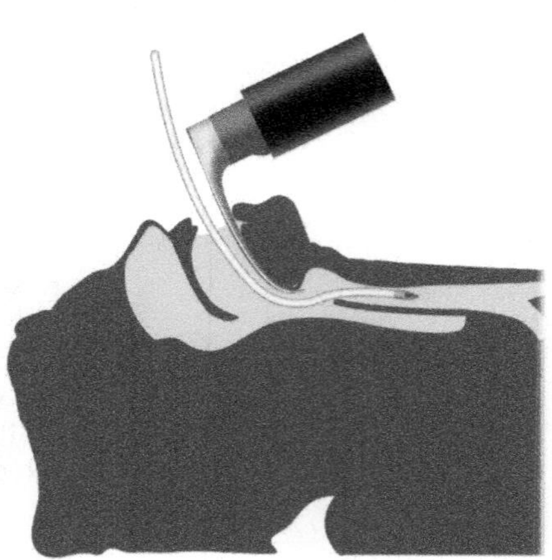

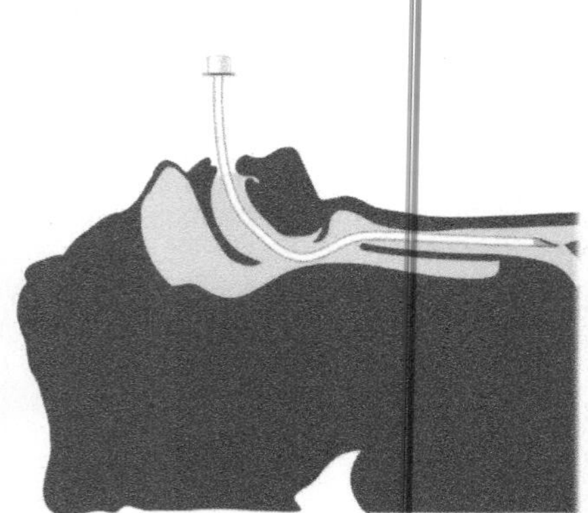

■ **Figure 7.11** Endotracheal intubation. First, a lighted scope is used to identify the trachea from the esophagus. Next, the tube is placed through the pharynx and into the trachea. Finally, the scope is removed, leaving the tube in place.

TERM	WORD PARTS	DEFINITION
intermittent positive pressure breathing (IPPB)		Method for assisting patients in breathing using a mask connected to a machine that produces an increased positive thoracic pressure.
nasal cannula (CAN-you-lah)	nas/o = nose -al = pertaining to	Two-pronged plastic device for delivering oxygen into the nose; one prong is inserted into each naris.
postural drainage	-al = pertaining to	Drainage of secretions from the bronchi by placing the patient in a position that uses gravity to promote drainage. Used for the treatment of cystic fibrosis and bronchiectasis.
supplemental oxygen therapy	-al = pertaining to	Providing a patient with additional concentration of oxygen to improve oxygen levels in the bloodstream. Oxygen may be provided by a mask or nasal cannula.
ventilator (VENT-ih-later)		Machine that provides artificial ventilation for a patient unable to breathe on his or her own. Also called a *respirator.*

Therapeutic Procedures *(continued)*

TERM	WORD PARTS	DEFINITION
Surgical Procedures		
bronchoplasty (BRONG-koh-plas-tee)	bronch/o = bronchus -plasty = surgical repair	Surgical repair of a bronchus.
laryngectomy (lair-in-JEK-toh-mee)	laryng/o = larynx -ectomy = surgical removal	Surgical removal of the larynx.
laryngoplasty (lair-RING-goh-plas-tee)	laryng/o = larynx -plasty = surgical repair	Surgical repair of the larynx.
lobectomy (loh-BEK-toh-mee)	lob/o = lobe -ectomy = surgical removal	Surgical removal of a lobe of a lung.
pleurectomy (ploor-EK-toh-mee)	pleur/o = pleura -ectomy = surgical removal	Surgical removal of the pleura.
pleurocentesis (ploor-oh-sen-TEE-sis)	pleur/o = pleura -centesis = puncture to withdraw fluid	Procedure involving insertion of a needle into the pleural space to withdraw fluid; may be a treatment for excess fluid accumulating or to obtain fluid for diagnostic examination.
rhinoplasty (RYE-noh-plas-tee)	rhin/o = nose -plasty = surgical repair	Surgical repair of the nose.
thoracentesis (thor-ah-sen-TEE-sis)	thorac/o = chest -centesis = puncture to withdraw fluid	Surgical puncture of the chest wall for the removal of fluids. Also called *thoracocentesis*.

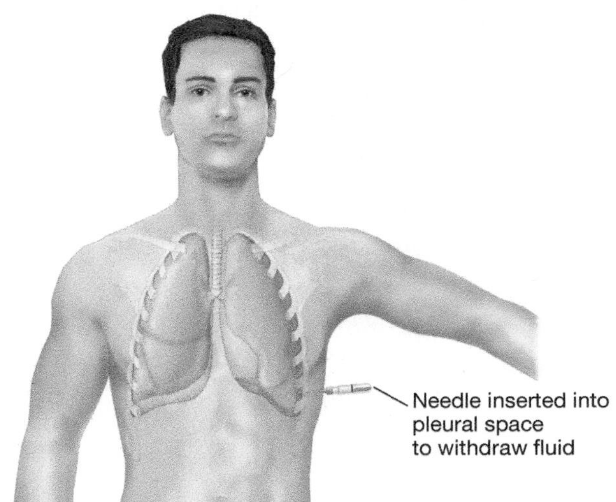

■ **Figure 7.12** Thoracentesis. A needle is inserted between the ribs to withdraw fluid from the pleural sac at the base of the left lung.

TERM	WORD PARTS	DEFINITION
thoracostomy (thor-ah-KOS-toh-mee)	thorac/o = chest -ostomy = surgically create an opening	Insertion of a tube into the chest cavity for the purpose of draining off fluid or air. Also called *chest tube.*
thoracotomy (thor-ah-KOT-oh-mee)	thorac/o = chest -otomy = cutting into	To cut into the chest cavity.

Therapeutic Procedures *(continued)*

TERM	WORD PARTS	DEFINITION
tracheotomy (tray-kee-OTT-oh-mee)	trache/o = trachea -otomy = cutting into	Surgical procedure often performed in an emergency that creates an opening directly into the trachea to allow the patient to breathe easier; also called *tracheostomy*.

■ **Figure 7.13** A tracheotomy tube in place, inserted through an opening in the front of the neck and anchored within the trachea.

Additional Procedures		
cardiopulmonary resuscitation (CPR) (car-dee-oh-PULL-mon-air-ee / ree-suss-ih-TAY-shun)	cardi/o = heart pulmon/o = lung -ary = pertaining to	Emergency treatment provided by persons trained in CPR and given to patients when their respirations and heart stop. CPR provides oxygen to the brain, heart, and other vital organs until medical treatment can restore a normal heart and pulmonary function.
Heimlich maneuver (HYME-lik)		Technique for removing a foreign body from the trachea or pharynx by exerting diaphragmatic pressure. Named for Harry Heimlich, a U.S. thoracic surgeon.
percussion (per-KUH-shun)		Use of the fingertips to tap on a surface to determine the condition beneath the surface. Determined in part by the feel of the surface as it is tapped and the sound generated.

Pharmacology

CLASSIFICATION	WORD PARTS	ACTION	EXAMPLES
antibiotic (an-tih-bye-AW-tic)	anti- = against bi/o = life -tic = pertaining to	Kills bacteria causing respiratory infections.	ampicillin; amoxicillin, Amoxil; ciprofloxacin, Cipro
antihistamine (an-tih-HIST-ah-meen)	anti- = against	Blocks the effects of histamine that has been released by the body during an allergy attack.	fexofenadine, Allegra; loratadine, Claritin; diphenhydramine, Benadryl

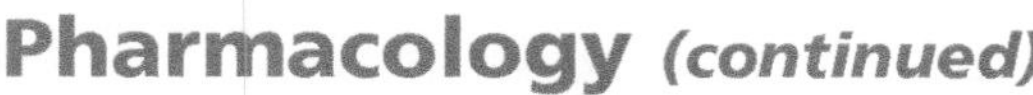

Pharmacology *(continued)*

CLASSIFICATION	WORD PARTS	ACTION	EXAMPLES
antitussive (an-tih-TUSS-ive)	anti- = without tuss/o = cough	Relieves the urge to cough.	hydrocodon, Hycodan; dextromethorphan, Vicks Formula 44
bronchodilator (BRONG-koh-dye-late-or)	bronch/o = bronchus	Relaxes muscle spasms in bronchial tubes. Used to treat asthma.	albuterol, Proventil, Ventolin; theophyllin, Theo-Dur
corticosteroids (core-tih-koh-STAIR-ryods)	cortic/o = outer region, cortex	Reduces inflammation and swelling in the respiratory tract.	fluticasone, Flonase; mometasone, Nasonex; triamcinolone, Azmacort
decongestant (dee-kon-JES-tant)	de- = without	Reduces stuffiness and congestion throughout the respiratory system.	oxymetazoline, Afrin, Dristan, Sinex; pseudoephedrine, Drixoral, Sudafed
expectorant (ek-SPEK-toh-rant)		Improves the ability to cough up mucus from the respiratory tract.	guaifenesin, Robitussin, Mucinex
mucolytic (myoo-koh-LIT-ik)	muc/o = mucus -lytic = destruction	Liquefies mucus so it is easier to cough and clear it from the respiratory tract.	N-acetyl-cysteine, Mucomyst

Abbreviations

ABGs	arterial blood gases
ARDS	adult (or acute) respiratory distress syndrome
Bronch	bronchoscopy
CO_2	carbon dioxide
COPD	chronic obstructive pulmonary disease
CPR	cardiopulmonary resuscitation
C&S	culture and sensitivity
CTA	clear to auscultation
CXR	chest X-ray
DOE	dyspnea on exertion
DPT	diphtheria, pertussis, tetanus injection
ENT	ear, nose, and throat
ERV	expiratory reserve volume
FRC	functional residual capacity
HMD	hyaline membrane disease
IC	inspiratory capacity
IPPB	intermittent positive pressure breathing
IRDS	infant respiratory distress syndrome
IRV	inspiratory reserve volume
LLL	left lower lobe
LUL	left upper lobe
MDI	metered-dose inhaler
O_2	oxygen
PCP	pneumocystis pneumonia
PFT	pulmonary function test
PPD	purified protein derivative
R	respiration
RA	room air
RDS	respiratory distress syndrome
RLL	right lower lobe
RML	right middle lobe
RRT	registered respiratory therapist
RV	reserve volume
RUL	right upper lobe
SARS	severe acute respiratory syndrome
SIDS	sudden infant death syndrome
SOB	shortness of breath
TB	tuberculosis
TLC	total lung capacity
TPR	temperature, pulse, and respiration
TV	tidal volume
URI	upper respiratory infection
VC	vital capacity

Chapter Review

Real-World Applications

Medical Record Analysis

This Pulmonology Consultation Report contains 12 medical terms. Underline each term and write it in the list below the report. Then define each term.

Pulmonology Consultation Report

Reason for Consultation:	Evaluation of increasingly severe asthma.
History of Present Illness:	Patient is a 10-year-old male who first presented to the Emergency Room with dyspnea, coughing, and wheezing at 7 years of age. Attacks are increasing in frequency, and there do not appear to be any precipitating factors such as exercise. No other family members are asthmatics.
Results of Physical Examination:	Patient is currently in the ER with marked dyspnea, cyanosis around the lips, prolonged expiration, and a hacking cough producing thick phlegm. Auscultation revealed rhonchi throughout lungs. ABGs indicate hypoxemia. Spirometry reveals moderately severe airway obstruction during expiration. This patient responded to Proventil and he is beginning to cough less and breathe with less effort.
Assessment:	Acute asthma attack with severe airway obstruction. There is no evidence of infection. In view of increasing severity and frequency of attacks, all his medications should be reevaluated for effectiveness and all attempts to identify precipitating factors should be made.

	Term	Definition
1		
2		
3		
4		
5		
6		
7		
8		
9		
10		
11		
12		

Chart Note Transcription

The chart note below contains 11 phrases that can be reworded with a medical term that you learned in this chapter. Each phrase is identified with an underline. Determine the medical term and write your answers in the space provided.

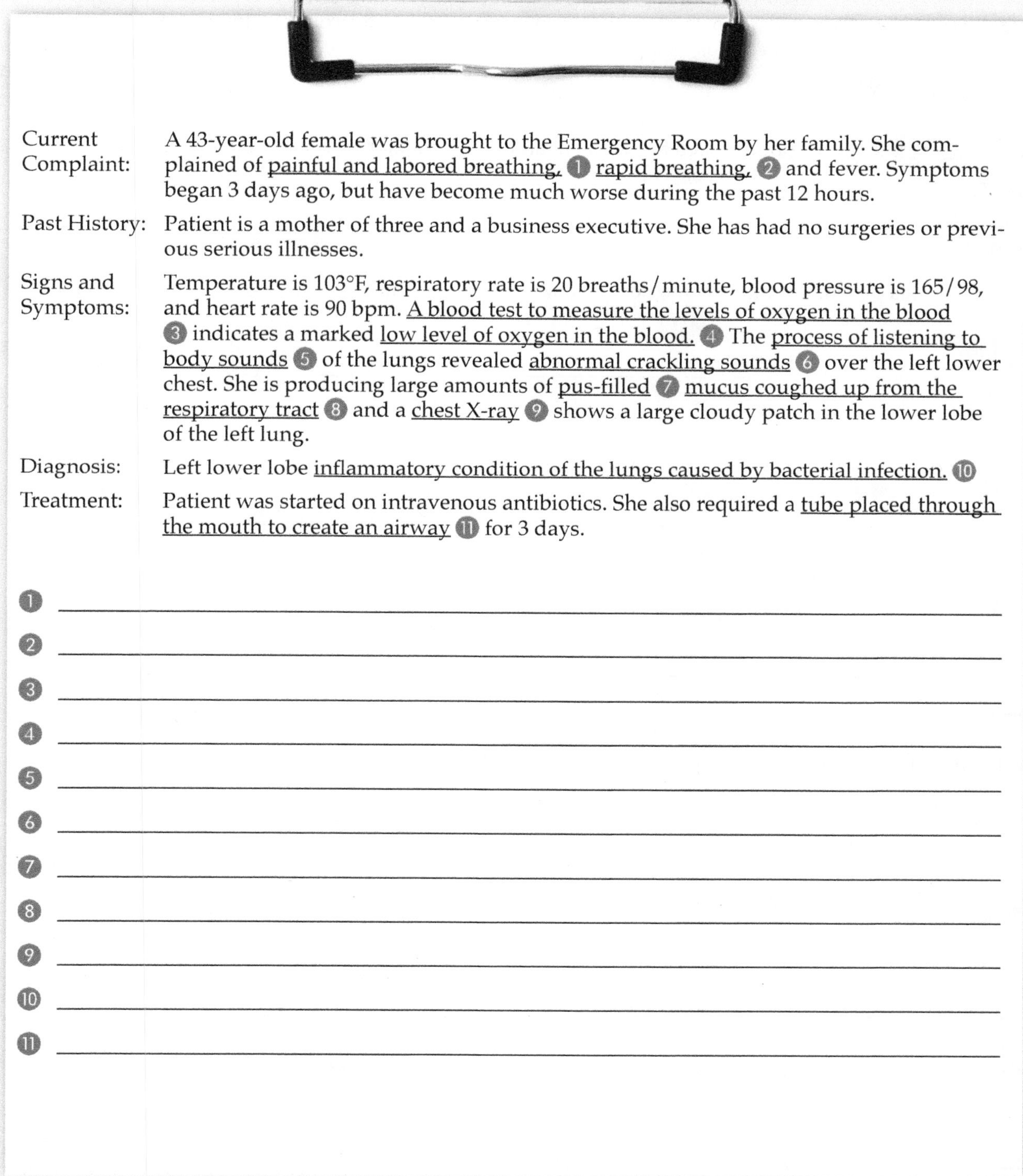

Current Complaint:	A 43-year-old female was brought to the Emergency Room by her family. She complained of painful and labored breathing, (1) rapid breathing, (2) and fever. Symptoms began 3 days ago, but have become much worse during the past 12 hours.
Past History:	Patient is a mother of three and a business executive. She has had no surgeries or previous serious illnesses.
Signs and Symptoms:	Temperature is 103°F, respiratory rate is 20 breaths/minute, blood pressure is 165/98, and heart rate is 90 bpm. A blood test to measure the levels of oxygen in the blood (3) indicates a marked low level of oxygen in the blood. (4) The process of listening to body sounds (5) of the lungs revealed abnormal crackling sounds (6) over the left lower chest. She is producing large amounts of pus-filled (7) mucus coughed up from the respiratory tract (8) and a chest X-ray (9) shows a large cloudy patch in the lower lobe of the left lung.
Diagnosis:	Left lower lobe inflammatory condition of the lungs caused by bacterial infection. (10)
Treatment:	Patient was started on intravenous antibiotics. She also required a tube placed through the mouth to create an airway (11) for 3 days.

(1) ____________________

(2) ____________________

(3) ____________________

(4) ____________________

(5) ____________________

(6) ____________________

(7) ____________________

(8) ____________________

(9) ____________________

(10) ____________________

(11) ____________________

Case Study

Below is a case study presentation of a patient with a condition discussed in this chapter. Read the case study and answer the questions below. Some questions will ask for information not included within this chapter. Use your text, a medical dictionary, journals, technical materials, multimedia resources, electronic media, or any other reference material you choose to answer these questions.

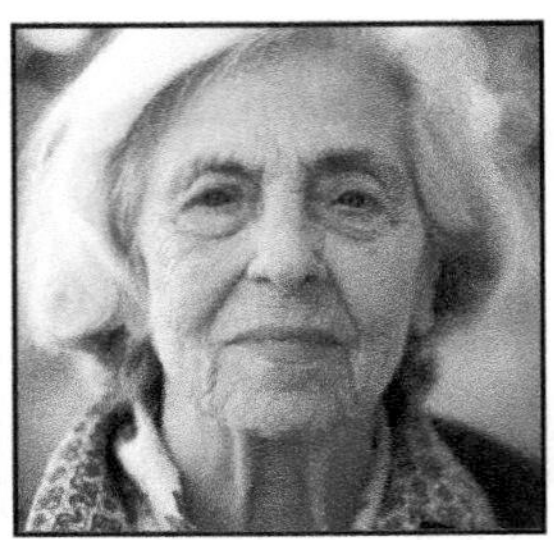

(© Francesco De Napoli/istockphoto.com)

An 88-year-old female was seen in the physician's office complaining of dyspnea, dizziness, orthopnea, elevated temperature, and a cough. Lung auscultation revealed crackles over the right bronchus. CXR revealed fluid in the RUL. The patient was sent to the hospital with an admitting diagnosis of pneumonia. Vital signs upon admission were temperature 102°F, pulse 100 BPM and rapid, respirations 24 breaths/min and labored, blood pressure 180/110. She was treated with IV antibiotics and IPPB. She responded well to treatment and was released home to her family with oral antibiotics on the third day.

1. What was this patient's admitting diagnosis? Look this condition up in a reference source and include a short description of it.

____

____

2. List and define each of the patient's presenting symptoms in your own words.

____

____

3. Define auscultation and CXR. Describe what each revealed in your own words.

____

____

4. What does the term "vital signs" mean? Describe this patient's vital signs.

____

____

5. Describe the treatments this patient received while in the hospital in your own words.

____

____

6. Explain the change in the patient's medication when she was discharged home.

____

____

Practice Exercises

A. Complete the Statement

1. The primary function of the respiratory system is ______________________.
2. The movement of air in and out of the lungs is called ______________________.
3. Define external respiration: ______________________.
4. Define internal respiration: ______________________.
5. The organs of the respiratory system are ______________________, ______________________, ______________________, ______________________, ______________________, and ______________________.
6. The passageway for food, liquids, and air is the ______________________.
7. The ______________________ helps to keep food out of the respiratory tract.
8. The function of the cilia in the nose is to ______________________.
9. The muscle that divides the thoracic cavity from the abdominal cavity is the ______________________.
10. The respiratory rate for an adult is ______________________ to ______________________ respirations per minute.
11. The respiratory rate for a newborn is ______________________ to ______________________ respirations per minute.
12. The right lung has ______________________ lobes; the left lung has ______________________ lobes.
13. The air sacs at the ends of the bronchial tree are called ______________________.
14. The term for the double membrane around the lungs is ______________________.
15. The nasal cavity is separated from the mouth by the ______________________.
16. The small branches of the bronchi are the ______________________.

B. Define the Suffix

	Definition	Example from Chapter
1. -ectasis	______________________	______________________
2. -capnia	______________________	______________________
3. -phonia	______________________	______________________
4. -thorax	______________________	______________________
5. -pnea	______________________	______________________
6. -ptysis	______________________	______________________
7. -osmia	______________________	______________________

C. Combining Form Practice

The combining form **rhin/o** refers to the nose. Use it to write a term that means:

1. inflammation of the nose ____________________
2. abnormal flow from the nose ____________________
3. discharge from the nose ____________________
4. surgical repair of the nose ____________________

The combining form **laryng/o** refers to the larynx or voice box. Use it to write a term that means:

5. inflammation of the larynx ____________________
6. spasm of the larynx ____________________
7. visual examination of the larynx ____________________
8. pertaining to the larynx ____________________
9. cutting into the larynx ____________________
10. removal of the larynx ____________________
11. surgical repair of the larynx ____________________
12. paralysis of the larynx ____________________

The combining form **bronch/o** refers to the bronchus. Use it to write a term that means:

13. pertaining to bronchus ____________________
14. inflammation of the bronchus ____________________
15. visually examine the interior of the bronchus ____________________
16. produced by bronchus ____________________
17. spasm of the bronchus ____________________

The combining form **thorac/o** refers to the chest. Use it to write a term that means:

18. surgical repair of the chest ____________________
19. cutting into the chest ____________________
20. chest pain ____________________
21. pertaining to chest ____________________

The combining form **trache/o** refers to the trachea. Use it to write a term that means:

22. cutting into the trachea ____________________

23. surgical repair of the trachea ______

24. narrowing of the trachea ______

25. pertaining to inside the trachea ______

26. inflammation of the trachea ______

D. Define the Combining Form

	Definition	Example from Chapter
1. trache/o	______	______
2. laryng/o	______	______
3. bronch/o	______	______
4. spir/o	______	______
5. pneum/o	______	______
6. rhin/o	______	______
7. coni/o	______	______
8. pleur/o	______	______
9. epiglott/o	______	______
10. alveol/o	______	______
11. pulmon/o	______	______
12. ox/o	______	______
13. sinus/o	______	______
14. lob/o	______	______
15. nas/o	______	______

E. Suffix Practice

The suffix -pnea means breathing. Use this suffix to write a medical term that means:

1. normal breathing ______
2. difficult or labored breathing ______
3. rapid breathing ______
4. can breathe only in an upright position ______
5. lack of breathing ______

F. Name That Term

1. the process of breathing in ______________________
2. spitting up of blood ______________________
3. blood clot in the pulmonary artery ______________________
4. inflammation of a sinus ______________________
5. sore throat ______________________
6. air in the pleural cavity ______________________
7. whooping cough ______________________
8. cutting into the pleura ______________________
9. pain in the pleural region ______________________
10. common cold ______________________

G. What's the Abbreviation?

1. upper respiratory infection ______________
2. pulmonary function test ______________
3. left lower lobe ______________
4. oxygen ______________
5. carbon dioxide ______________
6. intermittent positive pressure breathing ______________
7. chronic obstructive pulmonary disease ______________
8. bronchoscopy ______________
9. total lung capacity ______________
10. tuberculosis ______________
11. infant respiratory distress syndrome ______________

H. What Does it Stand For?

1. CXR ______________________
2. TV ______________________
3. TPR ______________________
4. ABGs ______________________

5. DOE ____________________

6. RUL ____________________

7. SIDS ____________________

8. TLC ____________________

9. ARDS ____________________

10. MDI ____________________

11. CTA ____________________

12. SARS ____________________

I. Terminology Matching

Match each term to its definition.

1.	_______ inhaling environmental particles	a.	polysomnography
2.	_______ whooping cough	b.	Mantoux test
3.	_______ may result in collapsed lung	c.	oximetry
4.	_______ test to identify sleep apnea	d.	epistaxis
5.	_______ respiratory tract mucus	e.	pneumoconiosis
6.	_______ sweat test	f.	emphysema
7.	_______ measures oxygen levels in blood	g.	walking pneumonia
8.	_______ *Mycoplasma* pneumonia	h.	pneumothorax
9.	_______ disease with overexpanded air sacs	i.	empyema
10.	_______ tuberculin test	j.	phlegm
11.	_______ nosebleed	k.	pertussis
12.	_______ pus in the pleural space	l.	test for cystic fibrosis

J. Define the Term

1. total lung capacity ____________________

2. tidal volume ____________________

3. residual volume ____________________

K. Fill in the Blank

anthracosis	sputum cytology	cardiopulmonary resuscitation	patent
thoracentesis	respirator	ventilation-perfusion scan	rhonchi
supplemental oxygen	hyperventilation		

1. When the patient's breathing and heart stopped, the paramedics began ______________________.
2. The physician performed a ______________________ to remove fluid from the chest.
3. A ______________________ is also called a ventilator.
4. The patient received ______________________ through a nasal cannula.
5. An endotracheal intubation was performed to establish a ______________________ airway.
6. A ______________________ is a particularly useful test to identify a pulmonary embolus.
7. The result of the ______________________ was negative for cancer.
8. ______________________ involves tachypnea and hyperpnea.
9. ______________________ are wheezing lung sounds.
10. Miners are at risk of developing ______________________.

L. Pharmacology Challenge

Fill in the classification for each drug description, then match the brand name.

	Drug Description	Classification	Brand Name
1.	_______ Reduces stuffiness and congestion	______________________	a. Hycodan
2.	_______ Relieves the urge to cough	______________________	b. Flonase
3.	_______ Kills bacteria	______________________	c. Cipro
4.	_______ Improves ability to cough up mucus	______________________	d. Ventolin
5.	_______ Liquefies mucus	______________________	e. Allegra
6.	_______ Relaxes bronchial muscle spasms	______________________	f. Afrin
7.	_______ Blocks allergy attack	______________________	g. Robitussin
8.	_______ Reduces inflammation and swelling	______________________	h. Mucomyst

Labeling Exercise

Image A

Write the labels for this figure on the numbered lines provided.

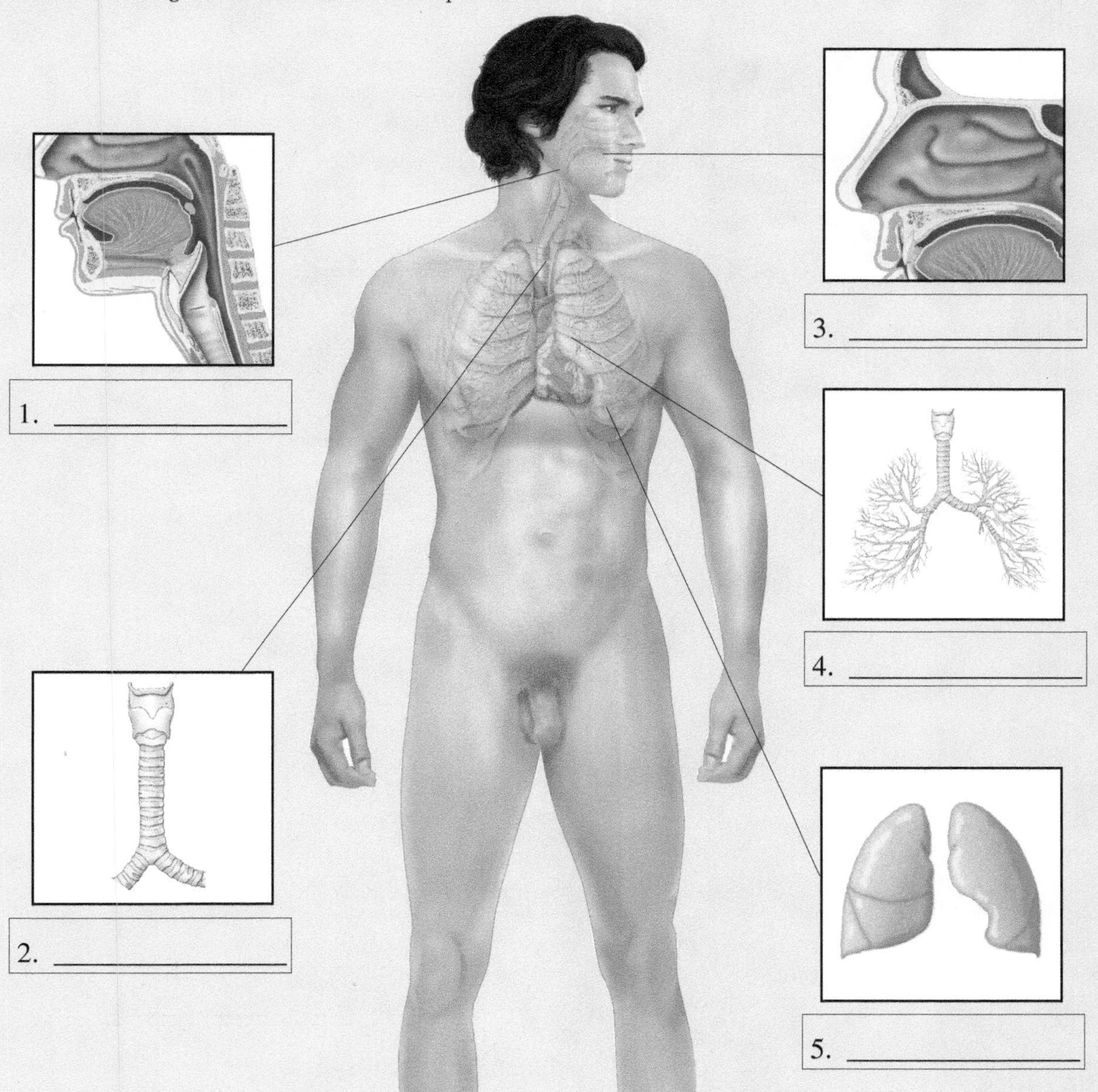

Image B

Write the labels for this figure on the numbered lines provided.

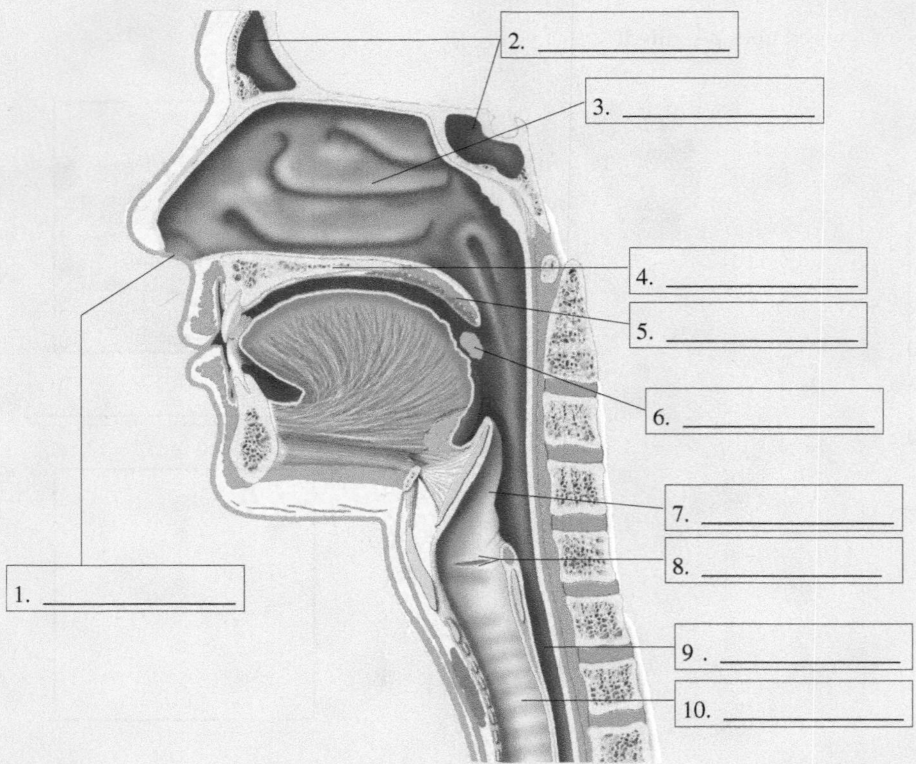

Image C

Write the labels for this figure on the numbered lines provided.

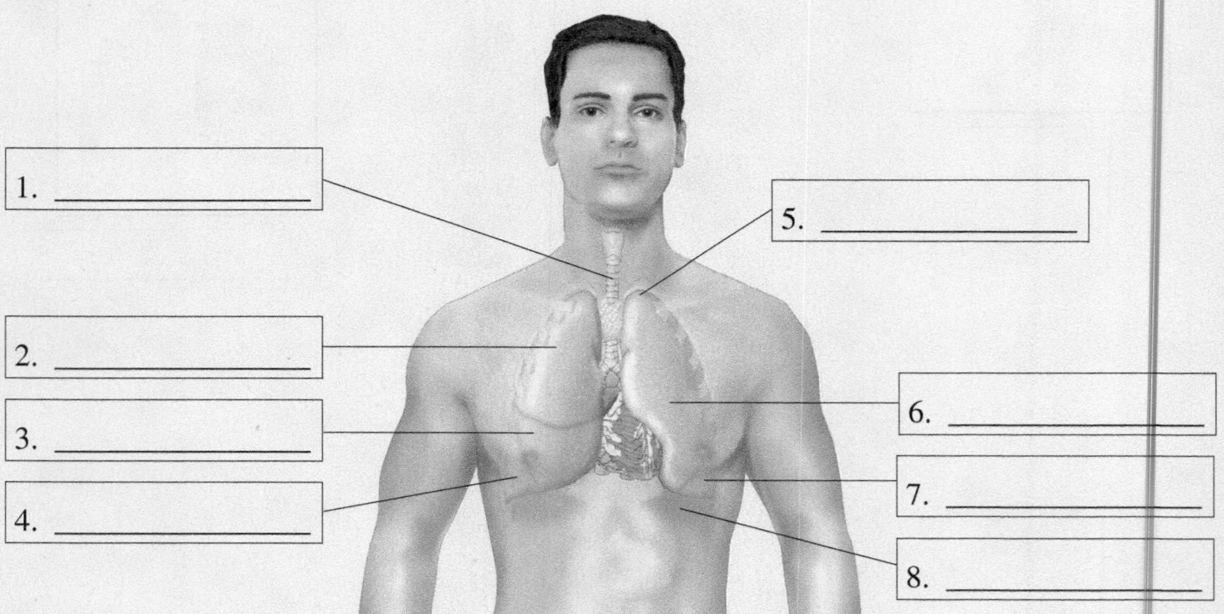

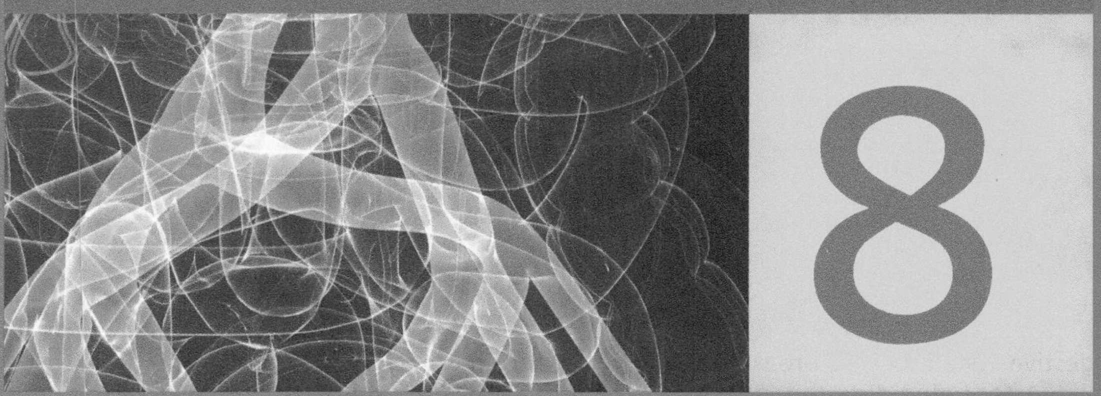

8

DIGESTIVE SYSTEM

Learning Objectives

Upon completion of this chapter, you will be able to

- Identify and define the combining forms and suffixes introduced in this chapter.
- Correctly spell and pronounce medical terms and major anatomical structures relating to the digestive system.
- Locate and describe the major organs of the digestive system and their functions.
- Describe the function of the accessory organs of the digestive system.
- Identify the shape and function of each type of tooth.
- Identify and define digestive system anatomical terms.
- Identify and define selected digestive system pathology terms.
- Identify and define selected digestive system diagnostic procedures.
- Identify and define selected digestive system therapeutic procedures.
- Identify and define selected medications relating to the digestive system.
- Define selected abbreviations associated with the digestive system.

Digestive System at a Glance

Function

The digestive system begins breaking down food through mechanical and chemical digestion. After being digested, nutrient molecules are absorbed into the body and enter the bloodstream; any food not digested or absorbed is eliminated as solid waste.

Structures

Here are the primary structures that comprise the digestive system.

colon
esophagus
gallbladder (GB)
liver
oral cavity
pancreas
pharynx
salivary glands
small intestine
stomach

Word Parts

Here are the most common word parts (with their meanings) used to build digestive system terms. For a more comprehensive list, refer to the Terminology section of this chapter.

Combining Forms

an/o	anus
append/o	appendix
appendic/o	appendix
bar/o	weight
bucc/o	cheek
cec/o	cecum
cholangi/o	bile duct
chol/e	bile, gall
cholecyst/o	gallbladder
choledoch/o	common bile duct
cirrh/o	yellow
col/o	colon
colon/o	colon
dent/o	tooth
diverticul/o	pouch
duoden/o	duodenum
enter/o	small intestine
esophag/o	esophagus
gastr/o	stomach
gingiv/o	gums
gloss/o	tongue
hepat/o	liver
ile/o	ileum
jejun/o	jejunum
labi/o	lip
lapar/o	abdomen
lingu/o	tongue
lith/o	stone
odont/o	tooth
or/o	mouth
palat/o	palate
pancreat/o	pancreas
pharyng/o	pharynx (throat)
polyp/o	polyp
proct/o	anus and rectum
pylor/o	pylorus
pyr/o	fire
rect/o	rectum
sialaden/o	salivary gland
sigmoid/o	sigmoid colon

Suffixes

-emesis	vomit
-istry	specialty of
-lithiasis	condition of stones
-orexia	appetite
-pepsia	digestion
-phagia	eat, swallow
-prandial	pertaining to a meal
-tripsy	surgical crushing

Digestive System Illustrated

salivary glands, p. 264

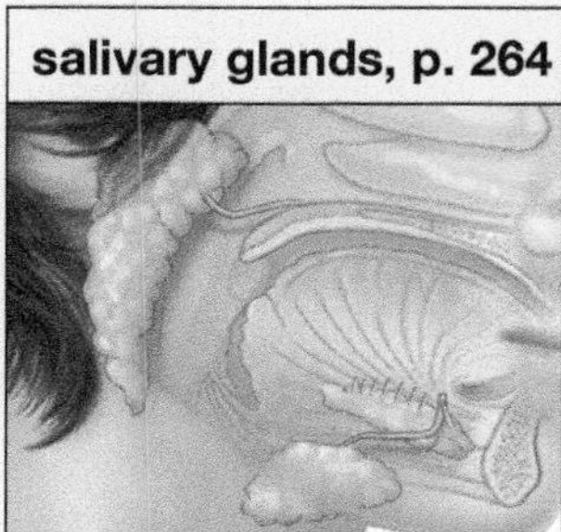

Produces saliva

oral cavity, p. 258

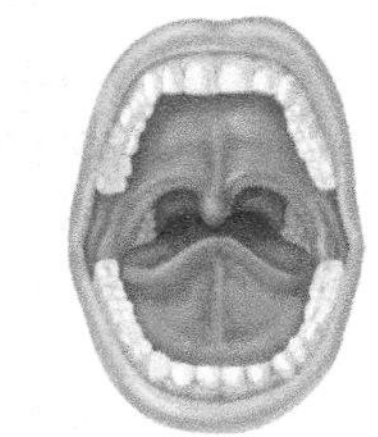

Ingests, chews, and swallows food

esophagus, p. 261

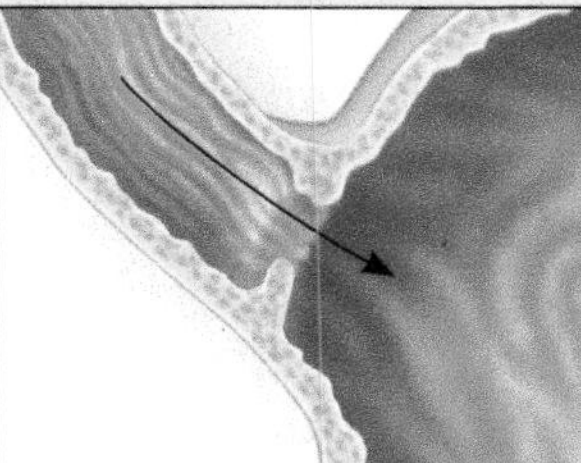

Transports food to the stomach

stomach, p. 262

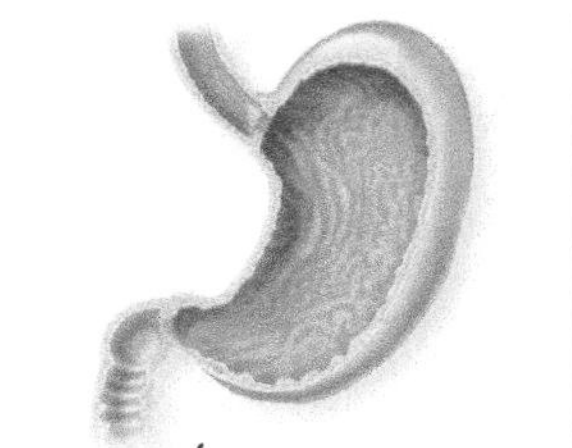

Secretes acid and mixes food to start digestion

pancreas, p. 265

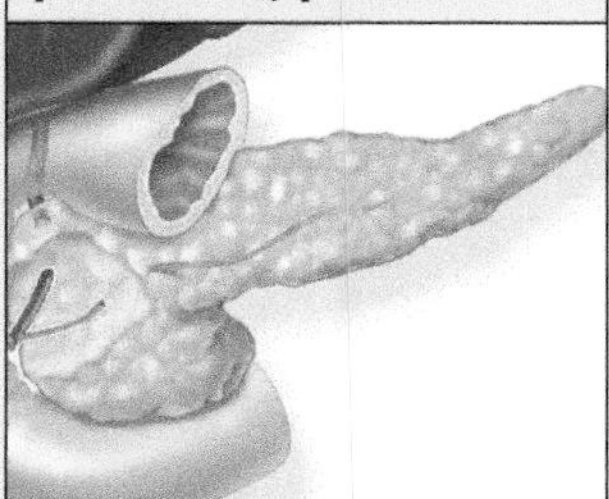

Secretes digestive enzymes and buffers

liver & gallbladder, p. 265

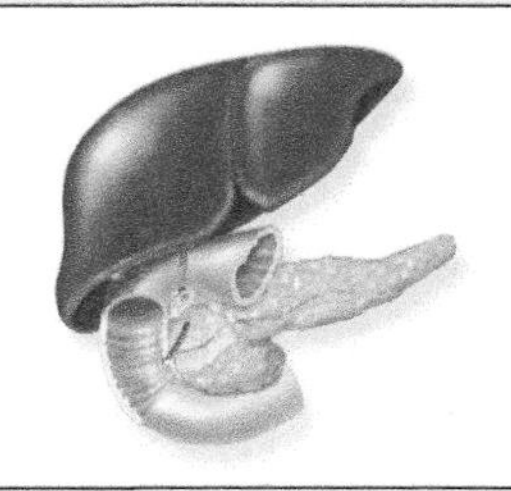

Produces and stores bile

small intestine, p. 262

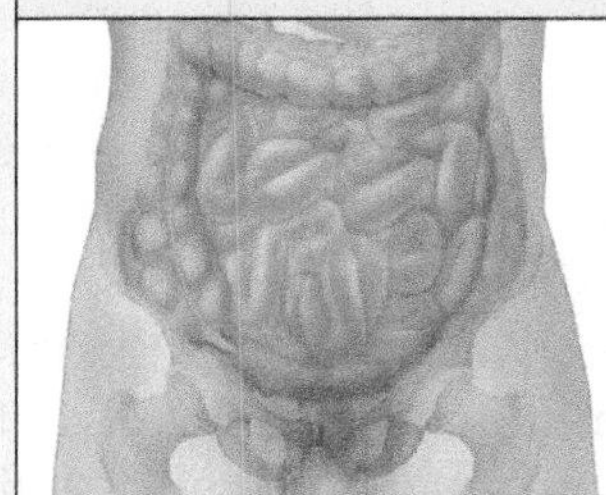

Digests and absorbs nutrients

colon, p. 263

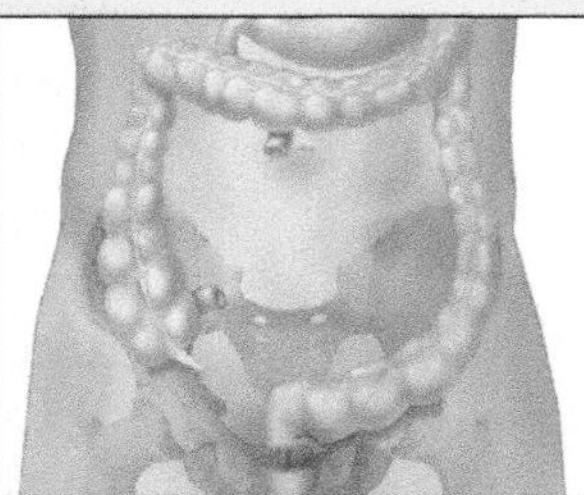

Reabsorbs water and stores feces

Anatomy and Physiology of the Digestive System

accessory organs
alimentary canal (al-ih-MEN-tar-ree)
colon (COH-lon)
esophagus (eh-SOFF-ah-gus)
gallbladder
gastrointestinal system (gas-troh-in-TESS-tih-nal)
gastrointestinal tract
gut
liver
oral cavity
pancreas (PAN-kree-ass)
pharynx (FAIR-inks)
salivary glands (SAL-ih-vair-ee)
small intestine
stomach (STUM-ak)

MED TERM TIP

The term *alimentary* comes from the Latin term *alimentum* meaning "nourishment."

The digestive system, also known as the **gastrointestinal (GI) system,** includes approximately 30 feet of a continuous muscular tube called the **gut, alimentary canal,** or **gastrointestinal tract** that stretches between the mouth and the anus. Most of the organs in this system are actually different sections of this tube. In order, beginning at the mouth and continuing to the anus, these organs are the **oral cavity, pharynx, esophagus, stomach, small intestine, colon, rectum,** and **anus.** The **accessory organs** of digestion are those that participate in the digestion process, but are not part of the continuous alimentary canal. These organs, which are connected to the gut by a duct, are the **liver, pancreas, gallbladder,** and **salivary glands.**

The digestive system has three main functions: digesting food, absorbing nutrients, and eliminating waste. Digestion includes the physical and chemical breakdown of large food particles into simple nutrient molecules like glucose, triglycerides, and amino acids. These simple nutrient molecules are absorbed from the intestines and circulated throughout the body by the cardiovascular system. They are used for growth and repair of organs and tissues. Any food that cannot be digested or absorbed by the body is eliminated from the gastrointestinal system as a solid waste.

Oral Cavity

cheeks
gingiva (JIN-jih-veh)
gums
lips
palate (PAL-at)
saliva (suh-LYE-vah)
taste buds
teeth
tongue
uvula (YU-vyu-lah)

Digestion begins when food enters the mouth and is mechanically broken up by the chewing movements of the **teeth.** The muscular **tongue** moves the food within the mouth and mixes it with **saliva** (see Figure 8.1 ■). Saliva contains digestive enzymes to break down carbohydrates and slippery lubricants to make food easier to swallow. **Taste buds,** found on the surface of the tongue, can distinguish the bitter, sweet, sour, and salty flavors in our food. The roof of the oral cavity is known as the **palate** and is subdivided into the hard palate (the bony anterior portion) and the soft palate (the flexible posterior portion). Hanging down from the posterior edge of the soft palate is the **uvula.** The uvula serves two important functions. First, it has a role in speech production, and second, it is the location of the gag reflex. This reflex is stimulated when food enters the throat without swallowing (e.g., laughing with food in your mouth). It is important because swallowing also results in the epiglottis covering the larynx to prevent food from entering the lungs (see Figure 8.2 ■). The **cheeks** form the lateral walls of this

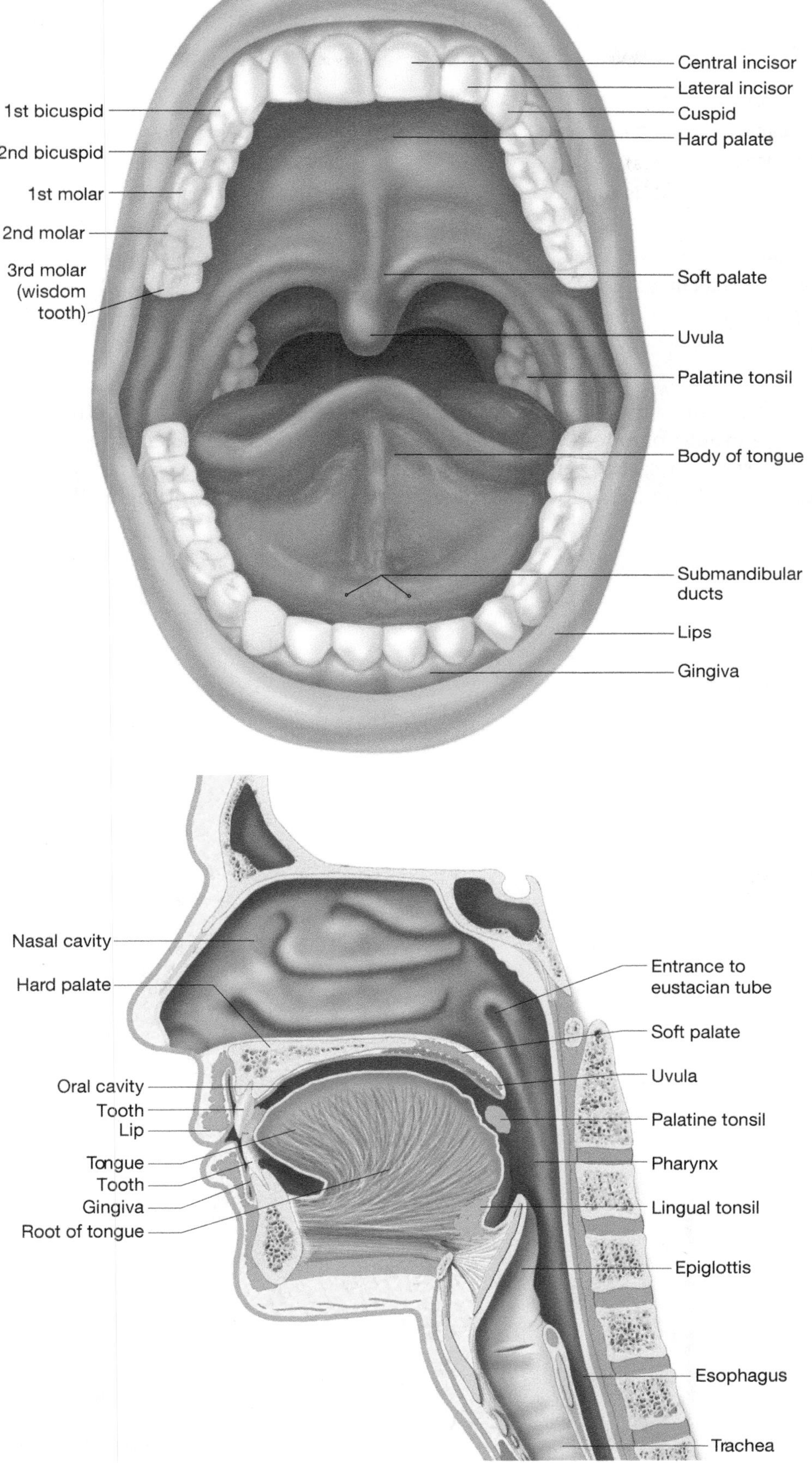

■ **Figure 8.1** Anatomy of structures of the oral cavity.

■ **Figure 8.2** Structures of the oral cavity, pharynx, and esophagus.

cavity and the **lips** are the anterior opening. The entire oral cavity is lined with mucous membrane, a portion of which forms the **gums,** or **gingiva,** that combine with connective tissue to cover the jaw bone and seal off the teeth in their bony sockets.

Teeth

bicuspids (bye-CUSS-pids)
canines (KAY-nines)
cementum (see-MEN-tum)
crown
cuspids (CUSS-pids)
deciduous teeth (dee-SID-yoo-us)
dentin (DEN-tin)
enamel
incisors (in-SIGH-zors)
molars (MOH-lars)
periodontal ligaments (pair-ee-on-DON-tal)
permanent teeth
premolars (pree-MOH-lars)
pulp cavity
root
root canal

MED TERM TIP

There are three different molars, simply referred to as the first, second, or third molars. However, the third molar has a more common name, the wisdom tooth. Not every person ever forms all four wisdom teeth. Unfortunately, most people do not have enough room in their jaws for the third molars to properly erupt through the gum, a condition requiring surgical removal of the third molar, referred to as an *impacted wisdom tooth.*

Teeth are an important part of the first stage of digestion. The teeth in the front of the mouth bite, tear, or cut food into small pieces. These cutting teeth include the **cuspids** (or **canines**) and the **incisors** (see Figure 8.3 ■). The remaining posterior teeth grind and crush food into even finer pieces. These grinding teeth include the

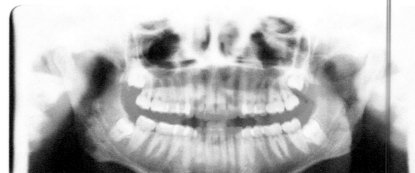

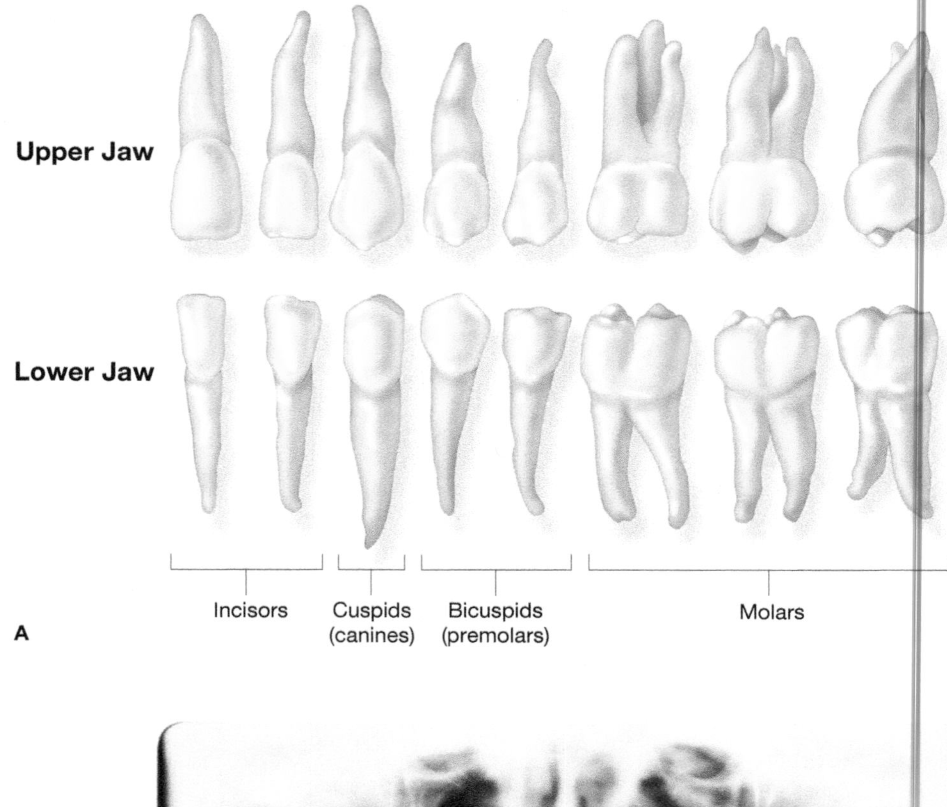

■ **Figure 8.3** (A) The name and shape of the adult teeth. These teeth represent those found in the right side of the mouth. Those of the left side would be a mirror image. The incisors and cuspids are cutting teeth. The bicuspids and molars are grinding teeth. (B) Color-enhanced X-ray of all teeth. Note the four wisdom teeth (third molars) that have not erupted.

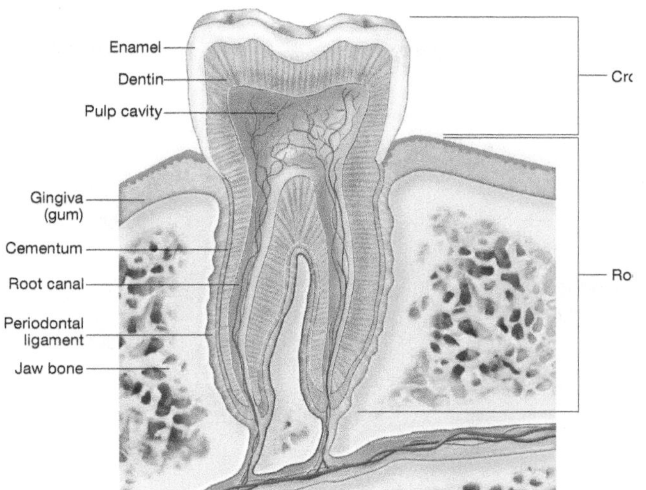

Figure 8.4 An adult tooth, longitudinal view showing internal structures of the crown and root.

bicuspids (or **premolars**) and the **molars.** A tooth can be subdivided into the **crown** and the **root.** The crown is that part of the tooth visible above the gum line; the root is below the gum line. The root is anchored in the bony socket of the jaw by **cementum** and tiny **periodontal ligaments.** The crown of the tooth is covered by a layer of **enamel,** the hardest substance in the body. Under the enamel layer is **dentin,** the substance that makes up the main bulk of the tooth. The hollow interior of a tooth is called the **pulp cavity** in the crown and the **root canal** in the root. These cavities contain soft tissue made up of blood vessels, nerves, and lymph vessels (see Figure 8.4 ■).

Humans have two sets of teeth. The first set, often referred to as baby teeth, are **deciduous teeth.** There are 20 teeth in this set that erupt through the gums between the ages of 6 and 28 months. At approximately 6 years of age, these teeth begin to fall out and are replaced by the 32 **permanent teeth.** This replacement process continues until about 18–20 years of age.

Often these permanent teeth erupt out of alignment, resulting in from minimal to severe malocclusion. This condition can affect the digestive system as well as appearance. Correction by an orthodontist is the recommended treatment. As with other medical conditions it is important that the patient clearly understand what is to take place. Communication in a conversational language will help with the understanding.

MED TERM TIP

The combining form *dent/o* means teeth. Hence we have terms such as dentist and dentistry. The combining form *odont/o* also means teeth and when combined with *orth/o,* which means straight, we have the specialty of *orthodontics,* or straightening teeth.

Pharynx

epiglottis (ep-ih-GLOT-iss)
oropharynx
laryngopharynx

When food is swallowed, it enters the **oropharynx** and then the **laryngopharynx** (see again Figure 8.2). Remember from your study of the respiratory system that air is also traveling through these portions of the pharynx. The **epiglottis** is a cartilaginous flap that folds down to cover the larynx and trachea so that food is prevented from entering the respiratory tract and instead continues into the esophagus.

Esophagus

peristalsis (pair-ih-STALL-sis)

The esophagus is a muscular tube of about 10 inches long in adults. Food entering the esophagus is carried through the thoracic cavity and diaphragm and into the abdominal cavity where it enters the stomach (see Figure 8.5 ■). Food is propelled along the esophagus by wavelike muscular contractions called **peristalsis.** In fact, peristalsis works to push food through the entire gastrointestinal tract.

MED TERM TIP

It takes about 10 seconds for swallowed food to reach the stomach.

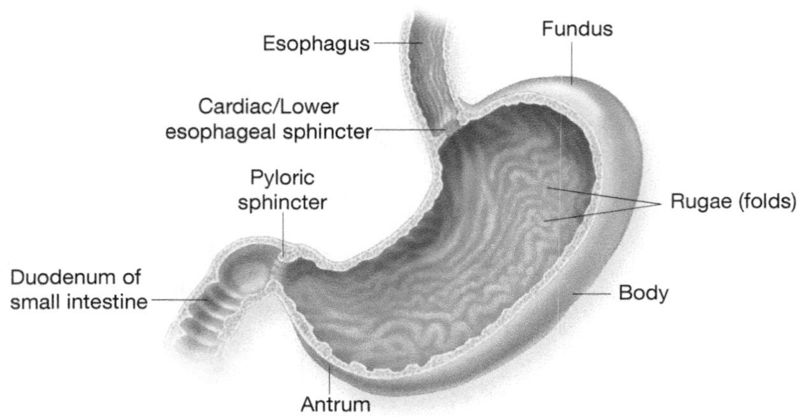

■ **Figure 8.5** The stomach. Longitudinal view showing regions and internal structures.

Stomach

antrum (AN-trum)
body
cardiac sphincter (CAR-dee-ak / SFINGK-ter)
chyme (KIGHM)
fundus (FUN-dus)
hydrochloric acid
lower esophageal sphincter (eh-soff-ah-JEE-al / SFINGK-ter)
pyloric sphincter (pigh-LOR-ik / SFINGK-ter)
rugae (ROO-gay)
sphincters (SFINGK-ters)

The stomach, a J-shaped muscular organ that acts as a bag or sac to collect and churn food with digestive juices, is composed of three parts: the **fundus** or upper region, the **body** or main portion, and the **antrum** or lower region (see again Figure 8.5). The folds in the lining of the stomach are called **rugae.** When the stomach fills with food, the rugae stretch out and disappear. **Hydrochloric acid** (HCl) is secreted by glands in the mucous membrane lining of the stomach. Food mixes with hydrochloric acid and other gastric juices to form a liquid mixture called **chyme,** which then passes through the remaining portion of the digestive system.

Entry into and exit from the stomach is controlled by muscular valves called **sphincters.** These valves open and close to ensure that food can only move forward down the gut tube. The **cardiac sphincter,** named for its proximity to the heart, is located between the esophagus and the fundus; also called the **lower esophageal sphincter** (LES), it keeps food from flowing backward into the esophagus.

The antrum tapers off into the **pyloric sphincter,** which regulates the passage of food into the small intestine. Only a small amount of the chyme is allowed to enter the small intestine with each opening of the sphincter for two important reasons. First, the small intestine is much narrower than the stomach and cannot hold as much as the stomach can. Second, the chyme is highly acidic and must be thoroughly neutralized as it leaves the stomach.

MED TERM TIP

It is easier to remember the function of the pyloric sphincter when you note that *pylor/o* means "gatekeeper." This gatekeeper controls the forward movement of food. Sphincters are rings of muscle that can be opened and closed to control entry and exit from hollow organs like the stomach, colon, and bladder.

Small Intestine

duodenum (doo-oh-DEE-num / doo-OD-eh-num)
ileocecal valve (ill-ee-oh-SEE-kal)
ileum (ILL-ee-um)
jejunum (jee-JOO-num)

The small intestine, or small bowel, is the major site of digestion and absorption of nutrients from food. It is located between the pyloric sphincter and the colon (see Figure 8.6 ■). Because the small intestine is concerned with absorption of food products, an abnormality in this organ can cause malnutrition. The small intestine, with an average length of 20 feet, is the longest portion of the alimentary canal and has three sections: the **duodenum,** the **jejunum,** and the **ileum.**

MED TERM TIP

Word Watch: Be careful not to confuse the word root *ile/o* meaning "ileum," a portion of the small intestines, and *ili/o* meaning "ilium," a pelvic bone.

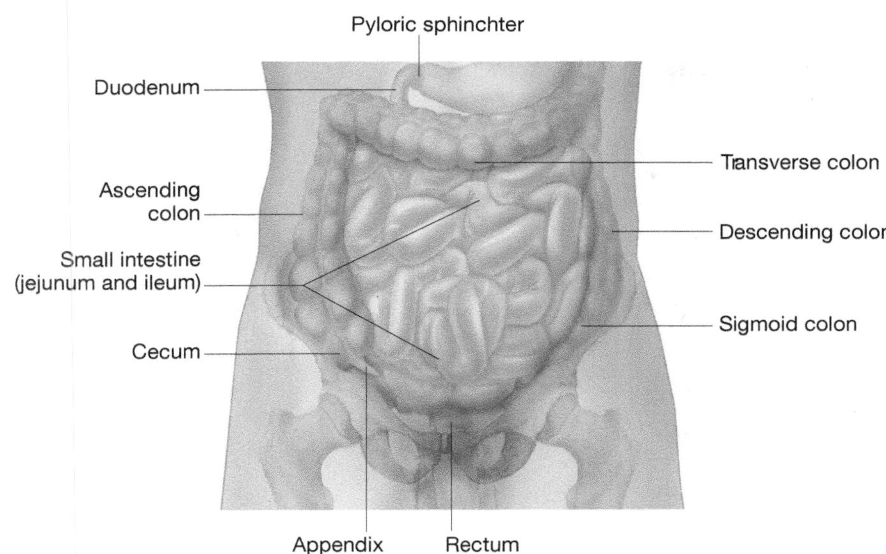

■ **Figure 8.6** The small intestine. Anterior view of the abdominopelvic cavity illustrating how the three sections of small intestine—duodenum, jejunum, and ileum—begin at the pyloric sphincter and end at the colon, but are not arranged in an orderly fashion.

- The duodenum extends from the pyloric sphincter to the jejunum, and is about 10–12 inches long. Digestion is completed in the duodenum after the liquid chyme from the stomach is mixed with digestive juices from the pancreas and gallbladder.
- The jejunum, or middle portion, extends from the duodenum to the ileum and is about 8 feet long.
- The ileum is the last portion of the small intestine and extends from the jejunum to the colon. At 12 feet in length, it is the longest portion of the small intestine. The ileum connects to the colon with a sphincter called the **ileocecal valve.**

MED TERM TIP

We can survive without a portion of the small intestine. For example, in cases of cancer, much of the small intestine and/or colon may have to be removed. The surgeon then creates an opening between the remaining intestine and the abdominal wall. The combining form for the section of intestine connected to the abdominal wall and the suffix *-ostomy* are used to describe this procedure. For example, if a person has a *jejunostomy,* the jejunum is connected to the abdominal wall and the ileum (and remainder of the gut tube) has been removed.

Colon

anal sphincter (AY-nal / SFINGK-ter)
anus (AY-nus)
ascending colon
cecum (SEE-kum)
defecation
descending colon
feces (FEE-seez)
rectum (REK-tum)
sigmoid colon (SIG-moyd)
transverse colon
vermiform appendix (VER-mih-form / ah-PEN-diks)

Fluid that remains after the complete digestion and absorption of nutrients in the small intestine enters the colon or large intestine (see Figure 8.7 ■). Most of this fluid is water that is reabsorbed into the body. The material that remains after absorption is solid waste called **feces** (or stool). This is the product evacuated in bowel movements (BM).

The colon is approximately 5 feet long and extends from the **cecum** to the **anus.** The cecum is a pouch or saclike area in the first 2–3 inches at the beginning of the colon. The **vermiform appendix** is a small worm-shaped outgrowth at the end of the cecum. The remaining colon consists of the **ascending colon, transverse colon, descending colon,** and **sigmoid colon.** The ascending colon on the right side extends from the cecum to the lower border of the liver. The transverse colon begins where the ascending colon leaves off and moves horizontally across the upper abdomen toward the spleen. The descending colon then travels down the left side of the body to where the sigmoid colon begins. The sigmoid colon curves in an S-shape back to the midline of the body and ends at the **rectum.** The rectum, where feces is stored, leads into the anus, which contains the **anal sphincter.** This sphincter consists of rings of voluntary and involuntary muscles to control the evacuation of feces or **defecation.**

MED TERM TIP

The term *colon* refers to the large intestine. However, you should be aware that many people use it incorrectly as a general term referring to the entire intestinal system, both small and large intestines.

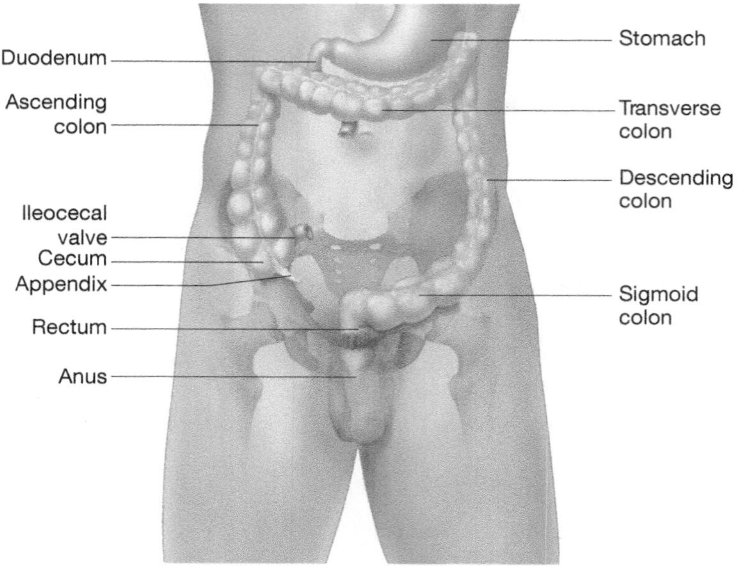

■ **Figure 8.7** The regions of the colon beginning with the cecum and ending at the anus.

Accessory Organs of the Digestive System

MED TERM TIP

In anatomy the term *accessory* generally means that the structure is auxiliary to a more important structure. This is not true for these organs. Digestion would not be possible without the digestive juices produced by these organs.

As described earlier, the accessory organs of the digestive system are the salivary glands, the liver, the pancreas, and the gallbladder. In general, these organs function by producing much of the digestive fluids and enzymes necessary for the chemical breakdown of food. Each is attached to the gut tube by a duct.

Salivary Glands

amylase (AM-ill-ace)
bolus
parotid glands (pah-ROT-id)
sublingual glands (sub-LING-gwal)
submandibular glands (sub-man-DIB-yoo-lar)

Salivary glands in the oral cavity produce saliva. This very watery and slick fluid allows food to be swallowed with less danger of choking. Saliva mixed with food in the mouth forms a **bolus,** chewed food that is ready to swallow. Saliva also contains the digestive enzyme **amylase** that begins the digestion of carbohydrates. There are three pairs of salivary glands. The **parotid glands** are in front of the ears, and the **submandibular glands** and **sublingual glands** are in the floor of the mouth (see Figure 8.8 ■).

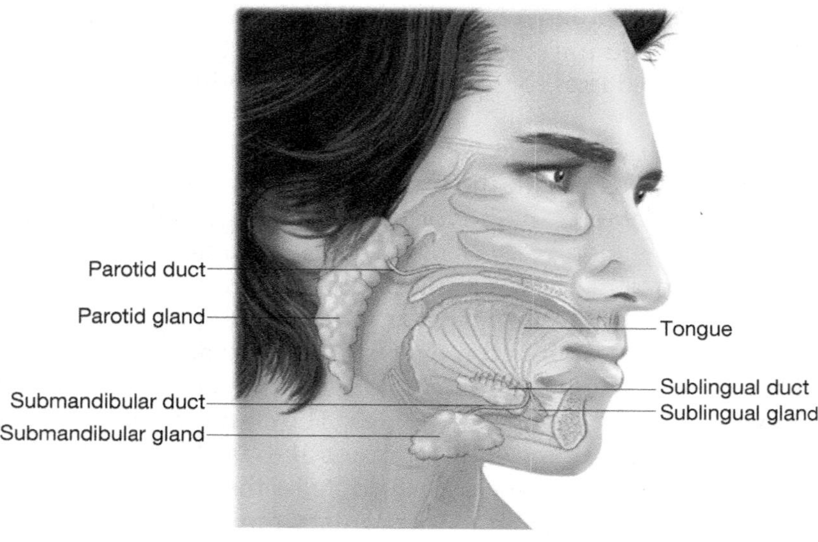

■ **Figure 8.8** The salivary glands, parotid, sublingual, and submandibular. This image shows the position of each gland and its duct emptying into the oral cavity.

Liver

bile (BYE-al) **emulsification** (ee-mull-sih-fih-KAY-shun)

The liver, a large organ located in the right upper quadrant of the abdomen, has several functions including processing the nutrients absorbed by the intestines, detoxifying harmful substances in the body, and producing **bile** (see Figure 8.9 ■). Bile is important for the digestion of fats and lipids because it breaks up large fat globules into much smaller droplets, making them easier to digest in the watery environment inside the intestines. The process is called **emulsification.**

MED TERM TIP

The liver weighs about 4 pounds and has so many important functions that people cannot live without it. It has become a major transplant organ. The liver is also able to regenerate itself. You can lose more than half of your liver, and it will regrow.

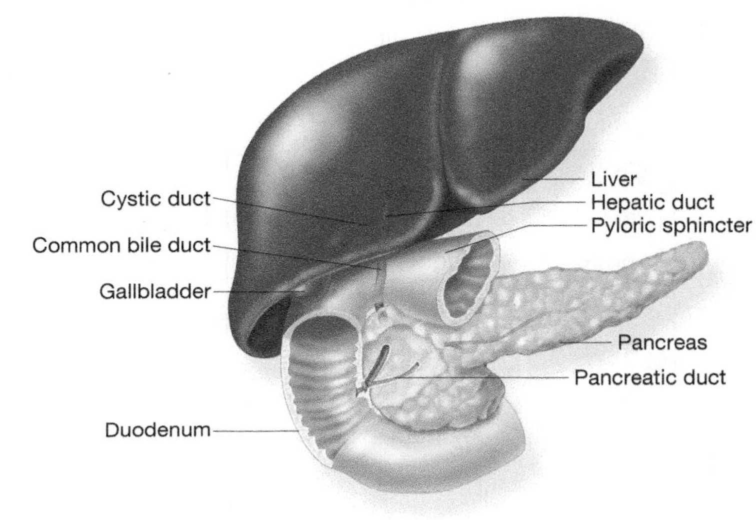

■ **Figure 8.9** The accessory organs of the digestive system: the liver, gallbladder, and pancreas. Image shows the relationship of these three organs and their ducts to the duodenum.

Gallbladder

common bile duct **cystic duct** (SIS-tik)
hepatic duct (hep-PAT-tik)

Bile produced by the liver is stored in the gallbladder (GB). As the liver produces bile, it travels down the **hepatic duct** and up the **cystic duct** into the gallbladder (see again Figure 8.9). In response to the presence of fat in the chyme, the muscular wall of the gallbladder contracts and sends bile back down the cystic duct and into the **common bile duct** (CBD), which carries bile to the duodenum where it is able to emulsify the fat in chyme.

Pancreas

buffers **pancreatic duct** (pan-kree-AT-ik)
pancreatic enzymes (pan-kree-AT-ik / EN-zimes)

The pancreas, connected to the duodenum by the **pancreatic duct,** produces two important secretions for digestion: **buffers** and **pancreatic enzymes** (see again Figure 8.9). Buffers neutralize acidic chyme that has just left the stomach, and pancreatic enzymes chemically digest carbohydrates, fats, and proteins. The pancreas is also an endocrine gland that produces the hormones insulin and glucagon, which play a role in regulating the level of glucose in the blood.

Terminology

Word Parts Used to Build Digestive System Terms

The following lists contain the combining forms, suffixes, and prefixes used to build terms in the remaining sections of this chapter.

Combining Forms

an/o	anus
append/o	appendix
appendic/o	appendix
bar/o	weight
bucc/o	cheek
carcin/o	cancer
cec/o	cecum
chol/e	bile
cholangi/o	bile duct
cholecyst/o	gallbladder
choledoch/o	common bile duct
cirrh/o	yellow
col/o	colon
colon/o	colon
cutane/o	skin
dent/o	tooth

diverticul/o	pouch
duoden/o	duodenum
enter/o	small intestine
esophag/o	esophagus
gastr/o	stomach
gingiv/o	gums
gloss/o	tongue
hem/o	blood
hemat/o	blood
hepat/o	liver
ile/o	ileum
jejun/o	jejunum
labi/o	lip
lapar/o	abdomen
lingu/o	tongue
lith/o	stone

nas/o	nose
odont/o	tooth
or/o	mouth
orth/o	straight
palat/o	palate
pancreat/o	pancreas
pharyng/o	pharynx
polyp/o	polyp
proct/o	anus and rectum
pylor/o	pylorus
pyr/o	fire
rect/o	rectum
sialaden/o	salivary gland
sigmoid/o	sigmoid colon
ven/o	vein

Suffixes

-al	pertaining to
-algia	pain
-centesis	process of removing fluid
-eal	pertaining to
-ectomy	surgical removal
-emesis	vomiting
-gram	record
-graphy	process of recording
-ic	pertaining to
-istry	specialty of

-itis	inflammation
-lithiasis	condition of stones
-logy	study of
-oma	tumor
-orexia	appetite
-osis	abnormal condition
-ostomy	create a new opening
-otomy	cutting into
-ous	pertaining to
-pepsia	digestion

-pexy	surgical fixation
-phagia	eating
-plasty	surgical repair
-plegia	paralysis
-prandial	a meal
-ptosis	drooping
-scope	instrument to view
-scopy	process of viewing
-tic	pertaining to
-tripsy	surgical crushing

Prefixes

a-	without
an-	without
anti-	against
brady-	slow
dys-	abnormal
endo-	within
hyper-	excessive
hypo-	under
intra-	within
per-	through
peri-	around
poly-	many
post-	after
retro-	backwards
sub-	under
trans-	across

Anatomical Terms

TERM	WORD PARTS	DEFINITION
anal	an/o = anus -al = pertaining to	Pertaining to the anus. MED TERM TIP Word Watch: Be careful when using the combining form *an/o* meaning "anus" and the prefix *an* meaning "none."
buccal (BYOO-kal)	bucc/o = cheek -al = pertaining to	Pertaining to the cheeks.
buccolabial (BYOO-koh-labe-ee-all)	bucc/o = cheek labi/o = lip -al = pertaining to	Pertaining to the cheeks and lips.
cecal (SEE-kal)	cec/o = cecum -al = pertaining to	Pertaining to the cecum.
cholecystic (koh-lee-SIS-tik)	cholecyst/o = gallbladder -ic = pertaining to	Pertaining to the gallbladder.
colonic (koh-LON-ik)	colon/o = colon -ic = pertaining to	Pertaining to the colon.
colorectal (kohl-oh-REK-tall)	col/o = colon rect/o = rectum -al = pertaining to	Pertaining to the colon and rectum.
dental (DENT-all)	dent/o = tooth -al = pertaining to	Pertaining to the teeth.
duodenal (duo-DEN-all / do-ODD-in-all)	duoden/o = duodenum -al = pertaining to	Pertaining to the duodenum.
enteric (en-TARE-ik)	enter/o = small intestine -ic = pertaining to	Pertaining to the small intestine.
esophageal (eh-soff-ah-JEE-al)	esophag/o = esophagus -eal = pertaining to	Pertaining to the esophagus.
gastric (GAS-trik)	gastr/o = stomach -ic = pertaining to	Pertaining to the stomach.
gingival (JIN-jih-vul)	gingiv/o = gums -al = pertaining to	Pertaining to the gums.
glossal (GLOSS-all)	gloss/o = tongue -al = pertaining to	Pertaining to the tongue.

Anatomical Terms *(continued)*

TERM	WORD PARTS	DEFINITION
hepatic (hep-AT-ik)	hepat/o = liver -ic = pertaining to	Pertaining to the liver.
hypoglossal (high-poe-GLOSS-all)	hypo- = under gloss/o = tongue -al = pertaining to	Pertaining to under the tongue.
ileal (ILL-ee-all)	ile/o = ileum -al = pertaining to	Pertaining to the ileum.
jejunal (jih-JUNE-all)	jejun/o = jejunum -al = pertaining to	Pertaining to the jejunum.
nasogastric (nay-zoh-GAS-trik)	nas/o = nose gastr/o = stomach -ic = pertaining to	Pertaining to the nose and stomach.
oral (OR-ral)	or/o = mouth -al = pertaining to	Pertaining to the mouth.
pancreatic (pan-kree-AT-ik)	pancreat/o = pancreas -ic = pertaining to	Pertaining to the pancreas.
pharyngeal (fair-in-JEE-all)	pharyng/o = pharynx -eal = pertaining to	Pertaining to the pharynx.
pyloric (pie-LORE-ik)	pylor/o = pylorus -ic = pertaining to	Pertaining to the pylorus.
rectal (RECK-tall)	rect/o = rectum -al = pertaining to	Pertaining to the rectum.
sigmoidal (sig-MOYD-all)	sigmoid/o = sigmoid colon -al = pertaining to	Pertaining to the sigmoid colon.
sublingual (sub-LING-gwal)	sub- = under lingu/o = tongue -al = pertaining to	Pertaining to under the tongue.

Pathology

TERM	WORD PARTS	DEFINITION
Medical Specialties		
dentistry	dent/o = tooth -istry = specialty of	Branch of healthcare involved with the prevention, diagnosis, and treatment of conditions involving the teeth, jaw, and mouth. Practitioner is a *dentist.*
gastroenterology (gas-troh-en-ter-ALL-oh-jee)	gastr/o = stomach enter/o = small intestine -logy = study of	Branch of medicine involved in diagnosis and treatment of diseases and disorders of the digestive system. Physician is a *gastroenterologist.*
oral surgery	or/o = mouth -al = pertaining to	Branch of dentistry that uses surgical means to treat dental conditions. Specialist is an *oral surgeon.*

Pathology *(continued)*

TERM	WORD PARTS	DEFINITION
orthodontics (or-thoh-DON-tiks)	orth/o = straight odont/o = tooth -ic = pertaining to	Branch of dentistry concerned with correction of problems with tooth alignment. Specialist is an *orthodontist.*
periodontics (pair-ee-oh-DON-tiks)	peri- = around odont/o = tooth -ic = pertaining to	Branch of dentistry concerned with treating conditions involving the gums and tissues surrounding the teeth. Specialist is a *periodontist.*
proctology (prok-TOL-oh-jee)	proct/o = anus and rectum -logy = study of	Branch of medicine involved in diagnosis and treatment of diseases and disorders of the anus and rectum. Physician is a *proctologist.*
Signs and Symptoms		
anorexia (an-oh-REK-see-ah)	an- = without -orexia = appetite	General term meaning loss of appetite that may accompany other conditions. Also used to refer to *anorexia nervosa,* which is an eating disorder involving the refusal to eat.
aphagia (ah-FAY-jee-ah)	a- = without -phagia = eating	Being unable to swallow or eat.
ascites (ah-SIGH-teez)		Collection or accumulation of fluid in the peritoneal cavity.
bradypepsia (brad-ee-PEP-see-ah)	brady- = slow -pepsia = digestion	Having a slow digestive system.
cachexia (ka-KEK-see-ah)		Loss of weight and generalized wasting that occurs during a chronic disease.
cholecystalgia (koh-lee-sis-TAL-jee-ah)	cholecyst/o = gallbladder -algia = pain	Having gallbladder pain.
constipation (kon-stih-PAY-shun)		Experiencing difficulty in defecation or infrequent defecation.
dentalgia (dent-AL-gee-ah)	dent/o = tooth -algia = pain	Tooth pain.
diarrhea (dye-ah-REE-ah)		Passing of frequent, watery, or bloody bowel movements. Usually accompanies gastrointestinal (GI) disorders.
dysorexia (dis-oh-REKS-ee-ah)	dys- = abnormal -orexia = appetite	Abnormal appetite; usually a diminished appetite.
dyspepsia (dis-PEP-see-ah)	dys- = difficult -pepsia = digestion	"Upset stomach"; indigestion.
dysphagia (dis-FAY-jee-ah)	dys- = abnormal -phagia = eating	Having difficulty swallowing or eating.
emesis (EM-eh-sis)		Vomiting.
gastralgia (gas-TRAL-jee-ah)	gastr/o = stomach -algia = pain	Stomach pain.
hematemesis (hee-mah-TEM-eh-sis)	hemat/o = blood -emesis = vomiting	Vomiting blood.
hematochezia (he-mat-oh-KEY-zee-ah)	hemat/o = blood	Passing bright red blood in the stools.

Pathology *(continued)*

TERM	WORD PARTS	DEFINITION
hyperemesis (high-per-EM-eh-sis)	hyper- = excessive -emesis = vomiting	Excessive vomiting.
jaundice (JAWN-diss)		Yellow cast to the skin, mucous membranes, and the whites of the eyes caused by the deposit of bile pigment from too much bilirubin in the blood. Bilirubin is a waste product produced when worn-out red blood cells are broken down. May be a symptom of a disorder such as gallstones blocking the common bile duct or carcinoma of the liver. Also called *icterus.*
melena (me-LEE-nah)		Passage of dark tarry stools. Color is the result of digestive enzymes working on blood in the gastrointestinal tract.
nausea (NAW-see-ah)	MED TERM TIP The term *nausea* comes from the Greek word for "seasickness."	Urge to vomit.
obesity		Body weight that is above a healthy level. A person whose weight interferes with normal activity and body function has *morbid obesity.*
polyphagia (pall-ee-FAY-jee-ah)	poly- = many -phagia = eating	Excessive eating; eating too much.
postprandial (post-PRAN-dee-all)	post- = after -prandial = a meal	After a meal.
pyrosis (pie-ROW-sis)	pyr/o = fire -osis = abnormal condition	Pain and burning sensation usually caused by stomach acid splashing up into the esophagus. Commonly called *heartburn.*
regurgitation (ree-gur-jih-TAY-shun)		Return of fluids and solids from the stomach into the mouth.
Oral Cavity		
aphthous ulcers (AF-thus)		Painful ulcers in the mouth of unknown cause. Commonly called *canker sores.*
cleft lip (CLEFT)		Congenital anomaly in which the upper lip and jaw bone fail to fuse in the midline, leaving an open gap. Often seen along with a cleft palate. Corrected with surgery.
cleft palate (CLEFT / PAL-at)		Congenital anomaly in which the roof of the mouth has a split or fissure. Corrected with surgery.
dental caries (KAIR-eez)	dent/o = tooth -al = pertaining to	Gradual decay and disintegration of teeth caused by bacteria; may lead to abscessed teeth. Commonly called a *tooth cavity.*
gingivitis (jin-jih-VIGH-tis)	gingiv/o = gums -itis = inflammation	Inflammation of the gums.

Pathology *(continued)*

TERM	WORD PARTS	DEFINITION
herpes labialis (HER-peez / lay-bee-AL-iz)	labi/o = lip	Infection of the lip by the herpes simplex virus type 1 (HSV-1). Also called *fever blisters* or *cold sores.*
periodontal disease (pair-ee-oh-DON-tal)	peri- = around odont/o = tooth -al = pertaining to	Disease of the supporting structures of the teeth, including the gums and bones; the most common cause of tooth loss.
sialadenitis (sigh-al-add-eh-NIGH-tis)	sialaden/o = salivary gland -itis = inflammation	Inflammation of a salivary gland.
Pharynx and Esophagus		
esophageal varices (eh-soff-ah-JEE-al / VAIR-ih-seez)	esophag/o = esophagus -eal = pertaining to	Enlarged and swollen varicose veins in the lower end of the esophagus. If these rupture, serious hemorrhage results; often related to liver disease.
gastroesophageal reflux disease (GERD) (gas-troh-ee-sof-ah-GEE-all / REE-fluks)	gastr/o = stomach esophag/o = esophagus -eal = pertaining to	Acid from the stomach flows backward up into the esophagus causing inflammation and pain.
pharyngoplegia (fair-in-goh-PLEE-jee-ah)	pharyng/o = pharynx -plegia = paralysis	Paralysis of the throat muscles.
Stomach		
gastric carcinoma (GAS-trik / car-si-NOH-mah)	gastr/o = stomach -ic = pertaining to	Cancerous tumor in the stomach.
gastritis (gas-TRY-tis)	gastr/o = stomach -itis = inflammation	Stomach inflammation.
gastroenteritis (gas-troh-en-ter-EYE-tis)	gastr/o = stomach enter/o = small intestines -itis = inflammation	Inflammation of stomach and small intestine.
hiatal hernia (high-AY-tal / HER-nee-ah)	-al = pertaining to	Protrusion of the stomach through the diaphragm (also called a *diaphragmatocele*) and extending into the thoracic cavity; gastroesophageal reflux disease is a common symptom.

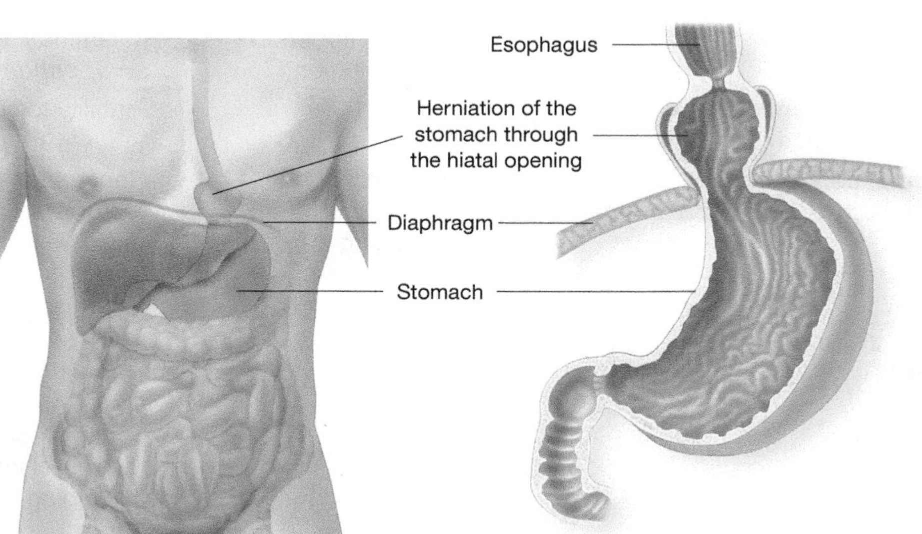

Figure 8.10 A hiatal hernia or diaphragmatocele. A portion of the stomach protrudes through the diaphragm into the thoracic cavity.

Pathology *(continued)*

TERM	WORD PARTS	DEFINITION
peptic ulcer disease (PUD) (PEP-tik / ULL-sir)	-ic = pertaining to	Ulcer occurring in the lower portion of the esophagus, stomach, and/or duodenum; thought to be caused by the acid of gastric juices. Initial damage to the protective lining of the stomach may be caused by a *Helicobacter pylori* (*H. pylori*) bacterial infection. If the ulcer extends all the way through the wall of the stomach, it is called a *perforated ulcer,* which requires immediate surgery to repair.

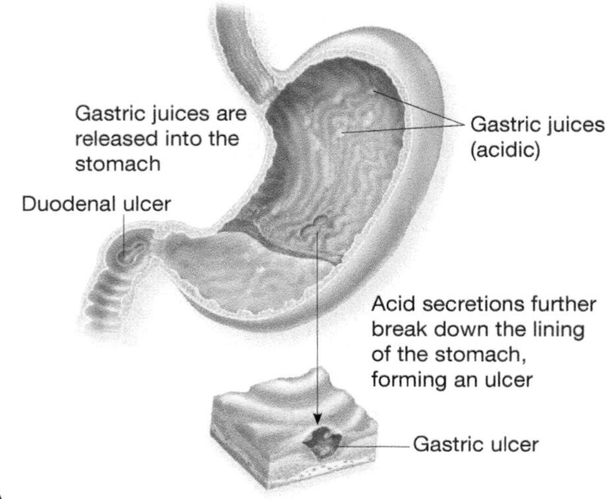
Gastric juices are released into the stomach
Gastric juices (acidic)
Duodenal ulcer
Acid secretions further break down the lining of the stomach, forming an ulcer
Gastric ulcer
A

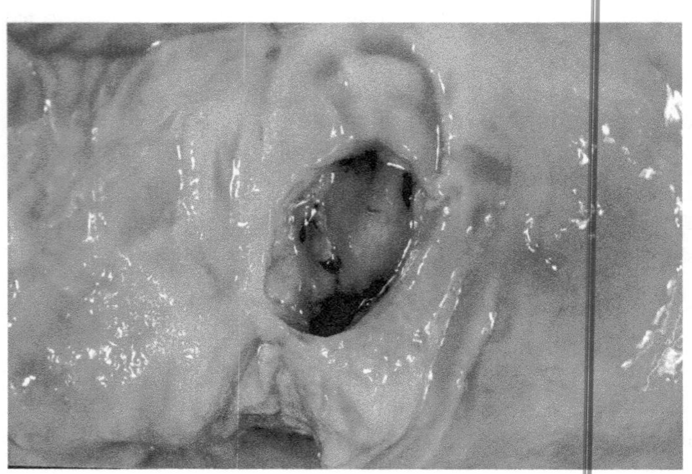
B

■ **Figure 8.11** (A) Figure illustrating the location and appearance of a peptic ulcer in both the stomach and the duodenum; (B) photomicrograph illustrating a gastric ulcer. *(Dr. E. Walker/Science Photo Library/Photo Researchers, Inc.)*

TERM	WORD PARTS	DEFINITION
Small Intestine and Colon		
anal fistula (FIH-styoo-lah)	-al = pertaining to	Abnormal tube-like passage from the surface around the anal opening directly into the rectum.
appendicitis (ah-pen-dih-SIGH-tis)	appendic/o = appendix -itis = inflammation	Inflammation of the appendix; may require an *appendectomy.*
bowel incontinence (in-CON-tih-nence)		Inability to control defecation.
colorectal carcinoma (kohl-oh-REK-tall / car-ci-NOH-mah)	col/o = colon rect/o = rectum -al = pertaining to carcin/o = cancer -oma = tumor	Cancerous tumor originating in the colon or rectum.
Crohn's disease (KROHNZ)		Form of chronic inflammatory bowel disease affecting primarily the ileum and/or colon. Also called *regional ileitis.* This autoimmune condition affects all the layers of the bowel wall and results in scarring and thickening of the gut wall.

Pathology *(continued)*

TERM	WORD PARTS	DEFINITION
diverticulitis (dye-ver-tik-yoo-LYE-tis)	diverticul/o = pouch -itis = inflammation	Inflammation of a *diverticulum* (an out-pouching off the gut), especially in the colon. Inflammation often results when food becomes within the pouch.

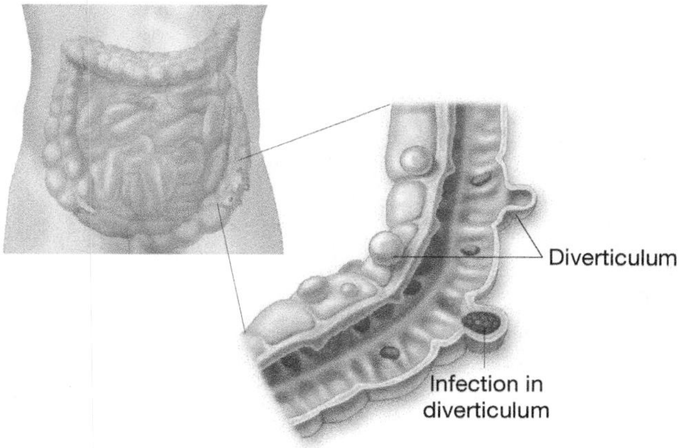

■ **Figure 8.12** Diverticulosis. Figure illustrates external and internal appearance of diverticula.

TERM	WORD PARTS	DEFINITION
diverticulosis (dye-ver-tik-yoo-LOW-sis)	diverticul/o = pouch -osis = abnormal condition	Condition of having diverticula (outpouches off the gut). May lead to *diverticulitis* if one becomes inflamed.
dysentery (dis-in-TARE-ee)		Disease characterized by diarrhea, often with mucus and blood, severe abdominal pain, fever, and dehydration. Caused by ingesting food or water contaminated by chemicals, bacteria, protozoans, or parasites.
enteritis (en-ter-EYE-tis)	enter/o = small intestine -itis = inflammation	Inflammation of the small intestines.
hemorrhoids (HEM-oh-roydz)	hem/o = blood	Varicose veins in the rectum and anus.
ileus (ILL-ee-us)		Severe abdominal pain, inability to pass stools, vomiting, and abdominal distension as a result of an intestinal blockage. The blockage can be a physical block such as a tumor or the failure of bowel contents to move forward due to loss of peristalsis (a nonmechanical blockage). May require surgery to reverse the blockage.
inguinal hernia (ING-gwih-nal / HER-nee-ah)	-al = pertaining to	Hernia or protrusion of a loop of small intestines into the inguinal (groin) region through a weak spot in the abdominal muscle wall that develops into a hole. May become *incarcerated* or *strangulated* if the muscle tightens down around the loop of intestines and cuts off its blood flow. See Figure 8.13 ■.

Pathology *(continued)*

TERM	WORD PARTS	DEFINITION

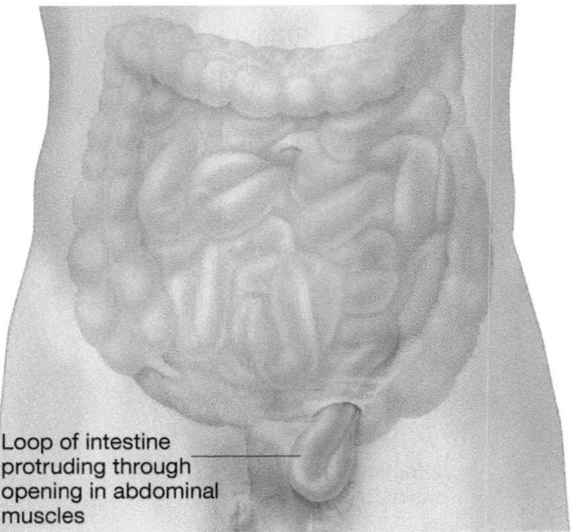

■ **Figure 8.13** An inguinal hernia. A portion of the small intestine is protruding through the abdominal muscles into the groin region.

TERM	WORD PARTS	DEFINITION
intussusception (in-tuh-suh-SEP-shun)		Result of the intestine slipping or telescoping into another section of intestine just below it. More common in children.

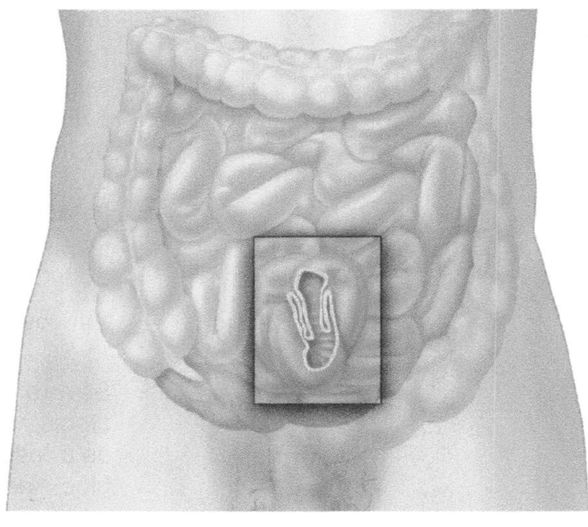

■ **Figure 8.14** Intussusception. A short length of small intestine has telescoped into itself.

TERM	WORD PARTS	DEFINITION
irritable bowel syndrome (IBS)		Disturbance in the functions of the intestine from unknown causes. Symptoms generally include abdominal discomfort and an alteration in bowel activity. Also called *spastic colon* or *functional bowel syndrome.*
polyposis (pall-ee-POH-sis)	polyp/o = polyp -osis = abnormal condition	Presence of small tumors, called **polyps,** containing a pedicle or stemlike attachment in the mucous membranes of the large intestine (colon); may be precancerous. See Figure 8.15 ■.

Pathology *(continued)*

TERM	WORD PARTS	DEFINITION
Figure 8.15 Endoscopic view of a polyp in the colon. Note the mushroom-like shape, an enlarged top growing at the end of a stem. It is being removed by means of a wire loop slipped over the polyp and then tightened to cut it off. *(David M. Martin, M.D./ Photo Researchers, Inc.)*	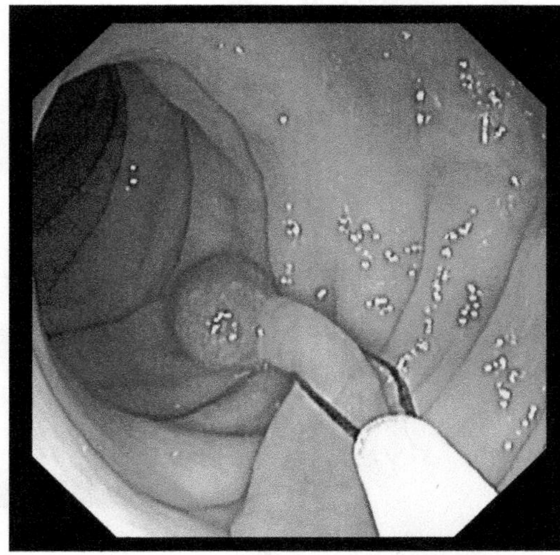	
proctoptosis (prok-top-TOH-sis)	proct/o = rectum and anus -ptosis = drooping	Prolapsed or drooping rectum.
ulcerative colitis (ULL-sir-ah-tiv / koh-LYE-tis)	col/o = colon -itis = inflammation	Chronic inflammatory condition resulting in numerous ulcers formed on the mucous membrane lining of the colon; the cause is unknown. Also known as *inflammatory bowel disease* (IBD).
volvulus (VOL-vyoo-lus)		Condition in which the bowel twists upon itself causing an obstruction; painful and requires immediate surgery.
Figure 8.16 Volvulus. A length of small intestine has twisted around itself, cutting off blood circulation to the twisted loop.	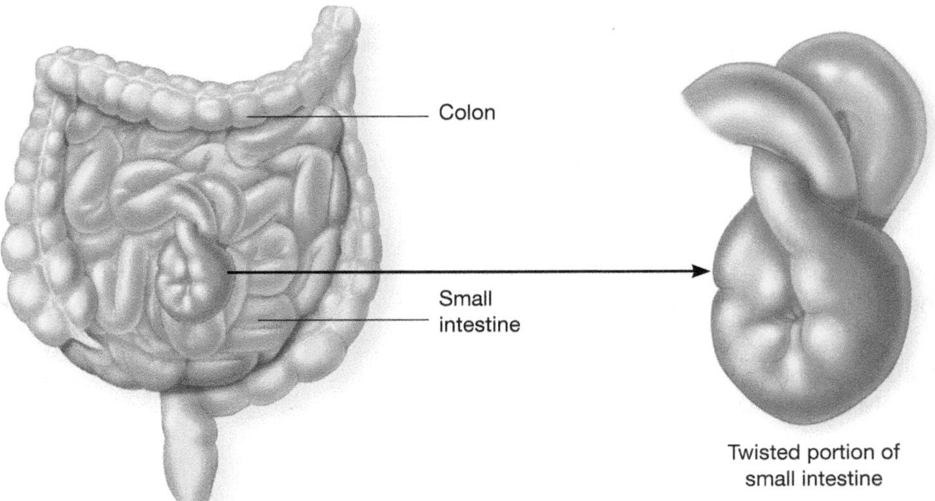	
Accessory Organs		
cholecystitis (koh-lee-sis-TYE-tis)	cholecyst/o = gallbladder -itis = inflammation	Inflammation of the gallbladder; most commonly caused by gallstones in the gallbladder or common bile duct that block the flow of bile.

Pathology *(continued)*

TERM	WORD PARTS	DEFINITION
cholelithiasis (koh-lee-lih-THIGH-ah-sis)	chol/e = bile -lithiasis = condition of stones	Presence of gallstones; may or may not cause symptoms such as *cholecystalgia*.

Figure 8.17 (A) Common sites for cholelithiasis; (B) a gallbladder specimen with multiple gallstones *(Biophoto Associates/Photo Researchers, Inc.).*

TERM	WORD PARTS	DEFINITION
cirrhosis (sih-ROH-sis)	cirrh/o = yellow -osis = abnormal condition	Chronic disease of the liver associated with failure of the liver to function properly.
hepatitis (hep-ah-TYE-tis)	hepat/o = liver -itis = inflammation	Inflammation of the liver, usually due to a viral infection. Different viruses are transmitted by different routes, such as sexual contact or from exposure to blood or fecally contaminated water or food.
hepatoma (hep-ah-TOH-mah)	hepat/o = liver -oma = tumor	Liver tumor.
pancreatitis (pan-kree-ah-TYE-tis)	pancreat/o = pancreas -itis = inflammation	Inflammation of the pancreas.

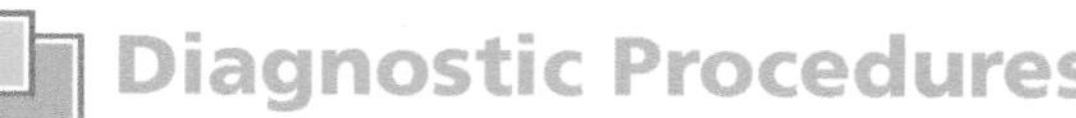

Diagnostic Procedures

TERM	WORD PARTS	DEFINITION
Clinical Laboratory Tests		
alanine transaminase (ALT) (AL-ah-neen / trans-AM-in-nase)		Enzyme normally present in the blood. Blood levels are increased in persons with liver disease.
aspartate transaminase (AST) (ass-PAR-tate / trans-AM-in-nase)		Enzyme normally present in the blood. Blood levels are increased in persons with liver disease.
fecal occult blood test (FOBT) (uh-CULT)	-al = pertaining to	Laboratory test on the feces to determine if microscopic amounts of blood are present. Also called *hemoccult* or *stool guaiac.*
ova and parasites (O&P) (OH-vah / PAR-ah-sights)		Laboratory examination of feces with a microscope for the presence of parasites or their eggs.
serum bilirubin (SEE-rum / BILLY-rubin)		Blood test to determine the amount of the waste product bilirubin in the bloodstream. Elevated levels indicate liver disease.

Diagnostic Procedures *(continued)*

TERM	WORD PARTS	DEFINITION
stool culture		Laboratory test of feces to determine if any pathogenic bacteria are present.
Diagnostic Imaging		
bite-wing X-ray		X-ray taken with a part of the film holder held between the teeth and parallel to the teeth.
cholecystogram (koh-lee-SIS-toh-gram)	cholecyst/o = gallbladder -gram = record	X-ray image of the gallbladder.
intravenous cholecystography (in-trah-VEE-nus / koh-lee-sis-TOG-rah-fee)	intra- = within ven/o = vein -ous = pertaining to cholecyst/o = gallbladder -graphy = process of recording	Dye is administered intravenously to the patient allowing for X-ray visualization of the gallbladder and bile ducts.
lower gastrointestinal series (lower GI series)	gastr/o = stomach -al = pertaining to	X-ray image of the colon and rectum is taken after the administration of barium (a radiopaque dye) by enema. Also called a *barium enema (BE).*

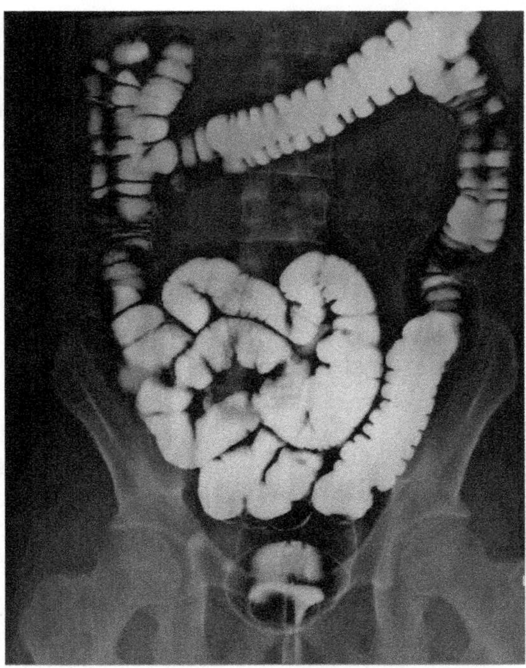

Figure 8.18 Color-enhanced X-ray of the colon taken during a barium enema.

TERM	WORD PARTS	DEFINITION
percutaneous transhepatic cholangiography (PTC) (per-kyoo-TAY-nee-us / trans-heh-PAT-ik / koh-lan-jee-OG-rah-fee)	per- = through cutane/o = skin -ous = pertaining to trans- = across hepat/o = liver -ic = pertaining to cholangi/o = bile duct -graphy = process of recording	Procedure in which contrast medium is injected directly into the liver to visualize the bile ducts. Used to detect obstructions such as gallstones in the common bile duct.

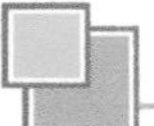

Diagnostic Procedures *(continued)*

TERM	WORD PARTS	DEFINITION
upper gastrointestinal (UGI) **series**	gastr/o = stomach -al = pertaining to	Patient is administered a barium contrast material orally and then X-rays are taken to visualize the esophagus, stomach, and duodenum. Also called a *barium swallow.*
Endoscopic Procedures		
colonoscope (koh-LON-oh-scope)	colon/o = colon -scope = instrument to view	Instrument used to view the colon.
colonoscopy (koh-lon-OSS-koh-pee)	colon/o = colon -scopy = process of viewing	Flexible fiberscope called a *colonoscope* is passed through the anus, rectum, and colon; used to examine the upper portion of the colon. Polyps and small growths can be removed during this procedure (see again Figure 8.15).
endoscopic retrograde cholangiopancreatography (ERCP) (en-doh-SKOP-ik / RET-roh-grayd / koh-lan-jee-oh-pan-kree-ah-TOG-rah-fee)	endo- = within -scopy = process of viewing -ic = pertaining to retro- = backwards cholangi/o = bile duct pancreat/o = pancreas -graphy = process of recording	Procedure using an endoscope to visually examine the hepatic duct, common bile duct, and pancreatic duct. First an endoscope is passed through the patient's mouth, esophagus, and stomach until it reaches the duodenum where the pancreatic and common bile ducts empty. Then a thin catheter is passed through the endoscope and into the ducts (in the retrograde direction). Contrast dye is then used to visualize these ducts on an X-ray.
esophagogastroduodenoscopy (EGD) (eh-soff-ah-go-gas-troh-duo-den-OS-koh-pee)	esophag/o = esophagus gastr/o = stomach duoden/o = duodenum -scopy = process of viewing	Use of a flexible fiberoptic endoscope to visually examine the esophagus, stomach, and beginning of the duodenum.
gastroscope (GAS-troh-scope)	gastr/o = stomach -scope = instrument to view	Instrument used to view inside the stomach.
gastroscopy (gas-TROS-koh-pee)	gastr/o = stomach -scopy = process of viewing	Procedure in which a flexible *gastroscope* is passed through the mouth and down the esophagus in order to visualize inside the stomach. Used to diagnose peptic ulcers and gastric carcinoma.
laparoscope (LAP-ah-roh-scope)	lapar/o = abdomen -scope = instrument to view	Instrument used to view inside the abdomen.
laparoscopy (lap-ar-OSS-koh-pee)	lapar/o = abdomen -scopy = process of viewing	*Laparoscope* is passed into the abdominal wall through a small incision. The abdominal cavity is then visually examined for tumors and other conditions with this lighted instrument. Also called *peritoneoscopy.*
sigmoidoscope (sig-MOYD-oh-scope)	sigmoid/o = sigmoid colon -scope = instrument to view	Instrument used to view inside the sigmoid colon.
sigmoidoscopy (sig-moid-OS-koh-pee)	sigmoid/o = sigmoid colon -scopy = process of viewing	Procedure using a flexible *sigmoidoscope* to visually examine the sigmoid colon. Commonly done to diagnose cancer and polyps.
Additional Diagnostic Procedures		
paracentesis (pair-ah-sin-TEE-sis)	-centesis = process of removing fluid	Insertion of a needle into the abdominal cavity to withdraw fluid. Tests to diagnose diseases may be conducted on the fluid.

Therapeutic Procedures

TERM	WORD PARTS	DEFINITION
Dental Procedures		
bridge		Dental appliance to replace missing teeth. It is attached to adjacent teeth for support.
crown		Artificial covering for a tooth that is created to replace the original enamel covering of the tooth.
denture (DEN-chur)	dent/o = tooth	Partial or complete set of artificial teeth that are set in plastic materials. Acts as a substitute for the natural teeth and related structures.
extraction	ex- = outward	Removing or "pulling" of teeth.
implant (IM-plant)		Prosthetic device placed in the jaw to which a tooth or denture may be anchored.
root canal	-al = pertaining to	Dental treatment involving the pulp cavity of the root of a tooth. Procedure is used to save a tooth that is badly infected or abscessed.
Medical Procedures		
gavage (guh-VAHZH)		Use of a nasogastric (NG) tube to place liquid nourishment directly into the stomach.
lavage (lah-VAHZH)		Use of a nasogastric (NG) tube to wash out the stomach. For example, after ingestion of dangerous substances.
nasogastric intubation (NG tube) (NAY-zo-gas-trik / in-two-BAY-shun)	nas/o = nose gastr/o = stomach -ic = pertaining to	Procedure in which a flexible catheter is inserted into the nose and down the esophagus to the stomach. May be used for feeding or to suction out stomach fluids.
total parenteral nutrition (TPN) (pair-in-TARE-all)	-al = pertaining to	Providing 100% of a patient's nutrition intravenously. Used when a patient is unable to eat.
Surgical Procedures		
anastomosis (ah-nas-toh-MOH-sis)		To surgically create a connection between two organs or vessels. For example, joining together two cut ends of the intestines after a section is removed.
appendectomy (ap-en-DEK-toh-mee)	append/o = appendix -ectomy = surgical removal	Surgical removal of the appendix.
bariatric surgery (bear-ee-AT-rik)	bar/o = weight	Group of surgical procedures such as stomach stapling and restrictive banding to reduce the size of the stomach. A treatment for morbid (extreme) obesity.
cholecystectomy (koh-lee-sis-TEK-toh-mee)	cholecyst/o = gallbladder -ectomy = surgical removal	Surgical removal of the gallbladder.
choledocholithotripsy (koh-led-oh-koh-LITH-oh-trip-see)	choledoch/o = common bile duct lith/o = stone -tripsy = surgical crushing	Crushing of a gallstone in the common bile duct.
colectomy (koh-LEK-toh-mee)	col/o = colon -ectomy = surgical removal	Surgical removal of the colon.

Therapeutic Procedures *(continued)*

TERM	WORD PARTS	DEFINITION
colostomy (koh-LOSS-toh-mee)	col/o = colon -ostomy = create a new opening	Surgical creation of an opening of some portion of the colon through the abdominal wall to the outside surface. Fecal material (stool) drains into a bag worn on the abdomen.

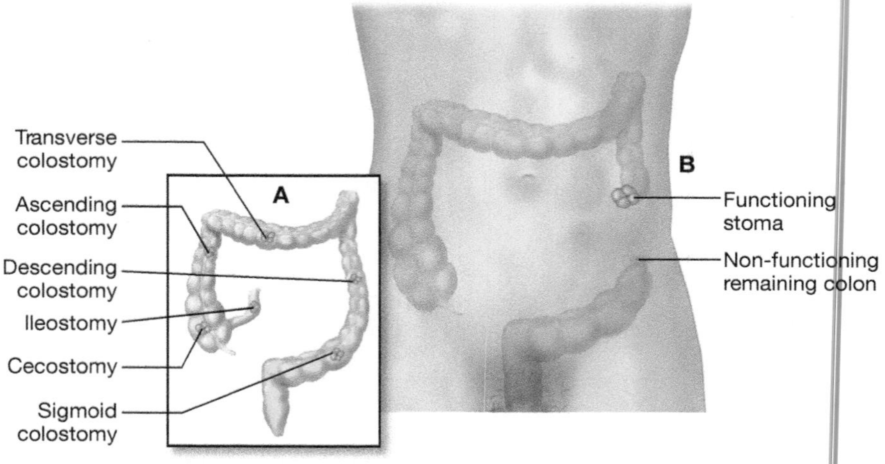

■ **Figure 8.19** (A) The colon illustrating various ostomy sites; (B) colostomy in the descending colon, illustrating functioning stoma and nonfunctioning distal sigmoid colon and rectum.

TERM	WORD PARTS	DEFINITION
diverticulectomy (dye-ver-tik-yoo-LEK-toh-mee)	diverticul/o = pouch -ectomy = surgical removal	Surgical removal of a diverticulum.
exploratory laparotomy (ek-SPLOR-ah-tor-ee / lap-ah-ROT-oh-mee)	lapar/o = abdomen -otomy = cutting into	Abdominal operation for the purpose of examining the abdominal organs and tissues for signs of disease or other abnormalities.
fistulectomy (fis-tyoo-LEK-toh-mee)	-ectomy = surgical removal	Removal of a fistula.
gastrectomy (gas-TREK-toh-mee)	gastr/o = stomach -ectomy = surgical removal	Surgical removal of the stomach.
gastric stapling	gastr/o = stomach -ic = pertaining to	Procedure that closes off a large section of the stomach with rows of staples. Results in a much smaller stomach to assist very obese patients to lose weight.
gastrostomy (gas-TROSS-toh-mee)	gastr/o = stomach -ostomy = create a new opening	Surgical procedure to create an opening in the stomach.
hemorrhoidectomy (hem-oh-royd-EK-toh-mee)	-ectomy = surgical removal	Surgical removal of hemorrhoids from the anorectal area.
hernioplasty (her-nee-oh-PLAS-tee)	-plasty = surgical repair	Surgical repair of a hernia. Also called *herniorrhaphy*.
ileostomy (ill-ee-OSS-toh-mee)	ile/o = ileum -ostomy = create a new opening	Surgical creation of an opening in the ileum.
laparoscopic cholecystectomy (lap-ar-oh-SKOP-ik / koh-lee-sis-TEK-toh-mee)	lapar/o = abdomen -scopy = process of viewing -ic = pertaining to cholecyst/o = gallbladder -ectomy = surgical removal	Surgical removal of the gallbladder through a very small abdominal incision with the assistance of a laparoscope.

Therapeutic Procedures *(continued)*

TERM	WORD PARTS	DEFINITION
laparotomy (lap-ah-ROT-oh-mee)	lapar/o = abdomen -otomy = cutting into	Surgical incision into the abdomen.
liver transplant		Transplant of a liver from a donor.
palatoplasty (pa-LOT-toh-plas-tee)	palat/o = palate -plasty = surgical repair	Surgical repair of the palate.
pharyngoplasty (fair-ING-oh-plas-tee)	pharyng/o = pharynx -plasty = surgical repair	Surgical repair of the throat.
proctopexy (PROK-toh-pek-see)	proct/o = rectum and anus -pexy = surgical fixation	Surgical fixation of the rectum and anus.

Pharmacology

CLASSIFICATION	WORD PARTS	ACTION	EXAMPLES
anorexiant (an-oh-REKS-ee-ant)	an- = without -orexia = appetite	Treats obesity by suppressing appetite.	phendimetrazine, Adipost, Obezine; phentermine, Zantryl, Adipex
antacid	anti- = against	Used to neutralize stomach acids.	calcium carbonate, Tums; aluminum hydroxide and magnesium hydroxide, Maalox, Mylanta
antidiarrheal (an-tee-dye-ah-REE-all)	anti- = against -al = pertaining to	Used to control diarrhea.	loperamide, Imodium; diphenoxylate and atropine, Lomotil; kaolin/pectin, Kaopectate
antiemetic (an-tye-ee-MEH-tik)	anti- = against -emesis = vomit -tic = pertaining to	Treats nausea, vomiting, and motion sickness.	prochlorperazine, Compazine; promethazine, Phenergan
antivirals	anti- = against	Treats herpes simplex infection.	valacyclovir, Valtrex; famcyclovir, Famvir; acyclovir, Zovirax
H_2-receptor antagonist	anti- = against	Used to treat peptic ulcers and gastroesophageal reflux disease. When stimulated, H_2-receptors increase the production of stomach acid. Using an antagonist to block these receptors results in a low acid level in the stomach.	ranitidine, Zantac; cimetidine, Tagamet; famotidine, Pepcid
laxative MED TERM TIP The term *laxative* refers to a medication to stimulate a bowel movement; comes from the Latin term meaning "to relax."		Treats constipation by stimulating a bowel movement.	senosides, Senokot; psyllium, Metamucil
proton pump inhibitors		Used to treat peptic ulcers and gastroesophageal reflux disease. Blocks the stomach's ability to secrete acid.	esomeprazole, Nexium; omeprazole, Prilosec

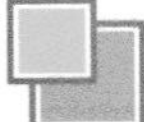

Abbreviations

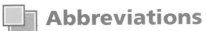

ac	before meals
ALT	alanine transaminase
AST	aspartate transaminase
Ba	barium
BE	barium enema
BM	bowel movement
BS	bowel sounds
CBD	common bile duct
EGD	esophagogastroduodenoscopy
ERCP	endoscopic retrograde cholangio-pancreatography
FOBT	fecal occult blood test
GB	gallbladder
GERD	gastroesophageal reflux disease
GI	gastrointestinal
HAV	hepatitis A virus
HBV	hepatitis B virus
HCl	hydrochloric acid
HCV	hepatitis C virus
HDV	hepatitis D virus
HEV	hepatitis E virus
HSV-1	herpes simplex virus type 1
IBD	inflammatory bowel disease
IBS	irritable bowel syndrome
IVC	intravenous cholangiography
n&v	nausea and vomiting
NG	nasogastric (tube)
NPO	nothing by mouth
O&P	ova and parasites
pc	after meals
PO	by mouth
pp	postprandial
PTC	percutaneous transhepatic cholangiography
PUD	peptic ulcer disease
TPN	total parenteral nutrition
UGI	upper gastrointestinal series

Chapter Review

Real-World Applications

Medical Record Analysis

This Gastroenterology Consultation Report contains 12 medical terms. Underline each term and write it in the list below the report. Then define each term.

Gastroenterology Consultation Report

Reason for Consultation:	Evaluation of recurrent epigastric pain with anemia and melena.
History of Present Illness:	Patient is a 56-year-old male. He reports a long history of mild dyspepsia characterized by burning epigastric pain, especially when his stomach is empty. This pain has been relieved by over-the-counter antacids. Approximately two weeks ago, the pain became significantly worse and he noted that his stools were dark and tarry.
Results of Physical Examination:	CBC indicates anemia, and a fecal occult blood test is positive for blood. A blood test for *Helicobacter pylori* is positive. Gastroscopy located an ulcer in the lining of the stomach. This ulcer is 1.5 cm in diameter and deep. There is evidence of active bleeding from the ulcer.
Assessment:	Peptic ulcer disease.

	Term	Definition
1	______________	______________________________
2	______________	______________________________
3	______________	______________________________
4	______________	______________________________
5	______________	______________________________
6	______________	______________________________
7	______________	______________________________
8	______________	______________________________
9	______________	______________________________
10	______________	______________________________
11	______________	______________________________
12	______________	______________________________

Chart Note Transcription

The chart note below contains 12 phrases that can be reworded with a medical term that you learned in this chapter. Each phrase is identified with an underline. Determine the medical term and write your answers in the space provided.

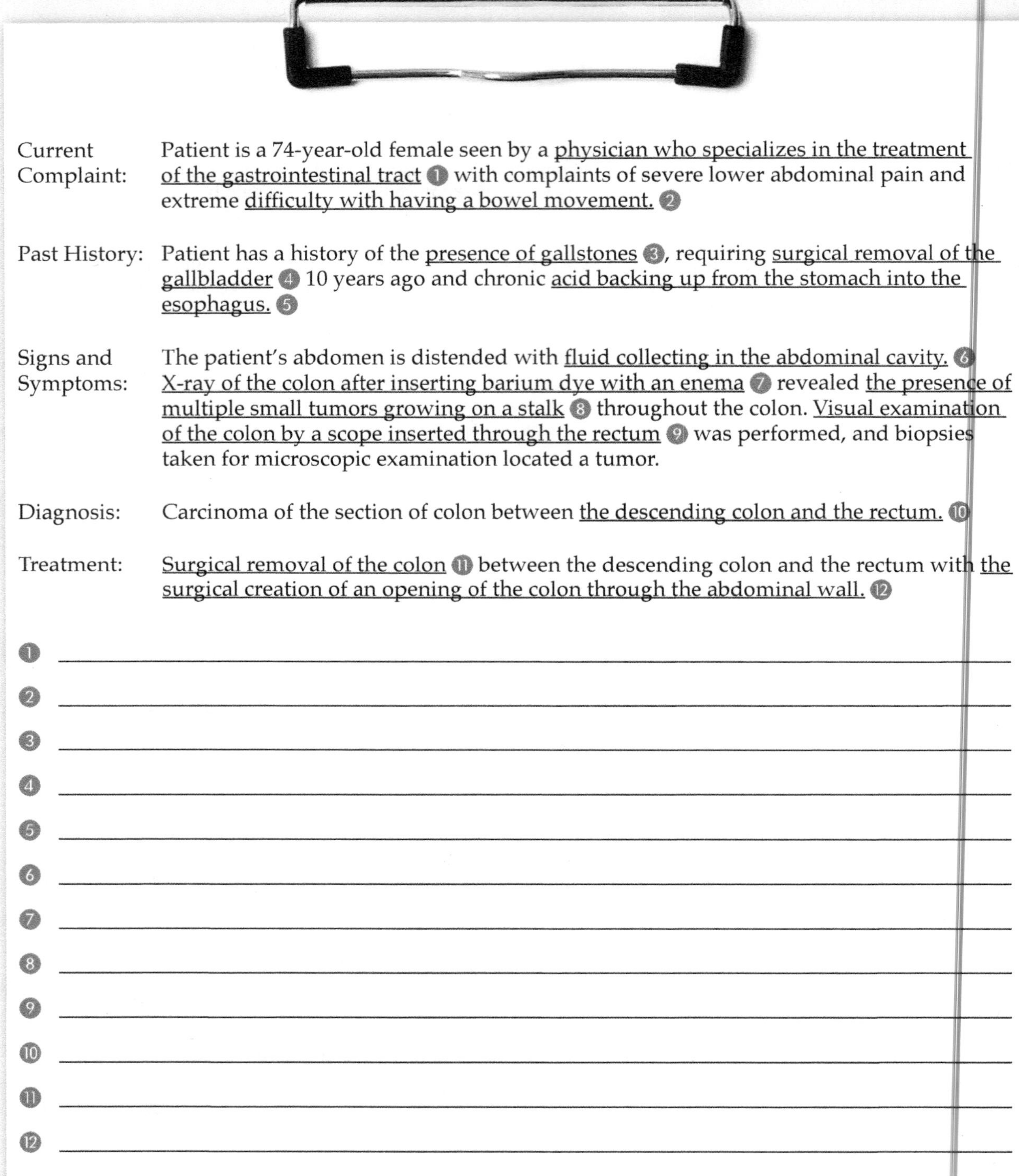

Current Complaint: Patient is a 74-year-old female seen by a physician who specializes in the treatment of the gastrointestinal tract (1) with complaints of severe lower abdominal pain and extreme difficulty with having a bowel movement. (2)

Past History: Patient has a history of the presence of gallstones (3), requiring surgical removal of the gallbladder (4) 10 years ago and chronic acid backing up from the stomach into the esophagus. (5)

Signs and Symptoms: The patient's abdomen is distended with fluid collecting in the abdominal cavity. (6) X-ray of the colon after inserting barium dye with an enema (7) revealed the presence of multiple small tumors growing on a stalk (8) throughout the colon. Visual examination of the colon by a scope inserted through the rectum (9) was performed, and biopsies taken for microscopic examination located a tumor.

Diagnosis: Carcinoma of the section of colon between the descending colon and the rectum. (10)

Treatment: Surgical removal of the colon (11) between the descending colon and the rectum with the surgical creation of an opening of the colon through the abdominal wall. (12)

(1) ______________________

(2) ______________________

(3) ______________________

(4) ______________________

(5) ______________________

(6) ______________________

(7) ______________________

(8) ______________________

(9) ______________________

(10) ______________________

(11) ______________________

(12) ______________________

Case Study

Below is a case study presentation of a patient with a condition discussed in this chapter. Read the case study and answer the questions below. Some questions will ask for information not included within this chapter. Use your text, a medical dictionary, journals, technical materials, multimedia resources, electronic media, or any other reference material you choose to answer these questions.

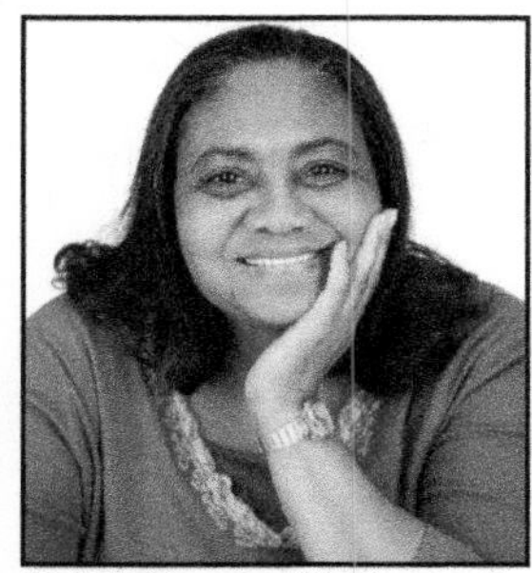

(© Rob Marmion/Shutterstock)

A 60-year-old obese female has come into the ER due to severe RUQ pain for the past 2 hours. Patient also reports increasing nausea but denies emesis. Patient states she has been told she has cholelithiasis by her family physician following a milder episode of this pain 2 years ago. In addition to severe pain, patient displays a moderate degree of scleral jaundice. Abdominal ultrasound identified acute cholecystitis and a large number of gallstones. Because of the jaundice a PTC was performed and confirmed choledocholithiasis. Patient was sent to surgery for laparoscopic cholecystectomy to remove the gallbladder and all gallstones. She recovered without incident.

1. Define each of the patient's symptoms.

____

____

2. The patient has severe RUQ pain. What organs are located in the RUQ?

____

____

3. After reading the definition of jaundice, what is most likely causing this patient to have it?

____

____

4. Describe the diagnostic imaging procedures this patient received.

____

____

5. What is the difference between cholelithiasis and cholecystitis?

____

____

6. The patient's gallbladder was removed laparoscopically. What does that mean?

____

____

Practice Exercises

A. Complete the Statement

1. The digestive system is also known as the ____________________ system.
2. The continuous muscular tube of the digestive system is called the ____________________ or ____________________ and stretches between the ____________________ and ____________________.
3. The accessory organs of the digestive system are the ____________________, ____________________, ____________________, and ____________________.
4. The three main functions of the digestive system are ____________________, ____________________, and ____________________.
5. The incisors are examples of ____________________ teeth and the molars are examples of ____________________ teeth.
6. Food is propelled through the gut by wavelike muscular contractions called ____________________.
7. Food in the stomach is mixed with ____________________ and other gastric juices to form a watery mixture called ____________________.
8. The three sections of small intestine in order are the ____________________, ____________________, and ____________________.
9. The S-shaped section of colon that curves back toward the rectum is called the ____________________ colon.
10. ____________________ produced by the liver is responsible for the ____________________ of fats. It is stored in the ____________________.

B. Combining Form Practice

The combining form **gastr/o** refers to the stomach. Use it to write a term that means:

1. inflammation of the stomach ____________________
2. study of the stomach and small intestines ____________________
3. removal of the stomach ____________________
4. visual exam of the stomach ____________________
5. stomach pain ____________________
6. enlargement of the stomach ____________________
7. cutting into the stomach ____________________

The combining form **esophag/o** refers to the esophagus. Use it to write a term that means:

8. inflammation of the esophagus ____________________
9. visual examination of the esophagus ____________________

10. surgical repair of the esophagus ______

11. pertaining to the esophagus ______

12. stretched-out esophagus ______

The combining form **proct/o** refers to the rectum and anus. Use it to write a term that means:

13. surgical fixation of the rectum and anus ______

14. drooping of the rectum and anus ______

15. inflammation of the rectum and anus ______

16. specialist in the study of the rectum and anus ______

The combining form **cholecyst/o** refers to the gallbladder. Use it to write a term that means:

17. removal of the gallbladder ______

18. condition of having gallbladder stones ______

19. gallbladder stone surgical crushing ______

20. gallbladder inflammation ______

The combining form **lapar/o** refers to the abdomen. Use it to write a term that means:

21. instrument to view inside the abdomen ______

22. cutting into the abdomen ______

23. visual examination of the abdomen ______

The combining form **hepat/o** refers to the liver. Use it to write a term that means:

24. liver tumor ______

25. enlargement of the liver ______

26. pertaining to the liver ______

27. inflammation of the liver ______

The combining form **pancreat/o** refers to the pancreas. Use it to write a term that means:

28. inflammation of the pancreas ______

29. pertaining to the pancreas ______

The combining form **col/o** refers to the colon. Use it to write a term that means:

30. create an opening in the colon ______

31. inflammation of the colon ______

C. Define the Combining Form

	Definition	Example from Chapter
1. esophag/o	______	______
2. hepat/o	______	______
3. ile/o	______	______
4. proct/o	______	______
5. gloss/o	______	______
6. labi/o	______	______
7. jejun/o	______	______
8. sigmoid/o	______	______
9. rect/o	______	______
10. gingiv/o	______	______
11. cholecyst/o	______	______
12. duoden/o	______	______
13. an/o	______	______
14. enter/o	______	______
15. dent/o	______	______

D. Suffix Practice

Use the following suffixes to create a medical term for the following definitions.

-orexia	-phagia	-pepsia	-prandial
-emesis	-lithiasis		

1. after meals ______
2. condition of having gallstones ______
3. no appetite ______
4. difficulty swallowing ______
5. vomiting blood ______
6. slow digestion ______

E. What Does it Stand For?

1. BM ______________________________
2. UGI ______________________________
3. BE ______________________________
4. BS ______________________________
5. n & v ______________________________
6. O & P ______________________________
7. PO ______________________________
8. CBD ______________________________
9. NPO ______________________________
10. pp ______________________________

F. Terminology Matching

Match each term to its definition.

1.	_______ dentures	a.	excess body weight
2.	_______ anorexia	b.	chronic liver disease
3.	_______ hematemesis	c.	heartburn
4.	_______ pyrosis	d.	small colon tumors
5.	_______ obesity	e.	fluid accumulation in abdominal cavity
6.	_______ constipation	f.	vomit blood
7.	_______ melena	g.	bowel twists on self
8.	_______ ascites	h.	set of artificial teeth
9.	_______ cirrhosis	i.	loss of appetite
10.	_______ spastic colon	j.	difficulty having BM
11.	_______ polyposis	k.	irritable bowel syndrome
12.	_______ volvulus	l.	black tarry stool
13.	_______ hiatal hernia	m.	yellow skin color
14.	_______ ulcerative colitis	n.	bloody diarrhea
15.	_______ dysentery	o.	diaphragmatocele
16.	_______ jaundice	p.	inflammatory bowel disease

G. What's the Abbreviation?

1. nasogastric ____________________
2. gastrointestinal ____________________
3. hepatitis B virus ____________________
4. fecal occult blood test ____________________
5. inflammatory bowel disease ____________________
6. herpes simplex virus type 1 ____________________
7. aspartate transaminase ____________________
8. after meals ____________________
9. peptic ulcer disease ____________________
10. gastroesophageal reflux disease ____________________

H. Define the Term

1. colonoscopy ____________________
2. bite wing X-ray ____________________
3. hematochezia ____________________
4. serum bilirubin ____________________
5. cachexia ____________________
6. lavage ____________________
7. hernioplasty ____________________
8. extraction ____________________
9. choledocholithotripsy ____________________
10. anastomosis ____________________

I. Fill in the Blank

colonoscopy	barium swallow	lower GI series
gastric stapling	colostomy	colectomy
total parenteral nutrition	choledocholithotripsy	liver biopsy
ileostomy	fecal occult blood test	intravenous cholecystography

1. Excising a small piece of hepatic tissue for microscopic examination is called a(n) ____________________.
2. When a surgeon performs a total or partial colectomy for cancer, she may have to create an opening on the surface of the skin for fecal matter to leave the body. This procedure is called a(n) ____________________.
3. Another name for an upper GI series is a(n) ____________________.
4. Mr. White has had a radiopaque material placed into his large bowel by means of an enema for the purpose of viewing his colon. This procedure is called a(n) ____________________.

5. A(n) ______________________ is the surgical removal of the colon.
6. Jessica has been on a red meat-free diet in preparation for a test of her feces for the presence of hidden blood. This test is called a(n) ______________________.
7. Dr. Mendez uses equipment to crush gallstones in the common bile duct. This procedure is called a(n) ______________.
8. Mrs. Alcazar required ______________________ because she could not eat following her intestinal surgery.
9. Mr. Bright had a(n) ______________________ to treat his morbid obesity.
10. Visualizing the gallbladder and bile ducts by injecting a dye into the patient's arm is called a(n) ______________________.
11. Passing an instrument into the anus and rectum in order to see the colon is called a(n) ______________________.
12. Ms. Fayne suffers from Crohn's disease, which has necessitated the removal of much of her small intestine. She has had a surgical passage created for the external disposal of waste material from the ileum. This is called a(n) ______________.

J. Terminology Matching

Match each term to its definition.

1. _______ dentures	a.	tooth decay
2. _______ cementum	b.	prosthetic device used to anchor a tooth
3. _______ root canal	c.	inflammation of the gums
4. _______ crown	d.	full set of artificial teeth
5. _______ bridge	e.	portion of the tooth covered by enamel
6. _______ implant	f.	replacement for missing teeth
7. _______ gingivitis	g.	anchors root in bony socket of jaw
8. _______ dental caries	h.	surgery on the tooth pulp

K. Pharmacology Challenge

Fill in the classification for each drug description, then match the brand name.

Drug Description	Classification	Brand Name
1. _______ Controls diarrhea	______________________	a. Pepcid
2. _______ Blocks stomach's ability to secrete acid	______________________	b. Obezine
3. _______ Treats motion sickness	______________________	c. Metamucil
4. _______ Blocks acid-producing receptors	______________________	d. Compazine
5. _______ Suppresses appetite	______________________	e. Maalox
6. _______ Stimulates a bowel movement	______________________	f. Imodium
7. _______ Neutralizes stomach acid	______________________	g. Nexium

Labeling Exercise

Image A

Write the labels for this figure on the numbered lines provided.

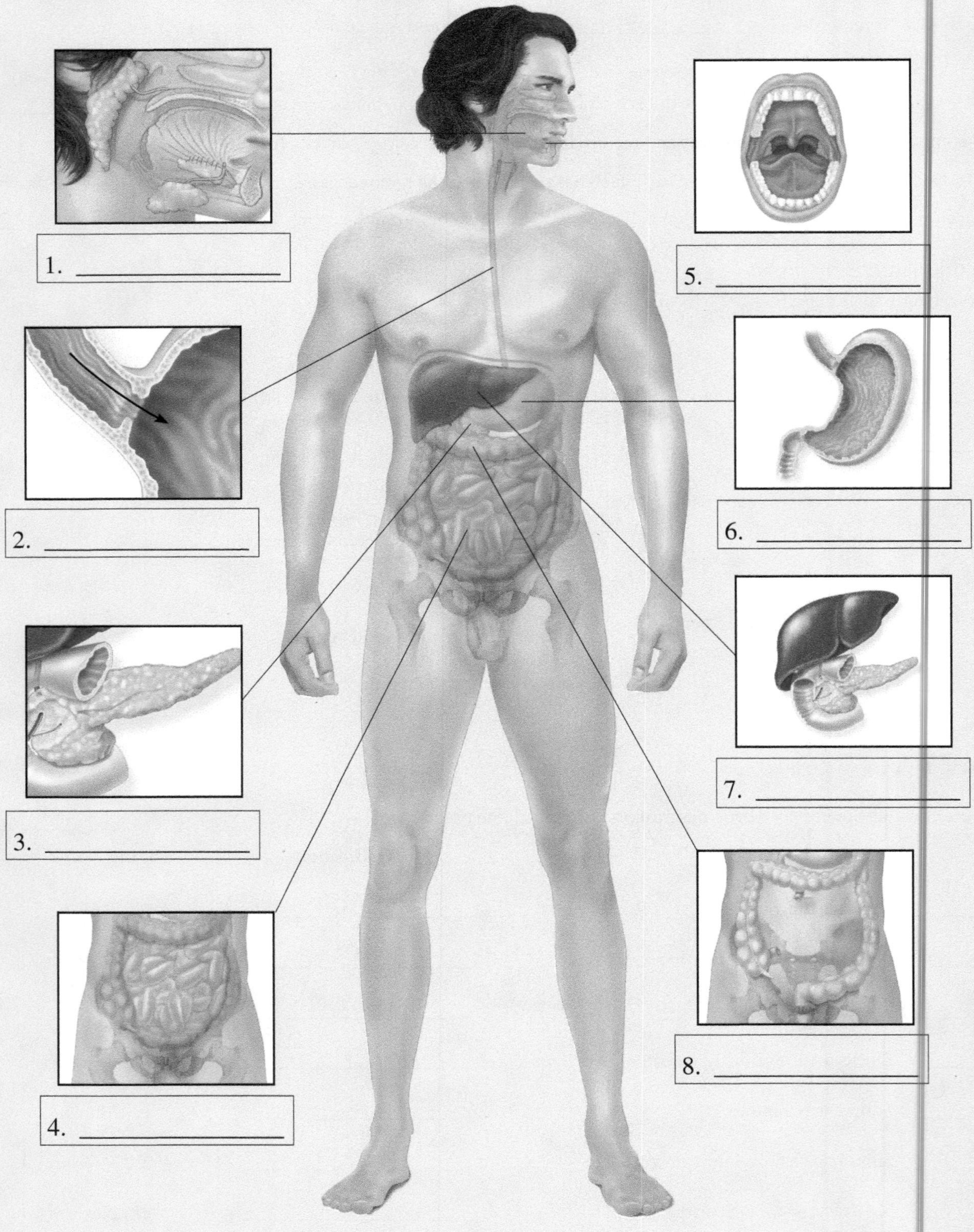

Image B

Write the labels for this figure on the numbered lines provided.

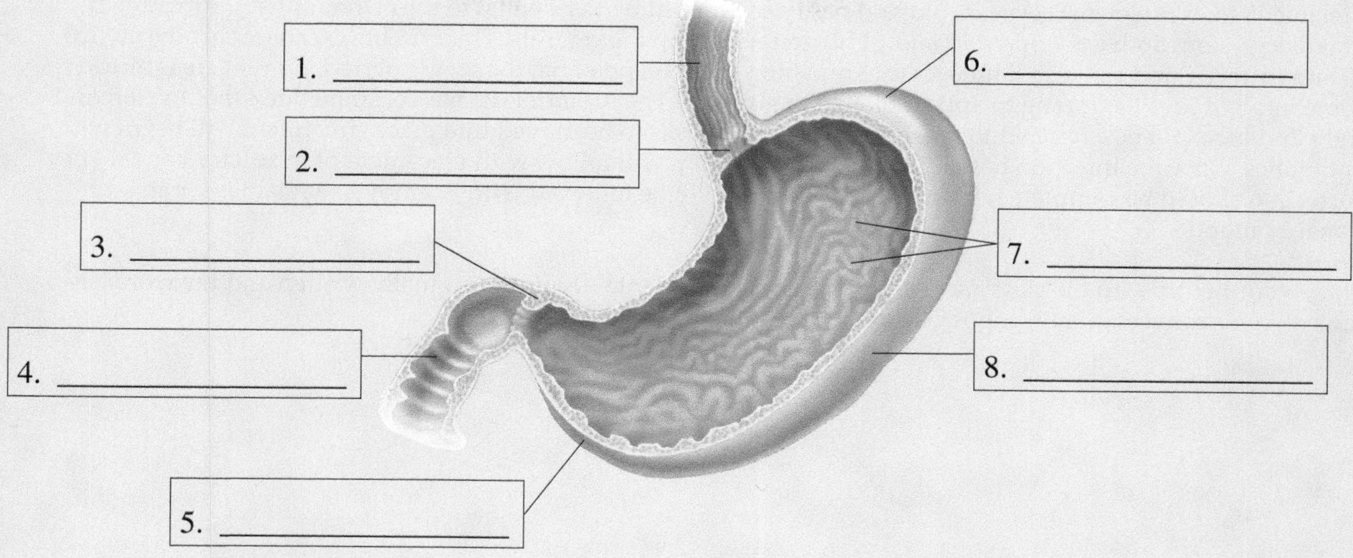

Image C

Write the labels for this figure on the numbered lines provided.

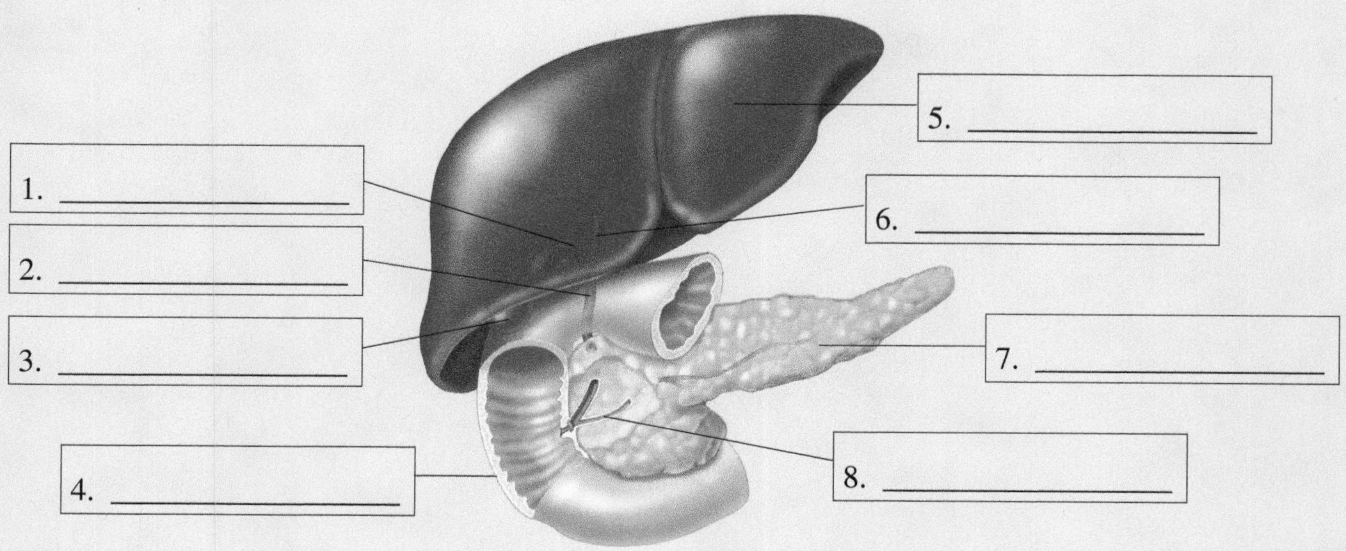

L. Scenario

On a separate piece of paper, re-write the following scenario by translating the dental terms into conversational language to facilitate communication. Use a dental dictionary or electronic media resource as needed to interpret the nomenclature.

Melanie Walker is eleven (11) years old and has been referred by her dentist to the orthodontist for treatment of malocclusion. Both the upper left and right lateral overlap the centrals. This condition can impact the ability to bite correctly and can also limit access to brushing with the potential for severe periodontia. There is already some infected area beginning to appear along the gingival. The orthodontist has recommended that the left and right 2nd bicuspid be extracted to make space for the laterals to be moved into place. Treatment will begin with antibiotics. Once the infection has cleared, corrective action will follow with placement of maxillary bands. The correction should be complete within a 24 month period to be followed with a removable retainer for an additional 24 months.

Share your report with the class carefully pronouncing the dental terms as originally written and the words as rewritten for conversational language communication.

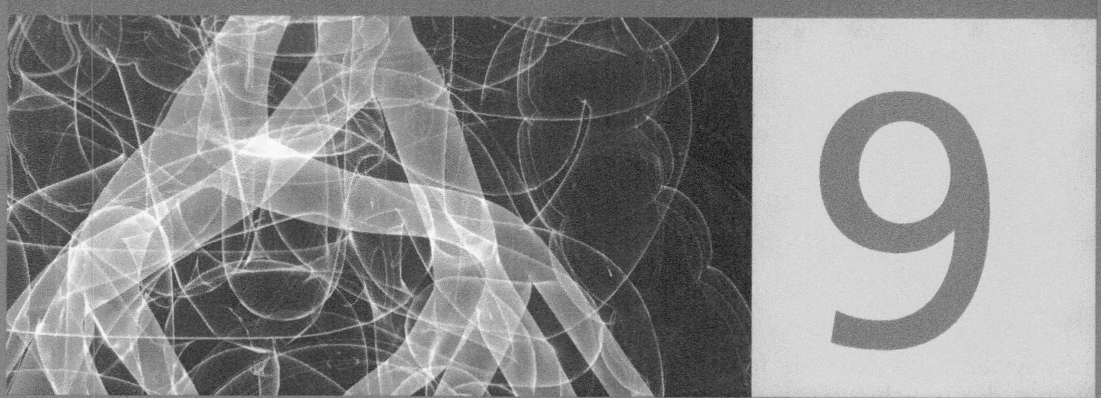

9

URINARY SYSTEM

Learning Objectives

Upon completion of this chapter, you will be able to

- Identify and define the combining forms and suffixes introduced in this chapter.
- Correctly spell and pronounce medical terms and major anatomical structures relating to the urinary system.
- Locate and describe the major organs of the urinary system and their functions.
- Describe the nephron and the mechanisms of urine production.
- Identify the characteristics of urine and a urinalysis.
- Identify and define urinary system anatomical terms.
- Identify and define selected urinary system pathology terms.
- Identify and define selected urinary system diagnostic procedures.
- Identify and define selected urinary system therapeutic procedures.
- Identify and define selected medications relating to the urinary system.
- Define selected abbreviations associated with the urinary system.

Urinary System at a Glance

Function

The urinary system is responsible for maintaining a stable internal environment for the body. In order to achieve this state, the urinary system removes waste products, adjusts water and electrolyte levels, and maintains the correct pH.

Structures

Here are the primary structures that comprise the urinary system.

kidneys
ureters
urethra
urinary bladder

Word Parts

Here are the most common word parts (with their meanings) used to build urinary system terms. For a more comprehensive list, refer to the Terminology section of this chapter.

Combining Forms

azot/o	nitrogenous waste
bacteri/o	bacteria
cyst/o	bladder, pouch
glomerul/o	glomerulus
glycos/o	sugar, glucose
keton/o	ketones
lith/o	stone
meat/o	meatus
nephr/o	kidney
noct/i	night
olig/o	scanty
protein/o	protein
pyel/o	renal pelvis
ren/o	kidney
ureter/o	ureter
urethr/o	urethra
urin/o	urine
ur/o	urine

Suffixes

-lith	stone
-lithiasis	condition of stones
-ptosis	drooping
-tripsy	surgical crushing
-uria	condition of the urine

Urinary System Illustrated

kidney, p. 298

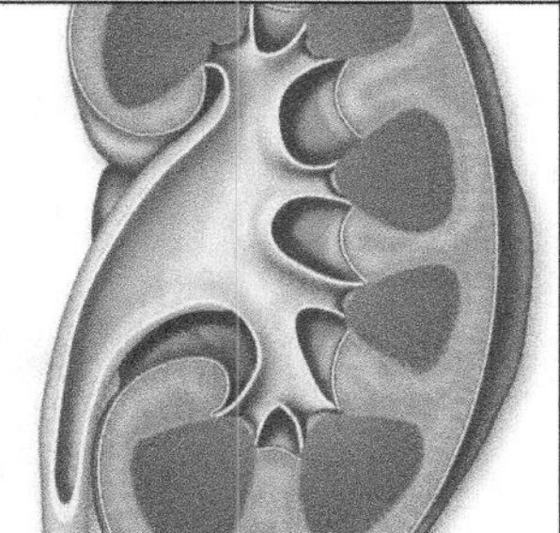

Filters blood and produces urine

ureter, p. 299

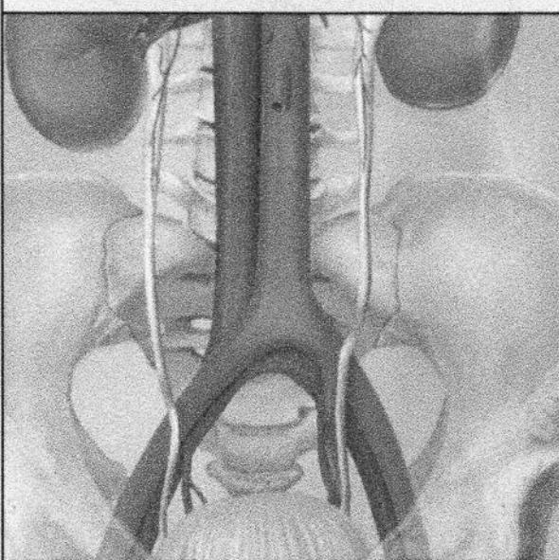

Transports urine to the bladder

urinary bladder, p. 300

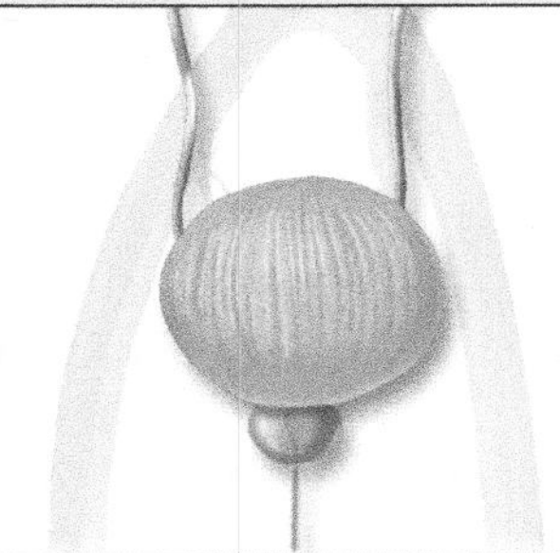

Stores urine

male urethra, p. 301

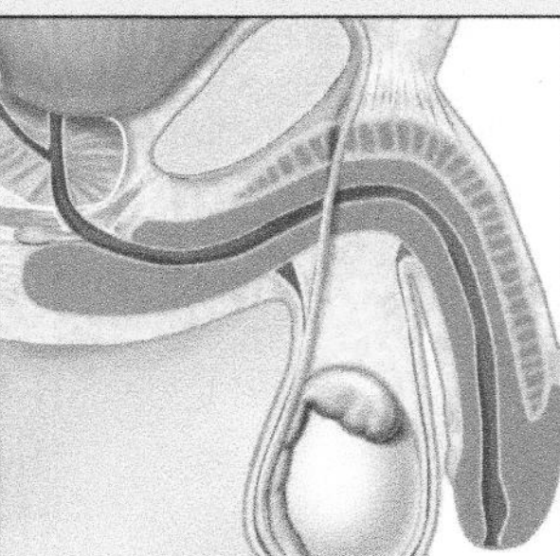

Transports urine to exterior

female urethra, p. 301

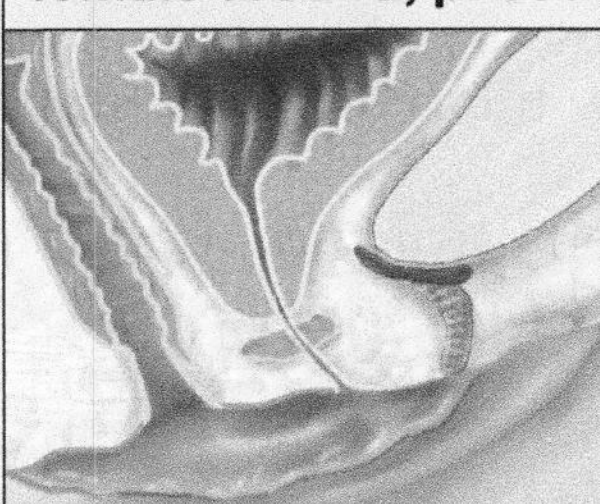

Transports urine to exterior

Anatomy and Physiology of the Urinary System

genitourinary system (jen-ih-toh-YOO-rih-nair-ee)
kidneys
nephrons (NEF-ronz)
uremia (yoo-REE-mee-ah)
ureters (YOO-reh-ters)
urethra (yoo-REE-thrah)
urinary bladder (YOO-rih-nair-ee)
urine (YOO-rin)

Think of the urinary system, sometimes referred to as the **genitourinary (GU) system,** as similar to a water filtration plant. Its main function is to filter and remove waste products from the blood. These waste materials result in the production and excretion of **urine** from the body.

The urinary system is one of the hardest working systems of the body. All the body's metabolic processes result in the production of waste products. These waste products are a natural part of life but quickly become toxic if they are allowed to build up in the blood, resulting in a condition called **uremia.** Waste products in the body are removed through a very complicated system of blood vessels and kidney tubules. The actual filtration of wastes from the blood takes place in millions of **nephrons,** which make up each of your two **kidneys.** As urine drains from each kidney, the **ureters** transport it to the **urinary bladder.** We are constantly producing urine, and our bladders can hold about one quart of this liquid. When the urinary bladder empties, urine moves from the bladder down the **urethra** to the outside of the body.

MED TERM TIP

The urinary system and the male reproductive system share some of the same organs, particularly the urethra. Hence the term *genitourinary* (GU) is sometimes used to describe the urinary system.

Kidneys

calyx (KAY-liks)
cortex (KOR-teks)
hilum (HIGH-lum)
medulla (meh-DULL-ah)
renal artery
renal papilla (pah-PILL-ah)
renal pelvis
renal pyramids
renal vein
retroperitoneal (ret-roh-pair-ih-toh-NEE-al)

MED TERM TIP

From the time of early man, there has been an interest in urine. Drawings on cave walls and hieroglyphics in Egyptian pyramids reveal interest in urine as a means of determining the physical state of the body. Some of the first doctors, called *pisse prophets,* believed that examining the urine would help treat a patient. Now urologists treat disorders of the urinary tract in both men and women, as well as disorders of the male reproductive tract.

The two kidneys are located in the lumbar region of the back above the waist on either side of the vertebral column. They are not inside the peritoneal sac, a location referred to as **retroperitoneal.** Each kidney has a concave or indented area on the edge toward the center that gives the kidney its bean shape. The center of this concave area is called the **hilum.** The hilum is where the **renal artery** enters and the **renal vein** leaves the kidney (see Figure 9.1 ■). The renal artery delivers the blood that is full of waste products to the kidney and the renal vein returns the now cleansed blood to the general circulation. The ureters also leave the kidneys at the hilum. The ureters are narrow tubes that lead from the kidneys to the bladder.

When a surgeon cuts into a kidney, several structures or areas are visible. The outer portion, called the **cortex,** is much like a shell for the kidney. The inner area is called the **medulla.** Within the medulla are a dozen or so triangular-shaped areas, the **renal pyramids,** which resemble their namesake, the Egyptian pyramids. The tip of each pyramid points inward toward the hilum. At its tip, called the **renal papilla,** each pyramid opens into a **calyx** (plural is *calyces*), which is continuous with the **renal pelvis.** The calyces and ultimately the renal pelvis collect urine as it is formed. The ureter for each kidney arises from the renal pelvis (see Figure 9.2 ■).

MED TERM TIP

At any one time, about 20% of your blood is being filtered by your kidneys. In this way, all your blood is cleansed every few minutes.

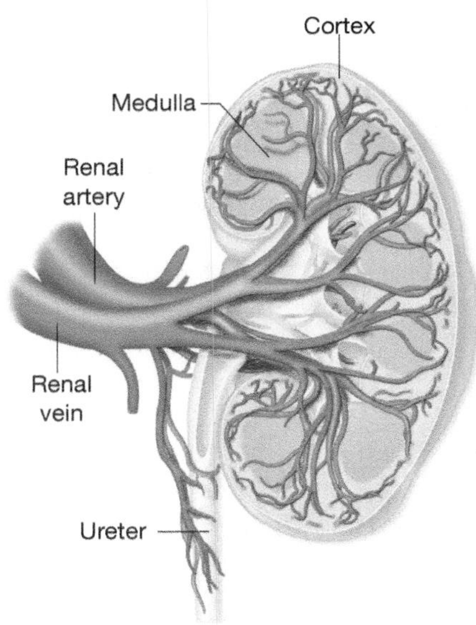

■ Figure 9.1 Kidney structure. Longitudinal section showing the renal artery entering and the renal vein and ureter exiting at the hilium of the kidney.

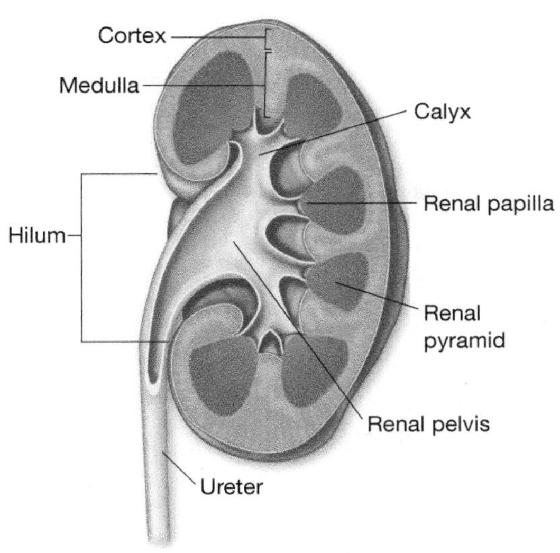

■ Figure 9.2 Longitudinal section of a kidney illustrating the internal structures.

Nephrons

afferent arteriole (AFF-er-ent)
Bowman's capsule
collecting tubule
distal convoluted tubule (DISS-tall / con-voh-LOOT-ed)
efferent arteriole (EF-er-ent)
glomerular capsule (glom-AIR-yoo-lar)
glomerulus (glom-AIR-yoo-lus)
loop of Henle
nephron (NEF-ron)
nephron loop
proximal convoluted tubule (PROK-sim-al / con-voh-LOOT-ed)
renal corpuscle (KOR-pus-ehl)
renal tubule

MED TERM TIP

The kidney bean is so named because it resembles a kidney in shape. Each organ weighs 4–6 ounces, is 2–3 inches wide and approximately 1 inch thick, and is about the size of your fist. In most people the left kidney is slightly higher and larger than the right kidney. Functioning kidneys are necessary for life, but it is possible to live with only one functioning kidney.

The functional or working unit of the kidney is the **nephron**. There are more than one million of these microscopic structures in each human kidney. Each nephron consists of the **renal corpuscle** and the **renal tubule** (see Figure 9.3 ■). The renal corpuscle is the blood-filtering portion of the nephron. It has a double-walled cuplike structure called the **glomerular capsule** (also known as **Bowman's capsule**) that encases a ball of capillaries called the **glomerulus.** An **afferent arteriole** carries blood to the glomerulus, and an **efferent arteriole** carries blood away from the glomerulus.

Water and substances that were removed from the bloodstream in the renal corpuscle flow into the renal tubules to finish the urine production process. This continuous tubule is divided into four sections: the **proximal convoluted tubule,** followed by the narrow **nephron loop** (also known as the **loop of Henle**), then the **distal convoluted tubule,** and finally the **collecting tubule.**

MED TERM TIP

Afferent, meaning moving toward, and *efferent,* meaning moving away from, are terms used when discussing moving either toward or away from the central point in many systems. For example, there are afferent and efferent nerves in the nervous system.

Ureters

As urine drains out of the renal pelvis it enters the ureter, which carries it down to the urinary bladder (see Figure 9.4 ■). Ureters are very narrow tubes measuring less than ¼-inch wide and 10–12 inches long that extend from the renal pelvis to the urinary bladder. Mucous membrane lines the ureters just as it lines most passages that open to the external environment.

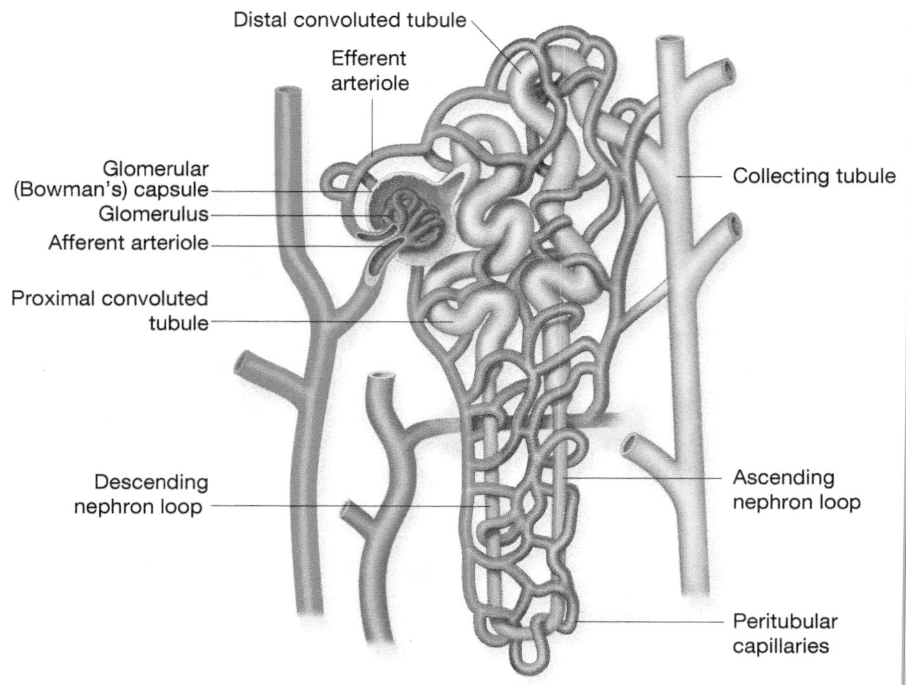

■ **Figure 9.3** The structure of a nephron, illustrating the nephron structure in relation to the circulatory system.

Urinary Bladder

external sphincter (SFINGK-ter)
internal sphincter
rugae (ROO-gay)
urination

The urinary bladder is an elastic muscular sac that lies in the base of the pelvis just behind the pubic symphysis (see Figure 9.5 ■). It is composed of three layers of smooth muscle tissue lined with mucous membrane containing **rugae** or folds that allow it to stretch. The bladder receives the urine directly from the ureters, stores it, and excretes it by **urination** through the urethra.

Generally, an adult bladder will hold 250 mL of urine. This amount then creates an urge to void or empty the bladder. Involuntary muscle action causes the bladder to contract and the **internal sphincter** to relax. The internal sphincter protects us from having our bladder empty at the wrong time. Voluntary action

MED TERM TIP

The terms *ureter* and *urethra* are frequently confused. Remember that there are two ureters carrying urine from the kidneys into the bladder. There is only one urethra, and it carries urine from the bladder to the outside of the body.

MED TERM TIP

Terms such as *micturition, voiding,* and *urination* all mean basically the same thing—the process of releasing urine from the body.

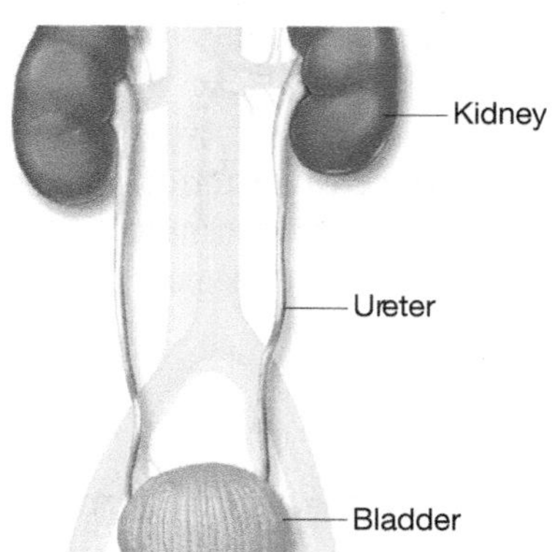

■ **Figure 9.4** The ureters extend from the kidneys to the urinary bladder.

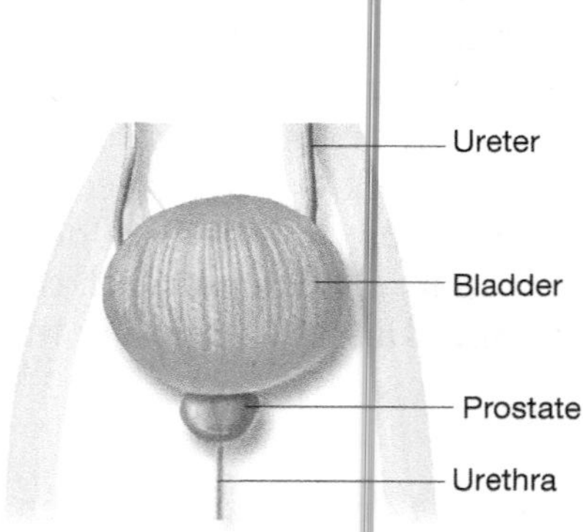

■ **Figure 9.5** The structure of the urinary bladder. (Note the prostate gland.)

controls the **external sphincter,** which opens on demand to allow the intentional emptying of the bladder. The act of controlling the emptying of urine is developed sometime after a child is 2 years of age.

Urethra

urinary meatus (mee-AY-tus)

The urethra is a tubular canal that carries the flow of urine from the bladder to the outside of the body (see Figure 9.6 ■ for the male urethra). The external opening through which urine passes out of the body is called the **urinary meatus.** Mucous membrane also lines the urethra as it does other structures of the urinary system. This is one of the reasons that infection spreads up the urinary tract. The urethra is 1–2 inches long in the female and 8 inches long in the male. In a woman it functions only as the outlet for urine and is in front of the vagina. In the male, however, it has two functions: an outlet for urine and the passageway for semen to leave the body.

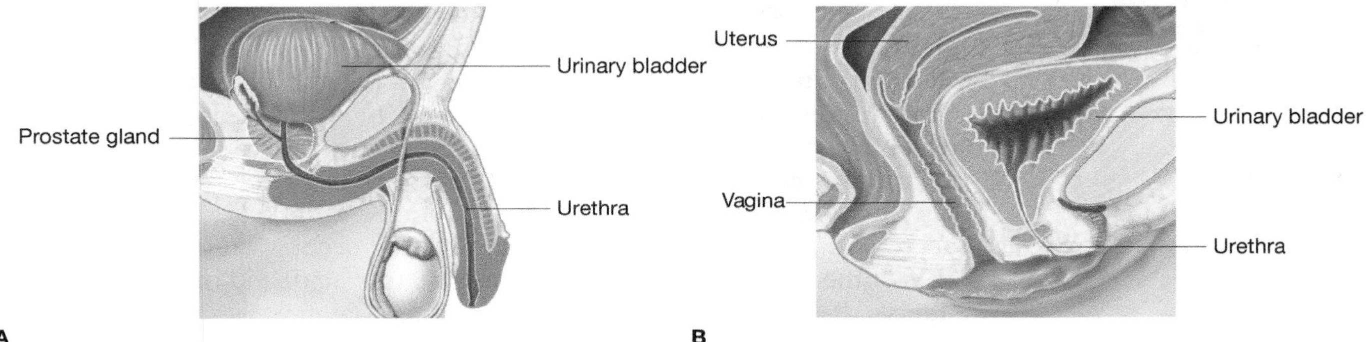

■ Figure 9.6 (A) The male urethra extends from the urinary bladder in the floor of the pelvis through the penis to the urinary meatus; (B) the much shorter female urethra extends from the urinary bladder to the floor of the pelvis and exits just in front of the vaginal opening.

Role of Kidneys in Homeostasis

electrolytes (ee-LEK-troh-lites) **homeostasis** (hoh-mee-oh-STAY-sis)

The kidneys are responsible for **homeostasis** or balance in the body. They continually adjust the chemical conditions in the body, allowing us to survive. Because of its interaction with the bloodstream and its ability to excrete substances from the body, the urinary system maintains the body's proper balance of water and chemicals. If the body is low on water, the kidneys conserve it, or in the opposite case, if there is excess water in the body, the kidneys excrete the excess. In adition to water, the kidneys regulate the level of **electrolytes**—small biologically important molecules such as sodium (Na^+), potassium (K^+), chloride (Cl^-), and bicarbonate (HCO_3^-). Finally, the kidneys play an important role in maintaining the correct pH range within the body, making sure we do not become too acidic or too alkaline. The kidneys accomplish these important tasks through the production of urine.

MED TERM TIP

Mucous membranes will carry infections up the urinary tract from the urinary meatus and urethra into the bladder and eventually up the ureters and the kidneys if not stopped. It is never wise to ignore a simple bladder infection or what is called *cystitis.*

Stages of Urine Production

filtration
glomerular filtrate
peritubular capillaries
reabsorption
secretion

As wastes and unnecessary substances are removed from the bloodstream by the nephrons, many desirable molecules are also removed initially. Waste products are eliminated from the body, but other substances such as water, electrolytes, and nutrients must be returned to the bloodstream. Urine, in its final form ready for elimination from the body, is the ultimate product of this entire process.

Urine production occurs in three stages: **filtration, reabsorption,** and **secretion.** Each of these steps is performed by a different section of the nephrons (see Figure 9.7 ■).

> **MED TERM TIP**
> The amount of water and other fluids processed by the kidneys each day is astonishing. Approximately 190 quarts of fluid are filtered out of the glomerular blood every day. Most of this fluid returns to the body through the reabsorption process. About 99% of the water that leaves the blood each day through the filtration process returns to the blood by proximal tubule reabsorption.

1. **Filtration.** The first stage is the filtering of particles, which occurs in the renal corpuscle. The pressure of blood flowing through the glomerulus forces material out of the bloodstream, through the wall of the glomerular capsule, and into the renal tubules. This fluid in the tubules is called the **glomerular filtrate** and consists of water, electrolytes, nutrients such as glucose and amino acids, wastes, and toxins.
2. **Reabsorption.** After filtration, the filtrate passes through the four sections of the tubule. As the filtrate moves along its twisted journey, most of the water and much of the electrolytes and nutrients are reabsorbed into the **peritubular capillaries,** a capillary bed that surrounds the renal tubules. They can then reenter the circulating blood.
3. **Secretion.** The final stage of urine production occurs when the special cells of the renal tubules secrete ammonia, uric acid, and other waste substances directly into the renal tubule. Urine formation is now finished; it passes into the collecting tubules, renal papilla, calyx, renal pelvis, and ultimately into the ureter.

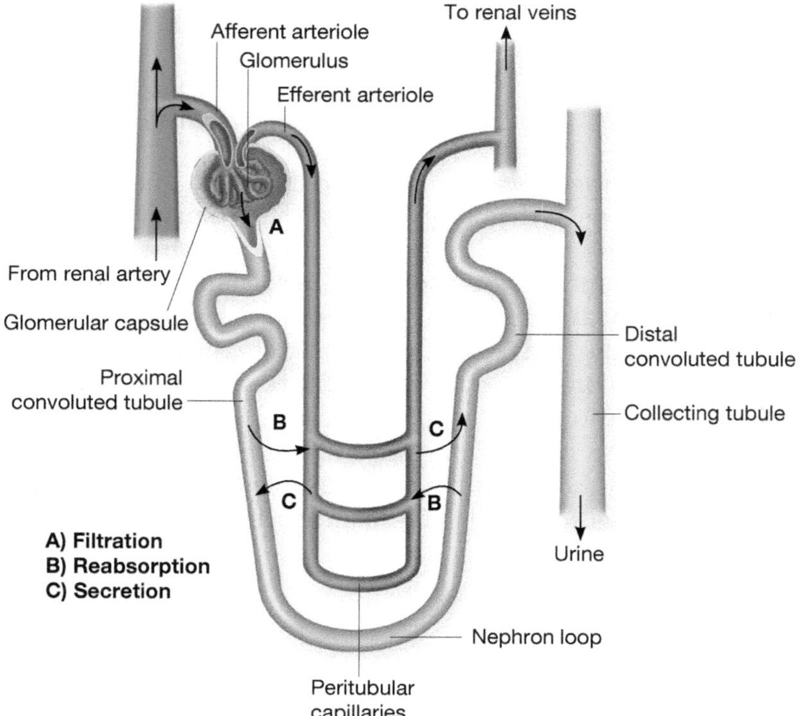

■ **Figure 9.7** The three stages of urine production: filtration, reabsorption, and secretion.

Urine

albumin (al-BEW-min)
nitrogenous wastes (nigh-TROJ-eh-nus)
specific gravity
urinalysis (yoo-rih-NAL-ih-sis)

Urine is normally straw-colored to clear, and sterile. Although it is 95% water, it also contains many dissolved substances, such as electrolytes, toxins, and **nitrogenous wastes,** the by-products of muscle metabolism. At times the urine also contains substances that should not be there, such as glucose, blood, or **albumin,** a protein that should remain in the blood. This is the reason for performing a **urinalysis,** a physical and chemical analysis of urine, which gives medical personnel important information regarding disease processes occurring in a patient. Normally, during a 24-hour period the output of urine will be 1,000–2,000 mL, depending on the amount of fluid consumed and the general health of the person. Normal urine is acidic because this is one way our bodies dispose of excess acids. **Specific gravity** indicates the amount of dissolved substances in urine. The specific gravity of pure water is 1.000. The specific gravity of urine varies from 1.001 to 1.030. Highly concentrated urine has a higher specific gravity, while the specific gravity of very dilute urine is close to that of water. See Table 9.1 ■ for the normal values for urine testing and Table 9.2 ■ for abnormal findings.

MED TERM TIP

The color, odor, volume, and sugar content of urine have been examined for centuries. Color charts for urine were developed by 1140, and "taste testing" was common in the late seventeenth century. By the nineteenth century, urinalysis was a routine part of a physical examination.

Table 9.1 Values for Urinalysis Testing

ELEMENT	NORMAL FINDINGS
Color	Straw-colored, pale yellow to deep gold
Odor	Aromatic
Appearance	Clear
Specific gravity	1.001–1.030
pH	5.0–8.0
Protein	Negative to trace
Glucose	None
Ketones	None
Blood	Negative

Table 9.2 Abnormal Urinalysis Findings

ELEMENT	IMPLICATIONS
Color	Color varies depending on the patient's fluid intake and output or medication. Brown or black urine color indicates a serious disease process.
Odor	A fetid or foul odor may indicate infection. While a fruity odor may be found in diabetes mellitus, dehydration, or starvation. Other odors may be due to medication or foods.
Appearance	Cloudiness may mean that an infection is present.
Specific gravity	Concentrated urine has a higher specific gravity. Dilute urine, such as can be found with diabetes insipidus, acute tubular necrosis, or salt-restricted diets, has a lower specific gravity.
pH	A pH value below 7.0 (acidic) is common in urinary tract infections, metabolic or respiratory acidosis, diets high in fruits or vegetables, or administration of some drugs. A pH higher than 7.0 (basic or alkaline) is common in metabolic or respiratory alkalosis, fever, high-protein diets, and taking ascorbic acid.
Protein	Protein may indicate glomerulonephritis or preeclampsia in a pregnant woman.
Glucose	Small amounts of glucose may be present as the result of eating a high-carbohydrate meal, stress, pregnancy, and taking some medications, such as aspirin or corticosteroids. Higher levels may indicate poorly controlled diabetes, Cushing's syndrome, or infection.
Ketones	The presence of ketones may indicate poorly controlled diabetes, dehydration, starvation, or ingestion of large amounts of aspirin.
Blood	Blood may indicate glomerulonephritis, cancer of the urinary tract, some types of anemia, taking of some medications (such as blood thinners), arsenic poisoning, reactions to transfusion, trauma, burns, and convulsions.

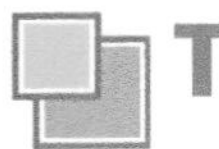

Terminology

Word Parts Used to Build Urinary System Terms

The following lists contain the combining forms, suffixes, and prefixes used to build terms in the remaining sections of this chapter.

Combining Forms

azot/o	nitrogenous waste
bacteri/o	bacteria
bi/o	life
carcin/o	cancer
corpor/o	body
cyst/o	bladder, pouch
glomerul/o	glomerulus
glycos/o	sugar
hem/o	blood
hemat/o	blood

keton/o	ketones
lith/o	stone
meat/o	meatus
necr/o	death
nephr/o	kidney
neur/o	nerve
noct/i	night
olig/o	scanty
peritone/o	peritoneum
protein/o	protein

py/o	pus
pyel/o	renal pelvis
ren/o	kidney
ur/o	urine
ureter/o	ureter
urethr/o	urethra
urin/o	urine
ven/o	vein

Suffixes

-al	pertaining to
-algia	pain
-ar	pertaining to
-ary	pertaining to
-cele	protrusion
-eal	pertaining to
-ectasis	dilated
-ectomy	surgical removal
-emia	blood condition
-genic	produced by
-gram	record
-graphy	process of recording
-ic	pertaining to
-itis	inflammation
-lith	stone

-lithiasis	condition of stones
-logist	one who studies
-logy	study of
-lysis	to destroy (to break down)
-malacia	softening
-megaly	enlarged
-meter	instrument to measure
-oma	tumor
-ory	pertaining to
-osis	abnormal condition
-ostomy	create a new opening
-otomy	cutting into
-ous	pertaining to

-pathy	disease
-pexy	surgical fixation
-plasty	surgical repair
-ptosis	drooping
-rrhagia	abnormal flow condition
-sclerosis	hardening
-scope	instrument to visually examine
-scopy	process of visually examining
-stenosis	narrowing
-tic	pertaining to
-tripsy	surgical crushing
-uria	urine condition

Prefixes

an-	without
anti-	against
dys-	abnormal, difficult

extra-	outside of
hydro-	water
intra-	within

poly-	many
retro-	backward

Anatomical Terms

TERM	WORD PARTS	DEFINITION
cystic (SIS-tik)	cyst/o = bladder -ic = pertaining to	Pertaining to the bladder.
renal (REE-nal)	ren/o = kidney -al = pertaining to	Pertaining to the kidney.
ureteral (yoo-REE-ter-all)	ureter/o = ureter -al = pertaining to	Pertaining to the ureter.
urethral (yoo-REE-thral)	urethr/o = urethra -al = pertaining to	Pertaining to the urethra.
urinary (yoo-rih-NAIR-ee)	urin/o = urine -ary = pertaining to	Pertaining to urine.

MED TERM TIP

Word Watch: Be particularly careful when using the three very similar combining forms: *uter/o* meaning "uterus," *ureter/o* meaning "ureter," and *urethr/o* meaning "urethra."

Pathology

TERM	WORD PARTS	DEFINITION
Medical Specialties		
nephrology (neh-FROL-oh-jee)	nephr/o = kidney -logy = study of	Branch of medicine involved in diagnosis and treatment of diseases and disorders of the kidney. Physician is a *nephrologist.*
urology (yoo-RAL-oh-jee)	ur/o = urine -logy = study of	Branch of medicine involved in diagnosis and treatment of diseases and disorders of the urinary system (and male reproductive system). Physician is a *urologist.*
Signs and Symptoms		
anuria (an-YOO-ree-ah)	an- = without -uria = urine condition	Complete suppression of urine formed by the kidneys and a complete lack of urine excretion.
azotemia (a-zo-TEE-mee-ah)	azot/o = nitrogenous waste -emia = blood condition	Accumulation of nitrogenous waste in the bloodstream. Occurs when the kidney fails to filter these wastes from the blood.
bacteriuria (back-teer-ree-YOO-ree-ah)	bacteri/o = bacteria -uria = urine condition	Presence of bacteria in the urine.

Pathology *(continued)*

TERM	WORD PARTS	DEFINITION
calculus (KAL-kew-lus)		Stone formed within an organ by an accumulation of mineral salts. Found in the kidney, renal pelvis, ureters, bladder, or urethra. Plural is *calculi*.
■ **Figure 9.8** Photograph of sectioned kidney specimen illustrating extensive renal calculi.	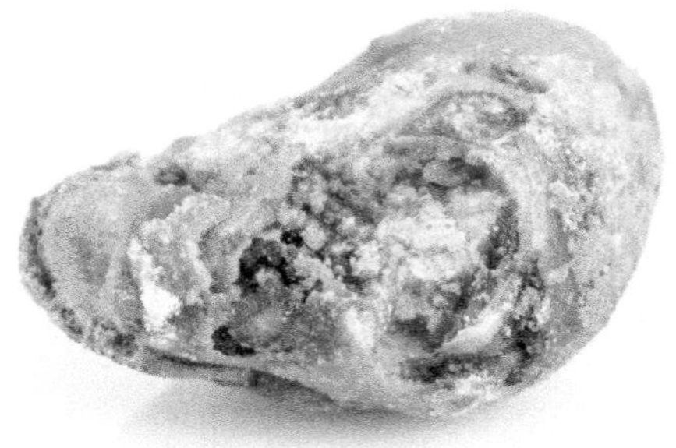	
cystalgia (sis-TAL-jee-ah)	cyst/o = bladder -algia = pain	Urinary bladder pain.
	MED TERM TIP Word Watch: Be careful using the combining forms *cyst/o* meaning "bladder" and *cyt/o* meaning "cell."	
cystolith (SIS-toh-lith)	cyst/o = bladder -lith = stone	Bladder stone.
cystorrhagia (sis-toh-RAH-jee-ah)	cyst/o = bladder -rrhagia = abnormal flow condition	Profuse bleeding from the urinary bladder.
diuresis (dye-yoo-REE-sis)		Increased formation and excretion of urine.
dysuria (dis-YOO-ree-ah)	dys- = abnormal, difficult -uria = urine condition	Difficult or painful urination.
enuresis (en-yoo-REE-sis)		Involuntary discharge of urine after the age by which bladder control should have been established. This usually occurs by the age of 5. *Nocturnal enuresis* refers to bed-wetting at night.
frequency		Greater-than-normal occurrence in the urge to urinate, without an increase in the total daily volume of urine. Frequency is an indication of inflammation of the bladder or urethra.
glycosuria (glye-kohs-YOO-ree-ah)	glycos/o = sugar -uria = urine condition	Presence of sugar in the urine.
hematuria (hee-mah-TOO-ree-ah)	hemat/o = blood -uria = urine condition	Presence of blood in the urine.

Pathology *(continued)*

TERM	WORD PARTS	DEFINITION
hesitancy		Decrease in the force of the urine stream, often with difficulty initiating the flow. It is often a symptom of a blockage along the urethra, such as an enlarged prostate gland.
ketonuria (key-tone-YOO-ree-ah)	keton/o = ketones -uria = urine condition	Presence of ketones in the urine. This occurs when the body burns fat instead of glucose for energy, such as in uncontrolled diabetes mellitus.
nephrolith (NEF-roh-lith)	nephr/o = kidney -lith = stone	Kidney stone.
nephromalacia (nef-roh-mah-LAY-she-ah)	nephr/o = kidney -malacia = softening	Kidney is abnormally soft.
nephromegaly (nef-roh-MEG-ah-lee)	nephr/o = kidney -megaly = enlarged	Kidney is enlarged.
nephrosclerosis (nef-roh-skleh-ROH-sis)	nephr/o = kidney -sclerosis = hardening	Kidney tissue has become hardened.
nocturia (nok-TOO-ree-ah)	noct/i = night -uria = urine condition	Having to urinate frequently during the night.
oliguria (ol-ig-YOO-ree-ah)	olig/o = scanty -uria = urine condition	Producing too little urine.
polyuria (pol-ee-YOO-ree-ah)	poly- = many -uria = urine condition	Producing an unusually large volume of urine.
proteinuria (pro-ten-YOO-ree-ah)	protein/o = protein -uria = urine condition	Presence of protein in the urine.
pyuria (pye-YOO-ree-ah)	py/o = pus -uria = urine condition	Presence of pus in the urine.
renal colic (KOL-ik)	ren/o = kidney -al = pertaining to -ic = pertaining to	Pain caused by a kidney stone. Can be an excruciating pain and generally requires medical treatment.
stricture (STRIK-chur)		Narrowing of a passageway in the urinary system.
uremia (yoo-REE-me-ah)	ur/o = urine -emia = blood condition	Accumulation of waste products (especially nitrogenous wastes) in the bloodstream. Associated with renal failure.
ureterectasis (yoo-ree-ter-EK-tah-sis)	ureter/o = ureter -ectasis = dilated	Ureter is stretched out or dilated.
ureterolith (yoo-REE-teh-roh-lith)	ureter/o = ureter -lith = stone	Stone in the ureter.
ureterostenosis (yoo-ree-ter-oh-sten-OH-sis)	ureter/o = ureter -stenosis = narrowing	Ureter has become narrow.
urethralgia (yoo-ree-THRAL-jee-ah)	urethr/o = urethra -algia = pain	Urethral pain.

Pathology (continued)

TERM	WORD PARTS	DEFINITION
urethrorrhagia (yoo-ree-throh-RAH-jee-ah)	urethr/o = urethra -rrhagia = abnormal flow condition	Profuse bleeding from the urethra.
urethrostenosis (yoo-ree-throh-steh-NOH-sis)	urethr/o = urethra -stenosis = narrowing	Urethra has become narrow.
urgency (ER-jen-see)		Feeling the need to urinate immediately.
urinary incontinence (in-CON-tin-ens)	urin/o = urine -ary = pertaining to	Involuntary release of urine. In some patients an indwelling catheter is inserted into the bladder for continuous urine drainage.

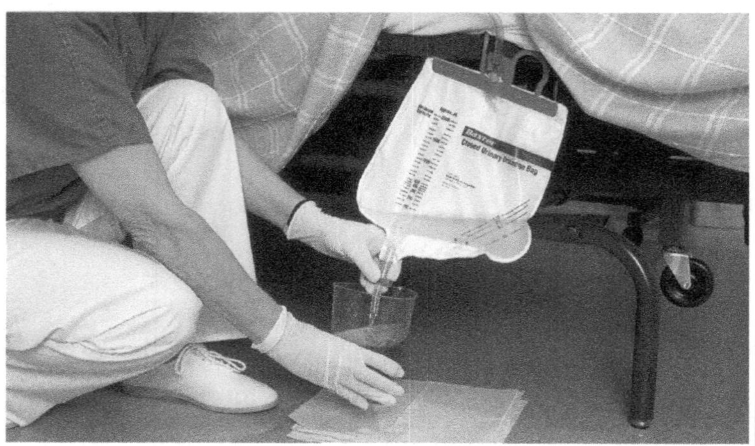

■ Figure 9.9 Healthcare worker draining urine from a bladder catheter bag.

TERM	WORD PARTS	DEFINITION
urinary retention	urin/o = urine -ary = pertaining to	Inability to fully empty the bladder, often indicates a blockage in the urethra.
Kidney		
acute tubular necrosis (ATN) (ne-KROH-sis)	-ar = pertaining to necr/o = death -osis = abnormal condition	Damage to the renal tubules due to presence of toxins in the urine or to ischemia. Results in oliguria.
diabetic nephropathy (ne-FROH-path-ee)	-ic = pertaining to nephr/o = kidney -pathy = disease	Accumulation of damage to the glomerulus capillaries due to the chronic high blood sugars of diabetes mellitus.
glomerulonephritis (gloh-mair-yoo-loh-neh-FRYE-tis)	glomerul/o = glomerulus nephr/o = kidney -itis = inflammation	Inflammation of the kidney (primarily of the glomerulus). Since the glomerular membrane is inflamed, it becomes more permeable and will allow protein and blood cells to enter the filtrate. Results in protein in the urine (proteinuria) and hematuria.
hydronephrosis (high-droh-neh-FROH-sis)	hydro- = water nephr/o = kidney -osis = abnormal condition	Distention of the renal pelvis due to urine collecting in the kidney; often a result of the obstruction of a ureter.
nephritis (neh-FRYE-tis)	nephr/o = kidney -itis = inflammation	Kidney inflammation.

Pathology *(continued)*

TERM	WORD PARTS	DEFINITION
nephrolithiasis (nef-roh-lith-EE-a-sis)	nephr/o = kidney -lithiasis = condition of stones	Presence of calculi in the kidney. Usually begins with the solidification of salts present in the urine.
nephroma (neh-FROH-ma)	nephr/o = kidney -oma = tumor	Kidney tumor.
nephropathy (neh-FROP-ah-thee)	nephr/o = kidney -pathy = disease	General term describing the presence of kidney disease.
nephroptosis (nef-rop-TOH-sis)	nephr/o = kidney -ptosis = drooping	Downward displacement of the kidney out of its normal location; commonly called a *floating kidney.*
nephrotic syndrome (NS)	nephr/o = kidney -tic = pertaining to	Damage to the glomerulus resulting in protein appearing in the urine, proteinuria, and the corresponding decrease in protein in the bloodstream. Also called *nephrosis.*
polycystic kidneys (POL-ee-sis-tik)	poly- = many cyst/o = pouch -tic = pertaining to	Formation of multiple cysts within the kidney tissue. Results in the destruction of normal kidney tissue and uremia.

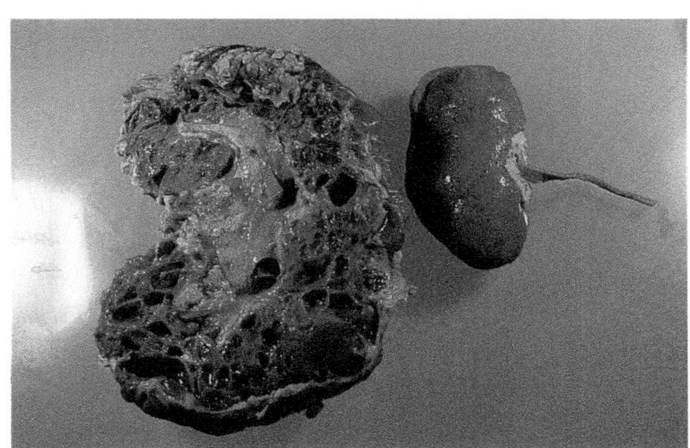

■ **Figure 9.10** Photograph of a polycystic kidney on the left compared to a normal kidney on the right. *(Simon Fraser/Royal Victoria Infirmary, Newcastle/Science Photo Library/Photo Researchers, Inc.)*

TERM	WORD PARTS	DEFINITION
pyelitis (pye-eh-LYE-tis)	pyel/o = renal pelvis -itis = inflammation	Renal pelvis inflammation.
pyelonephritis (pye-eh-loh-neh-FRYE-tis)	pyel/o = renal pelvis nephr/o = kidney -itis = inflammation	Inflammation of the renal pelvis and the kidney. One of the most common types of kidney disease. It may be the result of a lower urinary tract infection that moved up to the kidney by way of the ureters. There may be large quantities of white blood cells and bacteria in the urine. Blood (hematuria) may even be present in the urine in this condition. Can occur with any untreated or persistent case of cystitis.
renal cell carcinoma	ren/o = kidney -al = pertaining to carcin/o = cancer -oma = tumor	Cancerous tumor that arises from kidney tubule cells.

Pathology *(continued)*

TERM	WORD PARTS	DEFINITION
renal failure	ren/o = kidney -al = pertaining to	Inability of the kidneys to filter wastes from the blood resulting in uremia. May be acute or chronic. Major reason for a patient being placed on dialysis.
Wilm's tumor (VILMZ)		Malignant kidney tumor found most often in children.
Urinary Bladder		
bladder cancer		Cancerous tumor that arises from the cells lining the bladder; major sign is hematuria.
bladder neck obstruction (BNO)		Blockage of the bladder outlet. Often caused by an enlarged prostate gland in males.
cystitis (sis-TYE-tis)	cyst/o = bladder -itis = inflammation	Urinary bladder inflammation.
cystocele (SIS-toh-seel)	cyst/o = bladder -cele = protrusion	Hernia or protrusion of the urinary bladder into the wall of the vagina.
interstitial cystitis (in-ter-STISH-al / sis-TYE-tis)	-al = pertaining to cyst/o = bladder -itis = inflammation	Disease of unknown cause in which there is inflammation and irritation of the bladder. Most commonly seen in middle-aged women.
neurogenic bladder (noo-roh-JEN-ik)	neur/o = nerve -genic = produced by	Loss of nervous control that leads to retention; may be caused by spinal cord injury or multiple sclerosis.
urinary tract infection (UTI)	urin/o = urine -ary = pertaining to	Infection, usually from bacteria, of any organ of the urinary system. Most often begins with cystitis and may ascend into the ureters and kidneys. Most common in women because of their shorter urethra.

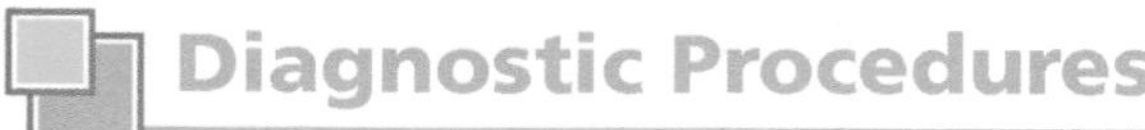

Diagnostic Procedures

TERM	WORD PARTS	DEFINITION
Clinical Laboratory Tests		
blood urea nitrogen (BUN) (yoo-REE-ah / NIGH-troh-jen)		Blood test to measure kidney function by the level of nitrogenous waste (urea) that is in the blood.
clean catch specimen (CC)		Urine sample obtained after cleaning off the urinary opening and catching or collecting a urine sample in midstream (halfway through the urination process) to minimize contamination from the genitalia.

Diagnostic Procedures *(continued)*

TERM	WORD PARTS	DEFINITION
creatinine clearance (kree-AT-tih-neen)		Test of kidney function. Creatinine is a waste product cleared from the bloodstream by the kidneys. For this test, urine is collected for 24 hours, and the amount of creatinine in the urine is compared to the amount of creatinine that remains in the bloodstream.
urinalysis (U/A, UA) (yoo-rih-NAL-ih-sis)	urin/o = urine -lysis = to destroy (to break down)	Laboratory test consisting of the physical, chemical, and microscopic examination of urine.
urine culture and sensitivity (C&S)		Laboratory test of urine for bacterial infection. Attempt to grow bacteria on a culture medium in order to identify it and determine which antibiotics it is sensitive to.
urinometer (yoo-rin-OH-meter)	urin/o = urine -meter = instrument to measure	Instrument to measure the specific gravity of urine; part of a urinalysis.
Diagnostic Imaging		
cystogram (SIS-toh-gram)	cyst/o = bladder -gram = record	X-ray record of the urinary bladder.
cystography (sis-TOG-rah-fee)	cyst/o = bladder -graphy = process of recording	Process of instilling a contrast material or dye into the bladder by catheter to visualize the urinary bladder on X-ray.
excretory urography (EU) (EKS-kreh-tor-ee / yoo-ROG-rah-fee)	-ory = pertaining to ur/o = urine -graphy = process of recording	Injecting dye into the bloodstream and then taking an X-ray to trace the action of the kidney as it excretes the dye.
intravenous pyelography (IVP) (in-trah-VEE-nus / pye-eh-LOG-rah-fee)	intra- = within ven/o = vein -ous = pertaining to pyel/o = renal pelvis -graphy = process of recording	Diagnostic X-ray procedure in which a dye is injected into a vein and then X-rays are taken to visualize the renal pelvis as the dye is removed by the kidneys.
kidneys, ureters, bladder (KUB)		X-ray taken of the abdomen demonstrating the kidneys, ureters, and bladder without using any contrast dye. Also called a *flat-plate abdomen*.
nephrogram (NEH-fro-gram)	nephr/o = kidney -gram = record	X-ray record of the kidney.
pyelogram (PYE-eh-loh-gram)	pyel/o = renal pelvis -gram = record	X-ray record of the renal pelvis.

Diagnostic Procedures *(continued)*

TERM	WORD PARTS	DEFINITION
retrograde pyelography (RP) (RET-roh-grayd/ pye-eh-LOG-rah-fee)	retro- = backward pyel/o = renal pelvis -graphy = process of recording	Diagnostic X-ray procedure in which dye is inserted through the urethra to outline the bladder, ureters, and renal pelvis.

■ **Figure 9.11** Color-enhanced retrograde pyelogram X-ray. Radiopaque dye outlines urinary bladder, ureters, and renal pelvis. *(Clinique Ste. Catherine/CNRI/ Science Photo Library/Photo Researchers, Inc.)*

TERM	WORD PARTS	DEFINITION
voiding cystourethrography (VCUG) (sis-toh-yoo-ree-THROG-rah-fee)	cyst/o = bladder urethr/o = urethra -graphy = process of recording	X-ray taken to visualize the urethra while the patient is voiding after a contrast dye has been placed in the bladder.
Endoscopic Procedure		
cystoscope (SIS-toh-scope)	cyst/o = bladder -scope = instrument to visually examine	Instrument used to visually examine the inside of the urinary bladder.
cystoscopy (cysto) (sis-TOSS-koh-pee)	cyst/o = bladder -scopy = process of visually examining	Visual examination of the urinary bladder using an instrument called a *cystoscope.*
urethroscope (yoo-REE-throh-scope)	urethr/o = urethra -scope = instrument to visually examine	Instrument to visually examine the inside of the urethra.

Therapeutic Procedures

TERM	WORD PARTS	DEFINITION
Medical Treatments		
catheter (KATH-eh-ter)		Flexible tube inserted into the body for the purpose of moving fluids into or out of the body. Most commonly used to refer to a tube threaded through the urethra into the bladder to withdraw urine (see again Figure 9.9).
catheterization (cath) (kath-eh-ter-ih-ZAY-shun)		Insertion of a tube through the urethra and into the urinary bladder for the purpose of withdrawing urine or inserting dye.

Therapeutic Procedures *(continued)*

TERM	WORD PARTS	DEFINITION
extracorporeal shockwave lithotripsy (ESWL) (eks-trah-cor-POR-ee-al / shockwave / LITH-oh-trip-see)	extra- = outside of corpor/o = body -eal = pertaining to lith/o = stone -tripsy = surgical crushing	Use of ultrasound waves to break up stones. Process does not require invasive surgery.

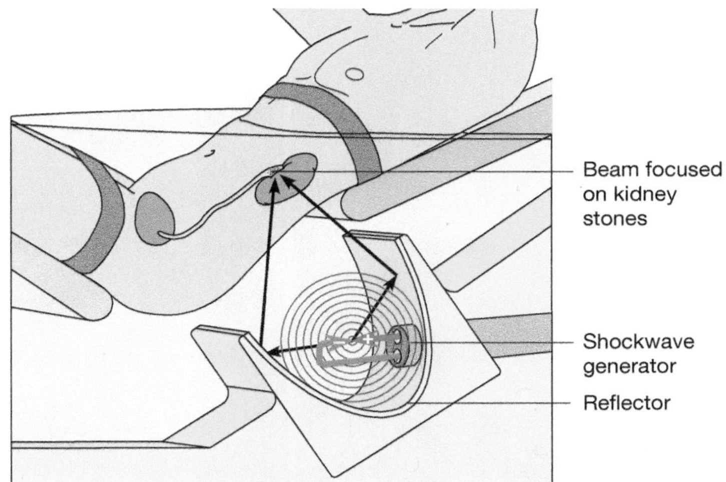

■ **Figure 9.12** Extracorporeal shockwave lithotripsy, a noninvasive procedure using high-frequency sound waves to shatter kidney stones.

TERM	WORD PARTS	DEFINITION
hemodialysis (HD) (hee-moh-dye-AL-ih-sis)	hem/o = blood	Use of an artificial kidney machine that filters the blood of a person to remove waste products. Use of this technique in patients who have defective kidneys is lifesaving.

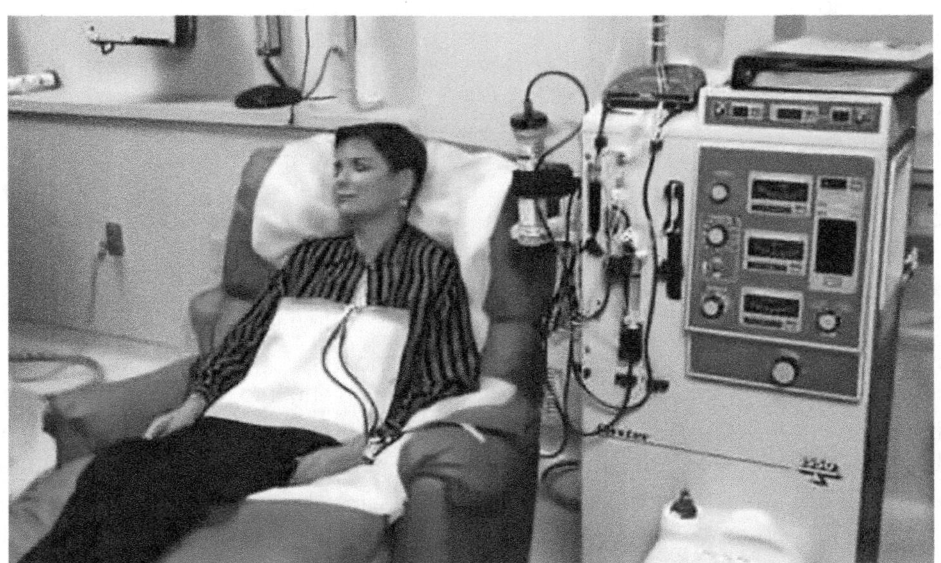

■ **Figure 9.13** Patient undergoing hemodialysis. Patient's blood passes through hemodialysis machine for cleansing and is then returned to her body.

Therapeutic Procedures *(continued)*

TERM	WORD PARTS	DEFINITION
peritoneal dialysis (pair-ih-TOH-nee-al / dye-AL-ih-sis)	peritone/o = peritoneum -eal = pertaining to	Removal of toxic waste substances from the body by placing warm chemically balanced solutions into the peritoneal cavity. Wastes are filtered out of the blood across the peritoneum. Used in treating renal failure and certain poisonings.

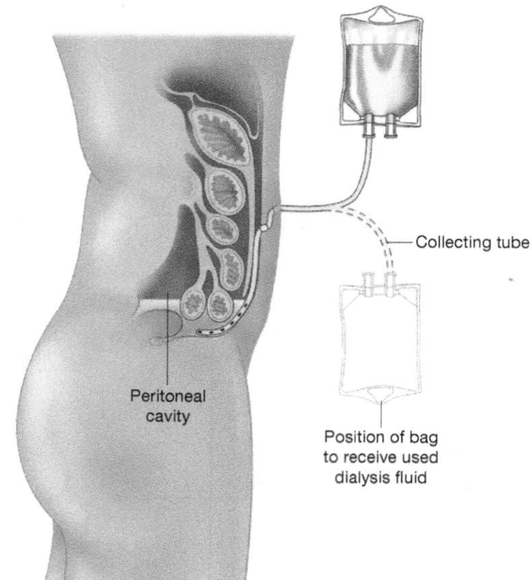

■ **Figure 9.14** Peritoneal dialysis. Chemically balanced solution is placed into the abdominal cavity to draw impurities out of the bloodstream. It is removed after several hours.

TERM	WORD PARTS	DEFINITION
Surgical Treatments		
cystectomy (sis-TEK-toh-me)	cyst/o = bladder -ectomy = surgical removal	Surgical removal of the urinary bladder.
cystopexy (SIS-toh-pek-see)	cyst/o = bladder -pexy = surgical fixation	Surgical fixation of the urinary bladder.
cystoplasty (SIS-toh-plas-tee)	cyst/o = bladder -plasty = surgical repair	To repair the urinary bladder by surgical means.
cystostomy (sis-TOSS-toh-mee)	cyst/o = bladder -ostomy = create a new opening	To create a new opening into the urinary bladder through the abdominal wall.
cystotomy (sis-TOT-oh-mee)	cyst/o = bladder -otomy = cutting into	To cut into the urinary bladder.
lithotomy (lith-OT-oh-me)	lith/o = stone -otomy = cutting into	To cut into an organ for the purpose of removing a stone.
lithotripsy (LITH-oh-trip-see)	lith/o = stone -tripsy = surgical crushing	Destroying or crushing stones in the bladder or urethra.
meatotomy (mee-ah-TOT-oh-me)	meat/o = meatus -otomy = cutting into	To cut into the meatus in order to enlarge the opening of the urethra.
nephrectomy (ne-FREK-toh-mee)	nephr/o = kidney -ectomy = surgical removal	Surgical removal of a kidney.
nephrolithotomy (nef-roh-lith-OT-oh-mee)	nephr/o = kidney lith/o = stone -otomy = cutting into	To cut into the kidney in order to remove stones.

Therapeutic Procedures *(continued)*

TERM	WORD PARTS	DEFINITION
nephropexy (NEF-roh-pek-see)	nephr/o = kidney -pexy = surgical fixation	Surgical fixation of a kidney; to anchor it in its normal anatomical position.
nephrostomy (neh-FROS-toh-mee)	nephr/o = kidney -ostomy = create a new opening	To create a new opening into the kidney through the abdominal wall.
nephrotomy (neh-FROT-oh-mee)	nephr/o = kidney -otomy = cutting into	To cut into the kidney.
pyeloplasty (PIE-ah-loh-plas-tee)	pyel/o = renal pelvis -plasty = surgical repair	To repair the renal pelvis by surgical means.
renal transplant	ren/o = kidney -al = pertaining to	Surgical placement of a donor kidney.

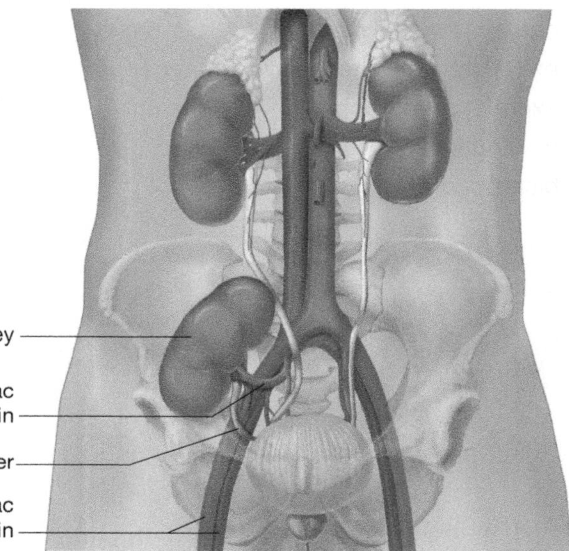

■ **Figure 9.15** Figure illustrates location utilized for implantation of donor kidney.

Pharmacology

CLASSIFICATION	WORD PARTS	ACTION	EXAMPLES
antibiotic	anti- = against bi/o = life -tic = pertaining to	Used to treat bacterial infections of the urinary tract.	ciprofloxacin, Cipro; nitrofurantoin, Macrobid
antispasmodic (an-tye-spaz-MAH-dik)	anti- = against -ic = pertaining to	Medication to prevent or reduce bladder muscle spasms.	oxybutynin, Ditropan; neostigmine, Prostigmine
diuretic (dye-yoo-REH-tiks)	-tic = pertaining to	Medication that increases the volume of urine produced by the kidneys. Useful in the treatment of edema, kidney failure, heart failure, and hypertension.	furosemide, Lasix; spironolactone, Aldactone

Abbreviations

AGN	acute glomerulonephritis	**HD**	hemodialysis
ARF	acute renal failure	**H_2O**	water
ATN	acute tubular necrosis	**I&O**	intake and output
BNO	bladder neck obstruction	**IPD**	intermittent peritoneal dialysis
BUN	blood urea nitrogen	**IVP**	intravenous pyelogram
CAPD	continuous ambulatory peritoneal dialysis	**K^+**	potassium
cath	catheterization	**KUB**	kidneys, ureters, bladder
CC	clean catch urine specimen	**mL**	milliliter
Cl^-	chloride	**Na^+**	sodium
CRF	chronic renal failure	**NS**	nephrotic syndrome
C&S	culture and sensitivity	**pH**	acidity or alkalinity of urine
cysto	cystoscopy	**RP**	retrograde pyelogram
ESRD	end-stage renal disease	**SG, sp. gr.**	specific gravity
ESWL	extracorporeal shockwave lithotripsy	**U/A, UA**	urinalysis
EU	excretory urography	**UC**	urine culture
GU	genitourinary	**UTI**	urinary tract infection
HCO_3^-	bicarbonate	**VCUG**	voiding cystourethrography

Chapter Review

Real-World Applications

Medical Record Analysis

This Discharge Summary contains 13 medical terms. Underline each term and write it in the list below the report. Then define each term.

Discharge Summary

Admitting Diagnosis:	Severe right side pain and hematuria.
Final Diagnosis:	Pyelonephritis right kidney, complicated by chronic cystitis.
History of Present Illness:	Patient has long history of frequent bladder infections, but denies any recent lower pelvic pain or dysuria. Earlier today he had rapid onset of severe right side pain and is unable to stand fully erect. His temperature was 101°F, and his skin was sweaty and flushed. He was admitted from the ER for further testing and diagnosis.
Summary of Hospital Course:	Clean catch urinalysis revealed gross hematuria and pyuria, but no albuminuria. A culture and sensitivity was ordered to identify the pathogen and an antibiotic was started. Cystoscopy showed evidence of chronic cystitis, bladder irritation, and a bladder neck obstruction. The obstruction appears to be congenital and the probable cause of the chronic cystitis. The patient was catheterized to ensure complete emptying of the bladder, and fluids were encouraged. Patient responded well to the antibiotic therapy and fluids, and his symptoms improved.
Discharge Plans:	Patient was discharged home after 3 days in the hospital. He was switched to an oral antibiotic for the pyelonephritis and chronic cystitis. A repeat urinalysis is scheduled for next week. After all inflammation is corrected, will repeat cystoscopy to reevaluate bladder neck obstruction.

	Term	Definition
1	______	______
2	______	______
3	______	______
4	______	______
5	______	______
6	______	______
7	______	______
8	______	______
9	______	______
10	______	______
11	______	______
12	______	______
13	______	______

Chart Note Transcription

The chart note below contains 11 phrases that can be reworded with a medical term that you learned in this chapter. Each phrase is identified with an underline. Determine the medical term and write your answers in the space provided.

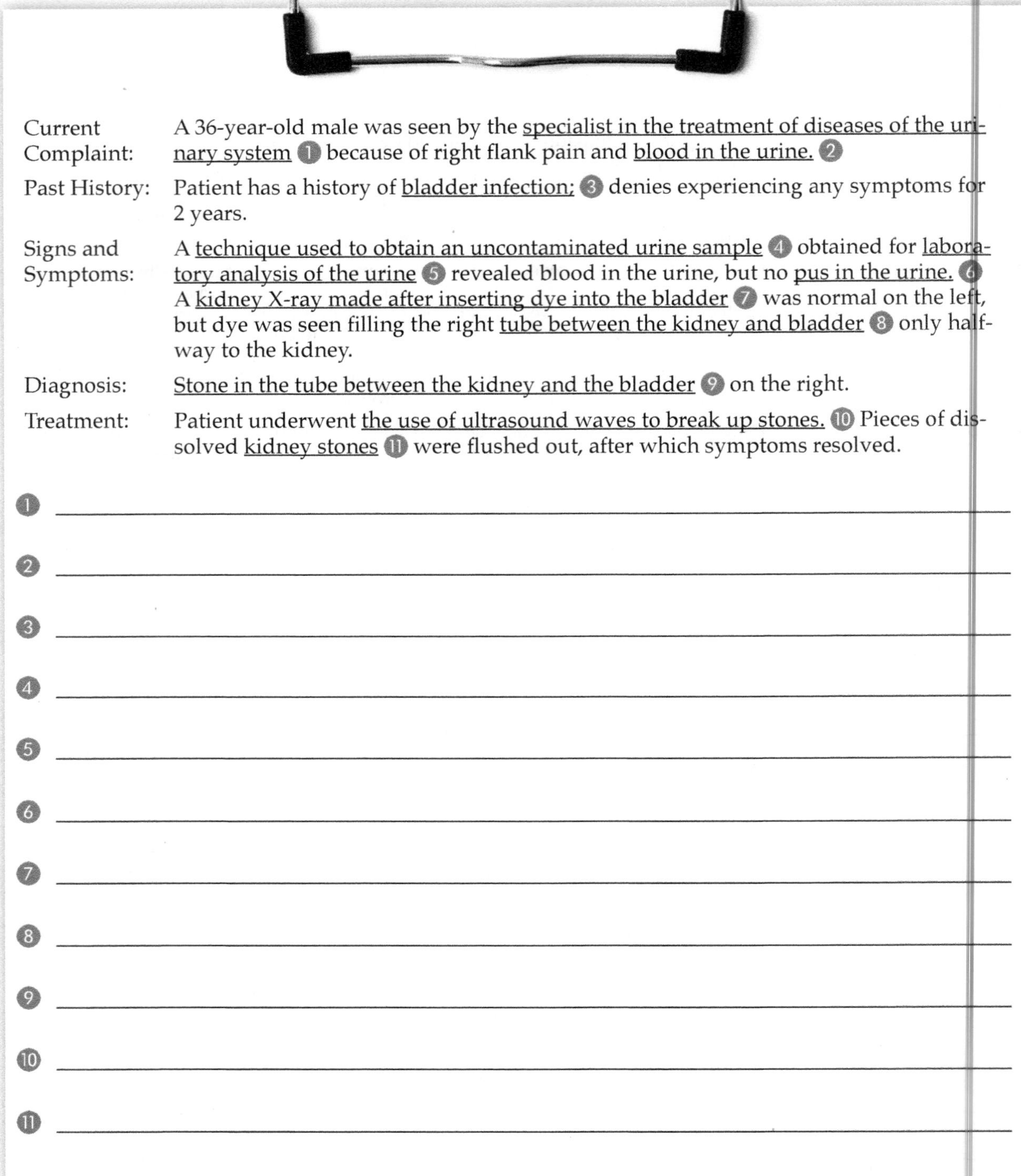

Current Complaint: A 36-year-old male was seen by the specialist in the treatment of diseases of the urinary system (1) because of right flank pain and blood in the urine. (2)

Past History: Patient has a history of bladder infection; (3) denies experiencing any symptoms for 2 years.

Signs and Symptoms: A technique used to obtain an uncontaminated urine sample (4) obtained for laboratory analysis of the urine (5) revealed blood in the urine, but no pus in the urine. (6) A kidney X-ray made after inserting dye into the bladder (7) was normal on the left, but dye was seen filling the right tube between the kidney and bladder (8) only halfway to the kidney.

Diagnosis: Stone in the tube between the kidney and the bladder (9) on the right.

Treatment: Patient underwent the use of ultrasound waves to break up stones. (10) Pieces of dissolved kidney stones (11) were flushed out, after which symptoms resolved.

1. ____________________
2. ____________________
3. ____________________
4. ____________________
5. ____________________
6. ____________________
7. ____________________
8. ____________________
9. ____________________
10. ____________________
11. ____________________

Case Study

Below is a case study presentation of a patient with a condition discussed in this chapter. Read the case study and answer the questions below. Some questions will ask for information not included within this chapter. Use your text, a medical dictionary, journals, technical materials, multimedia resources, electronic media, or any other reference material you choose to answer these questions.

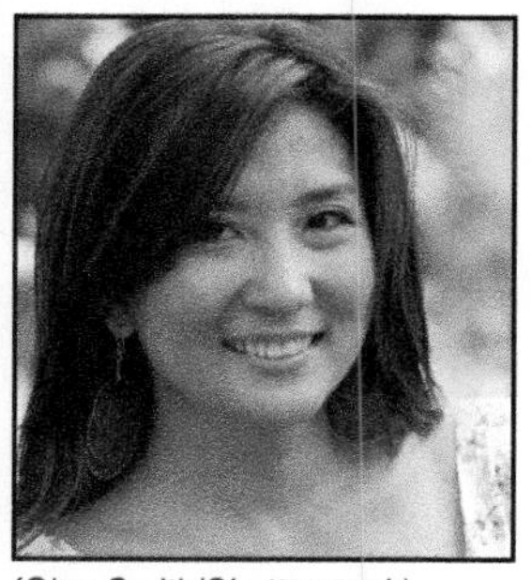

(Gina Smith/Shutterstock)

A 32-year-old female is seen in the urologist's office because of a fever, chills, and generalized fatigue. She also reported urgency, frequency, dysuria, and hematuria. In addition, she noticed that her urine was cloudy with a fishy odor. The physician ordered the following tests: a clean catch specimen for a U/A, a urine C&S, and a KUB. The U/A revealed pyuria, bacteriuria, and a slightly acidic pH. A common type of bacteria was grown in the culture. X-rays reveal acute pyelonephritis resulting from cystitis, which has spread up to the kidney from the bladder. The patient was placed on an antibiotic and encouraged to "push fluids" by drinking 2L of water a day.

Questions

1. This patient has two urinary system infections in different locations; name them. Which one caused the other and how?

____

____

2. List and define each of the patient's presenting symptoms in your own words.

____

____

3. What diagnostic tests did the urologist order? Describe them in your own words.

____

____

4. Explain the results of each diagnostic test in your own words.

____

____

5. What were the physician's treatment instructions for this patient? Explain the purpose of each treatment.

____

____

6. Describe the normal appearance of urine.

____

____

Practice Exercises

A. Complete the Statement

1. The functional or working units of the kidneys are the ________________________.
2. The three stages of urine production are ________________________, ________________________, and ________________________.
3. Na^+, K^+, and Cl^- are collectively known as ________________________.
4. The term that describes the location of the kidneys is ________________________.
5. The center of the concave side of the kidney is the ________________________.
6. The glomerular capsule surrounds the ________________________.
7. The tip of each renal pyramid opens into a(n) ________________________.
8. There are ________________________ ureters and ________________________ urethra.
9. Urination can also be referred to as ________________________ or ________________________.
10. A(n) ________________________ is the physical and chemical analysis of urine.

B. Combining Form Practice

The combining form **nephr/o** refers to the kidney. Use it to write a term that means:

1. surgical fixation of the kidney ________________________
2. X-ray record of the kidney ________________________
3. condition of kidney stones ________________________
4. removal of a kidney ________________________
5. inflammation of the kidney ________________________
6. kidney disease ________________________
7. hardening of the kidney ________________________

The combining form **cyst/o** refers to the urinary bladder. Use it to write a term that means:

8. inflammation of the bladder ________________________
9. abnormal flow condition from the bladder ________________________
10. surgical repair of the bladder ________________________
11. instrument to view inside the bladder ________________________
12. bladder pain ________________________

The combining form **pyel/o** refers to the renal pelvis. Use it to write a term that means:

13. surgical repair of the renal pelvis ____________________
14. inflammation of the renal pelvis ____________________
15. X-ray record of the renal pelvis ____________________

The combining form **ureter/o** refers to one or both of the ureters. Use it to write a term that means:

16. a ureteral stone ____________________
17. ureter dilation ____________________
18. ureter narrowing ____________________

The combining form **urethr/o** refers to the urethra. Use it to write a term that means:

19. urethra inflammation ____________________
20. instrument to view inside the urethra ____________________

C. Define the Combining Form

	Definition	Example from Chapter
1. **ur/o**	____________________	____________________
2. **meat/o**	____________________	____________________
3. **cyst/o**	____________________	____________________
4. **ren/o**	____________________	____________________
5. **pyel/o**	____________________	____________________
6. **glycos/o**	____________________	____________________
7. **noct/i**	____________________	____________________
8. **olig/o**	____________________	____________________
9. **ureter/o**	____________________	____________________
10. **glomerul/o**	____________________	____________________

D. Pharmacology Challenge

Fill in the classification for each drug description, then match the brand name.

	Drug Description	Classification	Brand Name
1.	_______ Reduces bladder muscle spasms	____________________	a. Lasix
2.	_______ Treats bacterial infections	____________________	b. Ditropan
3.	_______ Increases volume of urine produced	____________________	c. Cipro

E. Define the Term

1. micturition ____________________
2. diuretic ____________________
3. renal colic ____________________
4. catheterization ____________________
5. pyelitis ____________________
6. glomerulonephritis ____________________
7. lithotomy ____________________
8. enuresis ____________________
9. meatotomy ____________________
10. diabetic nephropathy ____________________
11. urinalysis ____________________
12. hesitancy ____________________

F. Name That Term

1. absence of urine ____________________
2. blood in the urine ____________________
3. kidney stone ____________________
4. crushing a stone ____________________
5. inflammation of the urethra ____________________
6. pus in the urine ____________________
7. bacteria in the urine ____________________
8. painful urination ____________________
9. ketones in the urine ____________________
10. protein in the urine ____________________
11. (too) much urine ____________________

G. What's the Abbreviation?

1. potassium ______________________________
2. sodium ______________________________
3. urinalysis ______________________________
4. blood urea nitrogen ______________________________
5. specific gravity ______________________________
6. intravenous pyelogram ______________________________
7. bladder neck obstruction ______________________________
8. intake and output ______________________________
9. acute tubular necrosis ______________________________
10. end stage renal disease ______________________________

H. What Does it Stand For?

1. KUB ______________________________
2. cath ______________________________
3. cysto ______________________________
4. GU ______________________________
5. ESWL ______________________________
6. UTI ______________________________
7. UC ______________________________
8. RP ______________________________
9. ARF ______________________________
10. BUN ______________________________
11. CRF ______________________________
12. H_2O ______________________________

I. Terminology Matching

Match each term to its definition.

1.	_______ Wilm's tumor	a.	kidney stones
2.	_______ electrolytes	b.	feeling the need to urinate immediately
3.	_______ nephrons	c.	childhood malignant kidney tumor
4.	_______ nephron loop	d.	swelling of the kidney due to urine collecting in the renal pelvis
5.	_______ calyx	e.	involuntary release of urine
6.	_______ incontinence	f.	collects urine as it is produced
7.	_______ hydronephrosis	g.	sodium and potassium
8.	_______ urgency	h.	functional unit of the kidneys
9.	_______ nephrolithiasis	i.	part of the renal tubule
10.	_______ polycystic kidneys	j.	multiple cysts in the kidneys

J. Define the Suffix

	Definition	Example from Chapter
1. -ptosis	______________________	______________
2. -uria	______________________	______________
3. -lith	______________________	______________
4. -tripsy	______________________	______________
5. -lithiasis	______________________	______________

K. Fill in the Blank

renal transplant	ureterectomy	intravenous pyelogram (IVP)
cystostomy	pyelolithectomy	nephropexy
renal biopsy	cystoscopy	urinary tract infection

1. Juan suffered from chronic renal failure. His sister, Maria, donated one of her normal kidneys to him, and he had a(n) ________________________.

2. Anesha's floating kidney needed surgical fixation. Her physician performed a surgical procedure known as ________________________.

3. Kenya's physician stated that she had a general infection that he referred to as a UTI. The full name for this infection is ________________________.

4. The surgeons operated on Robert to remove calculi from his renal pelvis. The name of this surgery is ________________________.

5. Charles had to have a small piece of his kidney tissue removed so that the physician could perform a microscopic evaluation. This procedure is called a(n) ________________________.

6. Naomi had to have one of her ureters removed due to a stricture. This procedure is called ________________________.

7. The physician had to create a temporary opening between Eric's bladder and his abdominal wall. This procedure is called ________________________.

8. Sally's bladder was visually examined using a special instrument. This procedure is called a(n) ________________________.

9. The doctors believe that Jacob has a tumor of the right kidney. They are going to do a test called a(n) ________________________ that requires them to inject a radiopaque contrast medium intravenously so that they can see the kidney on X-ray.

Labeling Exercise

Image A

Write the labels for this figure on the numbered lines provided.

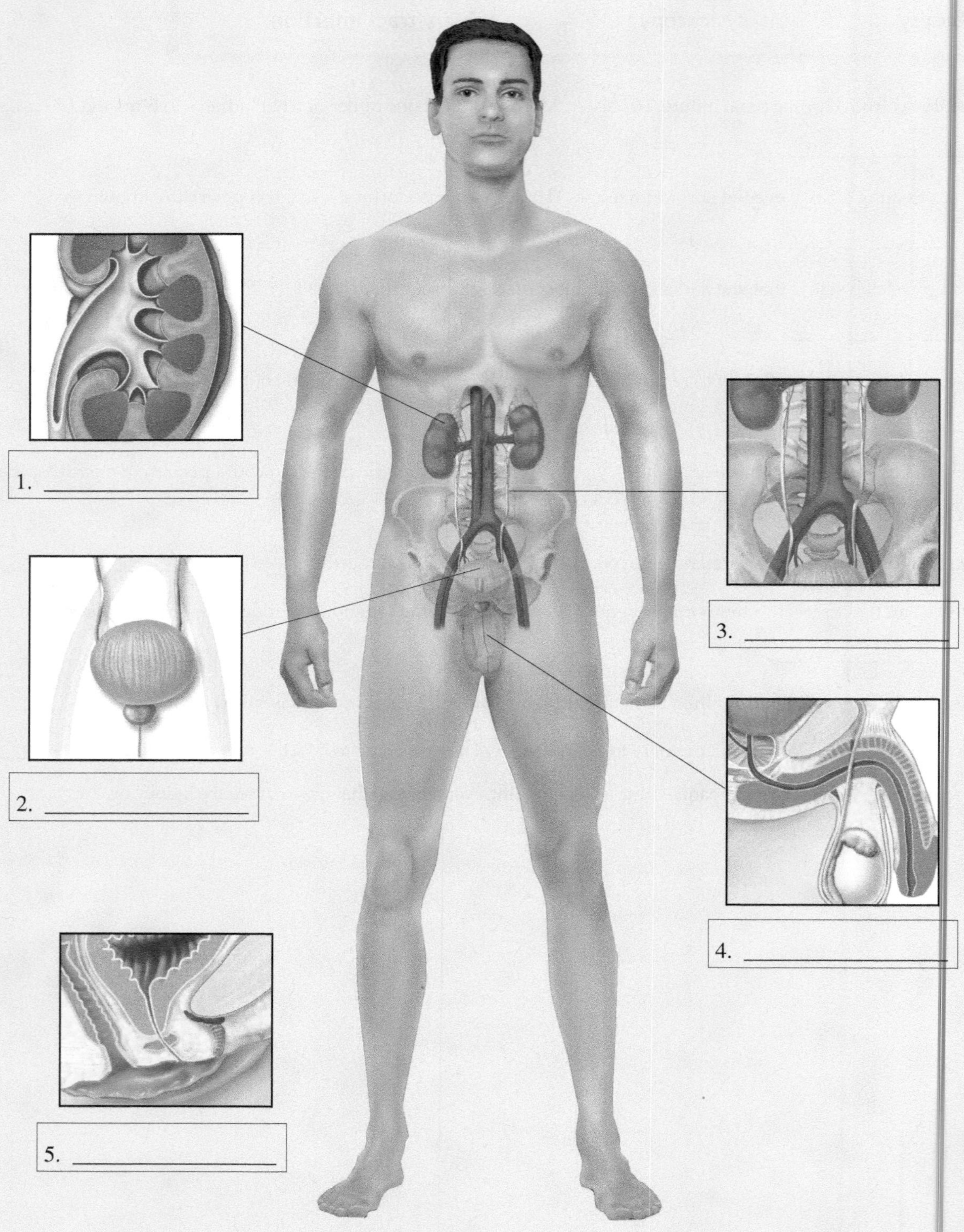

Image B

Write the labels for this figure on the numbered lines provided.

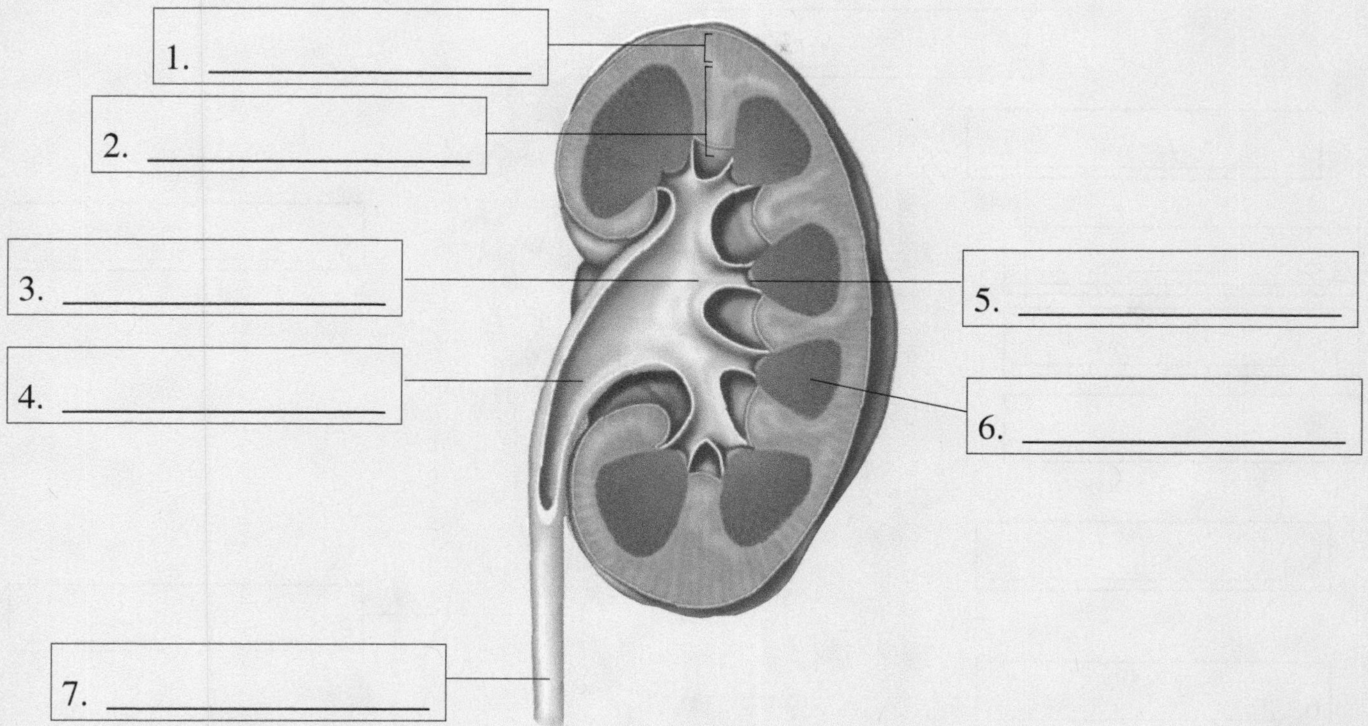

Image C

Write the labels for this figure on the numbered lines provided.

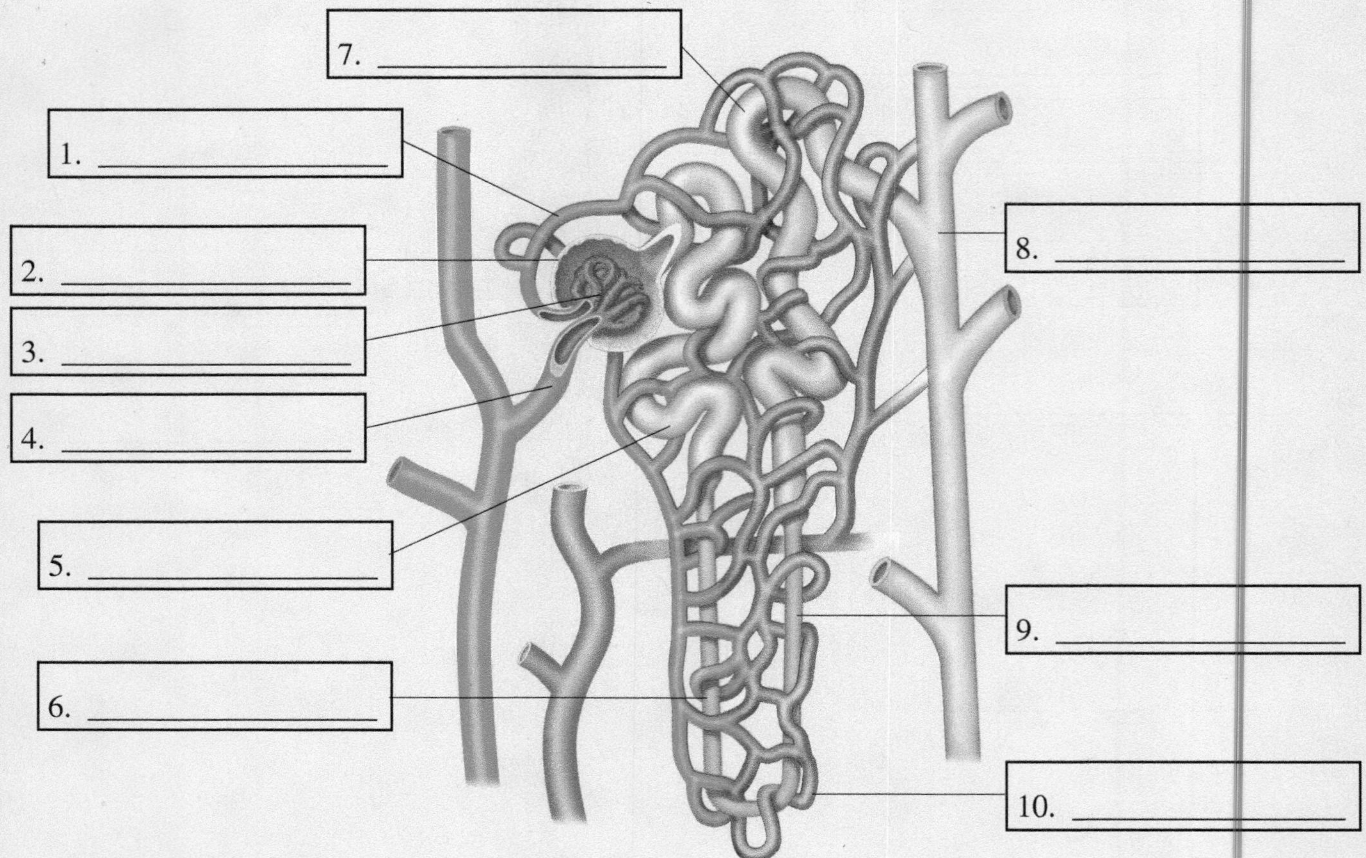

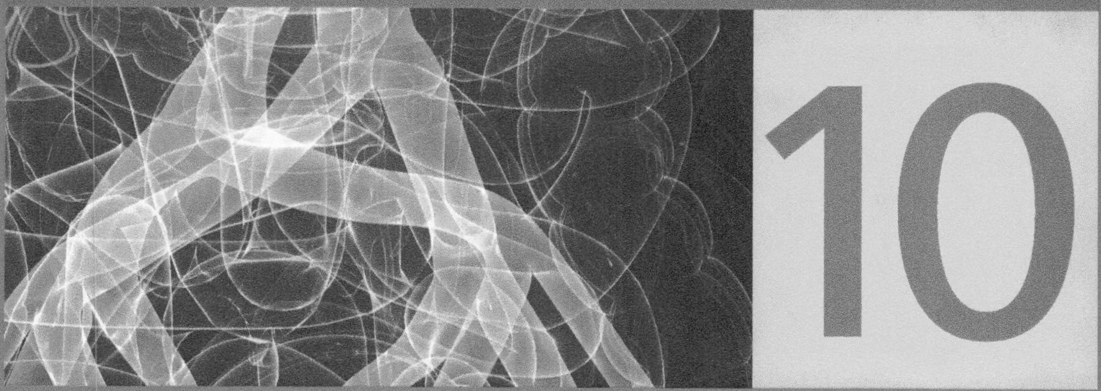

REPRODUCTIVE SYSTEM

Learning Objectives

Upon completion of this chapter, you will be able to

- Identify and define the combining forms and suffixes introduced in this chapter.
- Correctly spell and pronounce medical terms and major anatomical structures relating to the reproductive systems.
- Locate and describe the major organs of the reproductive systems and their functions.
- Use medical terms to describe circumstances relating to pregnancy.
- Identify the symptoms and origin of sexually transmitted diseases.
- Identify and define reproductive system anatomical terms.
- Identify and define selected reproductive system pathology terms.
- Identify and define selected reproductive system diagnostic procedures.
- Identify and define selected reproductive system therapeutic procedures.
- Identify and define selected medications relating to the reproductive systems.
- Define selected abbreviations associated with the reproductive systems.

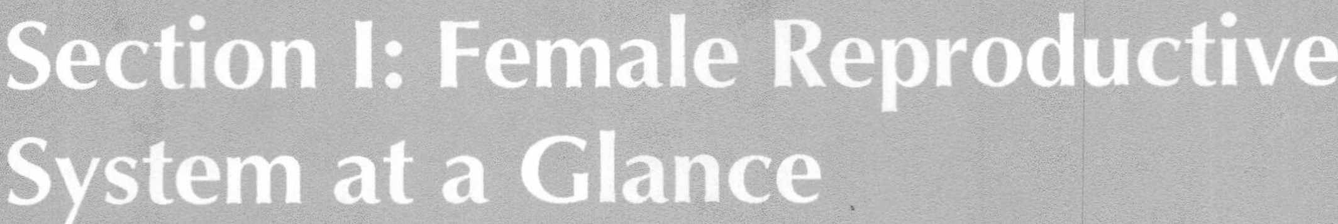

Section I: Female Reproductive System at a Glance

Function

The female reproductive system produces ova (the female reproductive cells), provides a location for fertilization and growth of a baby, and secretes female sex hormones. In addition, the breasts produce milk to nourish the newborn.

Structures

Here are the primary structures that comprise the female reproductive system.

breasts
uterine tubes
ovaries
uterus
vagina
vulva

Word Parts

Here are the most common word parts (with their meanings) used to build female reproductive system terms. For a more comprehensive list, refer to the Terminology section of this chapter.

Combining Forms

Combining Form	Meaning
amni/o	amnion
cervic/o	neck, cervix
chori/o	chorion
colp/o	vagina
culd/o	cul-de-sac
embry/o	embryo
episi/o	vulva
fet/o	fetus
gynec/o	woman, female
hymen/o	hymen
hyster/o	uterus
lact/o	milk
mamm/o	breast
mast/o	breast
men/o	menses, menstruation
metr/o	uterus
nat/o	birth
o/o	egg
oophor/o	ovary
ovari/o	ovary
perine/o	perineum
salping/o	uterine tubes, fallopian tubes
uter/o	uterus
vagin/o	vagina
vulv/o	vulva

Suffixes

Suffix	Meaning
-arche	beginning
-cyesis	state of pregnancy
-gravida	pregnancy
-para	to bear (offspring)
-partum	childbirth
-salpinx	uterine tube
-tocia	labor, childbirth

Female Reproductive System Illustrated

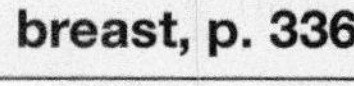

breast, p. 336

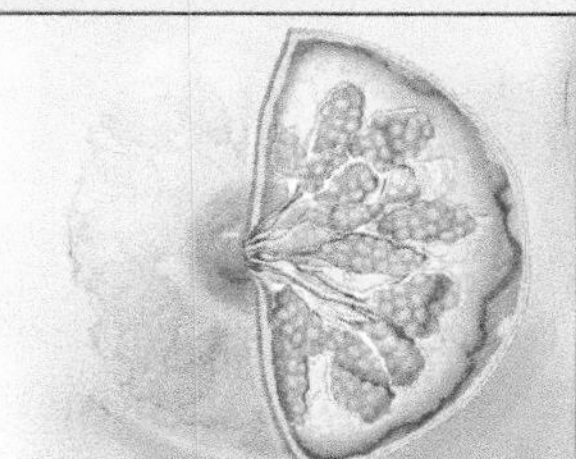

Produces milk

uterus, p. 334

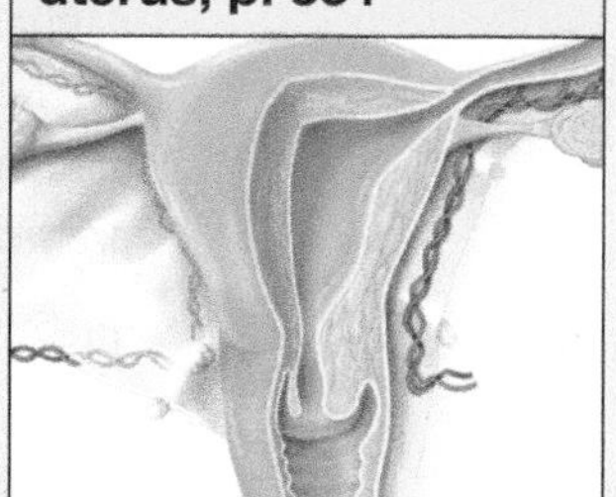

Site of development of fetus

uterine tube, p. 333

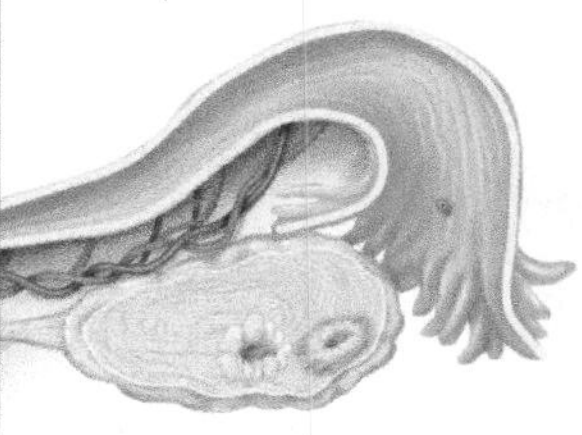

Transports ovum to uterus

ovary, p. 332

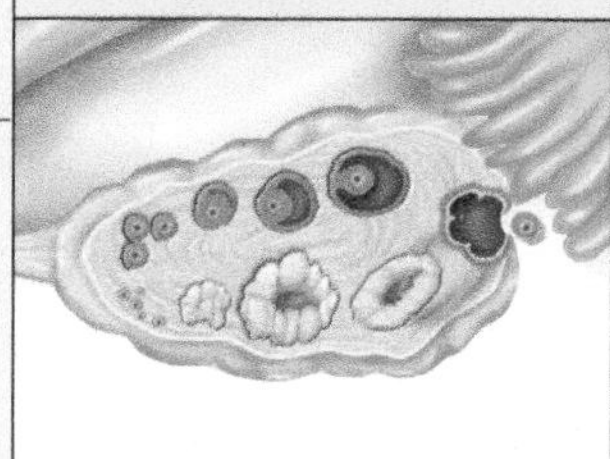

Produces ova and secretes estrogen and progesterone

vagina, p. 335

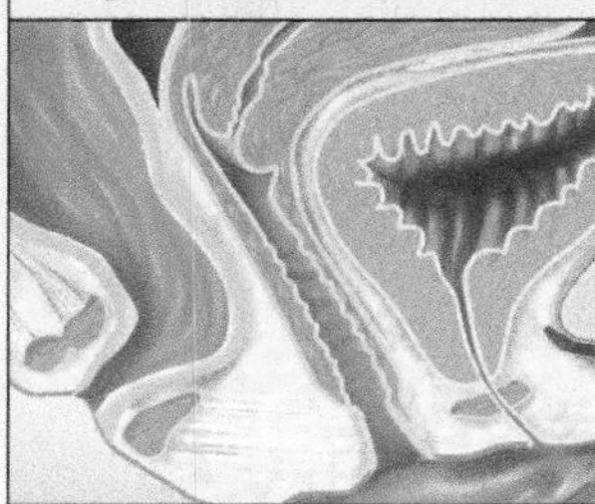

Receives semen during intercourse; birth canal

vulva, p. 335

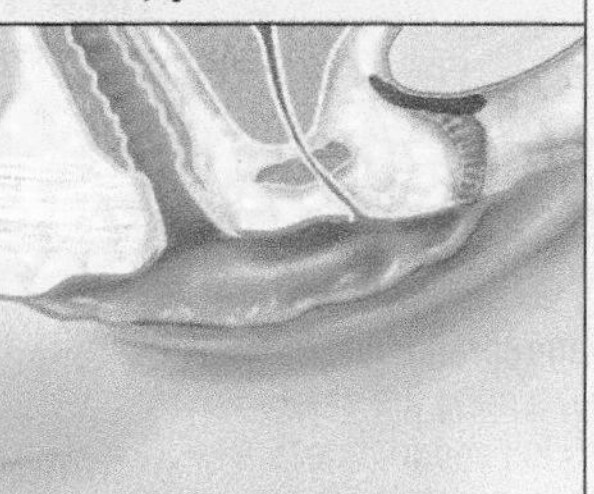

Protects vaginal orifice and urinary meatus

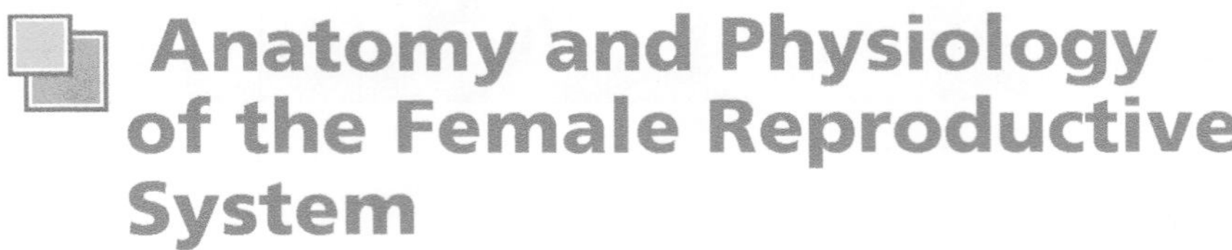

Anatomy and Physiology of the Female Reproductive System

breasts
fertilization
genitalia (jen-ih-TAY-lee-ah)
ova (OH-vah)
ovaries (OH-vah-reez)
pregnancy
sex hormones
uterine tubes (YOO-ter-in)
uterus (YOO-ter-us)
vagina (vah-JIGH-nah)
vulva (VULL-vah)

The female reproductive system plays many vital functions that ensure the continuation of the human race. First, it produces **ova,** the female reproductive cells. It then provides a place for **fertilization** to occur and for a baby to grow during **pregnancy.** The **breasts** provide nourishment for the newborn. Finally, this system secretes the female **sex hormones.**

This system consists of both internal and external **genitalia,** or reproductive organs (see Figure 10.1 ■). The internal genitalia are located in the pelvic cavity and consist of the **uterus,** two **ovaries,** two **uterine tubes,** and the **vagina,** which extends to the external surface of the body. The external genitalia are collectively referred to as the **vulva.**

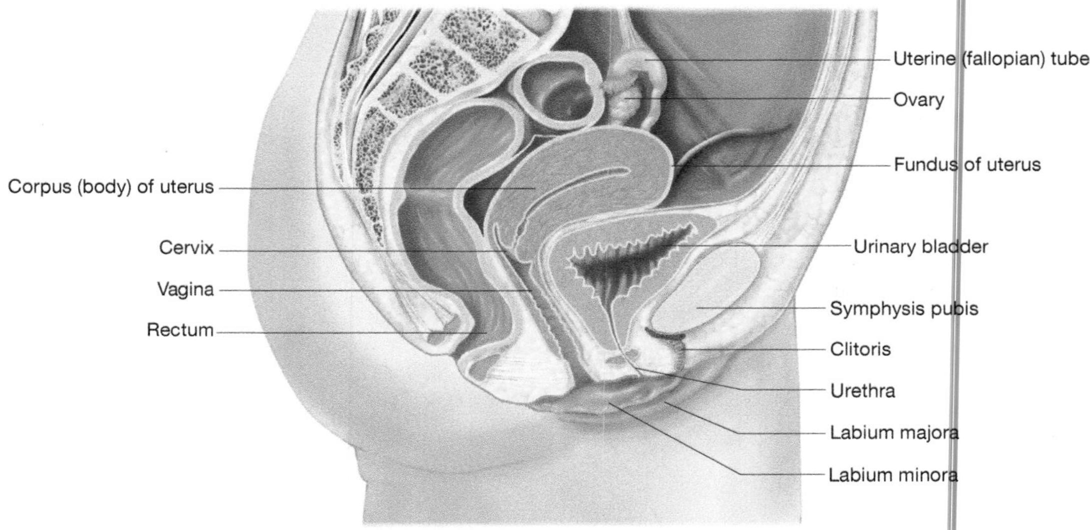

■ **Figure 10.1** The female reproductive system, sagittal view showing organs of the system in relation to the urinary bladder and rectum.

> **MED TERM TIP**
>
> The singular for egg is *ovum.* The plural term for many eggs is *ova.* The term *ova* is not used exclusively when discussing the human reproductive system. For instance, testing the stool for ova and parasites is used to detect the presence of parasites or their ova in the digestive tract, a common cause for severe diarrhea. Ova are produced in the ovary by a process called *oogenesis* (*o/o* = egg and *-genesis* = produced).

Internal Genitalia

Ovaries

estrogen (ESS-troh-jen)
follicle stimulating hormone (FOLL-ih-kl)
luteinizing hormone (loo-teh-NIGH-zing)
ovulation (ov-yoo-LAY-shun)
progesterone (proh-JES-ter-ohn)

There are two ovaries, one located on each side of the uterus within the pelvic cavity (see again Figure 10.1). These are small almond-shaped glands that produce ova (singular is *ovum*) and the female sex hormones (see Figure 10.2 ■). In humans approximately every 28 days hormones from the anterior pituitary, **follicle stimulating hormone** (FSH) and **luteinizing hormone** (LH), stimulate maturation of ovum and trigger **ovulation,** the process by which one ovary releases an ovum (see Figure 10.3 ■). The principal female sex hormones produced by the ovaries, **estrogen** and **progesterone,** stimulate the lining of the uterus to be prepared to receive a fertilized ovum. These hormones are also responsible for the female secondary sexual characteristics.

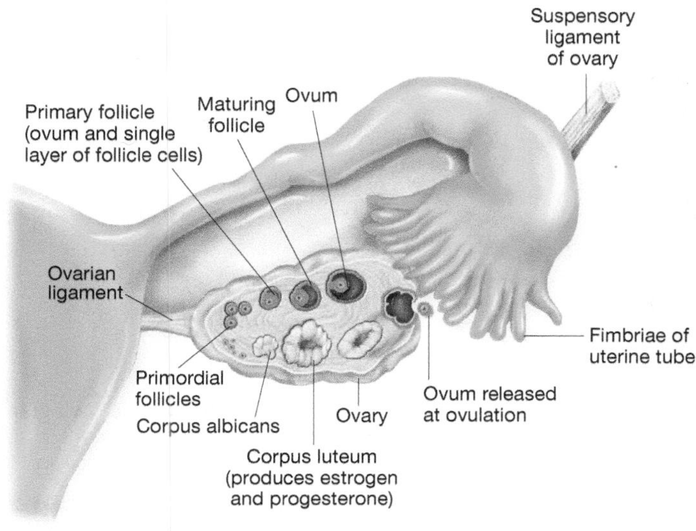

■ **Figure 10.2** Structure of the ovary and uterine (fallopian) tube. Figure illustrates stages of ovum development and the relationship of the ovary to the uterine tube.

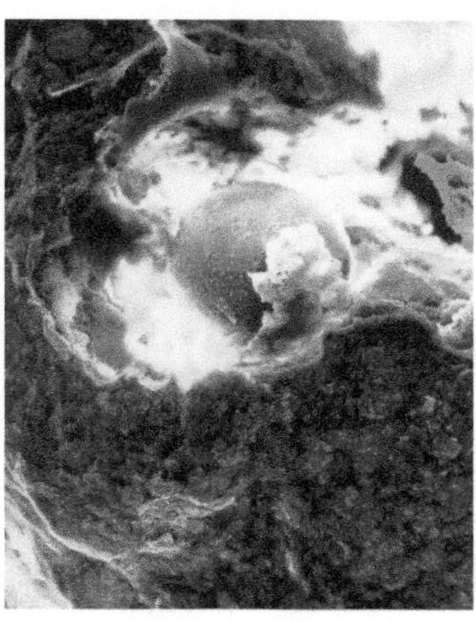

■ **Figure 10.3** Color-enhanced scanning electron micrograph showing an ovum (pink) released by the ovary at ovulation surrounded by follicle (white) tissue. The external surface of the ovary is brown in this photo. *(P.M. Motta and J. Van Blekrom/Science Photo Library/Photo Researchers, Inc.)*

Uterine Tubes

conception (con-SEP-shun)
fallopian tubes (fah-LOH-pee-an)
fimbriae (FIM-bree-ay)
oviducts (OH-vih-ducts)

The uterine tubes, also called the **fallopian tubes** or **oviducts,** are approximately 5 1/2 inches long and run from the area around each ovary to either side of the upper portion of the uterus (see Figures 10.4 ■ and 10.5 ■). As they near the ovaries,

MED TERM TIP

When the fertilized egg adheres or implants to the uterine tube instead of moving into the uterus, a condition called *tubal pregnancy* exists. There is not enough room in the uterine tube for the fetus to grow normally. Implantation of the fertilized egg in any location other than the uterus is called an *ectopic pregnancy. Ectopic* is a general term meaning "in the wrong place."

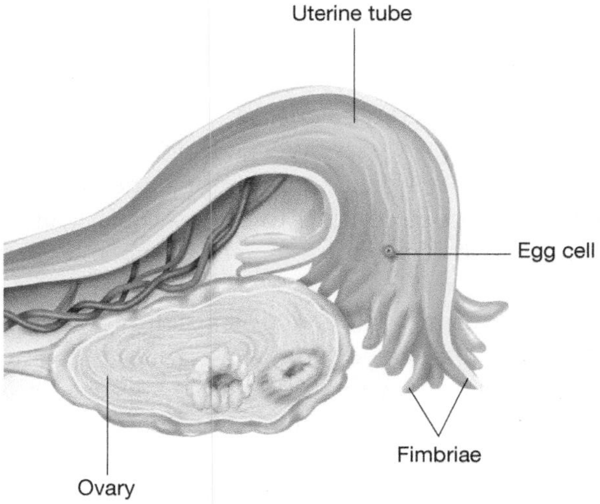

Uterine tube
Egg cell
Fimbriae
Ovary

■ **Figure 10.4** Uterine (fallopian) tube, showing released ovum within the uterine tube.

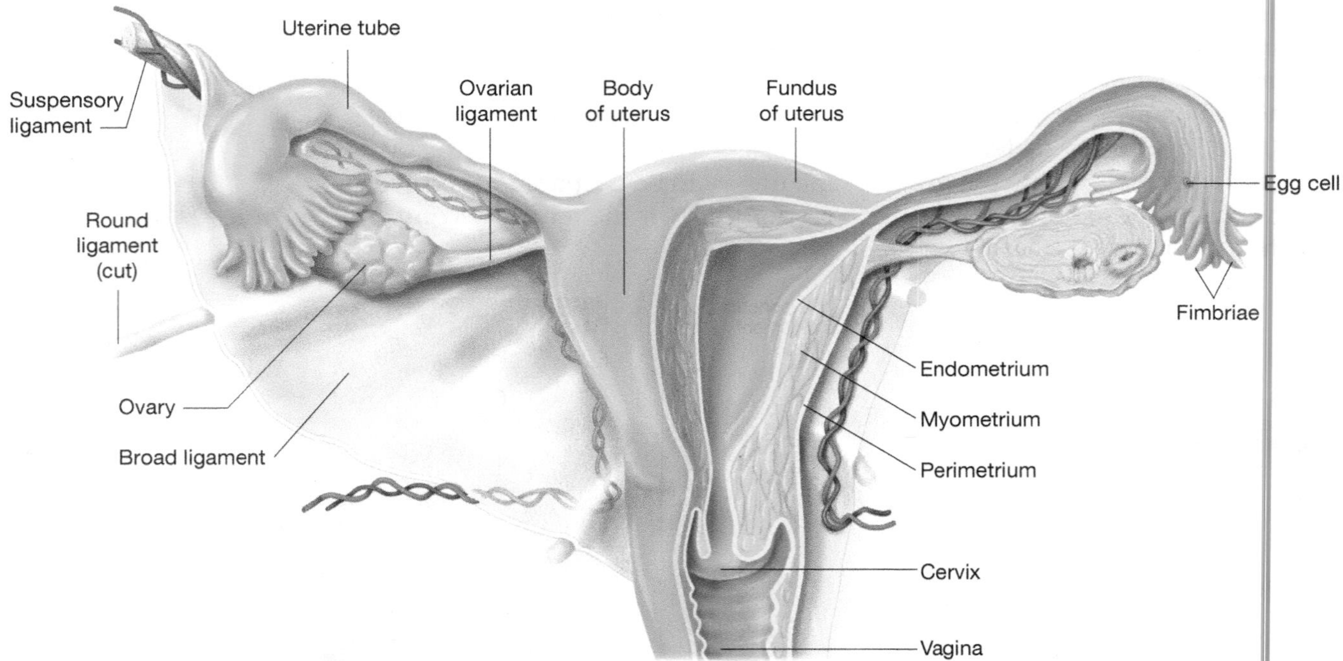

Figure 10.5 The uterus. Cutaway view shows regions of the uterus and cervix and its relationship to the uterine (fallopian) tubes and vagina.

the unattached ends of these two tubes expand into finger-like projections called **fimbriae.** The fimbriae catch an ovum after ovulation and direct it into the uterine tube. The uterine tube can then propel the ovum from the ovary to the uterus so that it can implant. The meeting of the egg and sperm, called fertilization or **conception,** normally takes place within the upper one-half of the uterine tubes.

Uterus

anteflexion (an-tee-FLEK-shun)
cervix (SER-viks)
corpus (KOR-pus)
endometrium (en-doh-MEE-tre-um)
fundus (FUN-dus)
menarche (men-AR-kee)
menopause (MEN-oh-pawz)
menstrual period (MEN-stroo-all)
menstruation (men-stroo-AY-shun)
myometrium (my-oh-MEE-tre-um)
perimetrium (pear-ee-MEE-tre-um)
puberty (PEW-ber-tee)

MED TERM TIP

During pregnancy, the height of the fundus is an important measurement for estimating the stage of pregnancy and the size of the fetus. Following birth, massaging the fundus with pressure applied in a circular pattern stimulates the uterine muscle to contract to help stop bleeding. Patients may be more familiar with a common term for uterus, *womb.* However, the correct medical term is uterus.

The uterus is a hollow, pear-shaped organ that contains a thick muscular wall, a mucous membrane lining, and a rich supply of blood (see again Figure 10.5). It lies in the center of the pelvic cavity between the bladder and the rectum. It is normally bent slightly forward, which is called **anteflexion,** and is held in position by strong fibrous ligaments anchored in the outer layer of the uterus, called the **perimetrium** (see again Figure 10.1). The uterus has three sections: the **fundus** or upper portion, between where the uterine tubes connect to the uterus; **corpus** or body, which is the central portion; and **cervix** (Cx), or lower portion, also called the neck of the uterus, which opens into the vagina.

The inner layer, or **endometrium,** of the uterine wall contains a rich blood supply. The endometrium reacts to hormonal changes every month that prepare it to receive a fertilized ovum. In a normal pregnancy the fertilized ovum implants in the endometrium, which can then provide nourishment and protection for the developing fetus. Contractions of the thick muscular walls of the uterus, called the **myometrium,** assist in propelling the fetus through the birth canal at delivery.

If a pregnancy is not established, the endometrium is sloughed off, resulting in **menstruation** or the **menstrual period.** During a pregnancy, the lining of the uterus does not leave the body but remains to nourish the fetus. A girl's first menstrual period occurs during **puberty** (the sequence of events by which a child becomes a young adult capable of reproduction) and is called **menarche** (*men/o* = menstruation, *-arche* = beginning), while the ending of menstrual activity and childbearing years is called **menopause.** This generally occurs between the ages of 40 and 55.

MED TERM TIP

Word Watch: Be careful using the combining forms *uter/o* meaning "uterus" and *ureter/o* meaning "ureter."

Vagina

Bartholin's glands (BAR-toh-linz)
hymen (HIGH-men)
vaginal orifice (VAJ-ih-nal / OR-ih-fis)

The vagina is a muscular tube lined with mucous membrane that extends from the cervix of the uterus to the outside of the body (see Figure 10.6 ■). The vagina allows for the passage of the menstrual flow. In addition, during intercourse, it receives the male's penis and semen, which is the fluid containing sperm. The vagina also serves as the birth canal through which the baby passes during a normal vaginal birth.

The **hymen** is a thin membranous tissue that partially covers the external vaginal opening or **vaginal orifice.** This membrane is broken by the use of tampons, during physical activity, or during sexual intercourse. A pair of glands (called **Bartholin's glands**) are located on either side of the vaginal orifice and secrete mucus for lubrication during intercourse.

MED TERM TIP

Word Watch: Be careful using the combining forms *colp/o* meaning "vagina" and *culd/o* meaning "cul-de-sac (rectouterine pouch)."

Vulva

clitoris (KLIT-oh-ris)
erectile tissue (ee-REK-tile)
labia majora (LAY-bee-ah / mah-JOR-ah)
labia minora (LAY-bee-ah / min-NOR-ah)
perineum (pair-ih-NEE-um)
urinary meatus (YOO-rih-nair-ee / mee-AY-tus)

The vulva is a general term that refers to the group of structures that make up the female external genitalia. The **labia majora** and **labia minora** are folds of skin that serve as protection for the genitalia, the vaginal orifice, and the **urinary meatus** (see Figure 10.7 ■). Since the urinary tract and the reproductive organs are located in proximity to one another and each contains mucous membranes that can transport infection, there is a danger of infection entering the urinary tract. The **clitoris**

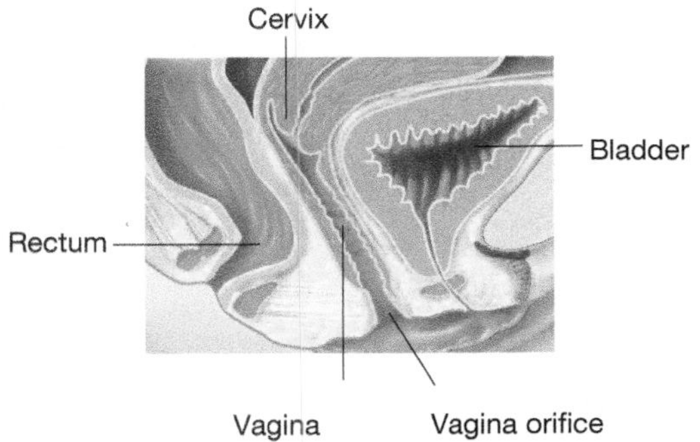

■ **Figure 10.6** The vagina, sagittal section showing the location of the vagina and its relationship to the cervix, uterus, rectum, and bladder.

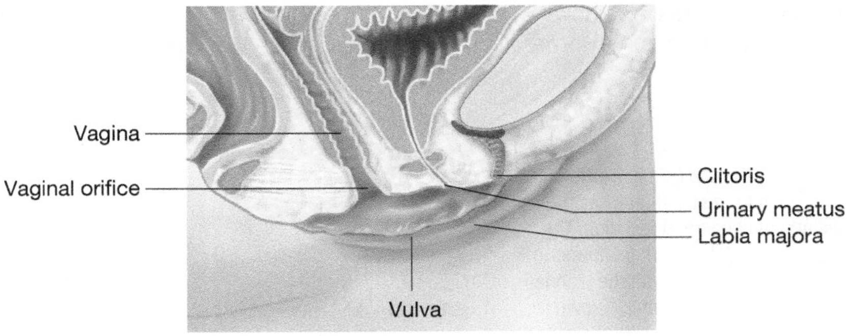

■ **Figure 10.7** The vulva, sagittal section illustrating how the labia majora and labia minora cover and protect the vaginal orifice, clitoris, and urinary meatus.

is a small organ containing sensitive **erectile tissue** that is aroused during sexual stimulation and corresponds to the penis in the male. The region between the vaginal orifice and the anus is referred to as the **perineum.**

Breast

areola (ah-REE-oh-la)
lactation (lak-TAY-shun)
lactiferous ducts (lak-TIF-er-us)
lactiferous glands (lak-TIF-er-us)
mammary glands (MAM-ah-ree)
nipple
nurse

The breasts, or **mammary glands,** play a vital role in the reproductive process because they produce milk, a process called **lactation,** to nourish the newborn. The size of the breasts, which varies greatly from woman to woman, has no bearing on the ability to **nurse** or feed a baby. Milk is produced by the **lactiferous glands** and is carried to the **nipple** by the **lactiferous ducts** (see Figure 10.8 ■). The **areola** is the pigmented area around the nipple. As long as the breast is stimulated by the nursing infant, the breast will continue to secrete milk.

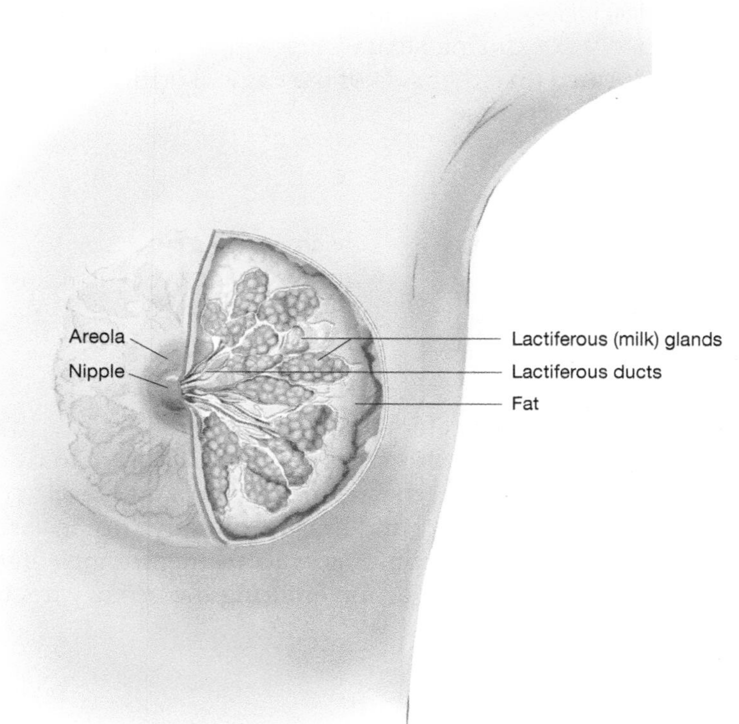

■ **Figure 10.8** The breast, cutaway view showing both internal and external features.

MED TERM TIP

The term *abortion* (AB) has different meanings for medical professionals and the general population. The general population equates the term *abortion* specifically with the planned termination of a pregnancy. However, to the medical community, abortion is a broader medical term meaning that a pregnancy has ended before a fetus is *viable*, meaning before it can live on its own.

Pregnancy

amnion (AM-nee-on)
amniotic fluid (am-nee-OT-ik)
chorion (KOR-ree-on)
embryo (EM-bree-oh)
fetus (FEE-tus)
gestation (jess-TAY-shun)
placenta (plah-SEN-tah)
premature
umbilical cord (um-BILL-ih-kal)

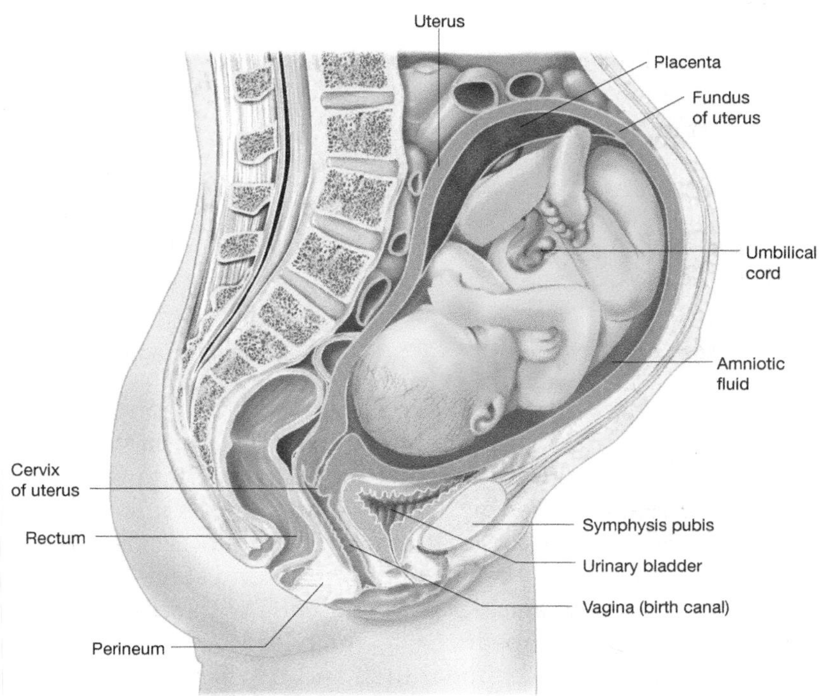

■ **Figure 10.9** A full-term pregnancy. Image illustrates position of the fetus and the structures associated with pregnancy.

Pregnancy refers to the period of time during which a fetus grows and develops in its mother's uterus (see Figure 10.9 ■). The normal length of time for a pregnancy (**gestation**) is 40 weeks. If a baby is born before completing at least 37 weeks of gestation, it is considered **premature.**

During pregnancy the female body undergoes many changes. In fact, all of the body systems become involved in the development of a healthy infant. From the time the fertilized egg implants in the uterus until approximately the end of the eighth week, the infant is referred to as an **embryo** (see Figure 10.10 ■). During this period all the major organs and body systems are formed. Following the embryo stage and lasting until birth, the infant is called a **fetus** (see Figure 10.11 ■). During this time, the longest period of gestation, the organs mature and begin to function.

MED TERM TIP

During the embryo stage of gestation, the organs and organ systems of the body are formed. Therefore, this is a very common time for *congenital anomalies*, or birth defects, to occur. This may happen before the woman is even aware of being pregnant.

The fetus receives nourishment from its mother by way of the **placenta,** which is a spongy, blood-filled organ that forms in the uterus next to the fetus. The placenta is commonly referred to as the afterbirth. The fetus is attached to the

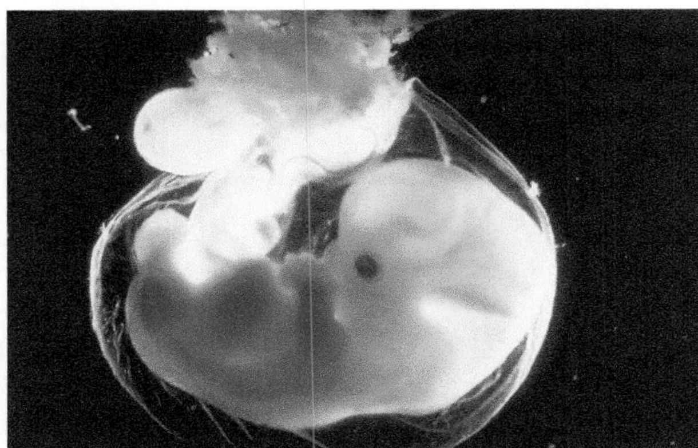

■ **Figure 10.10** Photograph illustrating the development of an embryo. *(Photo Researchers, Inc.)*

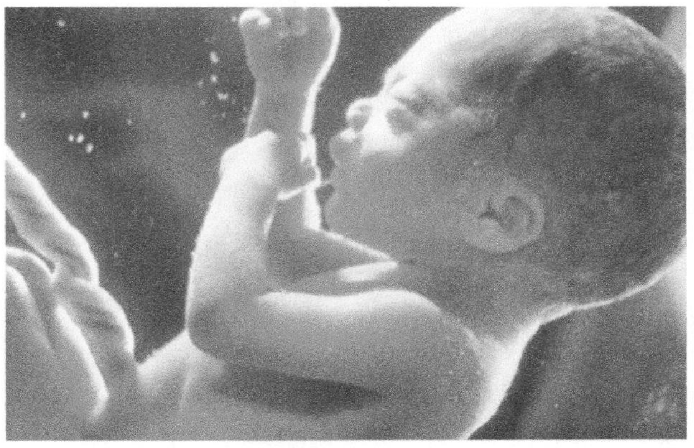

■ **Figure 10.11** Photograph illustrating the development of a fetus. *(Petit Format/Photo Researchers, Inc.)*

placenta by way of the **umbilical cord** and is surrounded by two membranous sacs, the **amnion** and the **chorion.** The amnion is the innermost sac, and it holds the **amniotic fluid** in which the fetus floats. The chorion is an outer, protective sac and also forms part of the placenta.

Labor and Delivery

breech presentation
crowning
delivery
dilation stage (dye-LAY-shun)
effacement (eh-FACE-ment)
expulsion stage (ex-PULL-shun)
labor
placental stage (plah-SEN-tal)

Labor is the actual process of expelling the fetus from the uterus and through the vagina. The first stage is referred to as the **dilation stage,** in which the uterine muscle contracts strongly to expel the fetus (see Figure 10.12A ■). During this process the fetus presses on the cervix and causes it to dilate or expand. As the cervix dilates, it also becomes thinner, referred to as **effacement.** When the cervix is completely dilated to 10 centimeters, the second stage of labor begins (see Figure 10.12B ■). This is the **expulsion stage** and ends with **delivery** of the baby. Generally, the head of the baby appears first, which is referred to as **crowning.** In some cases the baby's buttocks will appear first, and this is referred to as a **breech presentation** (see Figure 10.13 ■). The last stage of labor is the **placental stage** (see Figure 10.12C ■). Immediately after childbirth, the uterus continues to contract, causing the placenta to be expelled through the vagina.

A

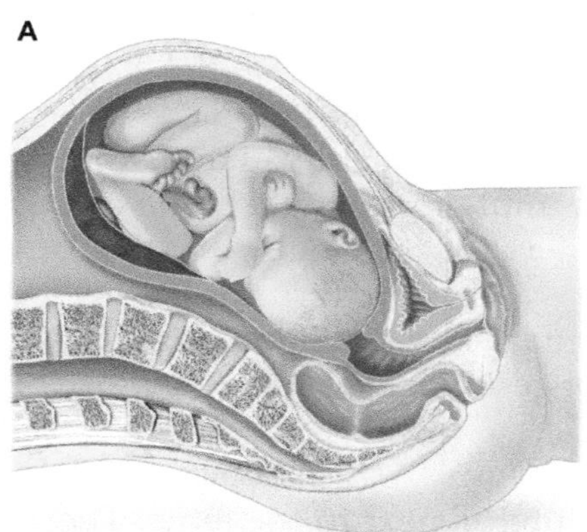

DILATION STAGE:
Uterine contractions dilate cervix

B

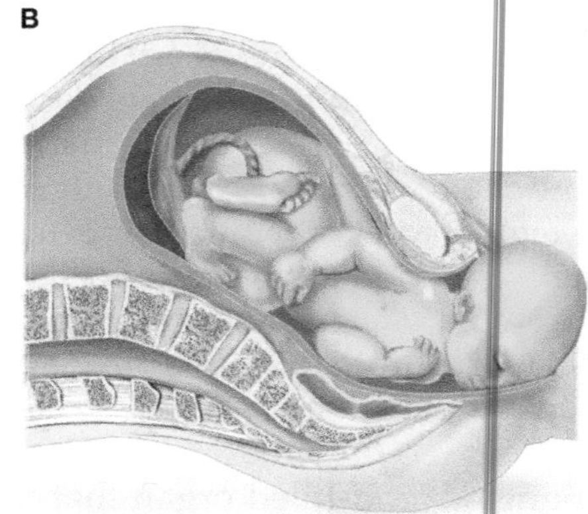

EXPULSION STAGE:
Birth of baby or expulsion

C

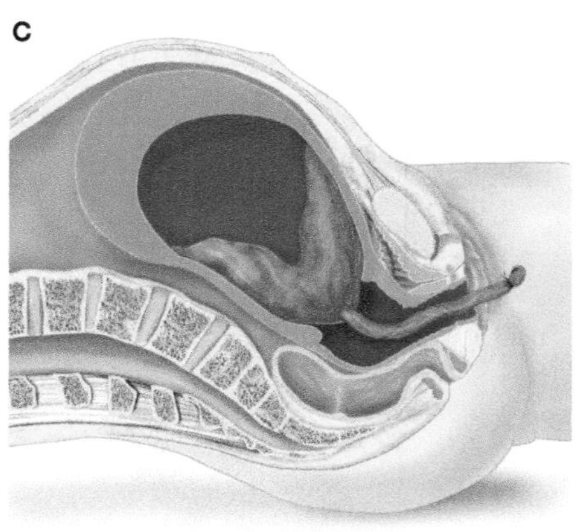

PLACENTAL STAGE:
Delivery of placenta

■ **Figure 10.12** The stages of labor and delivery. (A) During the dilation stage the cervix thins and dilates to 10 cm. (B) During the expulsion stage the infant is delivered. (C) During the placental stage the placenta is delivered.

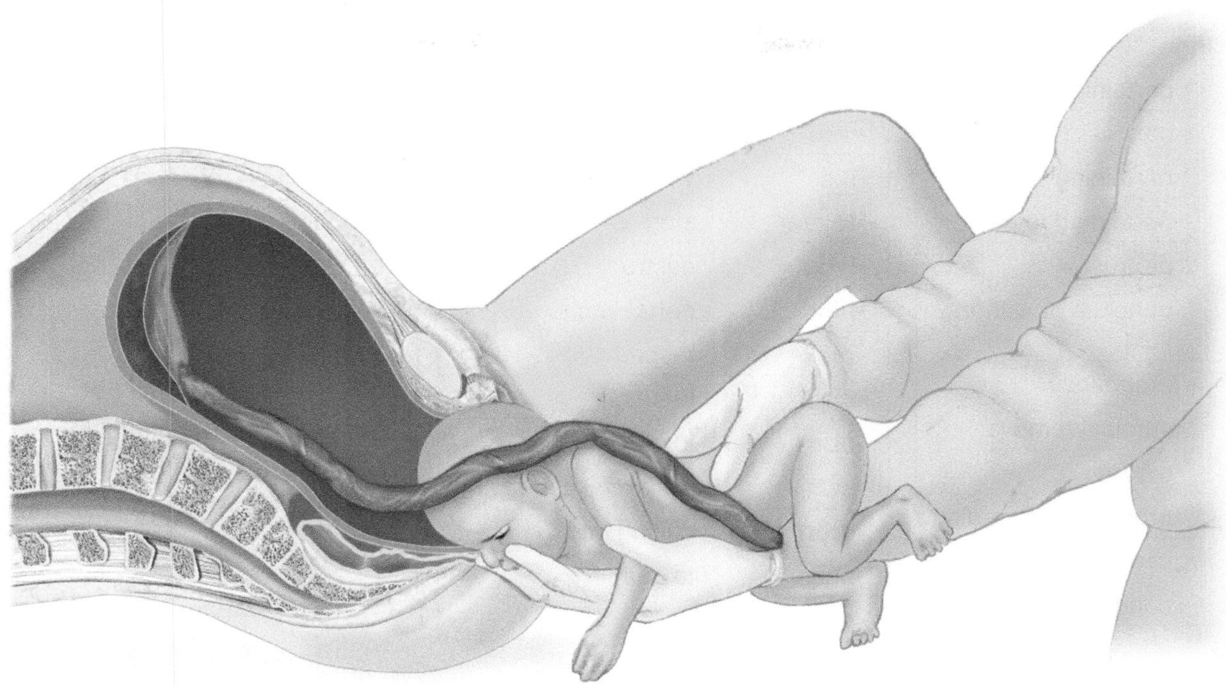

■ Figure 10.13 A breech birth. This image illustrates a newborn that has been delivered buttocks first.

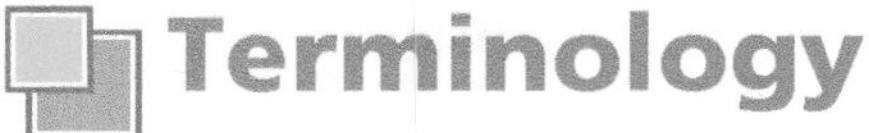

Terminology

Word Parts Used to Build Female Reproductive System Terms

The following lists contain the combining forms, suffixes, and prefixes used to build terms in the remaining sections of this chapter.

Combining Forms

abdomin/o	abdomen
amni/o	amnion
bi/o	life
carcin/o	cancer
cervic/o	cervix
chori/o	chorion
colp/o	vagina
culd/o	cul-de-sac
cyst/o	bladder, pouch
embry/o	embryo
episi/o	vulva
fet/o	fetus
fibr/o	fibers
gynec/o	woman

hem/o	blood
hemat/o	blood
hymen/o	hymen
hyster/o	uterus
lact/o	milk
lapar/o	abdomen
later/o	side
mamm/o	breast
mast/o	breast
men/o	menstruation
metr/o	uterus
nat/o	birth
olig/o	scanty
oophor/o	ovary

or/o	mouth
ovari/o	ovary
pelv/o	pelvis
perine/o	perineum
py/o	pus
rect/o	rectum
salping/o	uterine tube
son/o	sound
tox/o	poison
uter/o	uterus
vagin/o	vagina
vulv/o	vulva

Suffixes

-al	pertaining to
-algia	pain
-an	pertaining to
-ary	pertaining to
-cele	protrusion
-centesis	puncture to withdraw fluid
-cyesis	pregnancy
-ectomy	surgical removal
-gram	record
-graphy	process of recording
-gravida	pregnancy
-ia	condition
-iasis	abnormal condition

-ic	pertaining to
-ine	pertaining to
-itis	inflammation
-logy	study of
-lytic	destruction
-nic	pertaining to
-oid	resembling
-oma	tumor
-opsy	to view
-osis	abnormal condition
-otomy	cutting into
-para	to bear
-partum	childbirth

-pexy	surgical fixation
-plasty	surgical repair
-rrhagia	abnormal flow condition
-rrhaphy	suture
-rrhea	discharge
-rrhexis	rupture
-salpinx	uterine tube
-scope	instrument for viewing
-scopy	process of viewing
-tic	pertaining to
-tocia	labor and childbirth

Prefixes

a-	without
ante-	before
bi-	two
contra-	against
dys-	abnormal, difficult
endo-	within

in-	not
intra-	inside
multi-	many
neo-	new
nulli-	none
peri-	around

post-	after
pre-	before
primi-	first
pseudo-	false
ultra-	beyond

Anatomical Terms

TERM	WORD PARTS	DEFINITION
amniotic (am-nee-OT-ik)	amni/o = amnion -tic = pertaining to	Pertaining to the amnion.
cervical (SER-vih-kal)	cervic/o = cervix -al = pertaining to	Pertaining to the cervix.
chorionic (koh-ree-ON-ik)	chori/o = chorion -nic = pertaining to	Pertaining to the chorion.
embryonic (em-bree-ON-ik)	embry/o = embryo -nic = pertaining to	Pertaining to the embryo.
fetal (FEE-tall)	fet/o = fetus -al = pertaining to	Pertaining to the fetus.
lactic (LAK-tik)	lact/o = milk -ic = pertaining to	Pertaining to milk.
mammary (MAM-mah-ree)	mamm/o = breast -ary = pertaining to	Pertaining to the breast.

Anatomical Terms *(continued)*

TERM	WORD PARTS	DEFINITION
ovarian (oh-VAIR-ee-an)	ovari/o = ovary -an = pertaining to	Pertaining to the ovary.
perineal (per-ih-NEE-al)	perine/o = perineum -al = pertaining to	Pertaining to the perineum.
uterine (YOO-ter-in)	uter/o = uterus -ine = pertaining to	Pertaining to the uterus.
vaginal (VAJ-ih-nal)	vagin/o = vagina -al = pertaining to	Pertaining to the vagina.
vulvar (VUL-var)	vulv/o = vulva -ar = pertaining to	Pertaining to the vulva.

Pregnancy Terms

TERM	WORD PARTS	DEFINITION
antepartum (an-tee-PAR-tum)	ante- = before -partum = childbirth	Period of time before birth.
colostrum (kuh-LOS-trum)		Thin fluid first secreted by the breast after delivery. It does not contain much protein, but is rich in antibodies.
fraternal twins	-al = pertaining to	Twins that develop from two different ova fertilized by two different sperm. Although twins, these siblings do not have identical DNA.
identical twins	-al = pertaining to	Twins that develop from the splitting of one fertilized ovum. These siblings have identical DNA.
lactorrhea (lak-toh-REE-ah)	lact/o = milk -rrhea = flow	Discharge of milk from the breast.
meconium (meh-KOH-nee-um)		First bowel movement of a newborn. It is greenish-black in color and consists of mucus and bile.
multigravida (mull-tih-GRAV-ih-dah)	multi- = many -gravida = pregnancy	A woman who has been pregnant two or more times.
multipara (mull-TIP-ah-rah)	multi- = many -para = to bear	A woman who has given birth to a live infant two or more times.
neonate (NEE-oh-nayt)	neo- = new nat/o = birth	Term for a newborn baby.
nulligravida (null-ih-GRAV-ih-dah)	nulli- = none -gravida = pregnancy	A woman who has not been pregnant.
nullipara (null-IP-ah-rah)	nulli- = none -para = to bear	A woman who has not given birth to a live infant.
postpartum (post-PAR-tum)	post- = after -partum = childbirth	Period of time shortly after birth.
primigravida (prem-ih-GRAV-ih-dah)	primi- = first -gravida = pregnancy	A woman who is pregnant for the first time.
primipara (prem-IP-ah-rah)	primi- = first -para = to bear	A woman who has given birth to a live infant once.

Pathology

TERM	WORD PARTS	DEFINITION
Medical Specialties		
gynecology (GYN) (gigh-neh-KOL-oh-jee)	gynec/o = woman -logy = study of	Branch of medicine specializing in the diagnosis and treatment of conditions of the female reproductive system. Physician is called a *gynecologist.*
neonatology (nee-oh-nay-TALL-oh-jee)	neo- = new nat/o = birth -logy = study of	Branch of medicine specializing in the diagnosis and treatment of conditions involving newborns. Physician is called a *neonatologist.*
obstetrics (OB) (ob-STET-riks)		Branch of medicine specializing in the diagnosis and treatment of women during pregnancy and childbirth, and immediately after childbirth. Physician is called an *obstetrician.*
Signs and Symptoms		
amenorrhea (ah-men-oh-REE-ah)	a- = without men/o = menstruation -rrhea = flow	Condition of having no menstrual flow.
amniorrhea (am-nee-oh-REE-ah)	amni/o = amnion -rrhea = flow	Flow of amniotic fluid when the amnion ruptures.
dysmenorrhea (dis-men-oh-REE-ah)	dys- = abnormal, painful men/o = menstruation -rrhea = flow	Condition of having abnormal or painful menstrual flow.
dystocia (dis-TOH-she-ah)	dys- = abnormal, difficult -tocia = labor and childbirth	Difficult labor and childbirth.
hematosalpinx (hee-mah-toh-SAL-pinks)	hemat/o = blood -salpinx = uterine tube	Presence of blood in a uterine tube.
mastalgia (mas-TAL-jee-ah)	mast/o = breast -algia = pain	Breast pain.
menorrhagia (men-oh-RAY-jee-ah)	men/o = menstruation -rrhagia = abnormal flow condition	Condition of having abnormally heavy menstrual flow during normal menstruation time.
metrorrhagia (meh-troh-RAY-jee-ah)	metr/o = uterus -rrhagia = abnormal flow condition	Term is used to describe uterine bleeding between menstrual periods.
metrorrhea (meh-troh-REE-ah)	metr/o = uterus -rrhea = discharge	Having a discharge (such as mucus or pus) from the uterus that is not the menstrual flow.
oligomenorrhea (ol-lih-goh-men-oh-REE-ah)	olig/o = scanty men/o = menstruation -rrhea = flow	Condition of having light menstrual flow.
Ovary		
oophoritis (oh-off-oh-RIGH-tis)	oophor/o = ovary -itis = inflammation	Inflammation of the ovary.

Pathology *(continued)*

TERM	WORD PARTS	DEFINITION
ovarian carcinoma (oh-VAY-ree-an / kar-sih-NOH-mah)	ovari/o = ovary -an = pertaining to carcin/o = cancer -oma = tumor	Cancer of the ovary.
ovarian cyst (oh-VAY-ree-an / SIST)	ovari/o = ovary -an = pertaining to	Cyst that develops within the ovary. These may be multiple cysts and may rupture, causing pain and bleeding.
Uterine Tubes		
pyosalpinx (pie-oh-SAL-pinks)	py/o = pus -salpinx = uterine tube	Presence of pus in a uterine tube.
salpingitis (sal-ping-JIGH-tis)	salping/o = uterine tube -itis = inflammation	Inflammation of the uterine tube.
Uterus		
cervical cancer (SER-vih-kal)	cervic/o = cervix -al = pertaining to	Malignant growth in the cervix. Some cases are caused by the *human papilloma virus* (HPV), a sexually transmitted virus for which there is now a vaccine. An especially difficult type of cancer to treat that causes 5% of the cancer deaths in women. Pap smear tests have helped to detect early cervical cancer.
endocervicitis (en-doh-ser-vih-SIGH-tis)	endo- = within cervic/o = cervix -itis = inflammation	Inflammation that occurs within the cervix.
endometrial cancer (en-doh-MEE-tree-al)	endo- = within metr/o = uterus -al = pertaining to	Cancer of the endometrial lining of the uterus.
endometritis (en-doh-meh-TRY-tis) MED TERM TIP Word Watch: Be careful when using the combining form *metr/o* meaning "uterus" and the suffix *-metry* meaning "process of measuring."	endo- = within metr/o = uterus -itis = inflammation	Inflammation of the endometrium (inner layer of the uterine wall)
fibroid tumor (FIGH-broyd / TOO-mor)	fibr/o = fibers -oid = resembling	Benign tumor or growth that contains fiber-like tissue. Uterine fibroid tumors are the most common tumors in women.

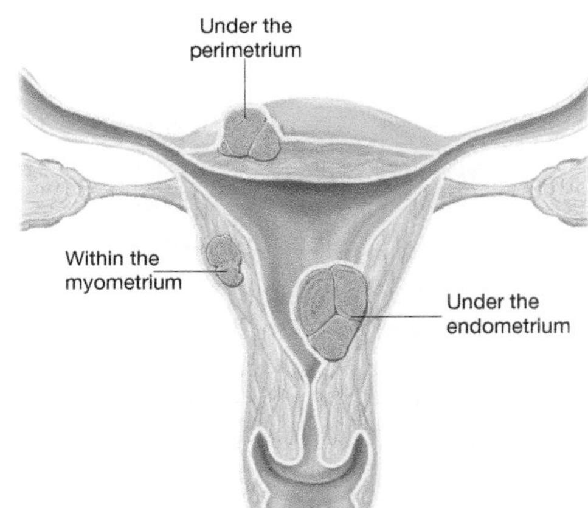

Figure 10.14 Common sites for the development of fibroid tumors.

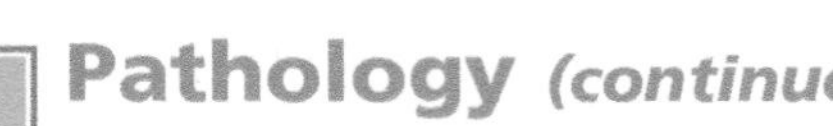

Pathology *(continued)*

TERM	WORD PARTS	DEFINITION
hysterorrhexis (hiss-ter-oh-REK-sis)	hyster/o = uterus -rrhexis = rupture	Rupture of the uterus; may occur during labor.
menometrorrhagia (men-oh-met-thro-RAY-jee-ah)	men/o = menstruation metr/o = uterus -rrhagia = abnormal flow condition	Excessive bleeding during the menstrual period and at intervals between menstrual periods.
premenstrual syndrome (PMS) (pre-MEN-stroo-al / SIN-drohm)	pre- = before men/o = menstruation -al = pertaining to	Symptoms that develop just prior to the onset of a menstrual period, which can include irritability, headache, tender breasts, and anxiety.
prolapsed uterus (pro-LAPS'D / YOO-ter-us)		Fallen uterus that can cause the cervix to protrude through the vaginal opening. Generally caused by weakened muscles from vaginal delivery or as the result of pelvic tumors pressing down.
Vagina		
candidiasis (kan-dih-DYE-ah-sis) MED TERM TIP The term *candida* comes from a Latin term meaning "dazzling white." Candida is the scientific name for yeast and refers to the very white discharge that is the hallmark of a yeast infection.	-iasis = abnormal condition	Yeast infection of the skin and mucous membranes that can result in white plaques on the tongue and vagina.
cystocele (SIS-toh-seel)	cyst/o = bladder -cele = protrusion	Hernia or outpouching of the bladder that protrudes into the vagina. This may cause urinary frequency and urgency.
rectocele (REK-toh-seel)	rect/o = rectum -cele = protrusion	Protrusion or herniation of the rectum into the vagina.
toxic shock syndrome (TSS)	tox/o = poison -ic = pertaining to	Rare and sometimes fatal staphylococcus infection that generally occurs in menstruating women. Initial infection of the vagina is associated with prolonged wearing of a super-absorbent tampon.
vaginitis (vaj-ih-NIGH-tis)	vagin/o = vagina -itis = inflammation	Inflammation of the vagina.
Pelvic Cavity		
endometriosis (en-doh-mee-tree-OH-sis)	endo- = within metr/o = uterus -osis = abnormal condition	Abnormal condition of endometrium tissue appearing throughout the pelvis or on the abdominal wall. This tissue is normally found within the uterus.
pelvic inflammatory disease (PID) (PELL-vik / in-FLAM-mah-toh-ree)	pelv/o = pelvis -ic = pertaining to	Chronic or acute infection, usually bacterial, that has ascended through the female reproductive organs and out into the pelvic cavity. May result in scarring that interferes with fertility.
perimetritis (pair-ih-meh-TRY-tis)	peri- = around metr/o = uterus -itis = inflammation	Inflammation in the pelvic cavity around the outside of the uterus.

Pathology *(continued)*

TERM	WORD PARTS	DEFINITION
Breast		
breast cancer		Malignant tumor of the breast. Usually forms in the milk-producing gland tissue or the lining of the milk ducts (see Figure 10.15A ■).
fibrocystic breast disease (figh-bro-SIS-tik)	fibr/o = fibers cyst/o = pouch -ic = pertaining to	Benign cysts forming in the breast (see Figure 10.15B ■).

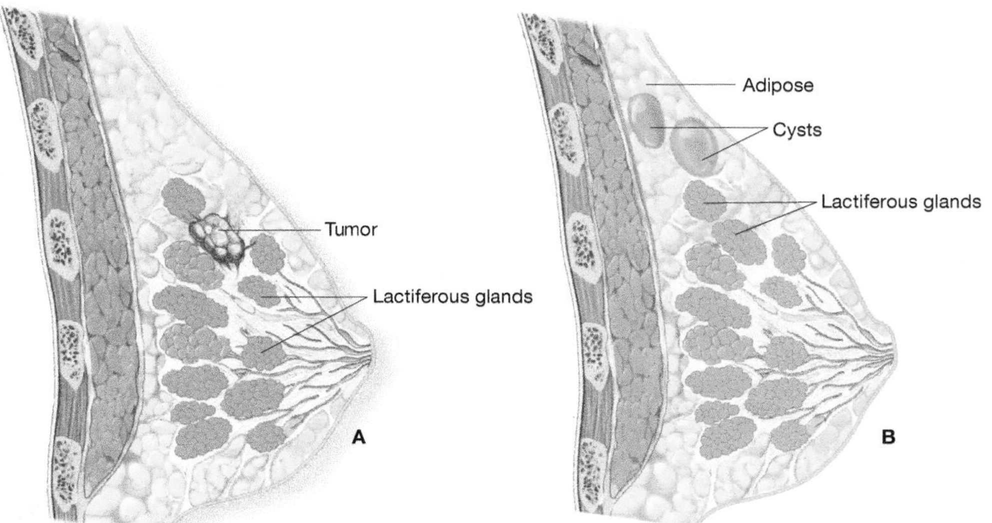

■ **Figure 10.15** Comparison of breast cancer and fibrocystic disease. (A) Breast with a malignant tumor growing in the lactiferous gland and duct; (B) the location of a fibrocystic lump in the adipose tissue covering the breast.

TERM	WORD PARTS	DEFINITION
mastitis (mas-TYE-tis)	mast/o = breast -itis = inflammation	Inflammation of the breast.
Pregnancy		
abruptio placentae (ah-BRUP-tee-oh / plah-SEN-tee)		Emergency condition in which the placenta tears away from the uterine wall prior to delivery of the infant. Requires immediate delivery of the baby.
eclampsia (eh-KLAMP-see-ah)	-ia = condition	Further worsening of preeclampsia symptoms with the addition of seizures and coma; may occur between the 20th week of pregnancy and up to 6 weeks postpartum.
hemolytic disease of the newborn (HDN) (hee-moh-LIT-ik)	hem/o = blood -lytic = destruction	Condition developing in the baby when the mother's blood type is Rh-negative and the baby's blood is Rh-positive. Antibodies in the mother's blood enter the fetus's bloodstream through the placenta and destroy the fetus's red blood cells, causing anemia, jaundice, and enlargement of the spleen. Treatment is early diagnosis and blood transfusion. Also called *erythroblastosis fetalis.*

Pathology *(continued)*

TERM	WORD PARTS	DEFINITION
infertility	in- = not	Inability to produce children. Generally defined as no pregnancy after properly timed intercourse for 1 year.
placenta previa (plah-SEN-tah / PREE-vee-ah)		A placenta that is implanted in the lower portion of the uterus and, in turn, blocks the birth canal.

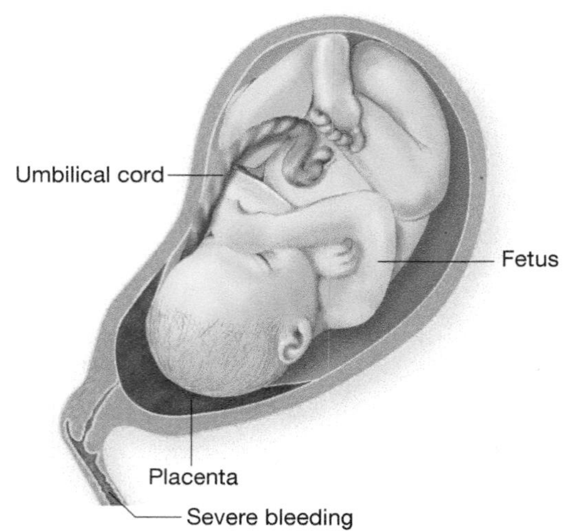

■ **Figure 10.16** Placenta previa, longitudinal section showing the placenta growing over the opening into the cervix.

TERM	WORD PARTS	DEFINITION
preeclampsia (pre-eh-KLAMP-see-ah)	pre- = before	Metabolic disease of pregnancy. If untreated, it may progress to eclampsia. Symptoms include hypertension, headaches, albumin in the urine, and edema. May occur between the 20th week of pregnancy and up to 6 weeks postpartum. Also called *toxemia* or pregnancy-induced hypertension (PIH)
prolapsed umbilical cord (pro-LAPS'D / um-BILL-ih-kal)		When the umbilical cord of the baby is expelled first during delivery and is squeezed between the baby's head and the vaginal wall. This presents an emergency situation since the baby's circulation is compromised.
pseudocyesis (soo-doh-sigh-EE-sis)	pseudo- = false -cyesis = pregnancy	Condition in which the body reacts as if there is a pregnancy (especially hormonal changes), but there is no pregnancy.
salpingocyesis (sal-ping-goh-sigh-EE-sis)	salping/o = uterine tube -cyesis = pregnancy	Pregnancy that occurs in the uterine tube instead of in the uterus.
spontaneous abortion		Unplanned loss of a pregnancy due to the death of the embryo or fetus before the time it is viable, commonly referred to as a *miscarriage.*
stillbirth		Birth in which a viable-aged fetus dies shortly before or at the time of delivery.

Diagnostic Procedures

TERM	WORD PARTS	DEFINITION
Clinical Laboratory Tests		
Pap (Papanicolaou) **smear** (pap-ah-NIK-oh-low)		Test for the early detection of cancer of the cervix named after the developer of the test, George Papanicolaou, a Greek physician. A scraping of cells is removed from the cervix for examination under a microscope.
pregnancy test (PREG-nan-see)		Chemical test that can determine a pregnancy during the first few weeks. Can be performed in a physician's office or with a home-testing kit.
Diagnostic Imaging		
hysterosalpingography (HSG) (hiss-ter-oh-sal-pin-GOG-rah-fee)	hyster/o = uterus salping/o = uterine tube -graphy = process of recording	Taking of an X-ray after injecting radiopaque material into the uterus and uterine tubes.
mammogram (MAM-moh-gram)	mamm/o = breast -gram = record	X-ray record of the breast.
mammography (mam-OG-rah-fee)	mamm/o = breast -graphy = process of recording	X-ray to diagnose breast disease, especially breast cancer.
pelvic ultrasonography (PELL-vik / ull-trah-son-OG-rah-fee)	pelv/o = pelvis -ic = pertaining to ultra- = beyond son/o = sound -graphy = process of recording	Use of high-frequency sound waves to produce an image or photograph of an organ, such as the uterus, ovaries, or fetus.
Endoscopic Procedures		
colposcope (KOL-poh-scope)	colp/o = vagina -scope = instrument for viewing	Instrument used to view inside the vagina.
colposcopy (kol-POS-koh-pee)	colp/o = vagina -scopy = process of viewing	Examination of vagina using an instrument called a *colposcope.*
culdoscopy (kul-DOS-koh-pee)	culd/o = cul-de-sac -scopy = process of viewing	Examination of the female pelvic cavity, particularly behind the uterus, by introducing an endoscope through the wall of the vagina.
laparoscope (LAP-ah-row-scope)	lapar/o = abdomen -scope = instrument for viewing	Instrument used to view inside the abdomen.
laparoscopy (lap-ar-OS-koh-pee)	lapar/o = abdomen -scopy = process of viewing	Examination of the peritoneal cavity using an instrument called a *laparoscope.* The instrument is passed through a small incision made by the surgeon into the abdominopelvic cavity.

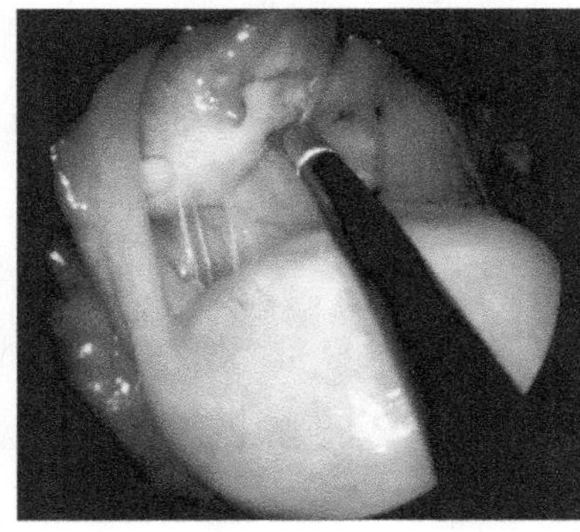

■ **Figure 10.17** Photograph taken during a laparoscopic procedure. The fundus of the uterus is visible below the probe, the ovary is at the tip of the probe, and the uterine tube extends along the left side of the photo. *(Southern Illinois University/ Photo Researchers, Inc.)*

Diagnostic Procedures *(continued)*

TERM	WORD PARTS	DEFINITION
Obstetrical Diagnostic Procedures		
amniocentesis (am-nee-oh-sen-TEE-sis)	amni/o = amnion -centesis = puncture to withdraw fluid	Puncturing of the amniotic sac using a needle and syringe for the purpose of withdrawing amniotic fluid for testing. Can assist in determining fetal maturity, development, and genetic disorders.
Apgar score (AP-gar)		Evaluation of a neonate's adjustment to the outside world. Observes color, heart rate, muscle tone, respiratory rate, and response to stimulus at 1 minute and 5 minutes after birth.
chorionic villus sampling (CVS) (kor-ree-ON-ik / vill-us)	chori/o = chorion -nic = pertaining to	Removal of a small piece of the chorion for genetic analysis. May be done at an earlier stage of pregnancy than amniocentesis.
fetal monitoring (FEE-tal)	fet/o = fetus -al = pertaining to	Using electronic equipment placed on the mother's abdomen or the fetus' scalp to check the fetal heart rate (FHR). Also called fetal heart tone (FHT) during labor. The normal heart rate of the fetus is rapid, ranging from 120 to 160 beats per minute. A drop in the fetal heart rate indicates the fetus is in distress.
Additional Diagnostic Procedures		
cervical biopsy (SER-vih-kal / BYE-op-see)	cervic/o = cervix -al = pertaining to bi/o = life -opsy = to view	Taking a sample of tissue from the cervix to test for the presence of cancer cells.
endometrial biopsy (EMB) (en-doh-MEE-tre-al BYE-op-see)	endo- = within metr/o = uterus -al = pertaining to bi/o = life -opsy = to view	Taking a sample of tissue from the lining of the uterus to test for abnormalities.
pelvic examination (PELL-vik)	pelv/o = pelvis -ic = pertaining to	Physical examination of the vagina and adjacent organs performed by a physician placing the fingers of one hand into the vagina. An instrument called a *speculum* is used to open the vagina.

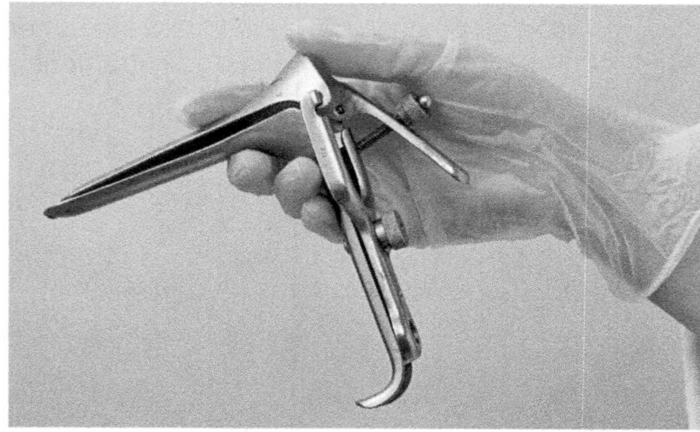

Figure 10.18 A speculum used to hold the vagina open in order to visualize the cervix.

Therapeutic Procedures

TERM	WORD PARTS	DEFINITION
Medical Procedures		
barrier contraception (kon-trah-SEP-shun)	contra- = against	Prevention of a pregnancy using a device to prevent sperm from meeting an ovum. Examples include condoms, diaphragms, and cervical caps.
hormonal contraception	-al = pertaining to contra- = against	Use of hormones to block ovulation and prevent conception. May be in the form of a pill, a patch, an implant under the skin, or an injection.
intrauterine device (IUD) (in-trah-YOO-ter-in)	intra- = inside uter/o = uterus -ine = pertaining to	Device inserted into the uterus by a physician for the purpose of contraception.

■ **Figure 10.19** Photographs illustrating the shape of two different intrauterine devices (IUDs). *(Jules Selmes and Debi Treloar/ Dorling Kindersley)*

TERM	WORD PARTS	DEFINITION
Surgical Procedures		
amniotomy (am-nee-OT-oh-mee)	amni/o = amnion -otomy = cutting into	Surgically cutting open the amnion; commonly referred to as "breaking the water."
cervicectomy (ser-vih-SEK-toh-mee)	cervic/o = cervix -ectomy = surgical removal	Surgical removal of the cervix.
cesarean section (CS, C-section) (see-SAYR-ee-an)		Surgical delivery of a baby through an incision into the abdominal and uterine walls. Legend has it that the Roman emperor, Julius Caesar, was the first person born by this method.
conization (kon-ih-ZAY-shun)		Surgical removal of a core of cervical tissue. Also refers to partial removal of the cervix.
dilation and curettage (D & C) (dye-LAY-shun / koo-reh-TAHZ)		Surgical procedure in which the opening of the cervix is dilated and the uterus is scraped or suctioned of its lining or tissue. Often performed after a spontaneous abortion and to stop excessive bleeding from other causes.
elective abortion		Legal termination of a pregnancy for nonmedical reasons.
episiorrhaphy (eh-peez-ee-OR-ah-fee)	episi/o = vulva -rrhaphy = suture	To suture the perineum; procedure to repair an episiotomy postpartum. Note that the combining form *episi/o* is used even though the perineum is not part of the vulva.
episiotomy (eh-peez-ee-OT-oh-mee)	episi/o = vulva -otomy = cutting into	Surgical incision of the perineum to facilitate the delivery process. Can prevent an irregular tearing of tissue during birth. Note that the combining form *episi/o* is used even though the perineum is not part of the vulva.

Therapeutic Procedures *(continued)*

TERM	WORD PARTS	DEFINITION
hymenectomy (high-men-EK-toh-mee)	hymen/o = hymen -ectomy = surgical removal	Surgical removal of the hymen.
hysterectomy (hiss-ter-EK-toh-mee)	hyster/o = uterus -ectomy = surgical removal	Surgical removal of the uterus.
hysteropexy (HISS-ter-oh-pek-see)	hyster/o = uterus -pexy = surgical fixation	To surgically anchor the uterus to its proper location in the pelvic cavity; a treatment for a prolapsed uterus.
laparotomy (lap-ah-ROT-oh-mee)	lapar/o = abdomen -otomy = cutting into	To cut open the abdomen; performed in order to complete other surgical procedures inside the abdomen or performed during a C-section.
lumpectomy (lump-EK-toh-mee)	-ectomy = surgical removal	Removal of only a breast tumor and the tissue immediately surrounding it.
mammoplasty (MAM-moh-plas-tee)	mamm/o = breast -plasty = surgical repair	Surgical repair or reconstruction of the breast.
mastectomy (mass-TEK-toh-mee)	mast/o = breast -ectomy = surgical removal	Surgical removal of the breast.
oophorectomy (oh-off-oh-REK-toh-mee)	oophor/o = ovary -ectomy = surgical removal	Surgical removal of the ovary.
radical mastectomy (mast-EK-toh-mee)	-al = pertaining to mast/o = breast -ectomy = surgical removal	Surgical removal of the breast tissue plus chest muscles and axillary lymph nodes.
salpingectomy (sal-ping-JECK-toh-mee)	salping/o = uterine tube -ectomy = surgical removal	Surgical removal of the uterine tube.
simple mastectomy (mast-EK-toh-mee)	mast/o = breast -ectomy = surgical removal	Surgical removal of the breast tissue.
therapeutic abortion		Termination of a pregnancy for the health of the mother or another medical reason.
total abdominal hysterectomy—bilateral salpingo-oophorectomy (TAH-BSO) (hiss-ter-EK-toh-me / sal-ping-goh / oh-oh-foe-REK-toh-mee)	abdomin/o = abdomen -al = pertaining to hyster/o = uterus -ectomy = surgical removal bi- = two later/o = side -al = pertaining to salping/o = uterine tube oophor/o = ovary -ectomy = surgical removal	Removal of the entire uterus, cervix, both ovaries, and both uterine tubes.
tubal ligation (TOO-bal / lye-GAY-shun)	-al = pertaining to	Surgical tying off of the uterine tubes to prevent conception from taking place. Results in sterilization of the female.
vaginal hysterectomy (VAJ-ih-nal / hiss-ter-EK-toh-me)	vagin/o = vagina -al = pertaining to hyster/o = uterus -ectomy = surgical removal	Removal of the uterus through the vagina rather than through an abdominal incision.

Pharmacology

CLASSIFICATION	WORD PARTS	ACTION	EXAMPLES
abortifacient (ah-bore-tih-FAY-shee-ent)		Medication that terminates a pregnancy.	mifepristone, Mifeprex; dinoprostone, Prostin E2
fertility drug		Medication that triggers ovulation. Also called *ovulation stimulant.*	clomiphene, Clomid; follitropin alfa, Gonal-F
hormone replacement therapy (HRT)		Menopause or the surgical loss of the ovaries results in the lack of estrogen production. Replacing this hormone may prevent some of the consequences of menopause, especially in younger women who have surgically lost their ovaries.	conjugated estrogens, Cenestin, Premarin
oral contraceptive pills (OCPs) (kon-trah-SEP-tive)	or/o = mouth -al = pertaining to contra- = against	Birth control medication that uses low doses of female hormones to prevent conception by blocking ovulation.	desogestrel/ethinyl estradiol, Ortho-Cept; ethinyl estradiol/norgestrel, Lo/Ovral
oxytocin (ox-ee-TOH-sin)		Oxytocin is a natural hormone that begins or improves uterine contractions during labor and delivery.	oxytocin, Pitocin, Syntocinon

Abbreviations

AB	abortion
AI	artificial insemination
BSE	breast self-examination
CS, C-section	cesarean section
CVS	chorionic villus sampling
Cx	cervix
D & C	dilation and curettage
EDC	estimated date of confinement
EMB	endometrial biopsy
ERT	estrogen replacement therapy
FEKG	fetal electrocardiogram
FHR	fetal heart rate
FHT	fetal heart tone
FSH	follicle-stimulating hormone
FTND	full-term normal delivery
GI, grav I	first pregnancy
GYN, gyn	gynecology
HCG, hCG	human chorionic gonadotropin
HDN	hemolytic disease of the newborn
HPV	human papilloma virus
HRT	hormone replacement therapy
HSG	hysterosalpingography
IUD	intrauterine device
IVF	*in vitro* fertilization
LBW	low birth weight
LH	luteinizing hormone
LMP	last menstrual period
NB	newborn
OB	obstetrics
OCPs	oral contraceptive pills
Pap	Papanicolaou test
PI, para I	first delivery
PID	pelvic inflammatory disease
PIH	pregnancy-induced hypertension
PMS	premenstrual syndrome
TAH-BSO	total abdominal hysterectomy–bilateral salpingo-oophorectomy
TSS	toxic shock syndrome
UC	uterine contractions

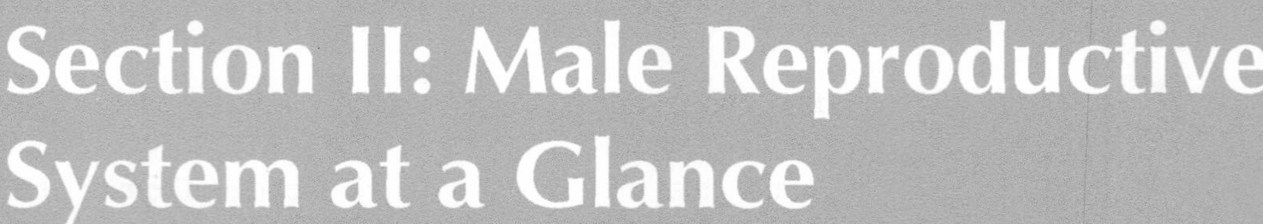

Section II: Male Reproductive System at a Glance

Function

Similar to the female reproductive system, the male reproductive system is responsible for producing sperm, the male reproductive cell, secreting the male sex hormones, and delivering sperm to the female reproductive tract.

Structures

Here are the primary structures that comprise the male reproductive system.

bulbourethral glands
epididymis
penis
prostate gland
seminal vesicles
testes
vas deferens

Word Parts

Here are the most common word parts (with their meanings) used to build male reproductive system terms. For a more comprehensive list, refer to the Terminology section of this chapter.

Combining Forms

andr/o	male
balan/o	glans penis
crypt/o	hidden
epididym/o	epididymis
genit/o	genitals
orch/o	testes
orchi/o	testes
orchid/o	testes
pen/o	penis
prostat/o	prostate
spermat/o	sperm
testicul/o	testes
vas/o	vas deferens
vesicul/o	seminal vesicle

Suffixes

-cide	to kill
-spermia	condition of sperm

Male Reproductive System Illustrated

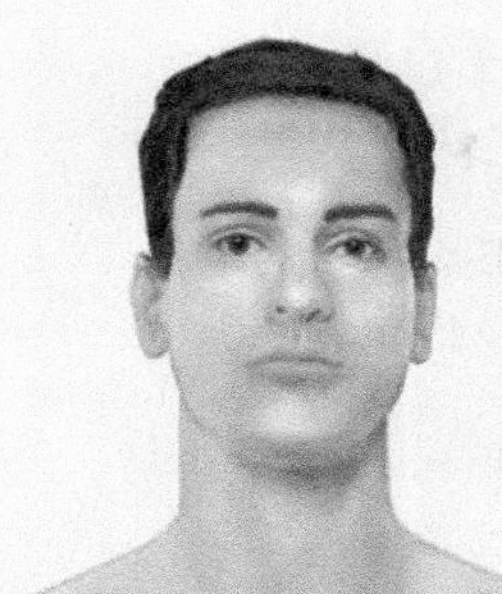

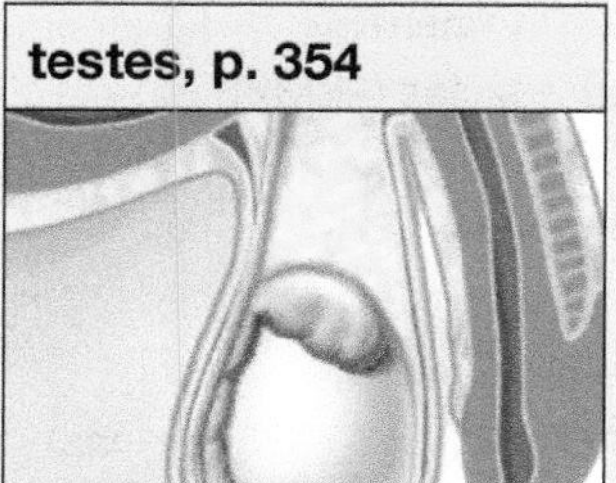

Produces sperm and secretes testosterone

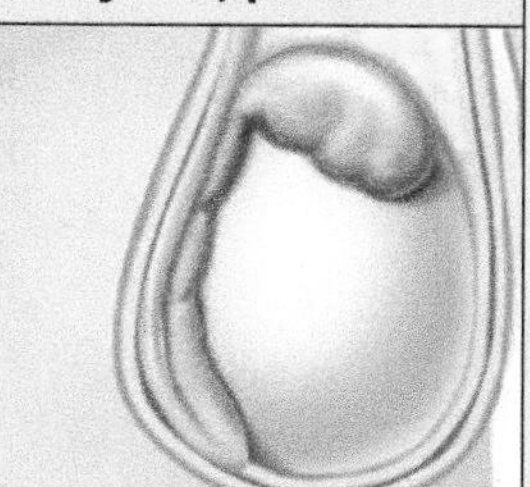

Stores sperm

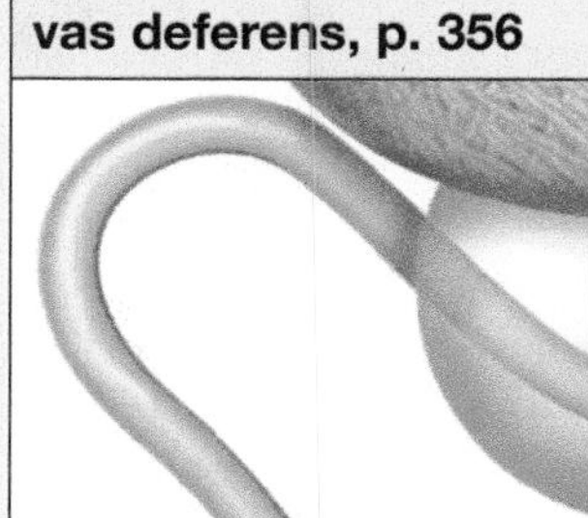

Transports sperm to urethra

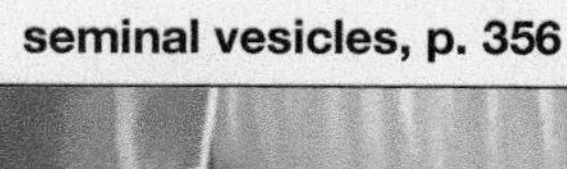

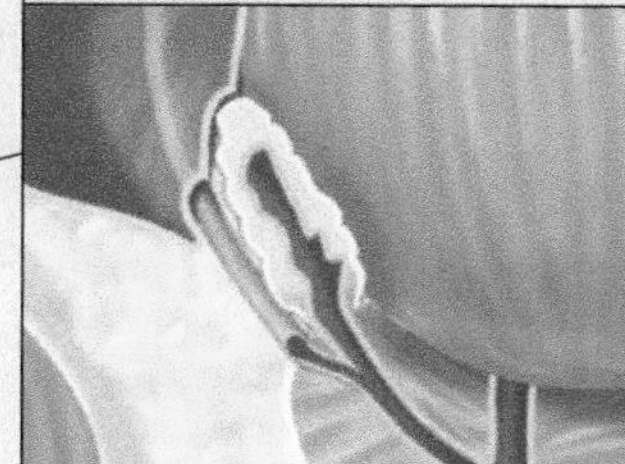

Secretes fluid for semen

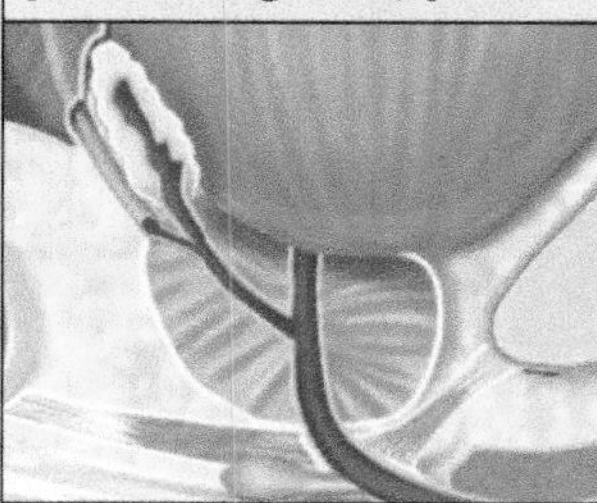

Secretes fluid for semen

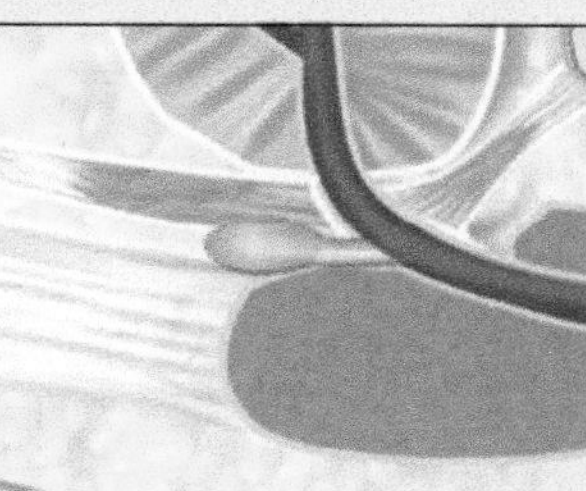

Secretes fluid for semen

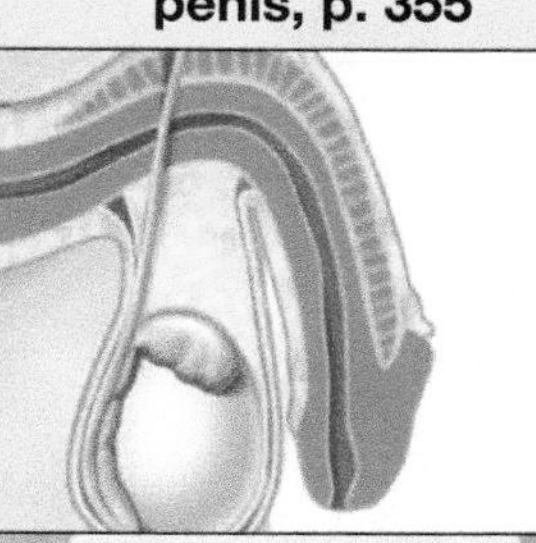

Delivers semen during intercourse

Anatomy and Physiology of the Male Reproductive System

bulbourethral glands (buhl-boh-yoo-REE-thral)
epididymis (ep-ih-DID-ih-mis)
genitourinary system (jen-ih-toh-YOO-rih-nair-ee)
penis (PEE-nis)
prostate gland (PROSS-tayt)
semen (SEE-men)
seminal vesicles (SEM-ih-nal / VESS-ih-kls)
sex hormones
sperm
testes (TESS-teez)
vas deferens (VAS / DEF-er-enz)

The male reproductive system has two main functions. The first is to produce **sperm,** the male reproductive cell; the second is to secrete the male **sex hormones.** In the male, the major organs of reproduction are located outside the body: the **penis,** and the two **testes,** each with an **epididymis** (see Figure 10.20 ■). The penis contains the urethra, which carries both urine and **semen** to the outside of the body. For this reason, this system is sometimes referred to as the **genitourinary system** (GU).

The internal organs of reproduction include two **seminal vesicles,** two **vas deferens,** the **prostate gland,** and two **bulbourethral glands.**

External Organs of Reproduction

Testes

perineum

scrotum (SKROH-tum)
seminiferous tubules (sem-ih-NIF-er-us / TOO-byools)
spermatogenesis (sper-mat-oh-JEN-eh-sis)
testicles (test-IH-kles)
testosterone (tess-TAHSS-ter-own)

The testes (singular is *testis*) or **testicles** are oval in shape and are

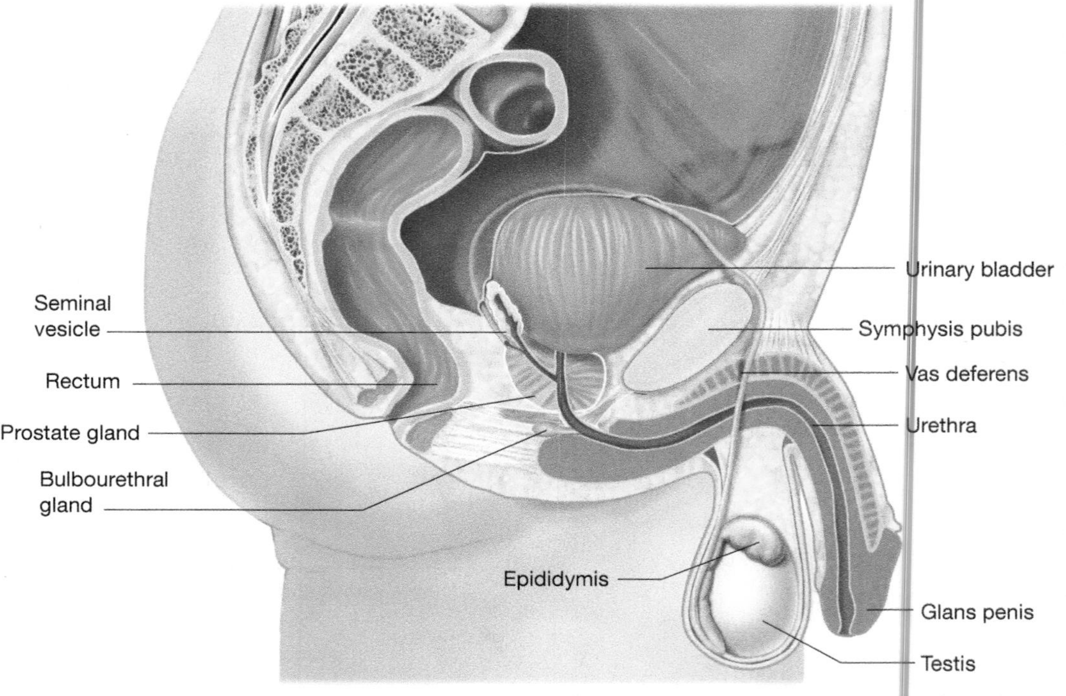

■ **Figure 10.20** The male reproductive system, sagittal section showing the organs of the system and their relation to the urinary bladder and rectum.

responsible for the production of sperm (see again Figure 10.20). This process, called **spermatogenesis,** takes place within the **seminiferous tubules** that make up the insides of the testes (see Figure 10.21 ■). The testes must be maintained at the proper temperature for the sperm to survive. This lower temperature level is achieved by the placement of the testes suspended in the **scrotum,** a sac outside the body. The **perineum** of the male is similar to that in the female and is the area between the scrotum and the anus. The male sex hormone **testosterone,** which is responsible for the development of the male reproductive organs, sperm, and secondary sex characteristics, is also produced by the testes.

MED TERM TIP

Spermatozoon and its plural form, *spermatozoa,* are other terms that mean "sperm." You have no doubt realized that there can be several terms with the same meaning in medical terminology. You must continue to remain flexible when working with these terms in your career. In some cases, one term will be more commonly used, depending on the type of medical specialty or even what part of the country you are in.

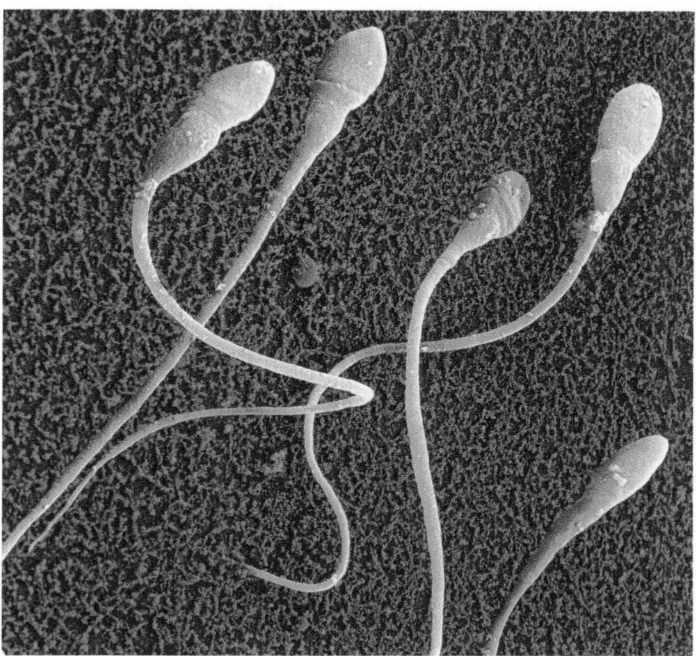

■ **Figure 10.21** Electronmicrograph of human sperm.
(Juergen Berger, Max-Planck Institute/Science Photo Library/Photo Researchers, Inc.)

Epididymis

Each epididymis is a coiled tubule that lies on top of the testes within the scrotum (see again Figure 10.20). This elongated structure serves as the location for sperm maturation and storage until they are ready to be released into the vas deferens.

Penis

circumcision (ser-kum-SIH-zhun)
ejaculation (ee-jak-yoo-LAY-shun)
erectile tissue (ee-REK-tile)
glans penis (GLANS / PEE-nis)
prepuce (PREE-pyoos)
sphincter (SFINGK-ter)
urinary meatus (YOO-rih-nair-ee / me-AY-tus)

The penis is the male sex organ containing **erectile tissue** that is encased in skin (see again Figure 10.20). This organ delivers semen into the female vagina. The soft tip of the penis is referred to as the **glans penis.** It is protected by a covering called the **prepuce** or foreskin. It is this covering of skin that is removed during the procedure known as **circumcision.** The penis becomes erect during sexual stimulation, which allows it to be placed within the female for the **ejaculation** of semen. The male urethra extends from the urinary bladder to the external opening in the penis, the **urinary meatus,** and serves a dual function: the elimination of urine and the ejaculation of semen. During the ejaculation process, a **sphincter** closes to keep urine from escaping.

MED TERM TIP

During sexual intercourse, which is also referred to as *coitus,* the male can eject up to 100 million sperm cells. The adult male produces nearly 200 million sperm daily.

Internal Organs of Reproduction

Vas Deferens

spermatic cord (sper-MAT-ik)

Each vas deferens carries sperm from the epididymis up into the pelvic cavity. They travel up in front of the urinary bladder, over the top, and then back down the posterior side of the bladder to empty into the urethra (see again Figure 10.20). They, along with nerves, arteries, veins, and lymphatic vessels running between the pelvic cavity and the testes, form the **spermatic cord.**

Seminal Vesicles

The two seminal vesicles are small glands located at the base of the urinary bladder (see again Figure 10.20). These vesicles are connected to the vas deferens just before it empties into the urethra. The seminal vesicles secrete a glucose-rich fluid that nourishes the sperm. This liquid, along with the sperm, constitutes semen, the fluid that is eventually ejaculated during sexual intercourse.

Prostate Gland

The single prostate gland is located just below the urinary bladder (see again Figure 10.20). It surrounds the urethra and when enlarged can cause difficulty in urination. The prostate is important for the reproductive process since it secretes an alkaline fluid that assists in keeping the sperm alive by neutralizing the pH of the urethra and vagina.

Bulbourethral Glands

Cowper's glands (KOW-perz)

The bulbourethral glands, also known as **Cowper's glands,** are two small glands located on either side of the urethra just below the prostate (see again Figure 10.20). They produce a mucus-like lubricating fluid that joins with semen to become a part of the ejaculate.

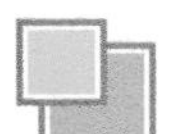

Terminology

Word Parts Used to Build Male Reproductive System Terms

The following lists contain the combining forms, suffixes, and prefixes used to build terms in the remaining sections of this chapter.

Combining Forms

andr/o	male
balan/o	glans penis
carcin/o	cancer
crypt/o	hidden
epididym/o	epididymis
genit/o	genital
hydr/o	water
immun/o	protection

olig/o	scanty
orch/o	testes
orchi/o	testes
orchid/o	testes
pen/o	penis
prostat/o	prostate gland
rect/o	rectum
spermat/o	sperm

testicul/o	testicle
ur/o	urine
urethr/o	urethra
varic/o	dilated vein
vas/o	vas deferens
vesicul/o	seminal vesicle

Suffixes

-al	pertaining to
-ar	pertaining to
-cele	protrusion
-cide	to kill
-ectomy	surgical removal
-gen	that which produces
-iasis	abnormal condition
-ic	pertaining to

-ile	pertaining to
-ism	state of
-itis	inflammation
-logy	study of
-lysis	destruction
-oid	resembling
-oma	tumor
-osis	abnormal condition

-ostomy	create a new opening
-otomy	cutting into
-pexy	surgical fixation
-plasia	growth
-plasty	surgical repair
-rrhea	discharge
-spermia	sperm condition

Prefixes

a-	without
an-	without
anti-	against

dys-	abnormal, difficult
epi-	upon

hyper-	excessive
hypo-	below

Anatomical Terms

TERM	WORD PARTS	DEFINITION
balanic (buh-LAN-ik)	balan/o = glans penis -ic = pertaining to	Pertaining to the glans penis.
epididymal (ep-ih-DID-ih-mal)	epididym/o = epididymis -al = pertaining to	Pertaining to the epididymis.
penile (PEE-nile)	pen/o = penis -ile = pertaining to	Pertaining to the penis.
prostatic (pross-TAT-ik)	prostat/o = prostate gland -ic = pertaining to	Pertaining to the prostate gland.
spermatic (sper-MAT-ik)	spermat/o = sperm -ic = pertaining to	Pertaining to sperm.
testicular (tes-TIK-yoo-lar)	testicul/o = testes -ar = pertaining to	Pertaining to the testes.
vasal (VAY-sal)	vas/o = vas deferens -al = pertaining to	Pertaining to the vas deferens.
vesicular (veh-SIC-yoo-lar)	vesicul/o = seminal vesicle -ar = pertaining to	Pertaining to the seminal vesicle.

MED TERM TIP

Word Watch: Be careful using the combining forms *vesic/o* meaning "bladder" and *vesicul/o* meaning "seminal vesicle."

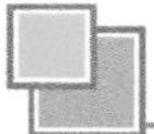

Pathology

TERM	WORD PARTS	DEFINITION
Medical Specialties		
urology (yoo-RAL-oh-jee)	ur/o = urine -logy = study of	Branch of medicine involved in diagnosis and treatment of diseases and disorders of the urinary system and male reproductive system. Physician is a *urologist.*
Signs and Symptoms		
aspermia (ah-SPER-mee-ah)	a- = without -spermia = sperm condition	Condition of having no sperm.
balanorrhea (bah-lah-noh-REE-ah)	balan/o = glans penis -rrhea = discharge	Discharge from the glans penis.
oligospermia (ol-ih-goh-SPER-mee-ah)	olig/o = scanty -spermia = sperm condition	Condition of having too few sperm, making the chances of fertilization very low.
spermatolysis (sper-mah-TOL-ih-sis)	spermat/o = sperm -lysis = destruction	Term that refers to anything that destroys sperm.
Testes		
anorchism (an-OR-kizm)	an- = without orch/o = testes -ism = condition	The absence of testes; may be congenital or as the result of an accident or surgery.
cryptorchidism (kript-OR-kid-izm)	crypt/o = hidden orchid/o = testes -ism = state of	Failure of the testes to descend into the scrotal sac before birth. Usually, the testes will descend before birth. A surgical procedure called orchidopexy may be required to bring the testes down into the scrotum permanently. Failure of the testes to descend could result in sterility in the male or an increased risk of testicular cancer.
hydrocele (HIGH-droh-seel)	hydr/o = water -cele = protrusion	Accumulation of fluid around the testes or along the spermatic cord. Common in infants.
sterility		Inability to father children due to a problem with spermatogenesis.
testicular carcinoma (kar-sih-NOH-mah)	testicul/o = testicle -ar = pertaining to carcin/o = cancer -oma = tumor	Cancer of one or both testicles; most common cancer in men under age 40.
testicular torsion	testicul/o = testicle -ar = pertaining to	Twisting of the spermatic cord.
varicocele (VAIR-ih-koh-seel)	varic/o = dilated vein -cele = protrusion	Enlargement of the veins of the spermatic cord that commonly occurs on the left side of adolescent males.
Epididymis		
epididymitis (ep-ih-did-ih-MYE-tis)	epididym/o = epididymis -itis = inflammation	Inflammation of the epididymis.

Pathology *(continued)*

TERM	WORD PARTS	DEFINITION
Prostate Gland		
benign prostatic hyperplasia (BPH) (bee-NINE / pross-TAT-ik / high-PER-troh-fee)	prostat/o = prostate gland -ic = pertaining to hyper- = excessive -plasia = growth	Noncancerous enlargement of the prostate gland commonly seen in males over age 50. Formerly called *benign prostatic hypertrophy.*
prostate cancer (PROSS-tayt)		Slow-growing cancer that affects a large number of males after age 50. The prostate-specific antigen (PSA) test is used to assist in early detection of this disease.
prostatitis (pross-tah-TYE-tis)	prostat/o = prostate gland -itis = inflammation	Inflammation of the prostate gland.
Penis		
balanitis (bal-ah-NYE-tis)	balan/o = glans penis -itis = inflammation	Inflammation of the glans penis.
epispadias (ep-ih-SPAY-dee-as)	epi- = upon	Congenital opening of the urethra on the dorsal surface of the penis.
erectile dysfunction (ED) (ee-REK-tile)	-ile = pertaining to dys- = abnormal, difficult	Inability to engage in sexual intercourse due to inability to maintain an erection. Also called *impotence.*
hypospadias (high-poh-SPAY-dee-as)	hypo- = below	Congenital opening of the male urethra on the underside of the penis.
phimosis (fih-MOH-sis)	-osis = abnormal condition	Narrowing of the foreskin over the glans penis resulting in difficulty with hygiene. This condition can lead to infection or difficulty with urination. The condition is treated with circumcision, the surgical removal of the foreskin.
priapism (pri-ah-pizm)	-ism = state of	A persistent and painful erection due to pathological causes, not sexual arousal.
Sexually Transmitted Diseases		
chancroid (SHANG-kroyd)	-oid = resembling	Highly infectious nonsyphilitic venereal ulcer.
chlamydia (klah-MID-ee-ah)		Bacterial infection causing genital inflammation in males and females. Can lead to pelvic inflammatory disease in females and eventual infertility.
genital herpes (JEN-ih-tal / HER-peez)	genit/o = genital -al = pertaining to	Spreading skin disease that can appear like a blister or vesicle on the genital region of males and females; may spread to other areas of the body. Caused by a sexually transmitted virus.

Pathology *(continued)*

TERM	WORD PARTS	DEFINITION
genital warts (JEN-ih-tal)	genit/o = genital -al = pertaining to	Growth of warts on the genitalia of both males and females that can lead to cancer of the cervix in females. Caused by the sexual transmission of the human papilloma virus (HPV).
gonorrhea (GC) (gon-oh-REE-ah)	-rrhea = discharge	Sexually transmitted bacterial infection of the mucous membranes of either sex. Can be passed on to an infant during the birth process.
human immunodeficiency virus (HIV)	immun/o = protection	Sexually transmitted virus that attacks the immune system.
sexually transmitted disease (STD)		Disease usually acquired as the result of sexual intercourse. Formerly referred to as *venereal disease* (VD).
syphilis (SIF-ih-lis)		Infectious, chronic, bacterial venereal disease that can involve any organ. May exist for years without symptoms, but is fatal if untreated. Treated with the antibiotic penicillin.
trichomoniasis (trik-oh-moh-NYE-ah-sis)	-iasis = abnormal condition	Genitourinary infection caused by a single-cell protist that is usually without symptoms (asymptomatic) in both males and females. In women the disease can produce itching and/or burning, a foul-smelling discharge, and result in vaginitis.

Diagnostic Procedures

TERM	WORD PARTS	DEFINITION
Clinical Laboratory Tests		
prostate-specific antigen (PSA) (PROSS-tayt-specific / AN-tih-jen)	anti- = against -gen = that which produces	Blood test to screen for prostate cancer. Elevated blood levels of PSA are associated with prostate cancer.
semen analysis (SEE-men / ah-NAL-ih-sis)		Procedure used when performing a fertility workup to determine if the male is able to produce sperm. Semen is collected by the patient after abstaining from sexual intercourse for a period of 3–5 days. The sperm in the semen are analyzed for number, swimming strength, and shape. Also used to determine if a vasectomy has been successful. After a period of 6 weeks, no further sperm should be present in a sample from the patient.
Additional Diagnostic Procedures		
digital rectal exam (DRE) (DIJ-ih-tal / REK-tal)	rect/o = rectum -al = pertaining to	Manual examination for an enlarged prostate gland performed by palpating (feeling) the prostate gland through the wall of the rectum.

Therapeutic Procedures

TERM	WORD PARTS	DEFINITION
Surgical Procedures		
balanoplasty (BAL-ah-noh-plas-tee)	balan/o = glans penis -plasty = surgical repair	Surgical repair of the glans penis.
castration (kass-TRAY-shun)		Removal of the testicles in the male or the ovaries in the female.
circumcision (ser-kum-SIH-zhun)		Surgical removal of the end of the prepuce or foreskin of the penis. Generally performed on the newborn male at the request of the parents. The primary reason is for ease of hygiene. Circumcision is also a ritual practice in some religions.
epididymectomy (ep-ih-did-ih-MEK-toh-mee)	epididym/o = epididymis -ectomy = surgical removal	Surgical removal of the epididymis.
orchidectomy (or-kid-EK-toh-mee)	orchid/o = testes -ectomy = surgical removal	Surgical removal of one or both testes.
orchidopexy (OR-kid-oh-peck-see)	orchid/o = testes -pexy = surgical fixation	Surgical fixation to move undescended testes into the scrotum and to attach them to prevent retraction. Used to treat cryptorchidism.
orchiectomy (or-kee-EK-toh-mee)	orchi/o = testes -ectomy = surgical removal	Surgical removal of one or both testes.
orchiotomy (or-kee-OT-oh-mee)	orchi/o = testes -otomy = cutting into	To cut into the testes.
orchioplasty (OR-kee-oh-plas-tee)	orchi/o = testes -plasty = surgical repair	Surgical repair of testes.
prostatectomy (pross-tah-TEK-toh-mee)	prostat/o = prostate gland -ectomy = surgical removal	Surgical removal of the prostate gland.
sterilization (ster-ih-lih-ZAY-shun)		Process of rendering a male or female sterile or unable to conceive children.
transurethral resection of the prostate (TUR, TURP) (trans-yoo-REE-thrall / REE-sek-shun / PROSS-tayt)	trans- = across urethr/o = urethra -al = pertaining to	Surgical removal of the part of the prostate gland that is blocking urine flow by inserting a device through the urethra and removing prostate tissue.
vasectomy (vas-EK-toh-mee)	vas/o = vas deferens -ectomy = surgical removal	Removal of a segment or all of the vas deferens to prevent sperm from leaving the male body. Used for contraception purposes. See Figure 10.22 ■.

MED TERM TIP

The vas deferens is the tubing that is severed during a procedure called a *vasectomy.* A vasectomy results in the sterilization of the male since the sperm are no longer able to travel into the urethra and out of the penis during sexual intercourse. The surgical procedure to reverse a vasectomy is a *vasovasostomy.* A new opening is created in order to reconnect one section of the vas deferens to another section of the vas deferens, thereby reestablishing an open tube for sperm to travel through.

Therapeutic Procedures *(continued)*

TERM	WORD PARTS	DEFINITION
vasovasostomy (vas-oh-vay-ZOS-toh-mee)	vas/o = vas deferens -ostomy = create a new opening	Surgical procedure to reconnect the vas deferens to reverse a vasectomy.

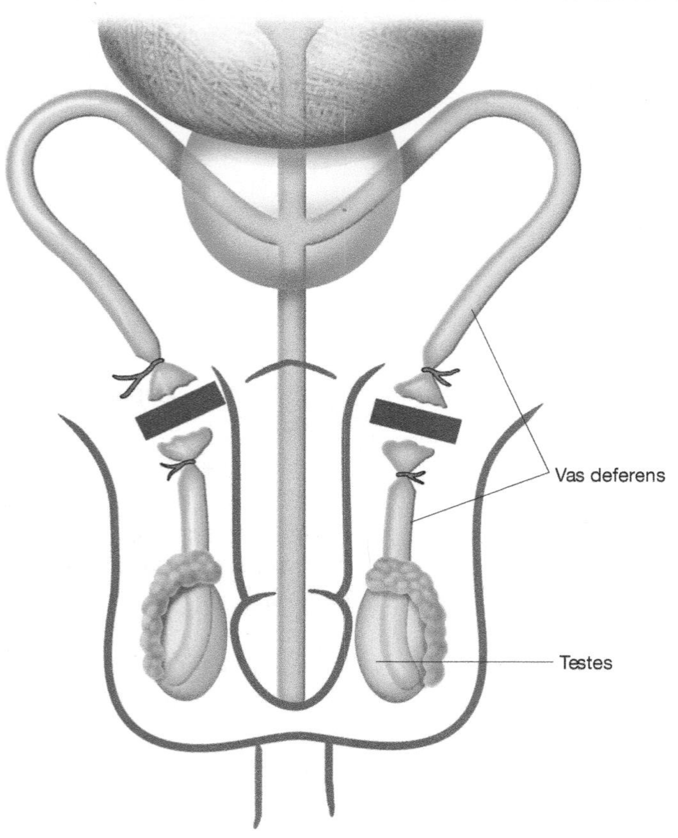

■ **Figure 10.22** A vasectomy, showing how each vas deferens is tied off in two places and then a section is removed from the middle. This prevents sperm from traveling through the vas deferens during ejaculation.

Pharmacology

CLASSIFICATION	WORD PARTS	ACTION	EXAMPLES
androgen therapy (AN-droh-jen)	andr/o = male -gen = that which produces	Replacement of male hormones to treat patients who produce insufficient hormone naturally.	testosterone cypionate, Andronate, depAndro
antiprostatic agents (an-tye-pross-TAT-ik)	anti- = against prostat/o = prostate gland -ic = pertaining to	Medication to treat early cases of benign prostatic hyperplasia. May prevent surgery for mild cases.	finasteride, Proscar; dutasteride, Avodart
erectile dysfunction agents (ee-REK-tile)	-ile = pertaining to dys- = abnormal, difficult	Medication that temporarily produces an erection in patients with erectile dysfunction.	sildenafil citrate, Viagra; tadalafil, Cialis
spermatocide (sper-mah-toh-LIT-ik)	spermat/o = sperm -cide = to kill	Destruction of sperm. One form of birth control is the use of spermatolytic creams.	octoxynol 9, Semicid, Ortho-Gynol

Abbreviations

BPH	benign prostatic hyperplasia	**RPR**	rapid plasma reagin (test for syphilis)
DRE	digital rectal exam	**SPP**	suprapubic prostatectomy
ED	erectile dysfunction	**STD**	sexually transmitted disease
GC	gonorrhea	**TUR**	transurethral resection
GU	genitourinary	**TURP**	transurethral resection of the prostate
PSA	prostate-specific antigen	**VD**	venereal disease

Chapter Review

Real-World Applications

Medical Record Analysis

This High-Risk Obstetrics Consultation Report contains 12 medical terms. Underline each term and write it in the list below the report. Then define each term.

High-Risk Obstetrics Consultation Report

Reason for Consultation:	High-risk pregnancy with late-term bleeding
History of Present Illness:	Patient is 23 years old. She is currently estimated to be at 175 days of gestation. Amniocentesis at 20 weeks shows a normally developing male fetus. She noticed a moderate degree of bleeding this morning but denies any cramping or pelvic pain. She immediately saw her obstetrician who referred her for high-risk evaluation.
Past Medical History:	This patient is multigravida but nullipara with three early miscarriages without obvious cause.
Results of Physical Examination:	Patient appears well nourished and abdominal girth appears consistent with length of gestation. Pelvic ultrasound indicates placenta previa with placenta almost completely overlying cervix. However, there is no evidence of abruptio placentae at this time. Fetal size estimate is consistent with 25 weeks of gestation. The fetal heartbeat is strong with a rate of 130 beats/minute.

Term

1. ______________________ ____
2. ______________________ ____
3. ______________________ ____
4. ______________________ ____
5. ______________________ ____
6. ______________________ ____
7. ______________________ ____
8. ______________________ ____
9. ______________________ ____
10. ______________________ ____
11. ______________________ ____
12. ______________________ ____

Chart Note Transcription

The chart note below contains 10 phrases that can be reworded with a medical term that you learned in this chapter. Each phrase is identified with an underline. Determine the medical term and write your answers in the space provided.

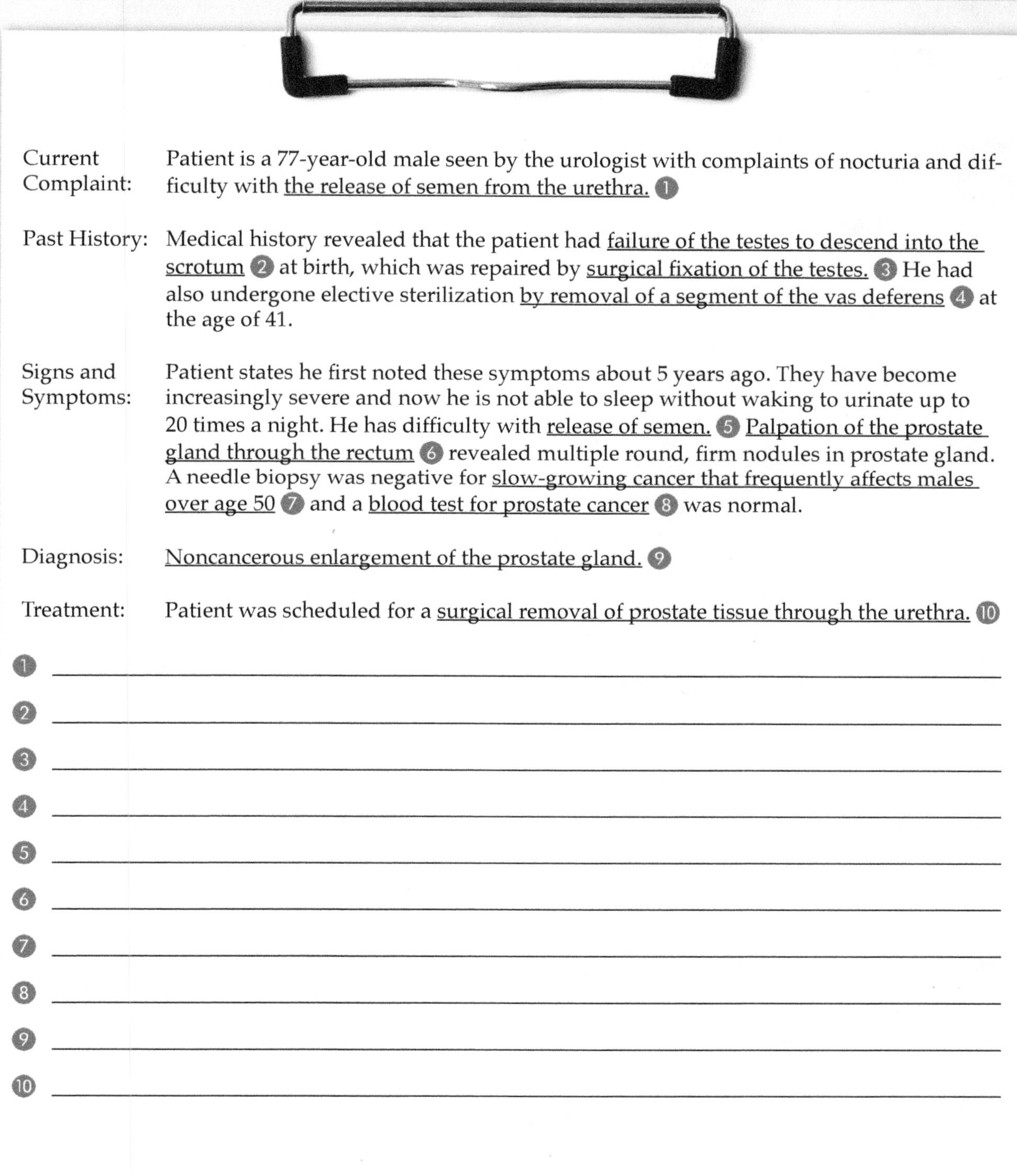

Current Complaint:	Patient is a 77-year-old male seen by the urologist with complaints of nocturia and difficulty with the release of semen from the urethra. (1)
Past History:	Medical history revealed that the patient had failure of the testes to descend into the scrotum (2) at birth, which was repaired by surgical fixation of the testes. (3) He had also undergone elective sterilization by removal of a segment of the vas deferens (4) at the age of 41.
Signs and Symptoms:	Patient states he first noted these symptoms about 5 years ago. They have become increasingly severe and now he is not able to sleep without waking to urinate up to 20 times a night. He has difficulty with release of semen. (5) Palpation of the prostate gland through the rectum (6) revealed multiple round, firm nodules in prostate gland. A needle biopsy was negative for slow-growing cancer that frequently affects males over age 50 (7) and a blood test for prostate cancer (8) was normal.
Diagnosis:	Noncancerous enlargement of the prostate gland. (9)
Treatment:	Patient was scheduled for a surgical removal of prostate tissue through the urethra. (10)

1. ______________________________
2. ______________________________
3. ______________________________
4. ______________________________
5. ______________________________
6. ______________________________
7. ______________________________
8. ______________________________
9. ______________________________
10. ______________________________

Case Study

Below is a case study presentation of a patient with a condition covered by this chapter. Read the case study and answer the questions below. Some questions will ask for information not included within this chapter. Use your text, a medical dictionary, journals, technical materials, multimedia resources, electronic media, or any other reference material you choose to answer these questions.

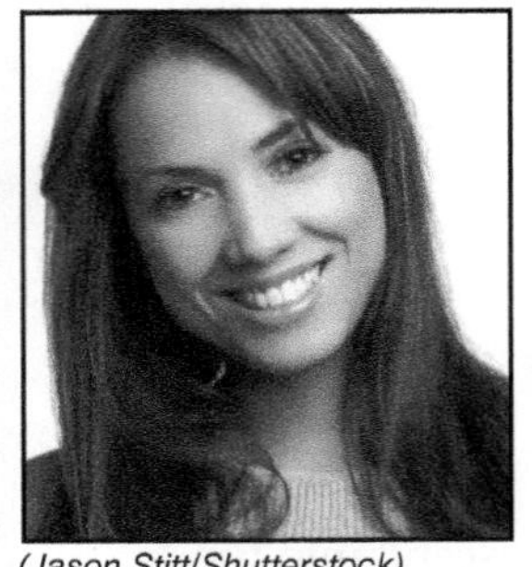

(Jason Stitt/Shutterstock)

A 22-year-old female has come into the gynecologist's office complaining of fever, malaise, dysuria, and vaginal leukorrhea. Upon examination the physician observes fluid-filled vesicles on her cervix, vulva, and perineum. Several have ruptured into ulcers with marked erythema and edema. Palpation revealed painful and enlarged inguinal lymph nodes. She also has an extragenital lesion on her mouth. Her diagnosis is genital herpes.

Questions

1. What pathological condition does this patient have? Look this condition up in a reference source and include a short description of it.

____

____

2. List and define each of the patient's presenting symptoms in your own words. Leukorrhea is a term you have not seen before. Can you give its meaning just from its word parts?

____

____

3. Describe the results of the physician's examination in your own words.

____

____

4. Explain what extragenital lesion means.

____

____

5. Explain what palpation means.

____

____

6. What is the potential effect of having this virus present in open genital lesions on the patient's future pregnancy and child birth?

____

____

Practice Exercises

A. Complete the Statement

1. The study of the female reproductive system is the medical specialty of ______________________.

2. A physician who specializes in the treatment of women is called a(n) ______________________.

3. The three stages of labor and delivery are the ______________________ stage, the ______________________ stage, and the ______________________ stage.

4. The time required for the development of a fetus is called ______________________.

5. The cessation of menstruation is called ______________________.

6. The female sex cell is a(n) ______________________.

7. The inner lining of the uterus is called the ______________________.

8. The organ in which the developing fetus resides is called the ______________________.

9. The tubes that extend from the outer edges of the uterus and assist in transporting the ova and sperm are called ______________________.

10. One of the longest terms used in medical terminology refers to the removal of the uterus, cervix, ovaries, and uterine tubes. This term is ______________________.

B. What Does it Stand For?

1. SPP ______________________

2. TUR ______________________

3. GU ______________________

4. BPH ______________________

5. DRE ______________________

6. PSA ______________________

C. Define the Term

1. spermatogenesis ______________________

2. hydrocele ______________________

3. transurethral resection of the prostate (TURP) ______________________

4. sterility ______________________

5. orchiectomy ______________________

6. vasectomy ______________________

7. castration ______________________

D. Combining Form Practice

The combining form **colp/o** refers to the vagina. Use it to write a term that means:

1. visual examination of the vagina __________
2. instrument used to examine the vagina __________

The combining form **cervic/o** refers to the cervix. Use it to write a term that means:

3. removal of the cervix __________
4. inflammation of the cervix __________
5. pertaining to the cervix __________

The combining form **hyster/o** also refers to the uterus. Use it to write a term that means:

6. surgical fixation of the uterus __________
7. removal of the uterus __________
8. rupture of the uterus __________

The combining form **oophor/o** refers to the ovaries. Use it to write a term that means:

9. inflammation of an ovary __________
10. removal of an ovary __________

The combining form **mamm/o** refers to the breasts. Use it to write a term that means:

11. pertaining to the breasts __________
12. record of breast __________
13. surgical repair of breast __________

The combining form **amni/o** refers to the amnion. Use it to write a term that means:

14. pertaining to the amnion __________
15. cutting into amnion __________
16. flow from amnion __________

E. What Does it Stand For?

1. Cx __________
2. LMP __________
3. FHR __________
4. PID __________
5. GYN __________

6. CS ____________________

7. NB ____________________

8. PMS ____________________

9. TSS ____________________

10. LBW ____________________

F. What's the Abbreviation?

1. first pregnancy ____________________
2. artificial insemination ____________________
3. uterine contractions ____________________
4. full-term normal delivery ____________________
5. intrauterine device ____________________
6. dilation and curettage ____________________
7. hormone replacement therapy ____________________
8. gynecology ____________________
9. abortion ____________________
10. oral contraception pills ____________________

G. Define the Combining Form

	Definition	Example from Chapter
1. metr/o	____________________	____________________
2. hyster/o	____________________	____________________
3. gynec/o	____________________	____________________
4. episi/o	____________________	____________________
5. oophor/o	____________________	____________________
6. ovari/o	____________________	____________________
7. salping/o	____________________	____________________
8. men/o	____________________	____________________
9. vagin/o	____________________	____________________
10. mast/o	____________________	____________________

H. Terminology Matching

Match each term to its definition.

1. _______ hemolytic disease of the newborn
2. _______ ovary
3. _______ vagina
4. _______ abruptio placentae
5. _______ placenta
6. _______ endometrium
7. _______ clitoris
8. _______ candidiasis
9. _______ Pap smear
10. _______ uterine tube
11. _______ dysmenorrhea
12. _______ breech presentation
13. _______ Apgar
14. _______ neonate
15. _______ eclampsia

a. seizures and coma during pregnancy
b. erythroblastosis fetalis
c. detached placenta
d. female erectile tissue
e. produces eggs
f. normal place for fertilization
g. buttocks first to appear in birth canal
h. birth canal
i. nourishes fetus
j. uterine lining
k. measures newborn's adjustment to outside world
l. test for cervical cancer
m. newborn
n. yeast infection
o. painful menstruation

I. Define the Suffix

	Definition	Example from Chapter
1. -tocia	______________________	______________
2. -gravida	______________________	______________
3. -arche	______________________	______________
4. -cyesis	______________________	______________
5. -partum	______________________	______________
6. -para	______________________	______________
7. -salpinx	______________________	______________
8. -spermia	______________________	______________

J. Fill in the Blank

premenstrual syndrome	stillbirth	conization	laparoscopy
D & C	puberty	endometriosis	eclampsia
fibroid tumor	cesarean section		

1. Kesha had a core of tissue from her cervix removed for testing. This is called ______________________________.
2. Joan delivered a baby that had died while still in the uterus. She had a(n) ______________________________.
3. Ashley has just started her first menstrual cycle. She is said to have entered ______________________________.
4. Kimberly is experiencing tender breasts, headaches, and some irritability just prior to her monthly menstrual cycle. This may be ______________________________.
5. Ana has been scheduled for an examination in which her physician will use an instrument to observe her abdominal cavity to rule out the diagnosis of severe endometriosis. The physician will insert the instrument through a small incision. This procedure is called a(n) ______________________________.
6. Lenora is scheduled to have a hysterectomy as a result of a long history of large benign growths in her uterus that have caused pain and bleeding. Lenora has a(n) ______________________________.
7. Tiffany's physician has recommended that she have a uterine scraping to stop excessive bleeding after a miscarriage. She will be scheduled for a(n) ______________________________.
8. Stacey is having frequent prenatal checkups to prevent the serious condition of pregnancy called ____________________.
9. Marion has experienced painful menstrual periods as a result of the lining of her uterus being displaced into her pelvic cavity. This is called ______________________________.
10. Because her cervix was not dilating, Shataundra was informed that she will probably require a(n) ____________________ for her baby's delivery.

K. Complete the Statement

1. The male reproductive system is a combination of the ____________________ and ____________________ systems.
2. The male's external organs of reproduction consist of the ____________________, ____________________, and the ____________________.
3. Another term for the prepuce is the ____________________.
4. The organs responsible for developing the sperm cells are the ____________________.
5. The glands of lubrication and fluid production at each side of the male urethra are the ____________________.
6. The male sex hormone is ____________________.
7. The area between the scrotum and the anus is called the ____________________.

L. Terminology Matching

Match each term to its definition.

1. _______ gonorrhea
2. _______ genital herpes
3. _______ human immunodeficiency virus
4. _______ syphilis
5. _______ venereal disease
6. _______ genital warts
7. _______ chancroid
8. _______ chlamydia
9. _______ trichomoniasis

a. also called STD
b. caused by parasitic microorganism
c. treated with penicillin
d. caused by human papilloma virus
e. can pass to infant during birth
f. genitourinary infection
g. venereal ulcer
h. attacks the immune system
i. skin disease with vesicles

M. Combining Form Practice

The combining form **prostat/o** refers to the prostate. Use this to write a term that means:

1. removal of prostate ____________________
2. pertaining to the prostate ____________________
3. inflammation of the prostate ____________________

The combining form **orchi/o** refers to the testes. Use this to write a term that means:

4. removal of the testes ____________________
5. surgical repair of the testes ____________________
6. incision into the testes ____________________

The suffix **-spermia** refers to a sperm condition. Use this to write a term that means:

7. condition of being without sperm ____________________
8. condition of having too few (scanty) sperm ____________________

The combining form **spermat/o** refers to sperm. Use this to write a term that means:

9. sperm forming ____________________
10. sperm destruction ____________________

N. Pharmacology Challenge

Fill in the classification for each drug description, then match the brand name.

	Drug Description	Classification		Brand Name
1.	_______ replacement male hormone	______________________	a.	Pitocin
2.	_______ improves uterine contractions	______________________	b.	Avodart
3.	_______ treats early BPH	______________________	c.	Clomid
4.	_______ blocks ovulation	______________________	d.	Semicid
5.	_______ kills sperm	______________________	e.	Mifeprex
6.	_______ produces an erection	______________________	f.	Andronate
7.	_______ replaces estrogen	______________________	g.	Ortho-Cept
8.	_______ terminates a pregnancy	______________________	h.	Viagra
9.	_______ triggers ovulation	______________________	i.	Premarin

Labeling Exercise

Image A

Write the labels for this figure on the numbered lines provided.

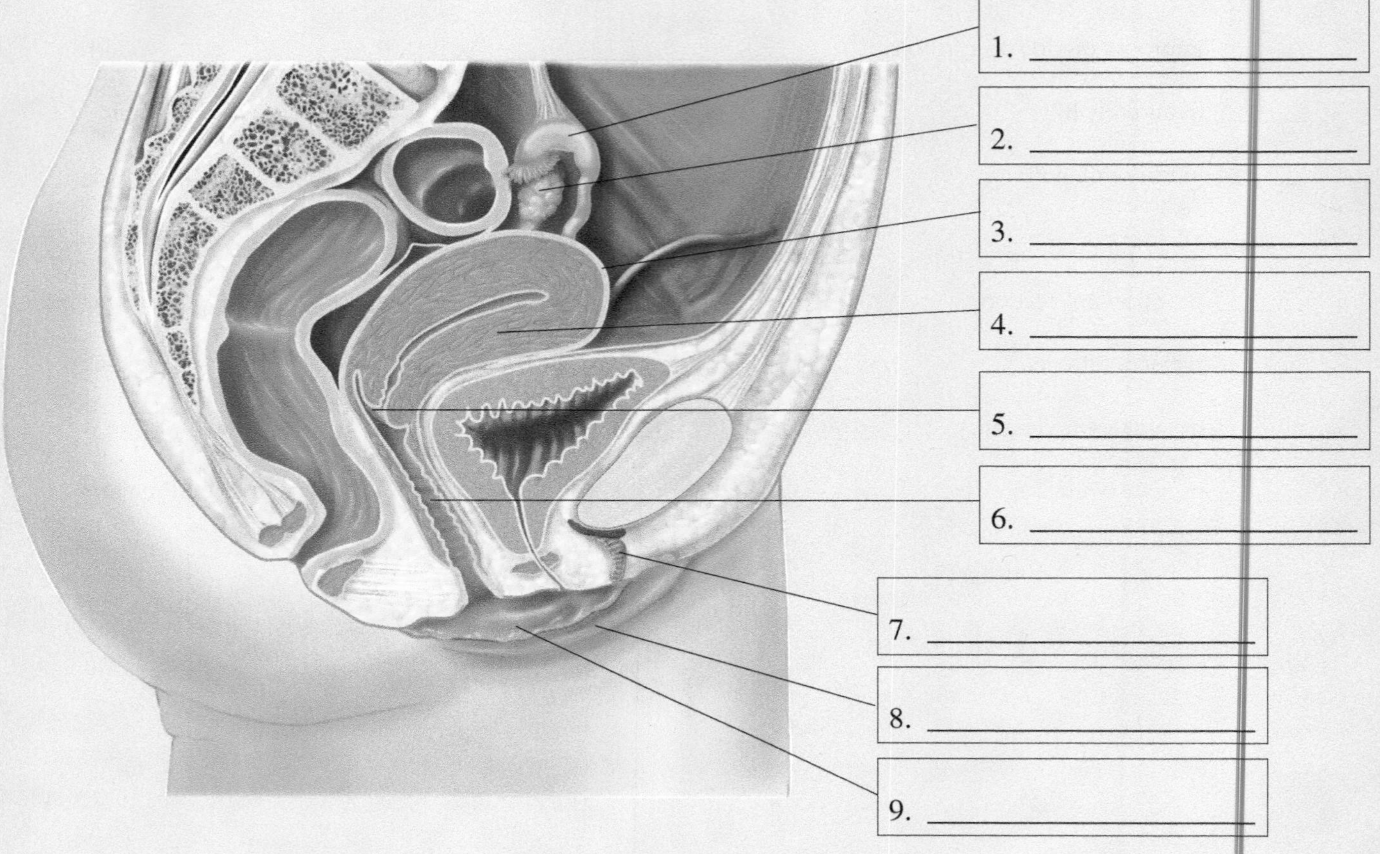

Image B

Write the labels for this figure on the numbered lines provided.

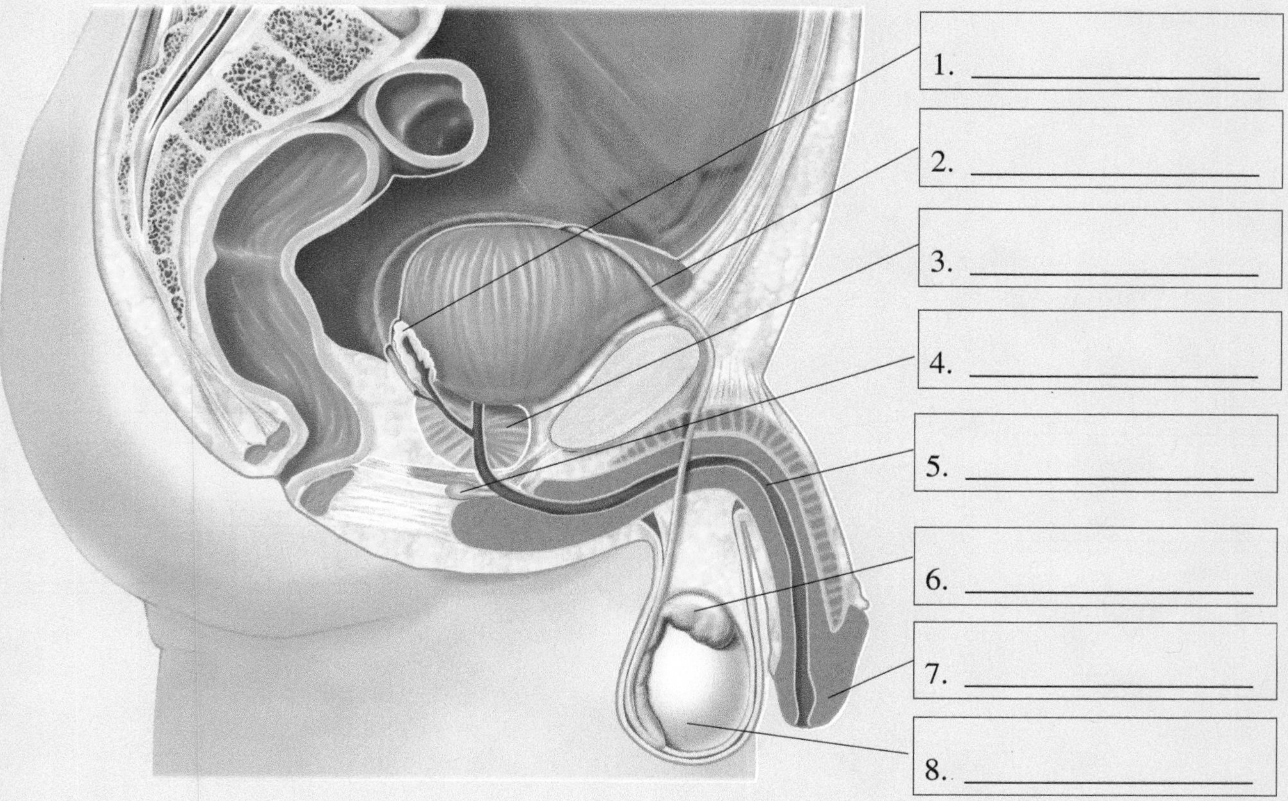

Image C

Write the labels for this figure on the numbered lines provided.

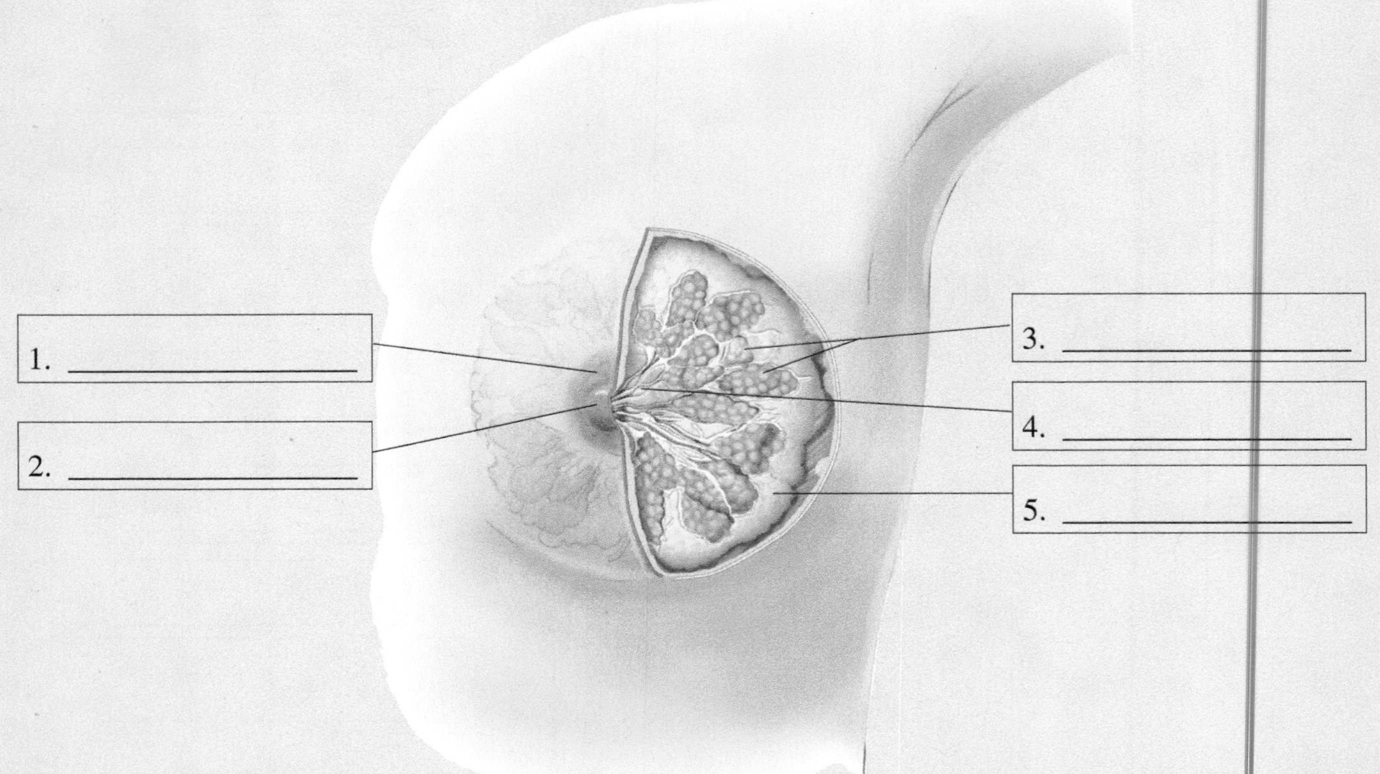

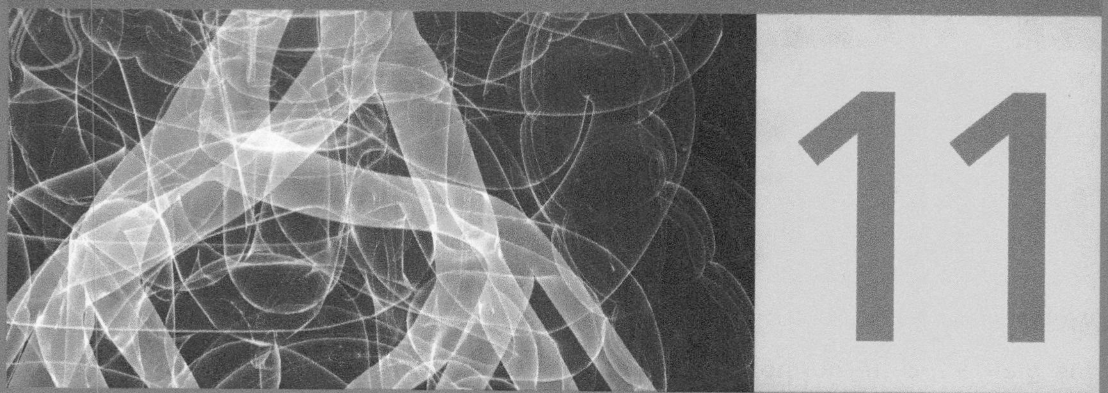

11

ENDOCRINE SYSTEM

Learning Objectives

Upon completion of this chapter, you will be able to

- Identify and define the combining forms and suffixes introduced in this chapter.
- Correctly spell and pronounce medical terms and major anatomical structures relating to the endocrine system.
- Locate and describe the major organs of the endocrine system and their functions.
- List the major hormones secreted by each endocrine gland and describe their functions.
- Identify and define endocrine system anatomical terms.
- Identify and define selected endocrine system pathology terms.
- Identify and define selected endocrine system diagnostic procedures.
- Identify and define selected endocrine system therapeutic procedures.
- Identify and define selected medications relating to the endocrine system.
- Define selected abbreviations associated with the endocrine system.

Endocrine System at a Glance

Function

Endocrine glands secrete hormones that regulate many body activities such as metabolic rate, water and mineral balance, immune system reactions, and sexual functioning.

Structures

Here are the primary structures that comprise the endocrine system.

adrenal glands
ovaries
pancreas (islets of Langerhans)
parathyroid glands
pineal gland
pituitary gland
testes
thymus gland
thyroid gland

Word Parts

Here are the most common word parts used to build endocrine system terms. For a more comprehensive list, refer to the Terminology section of this chapter.

Combining Forms

acr/o	extremities
adren/o	adrenal glands
adrenal/o	adrenal glands
andr/o	male
calc/o	calcium
crin/o	to secrete
estr/o	female
gluc/o	glucose
glyc/o	sugar
glycos/o	sugar
gonad/o	sex glands
home/o	sameness
iod/o	iodine
kal/i	potassium
ket/o	ketones
mineral/o	minerals, electrolytes
natr/o	sodium
ophthalm/o	eye
ovari/o	ovary
pancreat/o	pancreas
parathyroid/o	parathyroid gland
pineal/o	pineal gland
pituitar/o	pituitary gland
testicul/o	testes
thym/o	thymus gland
thyr/o	thyroid gland
thyroid/o	thyroid gland
toxic/o	poison

Suffixes

-dipsia	thirst
-prandial	relating to a meal
-pressin	to press down
-tropin	to stimulate

Endocrine System Illustrated

pineal gland, p. 384

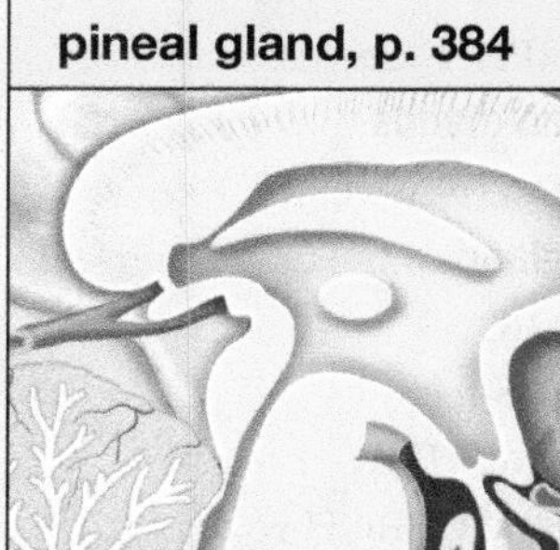

Regulates circadian rhythm

pituitary gland, p. 384

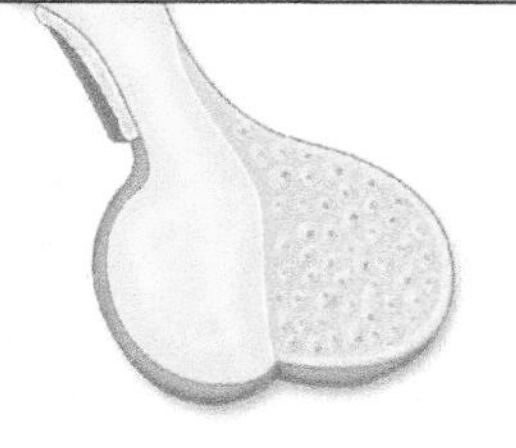

Regulates many other endocrine glands

thyroid gland, p. 387
parathyroid glands, p. 384

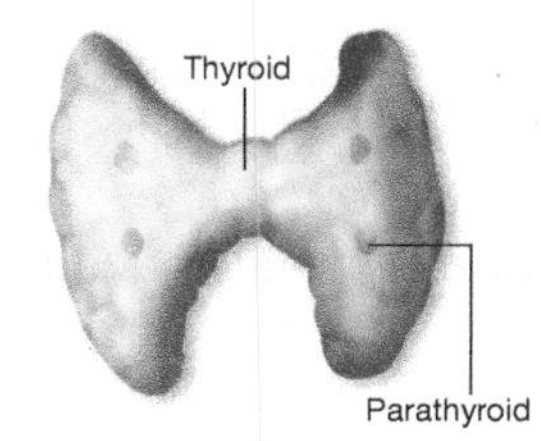

Regulates metabolic rate
Regulate blood calcium level

thymus gland, p. 387

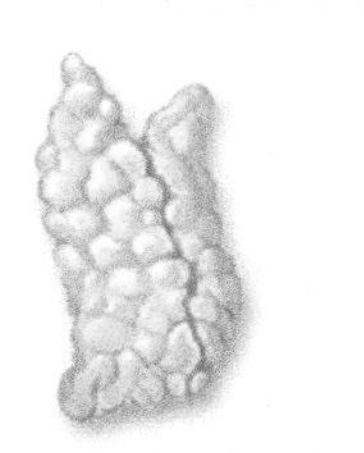

Development of immune system

adrenal glands, p. 382

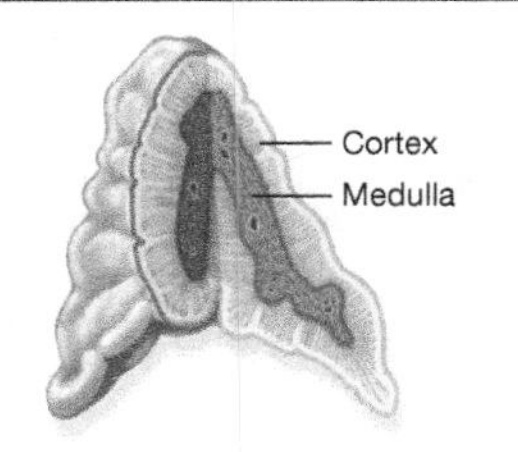

Regulate water and electrolyte levels

ovaries, p. 382

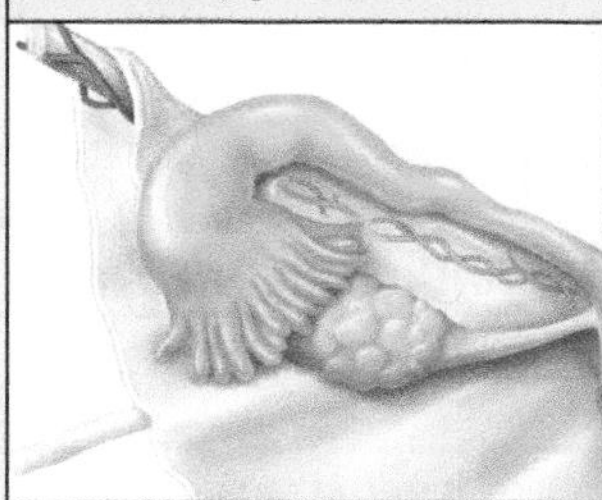

Regulate female reproductive system

pancreas, p. 383

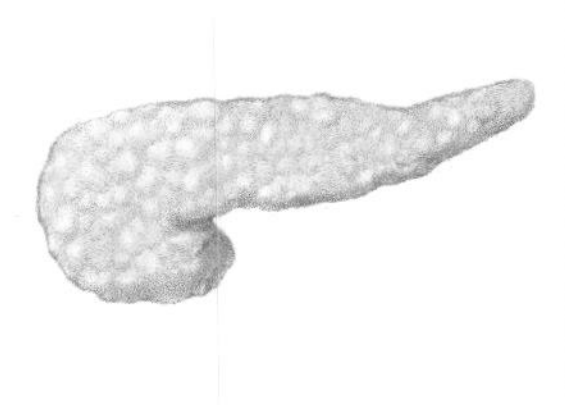

Regulates blood sugar levels

testes, p. 386

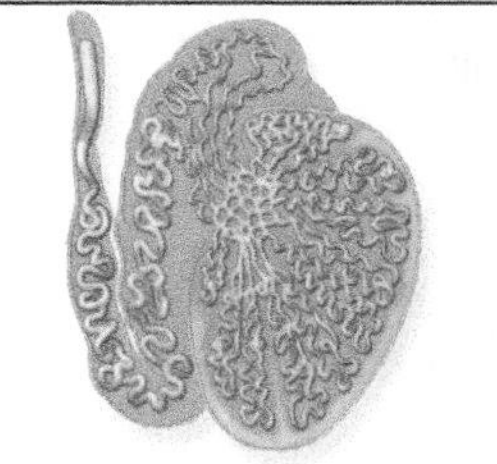

Regulate male reproductive system

Anatomy and Physiology of the Endocrine System

adrenal glands (ad-REE-nal)
endocrine glands (EN-doh-krin)
endocrine system
exocrine glands (EKS-oh-krin)
glands
homeostasis (hoe-me-oh-STAY-sis)
hormones (HOR-mohnz)
ovaries (OH-vah-reez)
pancreas (PAN-kree-ass)
parathyroid glands (pair-ah-THIGH-royd)
pineal gland (pih-NEAL)
pituitary gland (pih-TOO-ih-tair-ee)
target organs
testes (TESS-teez)
thymus gland (THIGH-mus)
thyroid gland (THIGH-royd)

MED TERM TIP

The terms *endocrine* and *exocrine* were constructed to reflect the function of each type of gland. As glands, they both secrete, indicated by the combining form *crin/o*. The prefix *exo-*, meaning "external" or "outward," tells us that exocrine gland secretions are carried to the outside of the body or to a passageway connected to the outside of the body. However, the prefix *endo-*, meaning "within" or "internal," indicates that endocrine gland secretions are carried to other internal body structures by the bloodstream.

The **endocrine system** is a collection of **glands** that secrete **hormones** directly into the bloodstream. Hormones are chemicals that act on their **target organs** to either increase or decrease the target's activity level. In this way the endocrine system is instrumental in maintaining **homeostasis** (*home/o* = sameness; *-stasis* = standing still)—that is, adjusting the activity level of most of the tissues and organs of the body to maintain a stable internal environment.

The body actually has two distinct types of glands: **exocrine glands** and **endocrine glands.** Exocrine glands release their secretions into a duct that carries them to the outside of the body or to a passageway connected to the outside of the body. For example, sweat glands release sweat into a sweat duct that travels to the surface of the body. Endocrine glands, however, release hormones directly into the bloodstream. For example, the thyroid gland secretes its hormones directly into the bloodstream. Because endocrine glands have no ducts, they are also referred to as *ductless glands.*

The endocrine system consists of the following glands: two **adrenal glands,** two **ovaries** in the female, four **parathyroid glands,** the **pancreas,** the **pineal gland,** the **pituitary gland,** two **testes** in the male, the **thymus gland,** and the **thyroid gland.** The endocrine glands as a whole affect the functions of the entire body. Table 11.1 ■ presents a description of the endocrine glands, their hormones, and their functions.

Table 11.1 Endocrine Glands and Their Hormones

GLAND AND HORMONE	WORD PARTS	FUNCTION
Adrenal cortex	adren/o = adrenal gland -al = pertaining to	
Glucocorticoids such as cortisol	gluc/o = glucose cortic/o = outer portion	Regulates carbohydrate levels in the body.
Mineralocorticoids such as aldosterone	mineral/o = minerals, electrolytes cortic/o = outer portion	Regulates electrolytes and fluid volume in body.
Steroid sex hormones such as androgen	andr/o = male -gen = that which produces	Male sex hormones from adrenal cortex may be converted to estrogens in the bloodstream. Responsible for reproduction and secondary sexual characteristics.
Adrenal medulla	adren/o = adrenal gland -al = pertaining to	
Epinephrine (adrenaline)	epi- = above nephr/o = kidney -ine = pertaining to	Intensifies response during stress; "fight-or-flight" response.
Norepinephrine	epi- = above nephr/o = kidney -ine = pertaining to	Chiefly a vasoconstrictor.

Table 11.1 Endocrine Glands and Their Hormones (continued)

GLAND AND HORMONE	WORD PARTS	FUNCTION
Ovaries		
Estrogen	estr/o = female -gen = that which produces	Stimulates development of secondary sex characteristics in females; regulates menstrual cycle.
Progesterone	pro- = before estr/o = female	Prepares for conditions of pregnancy.
Pancreas		
Glucagon		Stimulates liver to release glucose into the blood.
Insulin		Regulates and promotes entry of glucose into cells.
Parathyroid glands		
Parathyroid hormone (PTH)		Stimulates bone breakdown; regulates calcium level in the blood.
Pituitary anterior lobe		
Adrenocorticotropic hormone (ACTH)	adren/o = adrenal gland cortic/o = outer portion -tropin = to stimulate	Regulates function of adrenal cortex.
Gonadotropins	gonad/o = gonads -tropin = to stimulate	
Follicle-stimulating hormone (FSH)		Stimulates growth of eggs in female and sperm in males.
Luteinizing hormone (LH)		Regulates function of male and female gonads and plays a role in releasing ova in females.
Growth hormone (GH)		Stimulates growth of the body.
Melanocyte-stimulating hormone (MSH)	melan/o = black -cyte = cell	Stimulates pigment in skin.
Prolactin	pro- = before lact/o = milk	Stimulates milk production.
Thyroid-stimulating hormone (TSH)		Regulates function of thyroid gland.
Pituitary posterior lobe		
Antidiuretic hormone (ADH)	anti- = against -tic = pertaining to	Stimulates reabsorption of water by the kidneys.
Oxytocin		Stimulates uterine contractions and releases milk into ducts.
Testes		
Testosterone		Promotes sperm production and development of secondary sex characteristics in males.
Thymus		
Thymosin	thym/o = thymus gland	Promotes development of cells in immune system.
Thyroid gland		
Calcitonin (CT)		Stimulates deposition of calcium into bone.
Thyroxine (T_4)	thyr/o = thyroid gland -ine = pertaining to	Stimulates metabolism in cells.
Triiodothyronine (T_3)	tri- = three iod/o = iodine thyr/o = thyroid gland -ine = pertaining to	Stimulates metabolism in cells.

Adrenal Glands

adrenal cortex (KOR-tex)
adrenal medulla (meh-DOOL-lah)
adrenaline (ah-DREN-ah-lin)
aldosterone (al-DOSS-ter-ohn)
androgens (AN-druh-jenz)
corticosteroids (kor-tih-koh-STAIR-oydz)
cortisol (KOR-tih-sal)
epinephrine (ep-ih-NEF-rin)
estrogen (ESS-troh-jen)
glucocorticoids (gloo-koh-KOR-tih-koydz)
mineralocorticoids (min-er-al-oh-KOR-tih-koydz)
norepinephrine (nor-ep-ih-NEF-rin)
progesterone (proh-JESS-ter-ohn)
steroid sex hormones (STAIR-oyd)

The two adrenal glands are located above each of the kidneys (see Figure 11.1 ■). Each gland is composed of two sections: **adrenal cortex** and **adrenal medulla.**

The outer adrenal cortex manufactures several different families of hormones: **mineralocorticoids, glucocorticoids,** and **steroid sex hormones.** However, because they are all produced by the cortex, they are collectively referred to as **corticosteroids.** The mineralocorticoid hormone, **aldosterone,** regulates sodium (Na^+) and potassium (K^+) levels in the body. The glucocorticoid hormone, **cortisol,** regulates carbohydrates in the body. The adrenal cortex of both men and women secretes steroid sex hormones, **androgens** (which may be converted to **estrogen** once released into the bloodstream). These hormones regulate secondary sexual characteristics. All hormones secreted by the adrenal cortex are steroid hormones.

The inner adrenal medulla is responsible for secreting the hormones **epinephrine,** also called **adrenaline,** and **norepinephrine.** These hormones are critical during emergency situations because they increase blood pressure, heart rate, and respiration levels. This helps the body perform better during emergencies or otherwise stressful times.

MED TERM TIP

The term *cortex* is frequently used in anatomy to indicate the outer portion of an organ such as the adrenal gland or the kidney. The term *cortex* means "bark," as in the bark of a tree. The term *medulla* means "marrow." Because marrow is found in the inner cavity of bones, the term came to stand for the middle of an organ.

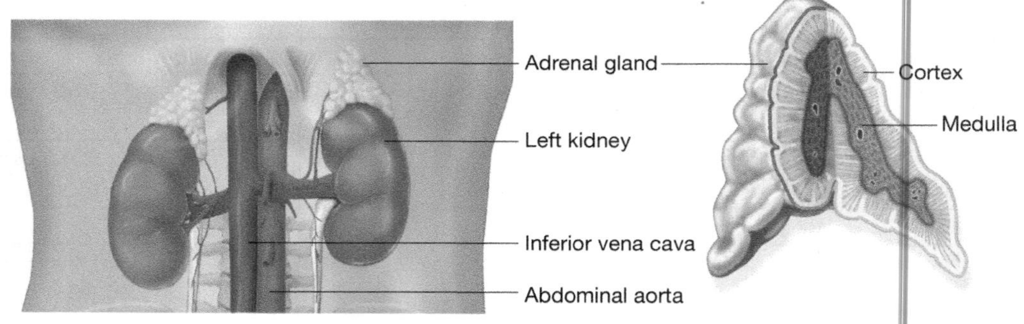

■ **Figure 11.1** The adrenal glands. These glands sit on top of each kidney. Each adrenal is subdivided into an outer cortex and an inner medulla. Each region secretes different hormones.

Ovaries

estrogen
gametes (GAM-eats)
gonads (GOH-nadz)
menstrual cycle (MEN-stroo-all)
ova
progesterone

The two ovaries are located in the lower abdominopelvic cavity of the female (see Figure 11.2 ■). They are the female **gonads.** Gonads are organs that produce **gametes** or the reproductive sex cells. In the case of females, the gametes are the **ova.** Of importance to the endocrine system, the ovaries produce the female sex hormones, **estrogen** and **progesterone.** Estrogen is responsible for the appearance of the female sexual characteristics and regulation of the **menstrual cycle.** Progesterone helps to maintain a suitable uterine environment for pregnancy.

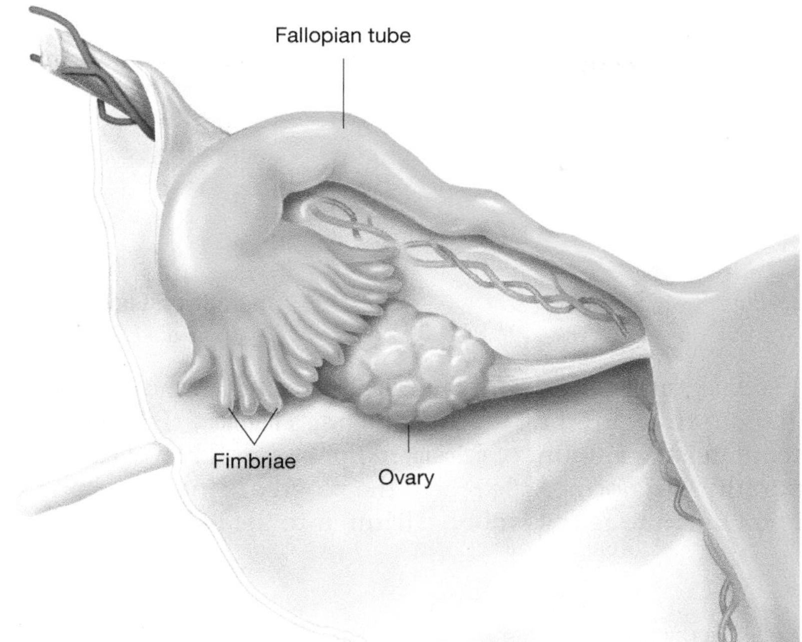

■ **Figure 11.2**
The ovaries. In addition to producing ova, the ovaries secrete the female sex hormones, estrogen and progesterone.

Pancreas

glucagon (GLOO-koh-gon)
insulin (IN-suh-lin)**w**
islets of Langerhans
(EYE-lets / of / LAHNG-er-hahnz)

The pancreas is located along the lower curvature of the stomach (see Figure 11.3A ■). It is the only organ in the body that has both endocrine and exocrine functions. The exocrine portion of the pancreas releases digestive enzymes through a duct into the duodenum of the small intestine. The endocrine sections of the pancreas, **islets of Langerhans,** are named after Dr. Paul Langerhans, a German anatomist. The islets cells produce two different hormones: **insulin** and **glucagon** (see Figure 11.3B ■). Insulin, produced by beta (β) islet cells, stimulates the cells of the body to take in glucose from the bloodstream, lowering the body's blood sugar level. This occurs after a meal has been eaten and the carbohydrates are absorbed into the bloodstream. In this way the cells obtain the glucose they need for cellular respiration.

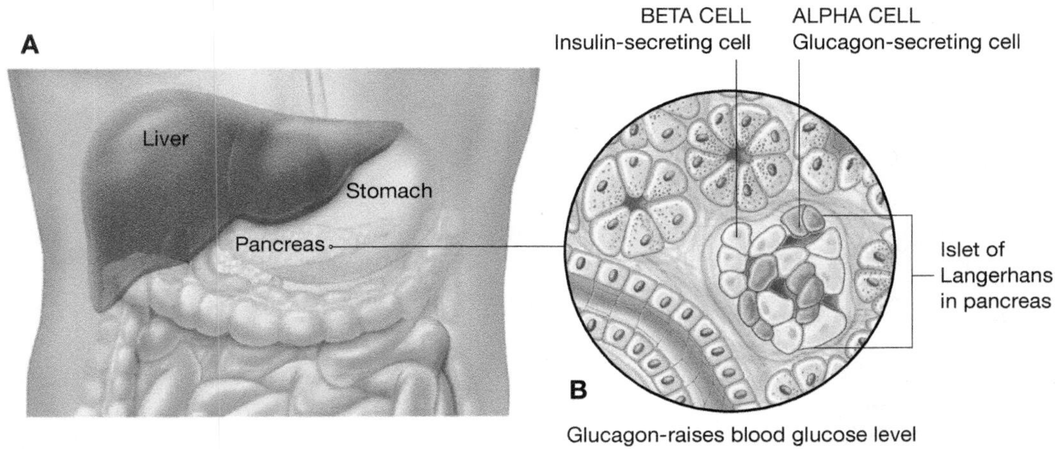

■ **Figure 11.3**
The pancreas. This organ sits just below the stomach and is both an exocrine and an endocrine gland. The endocrine regions of the pancreas are called the islets of Langerhans and they secrete insulin and glucagon.

Another set of islet cells, the alpha (α) cells, secrete a different hormone, glucagon, which stimulates the liver to release glucose, thereby raising the blood glucose level. Glucagon is released when the body needs more sugar, such as at the beginning of strenuous activity or several hours after the last meal has been digested. Insulin and glucagon have opposite effects on blood sugar level. Insulin will reduce the blood sugar level, while glucagon will increase it.

Parathyroid Glands

calcium

parathyroid hormone (pair-ah-THIGH-royd / HOR-mohn)

MED TERM TIP

A calcium deficiency in the system can result in a condition called *tetany*, or muscle excitability and tremors. If the parathyroid glands are removed during thyroid surgery, calcium replacement in the body is often necessary.

The four tiny parathyroid glands are located on the dorsal surface of the thyroid gland (see Figure 11.4 ■). The **parathyroid hormone** (PTH) secreted by these glands regulates the amount of **calcium** in the blood. If blood calcium levels fall too low, parathyroid hormone levels in the blood are increased and will stimulate bone breakdown to release more calcium into the blood.

Pineal Gland

circadian rhythm (seer-KAY-dee-an)
thalamus (THALL-mus)
melatonin (mel-ah-TOH-nin)

MED TERM TIP

The pineal gland is an example of an organ named for its shape. *Pineal* means "shaped like a pine cone."

The pineal gland is a small pine cone-shaped gland that is part of the **thalamus** region of the brain (see Figure 11.5 ■). The pineal gland secretes **melatonin,** a hormone not well understood, but that plays a role in regulating the body's **circadian rhythm.** This is the 24-hour clock that governs our periods of wakefulness and sleepiness.

Pituitary Gland

adrenocorticotropic hormone (ah-dree-noh-kor-tih-koh-TROH-pk)
anterior lobe
antidiuretic hormone (an-tye-dye-yoo-RET-ik)
follicle-stimulating hormone (FOLL-ih-kl / STIM-yoo-lay-ting)
gonadotropins (go-nad-oh-TROH-pins)
growth hormone
hypothalamus (high-poh-THAL-ah-mus)

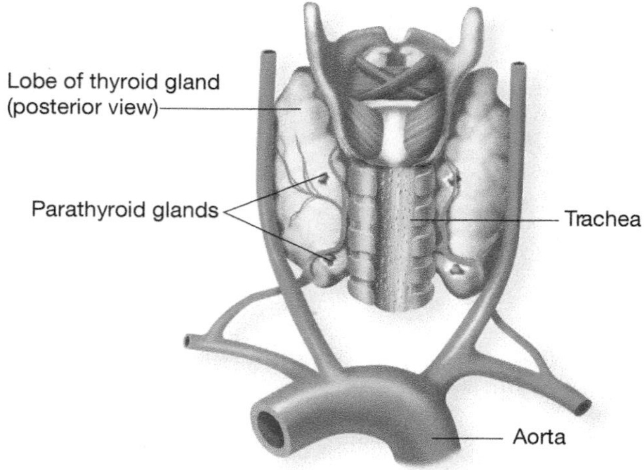

■ **Figure 11.4** The parathyroid glands. These four glands are located on the posterior side of the thyroid gland. They secrete parathyroid hormone.

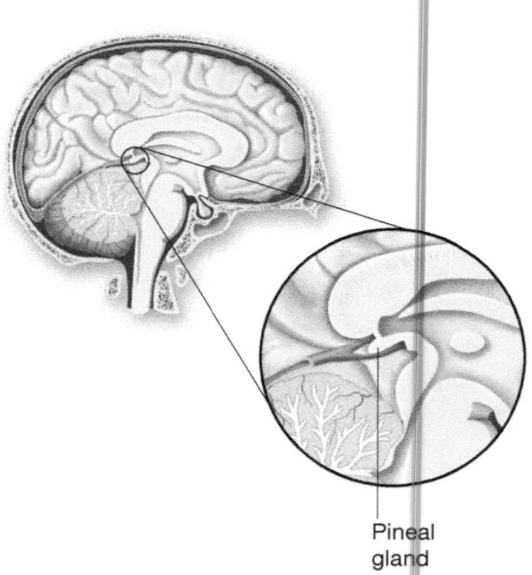

■ **Figure 11.5** The pineal gland is a part of the thalamus region of the brain. It secretes melatonin.

luteinizing hormone (LOO-tee-in-eye-zing)
melanocyte-stimulating hormone
oxytocin (ok-see-TOH-sin)
posterior lobe
prolactin (proh-LAK-tin)
somatotropin (so-mat-oh-TROH-pin)
thyroid-stimulating hormone

The pituitary gland is located underneath the brain (see Figure 11.6 ■). The small marble-shaped gland is divided into an **anterior lobe** and a **posterior lobe.** Both lobes are controlled by the **hypothalamus,** a region of the brain active in regulating automatic body responses.

The anterior pituitary secretes several different hormones (see Figure 11.7 ■). **Growth hormone** (GH), also called **somatotropin,** promotes growth of the body by stimulating cells to rapidly increase in size and divide. **Thyroid-stimulating hormone** (TSH) regulates the function of the thyroid gland. **Adrenocorticotropic hormone** (ACTH) regulates the function of the adrenal cortex. **Prolactin** (PRL) stimulates milk production in the breast following pregnancy and birth. **Follicle-stimulating hormone** (FSH) and **luteinizing hormone** (LH) both exert their influence on the male and female gonads. Therefore, these two hormones together are referred to as the **gonadotropins.** Follicle-stimulating hormone is responsible for the development of ova in ovaries and sperm in testes. It also stimulates the ovary to secrete estrogen. Luteinizing hormone stimulates secretion of sex hormones in both males and females and plays a role in releasing ova in females. **Melanocyte-stimulating hormone** (MSH) stimulates melanocytes to produce more melanin, thereby darkening the skin.

The posterior pituitary secretes two hormones, **antidiuretic hormone** (ADH) and **oxytocin.** Antidiuretic hormone promotes water reabsorption by the kidney tubules. Oxytocin stimulates uterine contractions during labor and delivery, and after birth the release of milk from the mammary glands.

MED TERM TIP

The pituitary gland is sometimes referred to as the "master gland" because several of its secretions regulate other endocrine glands.

MED TERM TIP

Many people use the term *diabetes* to refer to diabetes mellitus (DM). But there is another type of diabetes, called *diabetes insipidus* (DI), that is a result of the inadequate secretion of the antidiuretic hormone (ADH) from the pituitary gland.

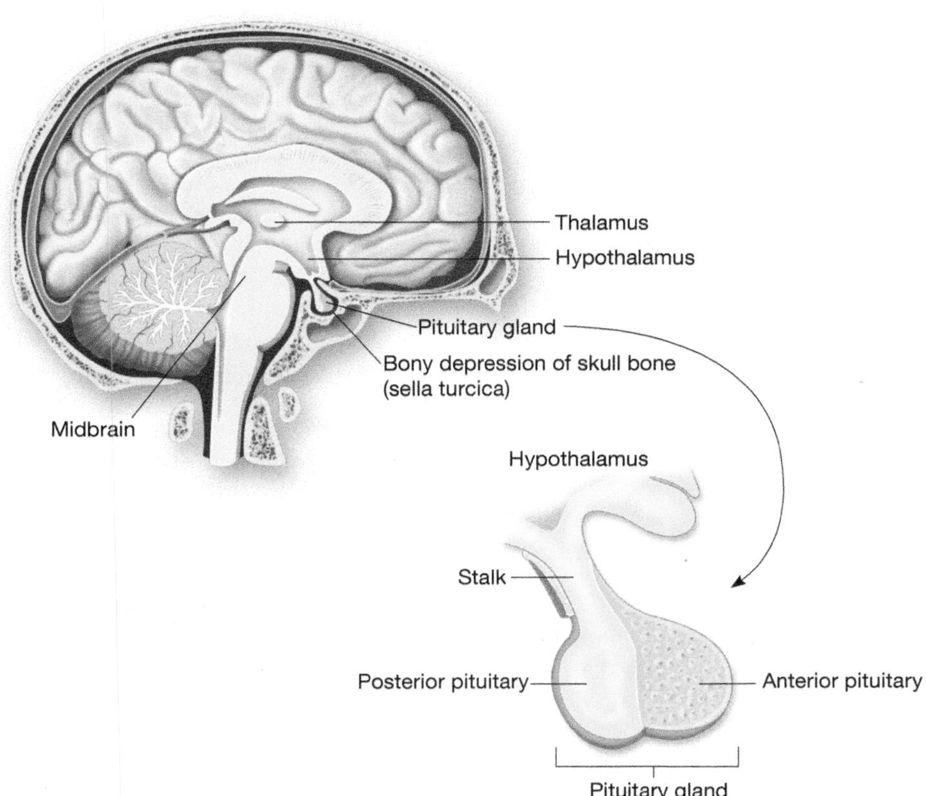

■ **Figure 11.6**
The pituitary gland lies just underneath the brain. It is subdivided into anterior and posterior lobes. Each lobe secretes different hormones.

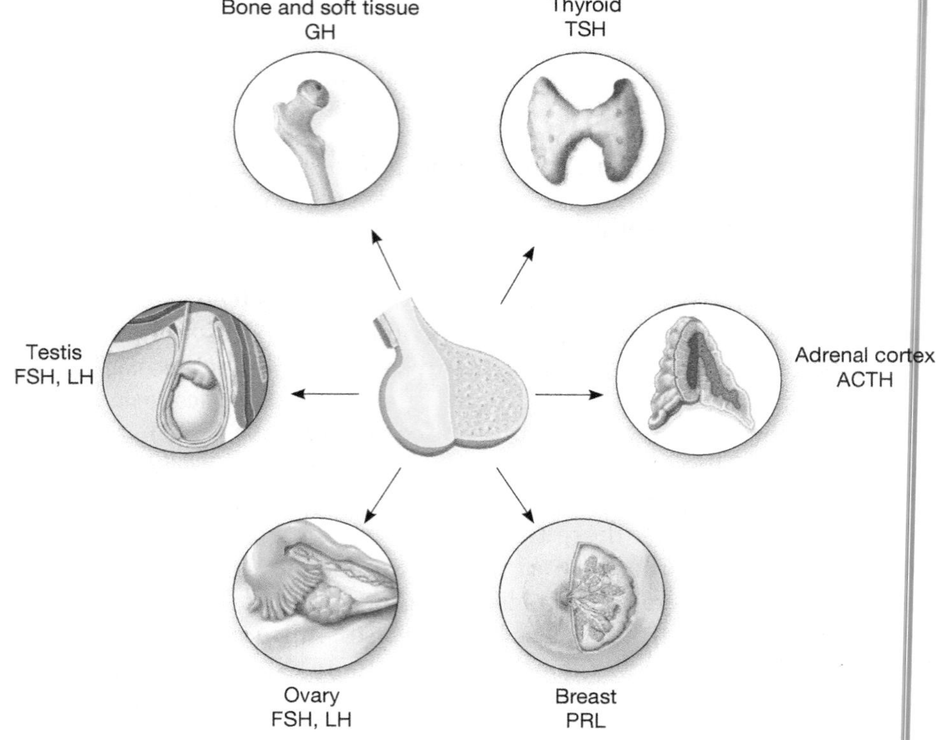

■ **Figure 11.7**
The anterior pituitary is sometimes called the master gland because it secretes many hormones that regulate other glands. This figure illustrates the different hormones and target tissues for the anterior pituitary.

Testes

sperm

testosterone (tess-TAHSS-ter-own)

The testes are two oval glands located in the scrotal sac of the male (see Figure 11.8 ■). They are the male gonads, which produce the male gametes, **sperm,** and the male sex hormone, **testosterone.** Testosterone produces the male secondary sexual characteristics and regulates sperm production.

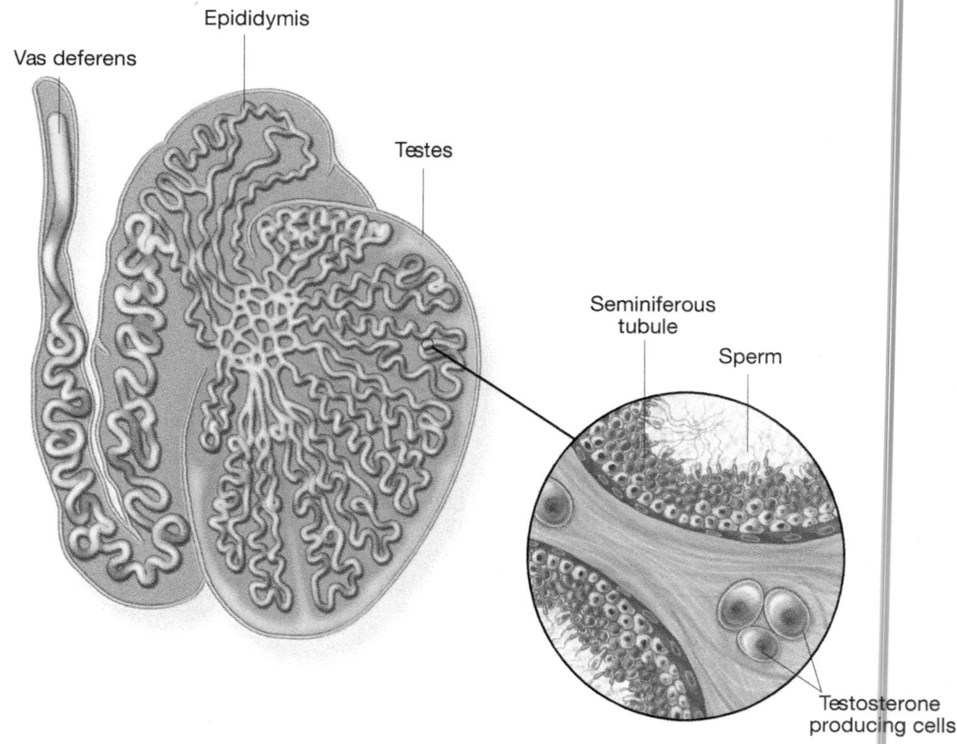

■ **Figure 11.8**
The testes. In addition to producing sperm, the testes secrete the male sex hormones, primarily testosterone.

Thymus Gland

T cells

thymosin (thigh-MOH-sin)

In addition to its role as part of the immune system, the thymus is also one of the endocrine glands because it secretes the hormone **thymosin.** Thymosin, like the rest of the thymus gland, is important for proper development of the immune system. The thymus gland is located in the mediastinal cavity anterior and superior to the heart (see Figure 11.9 ■). The thymus is present at birth and grows to its largest size during puberty. At puberty it begins to shrink and eventually is replaced with connective and adipose tissue.

The most important function of the thymus is the development of the immune system in the newborn. It is essential to the growth and development of thymic lymphocytes or **T cells,** which are critical for the body's immune system.

Thyroid Gland

calcitonin (kal-sih-TOH-nin)
iodine (EYE-oh-dine)
thyroxine (thigh-ROKS-in)
triiodothyronine (try-eye-oh-doh-THIGH-roh-neen)

The thyroid gland, which resembles a butterfly in shape, has right and left lobes (see Figure 11.10 ■). It is located on either side of the trachea and larynx. The thyroid cartilage, or Adam's apple, is located just above the thyroid gland. This gland produces the hormones **thyroxine** (T_4) and **triiodothyronine** (T_3). These hormones are produced in the thyroid gland from the mineral **iodine.** Thyroxine and triiodothyronine help to regulate the production of energy and heat in the body to adjust the body's metabolic rate.

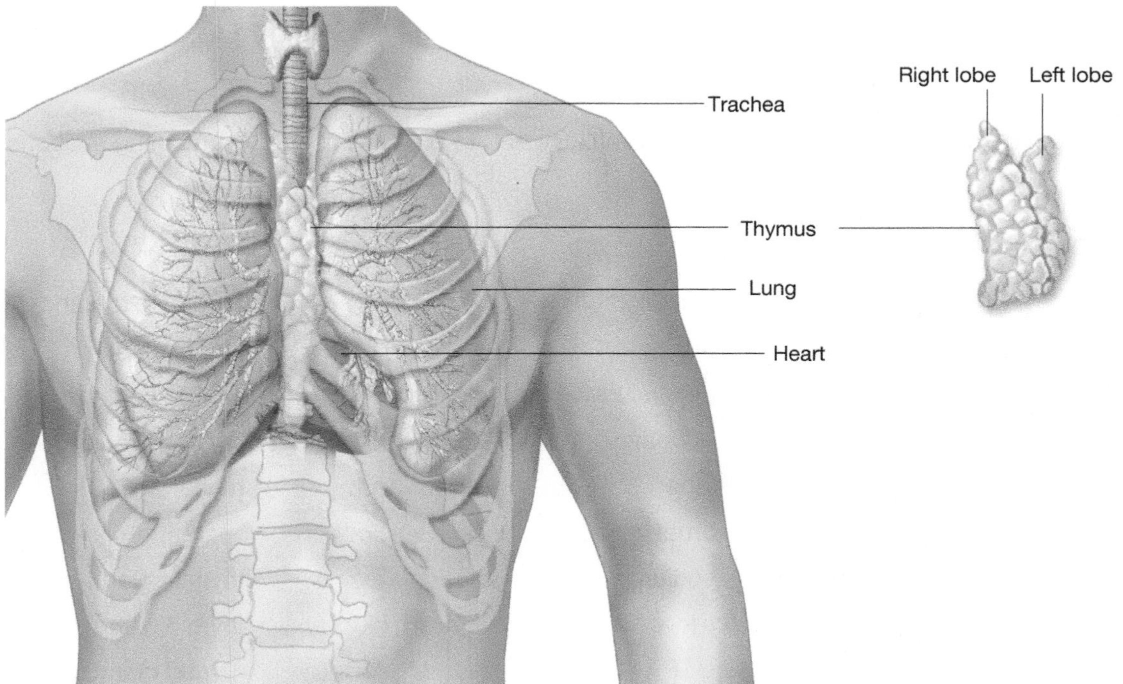

■ **Figure 11.9** The thymus gland. This gland lies in the mediastinum of the thoracic cavity, just above the heart. It secretes thymosin.

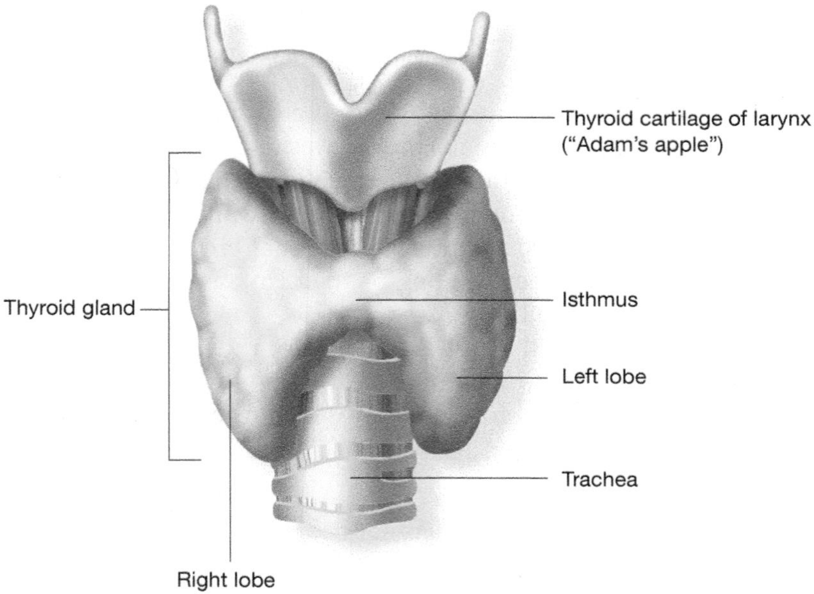

Figure 11.10 The thyroid gland is subdivided into two lobes, one on each side of the trachea.

MED TERM TIP

Iodine is found in many foods, including vegetables and seafood. It is also present in iodized salt, which is one of the best sources of iodine for people living in the Goiter Belt, composed of states located away from saltwater. A lack of iodine in the diet can lead to thyroid disorders, including *goiter.*

The thyroid gland also secretes **calcitonin** (CT) in response to hypercalcemia (too high blood calcium level). Its action is the opposite of parathyroid hormone and stimulates the increased deposition of calcium into bone, thereby lowering blood levels of calcium.

Terminology

Word Parts Used to Build Endocrine System Terms

The following lists contain the combining forms, suffixes, and prefixes used to build terms in the remaining sections of this chapter.

Combining Forms

acr/o	extremities
aden/o	gland
adren/o	adrenal gland
adrenal/o	adrenal gland
calc/o	calcium
carcin/o	cancer
chem/o	drug
cortic/o	outer portion
crin/o	to secrete
cyt/o	cell
glyc/o	sugar
glycos/o	sugar

gynec/o	female
immun/o	protection
kal/i	potassium
lapar/o	abdomen
lob/o	lobe
mast/o	breast
natr/o	sodium
neur/o	nerve
ophthalm/o	eye
or/o	mouth
ovari/o	ovary
pancreat/o	pancreas

parathyroid/o	parathyroid gland
pineal/o	pineal gland
pituitar/o	pituitary gland
radi/o	ray
retin/o	retina
testicul/o	testes
thym/o	thymus gland
thyr/o	thyroid gland
thyroid/o	thyroid gland
toxic/o	poison
vas/o	vessel

Suffixes

-al	pertaining to
-ary	pertaining to
-dipsia	thirst
-ectomy	surgical removal
-emia	blood condition
-emic	relating to a blood condition
-graphy	process of recording
-ia	condition

-ic	pertaining to
-ism	state of
-itis	inflammation
-logy	study of
-megaly	enlarged
-meter	instrument to measure
-oma	tumor
-osis	abnormal condition

-pathy	disease
-prandial	relating to a meal
-pressin	to press down
-scopy	procedure to visually examine
-tic	pertaining to
-uria	urine condition

Prefixes

anti-	against
endo-	within
ex-	outward

hyper-	excessive
hypo-	insufficient
pan-	all

poly-	many
post-	after

Anatomical Terms

TERM	WORD PARTS	DEFINITION
adrenal (ah-DREE-nall)	adren/o = adrenal gland -al = pertaining to	Pertaining to the adrenal glands.
ovarian (oh-VAIR-ee-an)	ovari/o = ovary -ian = pertaining to	Pertaining to the ovary.
pancreatic (pan-kree-AT-ik)	pancreat/o = pancreas -ic = pertaining to	Pertaining to the pancreas.
parathyroidal (pair-ah-THIGH-roy-dall)	parathyroid/o = parathyroid gland -al = pertaining to	Pertaining to the parathyroid gland.
pituitary (pih-TOO-ih-tair-ee)	pituitar/o = pituitary gland -ary = pertaining to	Pertaining to the pituitary gland.
testicular (tes-TIK-yoo-lar)	testicul/o = testes -ar = pertaining to	Pertaining to the testes.
thymic (THIGH-mik)	thym/o = thymus gland -ic = pertaining to	Pertaining to the thymus gland.
thyroidal (thigh-ROYD-all)	thyroid/o = thyroid gland -al = pertaining to	Pertaining to the thyroid gland.

Pathology

TERM	WORD PARTS	DEFINITION
Medical Specialties		
endocrinology (en-doh-krin-ALL-oh-jee)	endo- = within crin/o = to secrete -logy = study of	Branch of medicine involving diagnosis and treatment of conditions and diseases of endocrine glands. Physician is an *endocrinologist.*
Signs and Symptoms		
adrenomegaly (ad-ree-noh-MEG-ah-lee)	adren/o = adrenal gland -megaly = enlarged	Having one or both adrenal glands enlarged.
adrenopathy (ad-ren-OP-ah-thee)	adren/o = adrenal gland -pathy = disease	General term for adrenal gland disease.
edema (eh-DEE-mah)		Condition in which the body tissues contain excessive amounts of fluid.
endocrinopathy (en-doh-krin-OP-ah-thee)	endo- = within crin/o = to secrete -pathy = disease	General term for diseases of the endocrine system.
exophthalmos (eks-off-THAL-mohs)	ex- = outward ophthalm/o = eye	Condition in which the eyeballs protrude, such as in Graves' disease. This is generally caused by an overproduction of thyroid hormone.

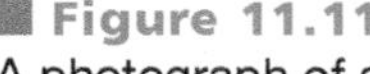
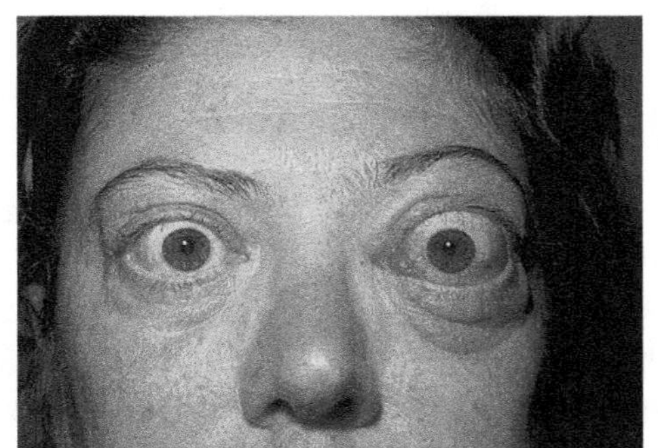

■ **Figure 11.11** A photograph of a woman with exophthalmos. This condition is associated with hypersecretion of the thyroid gland. *(Custom Medical Stock Photo, Inc.)*

TERM	WORD PARTS	DEFINITION
glycosuria (glye-kohs-YOO-ree-ah)	glycos/o = sugar -uria = urine condition	Having a high level of sugar excreted in the urine.
gynecomastia (gigh-neh-koh-MAST-ee-ah)	gynec/o = female mast/o = breast -ia = condition	Development of breast tissue in males. May be a symptom of adrenal feminization.
hirsutism (HER-soot-izm)	-ism = state of	Condition of having an excessive amount of hair. Term generally used to describe females who have the adult male pattern of hair growth. Can be the result of a hormonal imbalance.
hypercalcemia (high-per-kal-SEE-mee-ah)	hyper- = excessive calc/o = calcium -emia = blood condition	Condition of having a high level of calcium in the blood; associated with hypersecretion of parathyroid hormone.
hyperglycemia (high-per-glye-SEE-mee-ah)	hyper- = excessive glyc/o = sugar -emia = blood condition	Condition of having a high level of sugar in the blood; associated with diabetes mellitus.

Pathology *(continued)*

TERM	WORD PARTS	DEFINITION
hyperkalemia (high-per-kal-EE-mee-ah)	hyper- = excessive kal/i = potassium -emia = blood condition	The condition of having a high level of potassium in the blood.
hypersecretion	hyper- = excessive	Excessive hormone production by an endocrine gland.
hypocalcemia (high-poh-kal-SEE-mee-ah)	hypo- = insufficient calc/o = calcium -emia = blood condition	The condition of having a low level of calcium in the blood; associated with hyposecretion of parathyroid hormone. Hypocalcemia may result in tetany.
hypoglycemia (high-poh-glye-SEE-mee-ah)	hypo- = insufficient glyc/o = sugar -emia = blood condition	Condition of having a low level of sugar in the blood.
hyponatremia (high-poh-nah-TREE-mee-ah)	hypo- = insufficient natr/o = sodium -emia = blood condition	Condition of having a low level of sodium in the blood.
hyposecretion	hypo- = insufficient	Deficient hormone production by an endocrine gland.
obesity (oh-BEE-sih-tee)		Having an abnormal amount of fat in the body.
polydipsia (pall-ee-DIP-see-ah)	poly- = many -dipsia = thirst	Excessive feeling of thirst.
polyuria (pall-ee-YOO-ree-ah)	poly- = many -uria = urine condition	Condition of producing an excessive amount of urine.
syndrome (SIN-drohm)		Group of symptoms and signs that, when combined, present a clinical picture of a disease or condition.
thyromegaly (thigh-roh-MEG-ah-lee)	thyr/o = thyroid gland -megaly = enlarged	Having an enlarged thyroid gland.
Adrenal Glands		
Addison's disease (AD-ih-sons)		Disease named for British physician Thomas Addison; results from a deficiency in adrenocortical hormones. There may be an increased pigmentation of the skin, generalized weakness, and weight loss.
adrenal feminization (ad-REE-nal / fem-ih-nigh-ZAY-shun)	adren/o = adrenal gland -al = pertaining to	Development of female secondary sexual characteristics (such as breasts) in a male. Often as a result of increased estrogen secretion by the adrenal cortex.
adrenal virilism (ad-REE-nal / VIR-ill-izm)	adren/o = adrenal gland -al = pertaining to -ism = state of	Development of male secondary sexual characteristics (such as deeper voice and facial hair) in a female. Often as a result of increased androgen secretion by the adrenal cortex.
adrenalitis (ad-ree-nal-EYE-tis)	adrenal/o = adrenal gland -itis = inflammation	Inflammation of one or both adrenal glands.

Pathology *(continued)*

TERM	WORD PARTS	DEFINITION
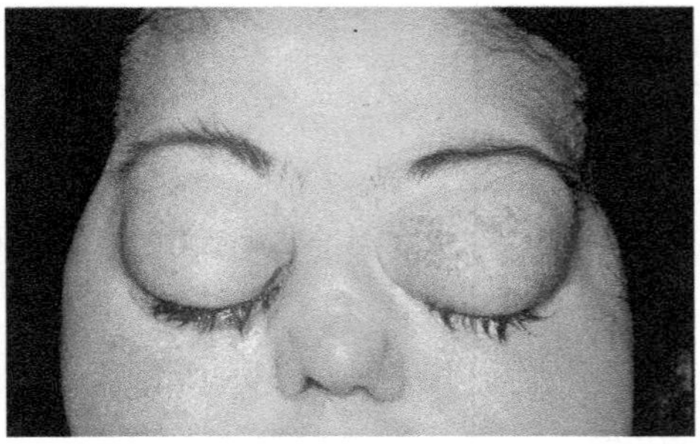 **Cushing's syndrome** (CUSH-ings / SIN-drohm)		Set of symptoms caused by excessive levels of cortisol due to high doses of corticosteroid drugs and adrenal tumors. The syndrome may present symptoms of weakness, edema, excess hair growth, skin discoloration, and osteoporosis.
Figure 11.12 Cushing's syndrome. A photograph of a woman with the characteristic facial features of Cushing's syndrome. *(Biophoto Photo Associates/Photo Researchers, Inc.)*		
pheochromocytoma (fee-oh-kroh-moh-sigh-TOH-ma)	cyt/o = cell -oma = tumor	Usually benign tumor of the adrenal medulla that secretes epinephrine. Symptoms include anxiety, heart palpitations, dyspnea, profuse sweating, headache, and nausea.
Pancreas		
diabetes mellitus (DM) (dye-ah-BEE-teez / MELL-ih-tus)		Chronic disorder of carbohydrate metabolism resulting in hyperglycemia and glycosuria. There are two distinct forms of diabetes mellitus: *insulin-dependent diabetes mellitus* (IDDM) or *type 1,* and *non-insulin-dependent diabetes mellitus* (NIDDM) or *type 2.*
diabetic retinopathy (dye-ah-BET-ik / ret-in-OP-ah-thee)	-tic = pertaining to retin/o = retina -pathy = disease	Secondary complication of diabetes that affects the blood vessels of the retina, resulting in visual changes and even blindness.
insulin-dependent diabetes mellitus (IDDM) (dye-ah-BEE-teez / MELL-ih-tus)		Also called *type 1 diabetes mellitus.* It develops early in life when the pancreas stops insulin production. Patient must take daily insulin injections.
insulinoma (in-sue-lin-OH-mah)	-oma = tumor	Tumor of the islets of Langerhans cells of the pancreas that secretes an excessive amount of insulin.
ketoacidosis (KEE-toh-ass-ih-DOH-sis)	ket/o = ketones -osis = abnormal condition	Acidosis due to an excess of acidic ketone bodies (waste products). A serious condition requiring immediate treatment that can result in death for the diabetic patient if not reversed. Also called *diabetic acidosis.*
non-insulin-dependent diabetes mellitus (dye-ah-BEE-teez / MELL-ih-tus)		Also called *type 2 diabetes mellitus.* It typically develops later in life. The pancreas produces normal to high levels of insulin, but the cells fail to respond to it. Patients may take oral hypoglycemics to improve insulin function, or may eventually have to take insulin.
peripheral neuropathy (per-IF-eh-rall / new-ROP-ah-thee)	-al = pertaining to neur/o = nerve -pathy = disease	Damage to the nerves in the lower legs and hands as a result of diabetes mellitus. Symptoms include either extreme sensitivity or numbness and tingling.

Pathology *(continued)*

TERM	WORD PARTS	DEFINITION
Parathyroid Glands		
hyperparathyroidism (HIGH-per-pair-ah-THIGH-royd-izm)	hyper- = excessive parathyroid/o = parathyroid gland -ism = state of	Hypersecretion of parathyroid hormone; may result in hypercalcemia and Recklinghausen disease.
hypoparathyroidism (HIGH-poh-pair-ah-THIGH-royd-izm)	hypo- = insufficient parathyroid/o = parathyroid gland -ism = state of	Hyposecretion of parathyroid hormone; may result in hypocalcemia and tetany.
Recklinghausen disease (REK-ling-how-zenz)		Excessive production of parathyroid hormone resulting in degeneration of the bones.
tetany (TET-ah-nee)		Nerve irritability and painful muscle cramps resulting from hypocalcemia. Hypoparathyroidism is one cause of tetany.
Pituitary Gland		
acromegaly (ak-roh-MEG-ah-lee) 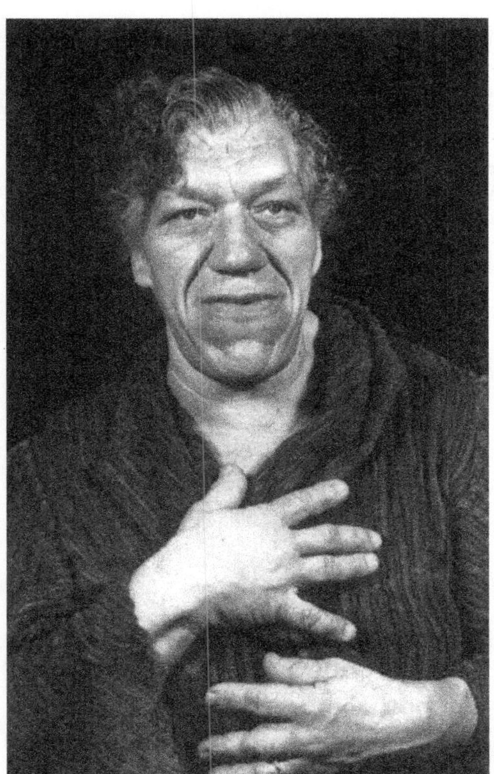 ■ **Figure 11.13** Acromegaly. Photo of a woman illustrating the enlarged skull, jaw, and hands typical of acromegaly. *(Reprinted from American Journal of Medicine, Vol 20, Dr. William H. Daughaday, University of California/Irvine, ©1956. With permission from Excerpta Medica Inc.)*	acr/o = extremities -megaly = enlarged	Chronic disease of adults that results in an elongation and enlargement of the bones of the head and extremities. There can also be mood changes. Due to an excessive amount of growth hormone in an adult.
diabetes insipidus (DI) (dye-ah-BEE-teez / in-SIP-ih-dus)		Disorder caused by the inadequate secretion of antidiuretic hormone by the posterior lobe of the pituitary gland. There may be polyuria and polydipsia.
dwarfism (DWARF-izm)	-ism = state of	Condition of being abnormally short in height. It may be the result of a hereditary condition or a lack of growth hormone.

Pathology (continued)

TERM	WORD PARTS	DEFINITION
gigantism (JYE-gan-tizm)	-ism = state of	Excessive development of the body due to the overproduction of the growth hormone by the pituitary gland in a child or teenager. The opposite of *dwarfism*.
hyperpituitarism (HIGH-per-pih-TOO-ih-tuh-rizm)	hyper- = excessive pituitar/o = pituitary gland -ism = state of	Hypersecretion of one or more pituitary gland hormones.
hypopituitarism (HIGH-poh-pih-TOO-ih-tuh-rizm)	hypo- = insufficient pituitar/o = pituitary gland -ism = state of	Hyposecretion of one or more pituitary gland hormones.
panhypopituitarism (pan-high-poh-pih-TOO-ih-tair-izm)	pan- = all hypo- = insufficient pituitar/o = pituitary gland -ism = state of	Deficiency in all the hormones secreted by the pituitary gland. Often recognized because of problems with the glands regulated by the pituitary–adrenal cortex, thyroid, ovaries, and testes.
Thymus Gland		
thymitis (thigh-MY-tis)	thym/o = thymus gland -itis = inflammation	Inflammation of the thymus gland.
thymoma (thigh-MOH-mah)	thym/o = thymus gland -oma = tumor	A tumor in the thymus gland.
Thyroid Gland		
cretinism (KREE-tin-izm)	-ism = state of	Congenital condition in which a lack of thyroid hormones may result in arrested physical and mental development.
goiter (GOY-ter) ■ **Figure 11.14** Goiter. A photograph of a male with an extreme goiter or enlarged thyroid gland.		Enlargement of the thyroid gland.
Graves' disease		Condition named for Irish physician Robert Graves that results in overactivity of the thyroid gland and can cause a crisis situation. Symptoms include exophthalmos and goiter. A type of *hyperthyroidism*.
Hashimoto's thyroiditis (hash-ee-MOH-tohz / thigh-roy-DYE-tis)	thyroid/o = thyroid gland -itis = inflammation	Chronic autoimmune form of thyroiditis; results in hyposecretion of thyroid hormones.

Pathology *(continued)*

TERM	WORD PARTS	DEFINITION
hyperthyroidism (hi-per-THIGH-royd-izm)	hyper- = excessive thyroid/o = thyroid gland -ism = state of	Hypersecretion of thyroid gland hormones.
hypothyroidism (high-poh-THIGH-royd-izm)	hypo- = insufficient thyroid/o = thyroid gland -ism = state of	Hyposecretion of thyroid gland hormones.
myxedema (miks-eh-DEE-mah)		Condition resulting from a hyposecretion of the thyroid gland in an adult. Symptoms can include anemia, slow speech, swollen facial features, edematous skin, drowsiness, and mental lethargy.
thyrotoxicosis (thigh-roh-toks-ih-KOH-sis)	thyr/o = thyroid gland toxic/o = poison -osis = abnormal condition	Condition resulting from marked overproduction of the thyroid gland. Symptoms include rapid heart action, tremors, enlarged thyroid gland, exophthalmos, and weight loss.
All Glands		
adenocarcinoma (ad-eh-no-car-sih-NO-mah)	aden/o = gland carcin/o = cancer -oma = tumor	Cancerous tumor in a gland that is capable of producing the hormones secreted by that gland. One cause of hypersecretion pathologies.

Diagnostic Procedures

TERM	WORD PARTS	DEFINITION
Clinical Laboratory Tests		
blood serum test		Blood test to measure the level of substances such as calcium, electrolytes, testosterone, insulin, and glucose. Used to assist in determining the function of various endocrine glands.
fasting blood sugar (FBS)		Blood test to measure the amount of sugar circulating throughout the body after a 12-hour fast.
glucose tolerance test (GTT) (GLOO-kohs)		Test to determine the blood sugar level. A measured dose of glucose is given to a patient either orally or intravenously. Blood samples are then drawn at certain intervals to determine the ability of the patient to use glucose. Used for diabetic patients to determine their insulin response to glucose.
protein-bound iodine test (PBI)		Blood test to measure the concentration of thyroxine (T_4) circulating in the bloodstream. The iodine becomes bound to the protein in the blood and can be measured. Useful in establishing thyroid function.

Diagnostic Procedures *(continued)*

TERM	WORD PARTS	DEFINITION
radioimmunoassay (RIA) (ray-dee-oh-im-yoo-noh-ASS-ay)	radi/o = ray immun/o = protection	Blood test that uses radioactively tagged hormones and antibodies to measure the quantity of hormone in the plasma.
thyroid function test (TFT) (THIGH-royd)		Blood test used to measure the levels of thyroxine, triiodothyronine, and thyroid-stimulating hormone in the bloodstream to assist in determining thyroid function.
total calcium		Blood test to measure the total amount of calcium to assist in detecting parathyroid and bone disorders.
two-hour postprandial glucose tolerance test (post-PRAN-dee-al)	post- = after -prandial = relating to a meal	Blood test to assist in evaluating glucose metabolism. The patient eats a high carbohydrate diet and then fasts overnight before the test. Then the blood sample is taken 2 hours after a meal.
Diagnostic Imaging		
thyroid echography (THIGH-royd / eh-KOG-rah-fee)	-graphy = process of recording	Ultrasound examination of the thyroid that can assist in distinguishing a thyroid nodule from a cyst.
thyroid scan (THIGH-royd)		Test in which radioactive iodine is administered that localizes in the thyroid gland. The gland can then be visualized with a scanning device to detect pathology such as tumors.

Therapeutic Procedures

TERM	WORD PARTS	DEFINITION
Medical Procedures		
chemical thyroidectomy (thigh-royd-EK-toh-mee)	chem/o = drug -al = pertaining to thyroid/o = thyroid gland -ectomy = surgical removal	Large dose of radioactive iodine is given in order to kill thyroid gland cells without having to actually do surgery.
glucometer	gluc/o = glucose -meter = instrument to measure	Device designed for a diabetic to use at home to measure the level of glucose in the bloodstream.
hormone replacement therapy		Artificial replacement of hormones in patients with hyposecretion disorders. May be oral pills, injections, or adhesive skin patches.
Surgical Procedures		
adrenalectomy (ad-ree-nal-EK-toh-mee)	adrenal/o = adrenal gland -ectomy = surgical removal	Surgical removal of one or both adrenal glands.
laparoscopic adrenalectomy (lap-row-SKOP-ik / ad-ree-nal-EK-toh-mee)	lapar/o = abdomen -scopy = procedure to visually examine -ic = pertaining to adren/o = adrenal gland -ectomy = surgical removal	Removal of the adrenal gland through a small incision in the abdomen and using endoscopic instruments.

Therapeutic Procedures *(continued)*

TERM	WORD PARTS	DEFINITION
lobectomy (lobe-EK-toh-mee)	lob/o = lobe -ectomy = surgical removal	Removal of a lobe from an organ. In this case, one lobe of the thyroid gland.
parathyroidectomy (pair-ah-thigh-royd-EK-toh-mee)	parathyroid/o = parathyroid gland -ectomy = surgical removal	Surgical removal of one or more of the parathyroid glands.
pinealectomy (PIN-ee-ah-LEK-toh-mee)	pineal/o = pineal gland -ectomy = surgical removal	Surgical removal of the pineal gland.
thymectomy (thigh-MEK-toh-mee)	thym/o = thymus gland -ectomy = surgical removal	Surgical removal of the thymus gland.
thyroidectomy (thigh-royd-EK-toh-mee)	thyroid/o = thyroid gland -ectomy = surgical removal	Surgical removal of the thyroid gland.

Pharmacology

CLASSIFICATION	WORD PARTS	ACTION	EXAMPLES
antithyroid agents	anti- = against	Medication given to block production of thyroid hormones in patients with hypersecretion disorders.	methimazole, Tapazole; propylthiouracil
corticosteroids (kor-tih-koh-STAIR-oydz)	cortic/o = outer portion	Although the function of these hormones in the body is to regulate carbohydrate metabolism, they also have a strong anti-inflammatory action. Therefore they are used to treat severe chronic inflammatory diseases such as rheumatoid arthritis. Long-term use of corticosteroids has adverse side effects such as osteoporosis and the symptoms of Cushing's disease. Also used to treat adrenal cortex hyposecretion disorders such as Addison's disease.	prednisone, Deltasone
human growth hormone therapy		Hormone replacement therapy with human growth hormone in order to stimulate skeletal growth. Used to treat children with abnormally short stature.	somatropin, Genotropin; somatrem, Protropin
insulin (IN-suh-lin)		Administered to replace insulin for type 1 diabetics or to treat severe type 2 diabetics.	human insulin, Humulin L
oral hypoglycemic agents (high-poh-glye-SEE-mik)	or/o = mouth -al = pertaining to hypo- = insufficient glyc/o = sugar -emic = relating to a blood condition	Medications taken by mouth that cause a decrease in blood sugar; not used for insulin-dependent patients.	metformin, Glucophage; glipizide, Glucotrol

Pharmacology *(continued)*

CLASSIFICATION	WORD PARTS	ACTION	EXAMPLES
thyroid replacement hormone		Hormone replacement therapy for patients with hypothyroidism or who have had a thyroidectomy.	levothyroxine, Levo-T; liothyronine, Cytomel
vasopressin (vaz-oh-PRESS-in)	vas/o = vessel -pressin = to press down	Given to control diabetes insipidus and promote reabsorption of water in the kidney tubules.	desmopressin acetate, Desmopressin; conivaptan, Vaprisol

Abbreviations

α	alpha	**LH**	luteinizing hormone
ACTH	adrenocorticotropic hormone	**MSH**	melanocyte-stimulating hormone
ADH	antidiuretic hormone	**Na^+**	sodium
β	beta	**NIDDM**	non-insulin-dependent diabetes mellitus
BMR	basal metabolic rate	**NPH**	neutral protamine Hagedorn (insulin)
CT	calcitonin	**PBI**	protein-bound iodine
DI	diabetes insipidus	**PRL**	prolactin
DM	diabetes mellitus	**PTH**	parathyroid hormone
FBS	fasting blood sugar	**RAI**	radioactive iodine
FSH	follicle-stimulating hormone	**RIA**	radioimmunoassay
GH	growth hormone	**T_3**	triiodothyronine
GTT	glucose tolerance test	**T_4**	thyroxine
IDDM	insulin-dependent diabetes mellitus	**TFT**	thyroid function test
K^+	potassium	**TSH**	thyroid-stimulating hormone

Chapter Review

Real-World Applications

Medical Record Analysis

This Discharge Summary below contains 10 medical terms. Underline each term and write it in the list below the report. Then define each term.

Discharge Summary

Admitting Diagnosis:	Hyperglycemia, ketoacidosis, glycosuria
Final Diagnosis:	New-onset type 1 diabetes mellitus
History of Present Illness:	A 12-year-old female patient presented to her physician's office with a 2-month history of weight loss, fatigue, polyuria, and polydipsia. Her family history is significant for a grandfather, mother, and older brother with type 1 diabetes mellitus. The pediatrician found hyperglycemia with a fasting blood sugar and glycosuria with a urine dipstick. She is being admitted at this time for management of new-onset diabetes mellitus.
Summary of Hospital Course:	At the time of admission, the FBS was 300 mg/100 mL and she was in ketoacidosis. She rapidly improved after receiving insulin; her blood glucose level normalized. The next day a glucose tolerance test confirmed the diagnosis of diabetes mellitus. The patient was started on insulin injections. Patient and family were instructed on diabetes mellitus, insulin, diet, exercise, and long-term complications.
Discharge Plans:	Patient was discharged to home with her parents. Her parents are to check her blood glucose levels twice daily and call the office for insulin dosage. She is to return to the office in 2 weeks.

	Term	Definition
1	______________	______________________________
2	______________	______________________________
3	______________	______________________________
4	______________	______________________________
5	______________	______________________________
6	______________	______________________________
7	______________	______________________________
8	______________	______________________________
9	______________	______________________________
10	______________	______________________________

Chart Note Transcription

The chart note below contains 11 phrases that can be reworded with a medical term that you learned in this chapter. Each phrase is identified with an underline. Determine the medical term and write your answers in the space provided.

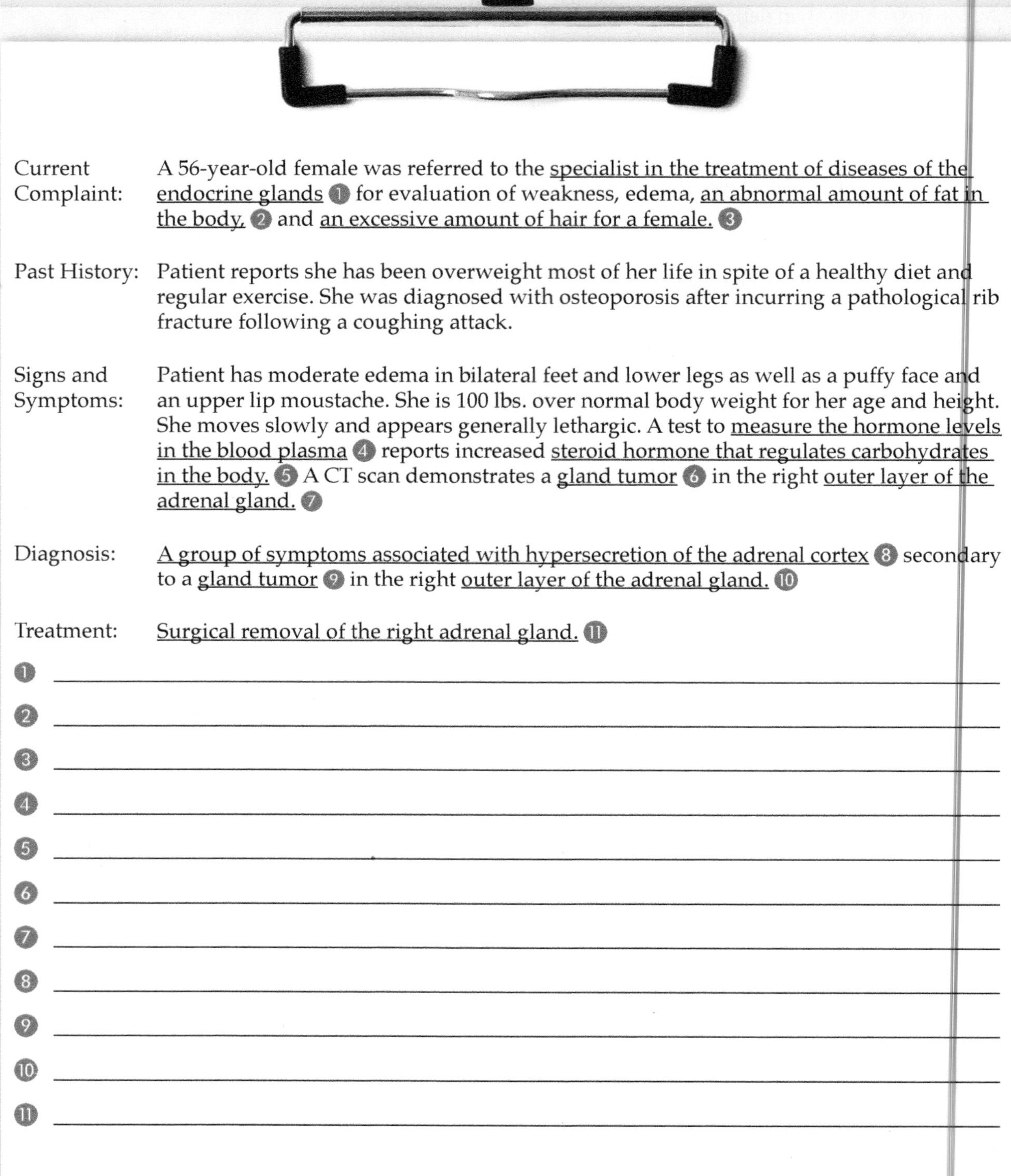

Current Complaint: A 56-year-old female was referred to the specialist in the treatment of diseases of the endocrine glands (1) for evaluation of weakness, edema, an abnormal amount of fat in the body, (2) and an excessive amount of hair for a female. (3)

Past History: Patient reports she has been overweight most of her life in spite of a healthy diet and regular exercise. She was diagnosed with osteoporosis after incurring a pathological rib fracture following a coughing attack.

Signs and Symptoms: Patient has moderate edema in bilateral feet and lower legs as well as a puffy face and an upper lip moustache. She is 100 lbs. over normal body weight for her age and height. She moves slowly and appears generally lethargic. A test to measure the hormone levels in the blood plasma (4) reports increased steroid hormone that regulates carbohydrates in the body. (5) A CT scan demonstrates a gland tumor (6) in the right outer layer of the adrenal gland. (7)

Diagnosis: A group of symptoms associated with hypersecretion of the adrenal cortex (8) secondary to a gland tumor (9) in the right outer layer of the adrenal gland. (10)

Treatment: Surgical removal of the right adrenal gland. (11)

(1) ______________________________

(2) ______________________________

(3) ______________________________

(4) ______________________________

(5) ______________________________

(6) ______________________________

(7) ______________________________

(8) ______________________________

(9) ______________________________

(10) ______________________________

(11) ______________________________

Case Study

Below is a case study presentation of a patient with a condition covered in this chapter. Read the case study and answer the questions below. Some questions will ask for information not included within this chapter. Use your text, a medical dictionary, journals, technical materials, multimedia resources, electronic media, or any other reference material you choose to answer these questions.

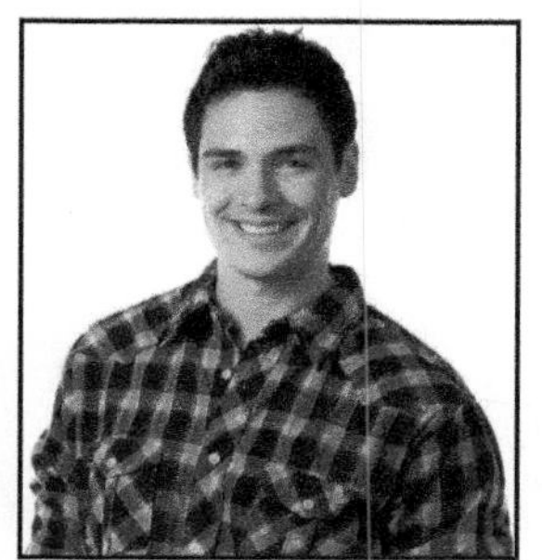

(Flashon Studio/Shutterstock)

A 22-year-old college student was admitted to the emergency room after his friends called an ambulance when he passed out in a bar. He had become confused, developed slurred speech, and had difficulty walking after having only one beer to drink. In the ER he was noted to have diaphoresis, rapid respirations and pulse, and was disoriented. Upon examination, needle marks were found on his abdomen and outer thighs. The physician ordered blood serum tests that revealed hyperglycemia and ketoacidosis. Unknown to his friends, this young man has had diabetes mellitus since early childhood. The patient quickly recovered following an insulin injection.

1. What pathological condition has this patient had since childhood? Look this condition up in a reference source and include a short description of it.

   ____

   ____

2. List and define each symptom noted in the ER in your own words.

   ____

   ____

3. What diagnostic test was performed? Describe it in your own words.

   ____

   ____

4. Explain the results of the test.

   ____

   ____

5. What specific type of diabetes does this young man probably have? Justify your answer.

   ____

   ____

6. Describe the other type of diabetes mellitus that this young man did not have.

   ____

   ____

Practice Exercises

A. Complete the Statement

1. The study of the endocrine system is called ____________________.

2. The master endocrine gland is the ____________________.

3. ____________________ is a general term for the sexual organs that produce gametes.

4. The term for the hormones produced by the outer portion of the adrenal cortex is ____________________.

5. The hormone produced by the testes is ____________________.

6. The two hormones produced by the ovaries are ____________________ and ____________________.

7. An inadequate supply of the hormone ____________________ causes diabetes insipidus.

8. The endocrine gland associated with the immune system is the ____________________.

9. The term for a protrusion of the eyeballs in Graves' disease is ____________________.

10. A general medical term for a hormone-secreting cancerous tumor is ____________________.

B. Combining Form Practice

The combining form **thyroid/o** refers to the thyroid. Use it to write a term that means:

1. removal of the thyroid ____________________
2. pertaining to the thyroid ____________________
3. state of excessive thyroid ____________________

The combining form **pancreat/o** refers to the pancreas. Use it to write a term that means:

4. pertaining to the pancreas ____________________
5. inflammation of the pancreas ____________________
6. removal of the pancreas ____________________
7. cutting into the pancreas ____________________

The combining form **adren/o** refers to the adrenal glands. Use it to write a term that means:

8. pertaining to the adrenal gland ____________________
9. enlargement of the adrenal glands ____________________
10. adrenal gland disease ____________________

The combining form **thym/o** refers to the thymus glands. Use it to write a term that means:

11. tumor of the thymus gland ____________________
12. removal of the thymus gland ____________________
13. pertaining to the thymus gland ____________________
14. inflammation of the thymus gland ____________________

C. Define the Combining Form

	Definition	Example from Chapter
1. natr/o	________________	________________
2. estr/o	________________	________________
3. pineal/o	________________	________________
4. pituitar/o	________________	________________
5. kal/i	________________	________________
6. calc/o	________________	________________
7. parathyroid/o	________________	________________
8. acr/o	________________	________________
9. glyc/o	________________	________________
10. gonad/o	________________	________________

D. Terminology Matching

Match the term to its definition.

1. ________ protein-bound iodine test
2. ________ fasting blood sugar
3. ________ radioimmunoassay
4. ________ thyroid scan
5. ________ 2-hour postprandial glucose tolerance test
6. ________ glucose tolerance test

a. measures levels of hormones in the blood
b. determines glucose metabolism after patient receives a measured dose of glucose
c. test of glucose metabolism 2 hours after eating a meal
d. measures blood sugar level after 12-hour fast
e. measures T4 concentration in the blood
f. uses radioactive iodine

E. What's the Abbreviation?

1. non-insulin-dependent diabetes mellitus ________________
2. insulin-dependent diabetes mellitus ________________
3. adrenocorticotropic hormone ________________
4. parathyroid hormone ________________
5. triiodothyronine ________________
6. thyroid-stimulating hormone ________________
7. fasting blood sugar ________________
8. prolactin ________________

F. Terminology Matching

Match each term to its definition.

1. _______ Cushing's disease
2. _______ goiter
3. _______ acromegaly
4. _______ gigantism
5. _______ cretinism
6. _______ myxedema
7. _______ diabetes mellitus
8. _______ diabetes insipidus
9. _______ Hashimoto's thyroiditis
10. _______ Graves' disease
11. _______ Addison's disease

a. enlarged thyroid
b. overactive adrenal cortex
c. hyperthyroidism
d. underactive adrenal cortex
e. enlarged bones of head and extremities
f. may cause polyuria and polydipsia
g. an autoimmune disease
h. arrested physical and mental development
i. disorder of carbohydrate metabolism
j. insufficient thyroid hormone in an adult
k. excessive growth hormone in a child

G. What Does it Stand For?

1. PBI ____________________
2. K^+ ____________________
3. T_4 ____________________
4. GTT ____________________
5. DM ____________________
6. BMR ____________________
7. Na^+ ____________________
8. ADH ____________________

H. Suffix Practice

Use the following suffixes to create medical terms for the following definitions.

-pressin	-uria	-tropin
-dipsia	-emia	-prandial

1. the presence of sugar or glucose in the urine ____________________
2. to press down a vessel ____________________

3. excessive urination ______

4. condition of excessive calcium in the blood ______

5. excessive thirst ______

6. stimulate adrenal cortex ______

7. after a meal ______

I. Define the Term

1. corticosteroid ______
2. hirsutism ______
3. tetany ______
4. diabetic retinopathy ______
5. hyperglycemia ______
6. hypoglycemia ______
7. adrenaline ______
8. insulin ______
9. thyrotoxicosis ______
10. hypersecretion ______

J. Fill in the Blank

insulinoma	ketoacidosis	pheochromocytoma
gynecomastia	panhypopituitarinism	Hashimoto's thyroiditis

1. The doctor found that Marsha's high level of insulin and hypoglycemia was caused by a(n) ______.
2. Kevin developed ______ as a result of his diabetes mellitus and required emergency treatment.
3. It was determined that Karen had ______ when doctors realized she had problems with her thyroid gland, adrenal cortex, and ovaries.
4. Luke's high epinephrine level was caused by a(n) ______.
5. When it was determined that Carl's thyroiditis was an autoimmune condition, it became obvious that he had ______.
6. Excessive sex hormones caused Jack to develop ______.

K. Pharmacology Challenge

Fill in the classification for each drug description, then match the brand name.

	Drug Description	Classification	Brand Name
1.	_______ strong anti-inflammatory	____________________	a. genotropin
2.	_______ stimulates skeletal growth	____________________	b. Desmopressin
3.	_______ treats type 1 diabetes mellitus	____________________	c. Tapazole
4.	_______ blocks production of thyroid hormone	____________________	d. glucophage
5.	_______ treats type 1 diabetes mellitus	____________________	e. Deltasone
6.	_______ controls diabetes insipidus	____________________	f. Humulin

Labeling Exercise

Image A

Write the labels for this figure on the numbered lines provided.

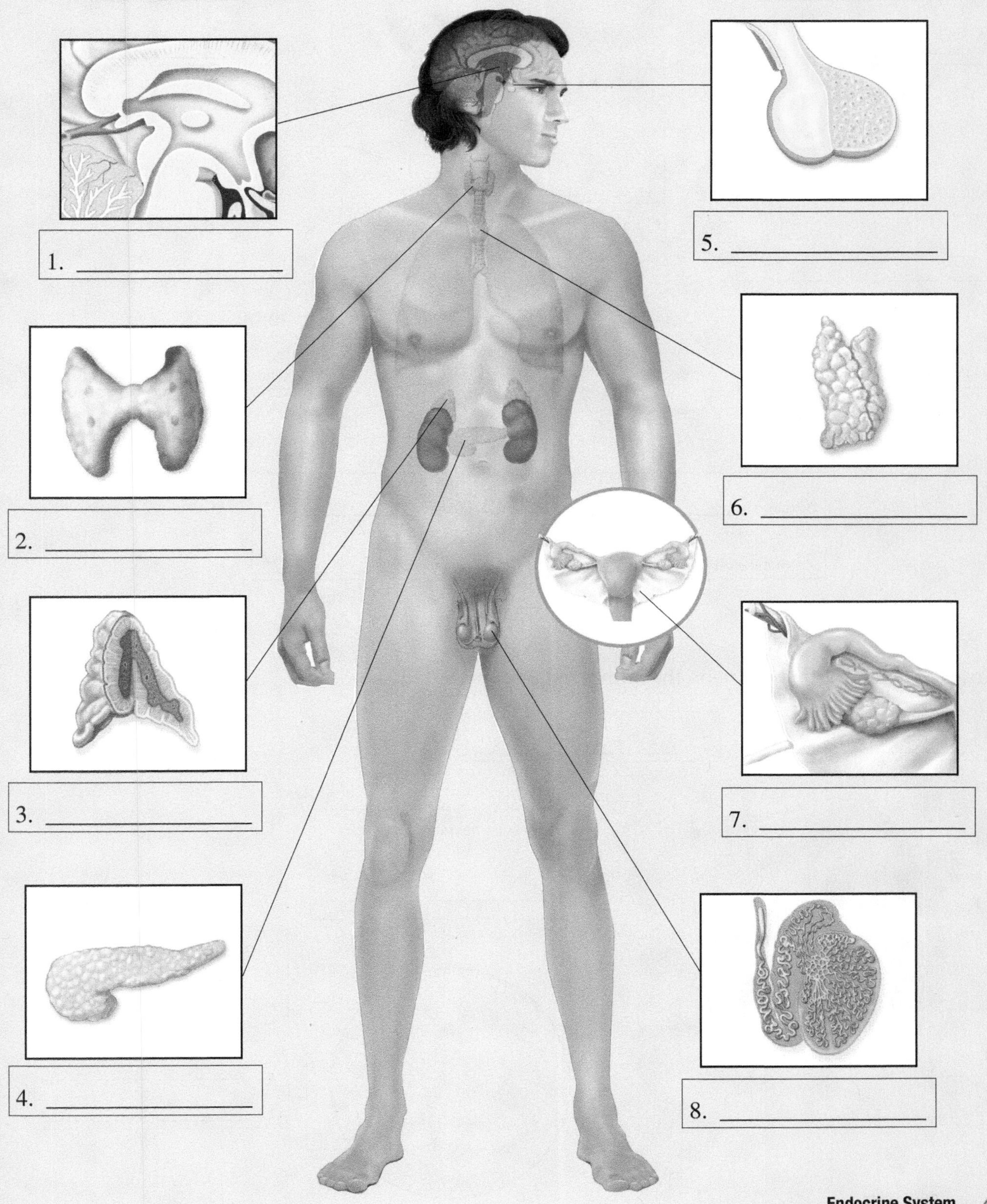

Image B

Write the labels for this figure on the numbered lines provided.

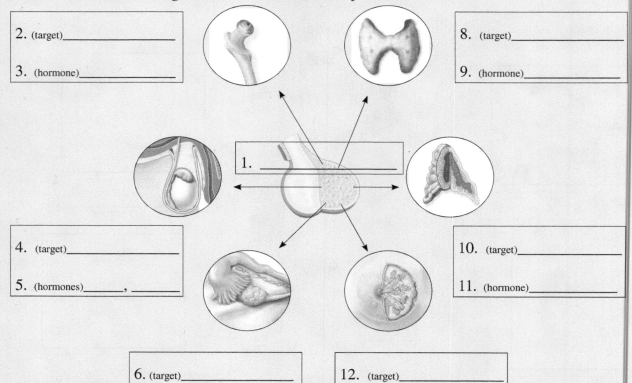

2. (target)________________

3. (hormone)________________

8. (target)________________

9. (hormone)________________

1. ________________

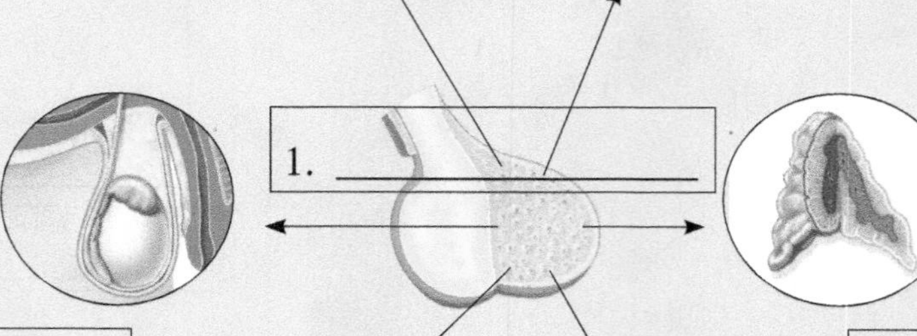

4. (target)________________

5. (hormones)_______, _______

10. (target)________________

11. (hormone)________________

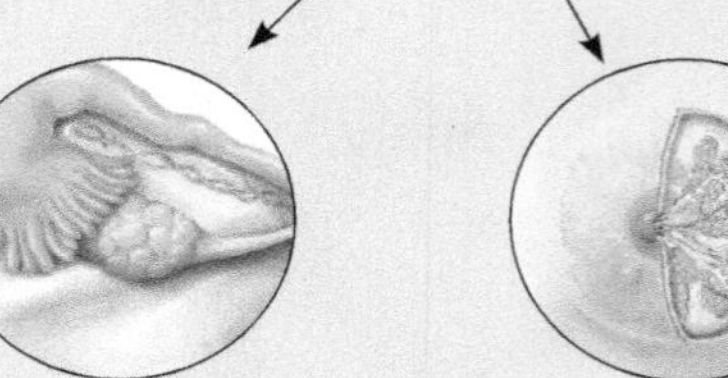

6. (target)________________

7. (hormones)_______, _______

12. (target)________________

13. (hormone)________________

Image C

Write the labels for this figure on the numbered lines provided.

1. ________________

2. ________________

3. ________________

4. Insulin-secreting cell ________________

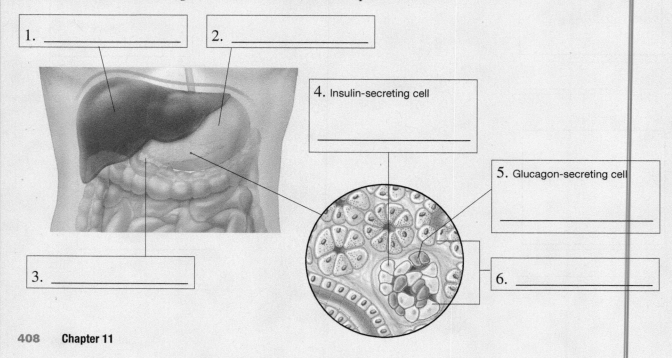

5. Glucagon-secreting cell ________________

6. ________________

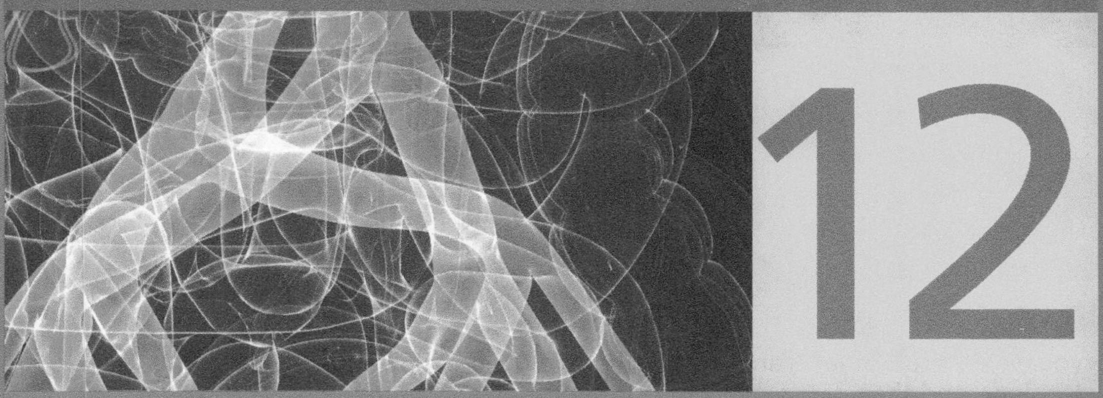

12 NERVOUS SYSTEM

Learning Objectives

Upon completion of this chapter, you will be able to

- Identify and define the combining forms and suffixes introduced in this chapter.
- Correctly spell and pronounce medical terms and major anatomical structures relating to the nervous system.
- Locate and describe the major organs of the nervous system and their functions.
- Describe the components of a neuron.
- Distinguish between the central nervous system, peripheral nervous system, and autonomic nervous system.
- Identify and define nervous system anatomical terms.
- Identify and define selected nervous system pathology terms.
- Identify and define selected nervous system diagnostic procedures.
- Identify and define selected nervous system therapeutic procedures.
- Identify and define selected medications relating to the nervous system.
- Define selected abbreviations associated with the nervous system.

Nervous System at a Glance

Function

The nervous system coordinates and controls body function. It receives sensory input, makes decisions, and then orders body responses.

Structures

Here are the primary structures that comprise the nervous system.

brain
nerves
spinal cord

Word Parts

Here are the most common word parts (with their meanings) used to build nervous system terms. For a more comprehensive list, refer to the Terminology section of this chapter.

Combining Forms

alges/o	sense of pain
astr/o	star
cephal/o	head
cerebell/o	cerebellum
cerebr/o	cerebrum
clon/o	rapid contracting and relaxing
dur/o	dura mater
encephal/o	brain
esthes/o	sensation, feeling
gli/o	glue
medull/o	medulla oblongata
mening/o	meninges
meningi/o	meninges
myel/o	spinal cord
neur/o	nerve
poli/o	gray matter
pont/o	pons
radicul/o	nerve root
thalam/o	thalamus
thec/o	sheath (meninges)
ton/o	tone
ventricul/o	ventricle

Suffixes

-paresis	weakness
-phasia	speech
-plegia	paralysis
-taxia	muscle coordination
-trophic	pertaining to development

Nervous System Illustrated

brain, p. 414

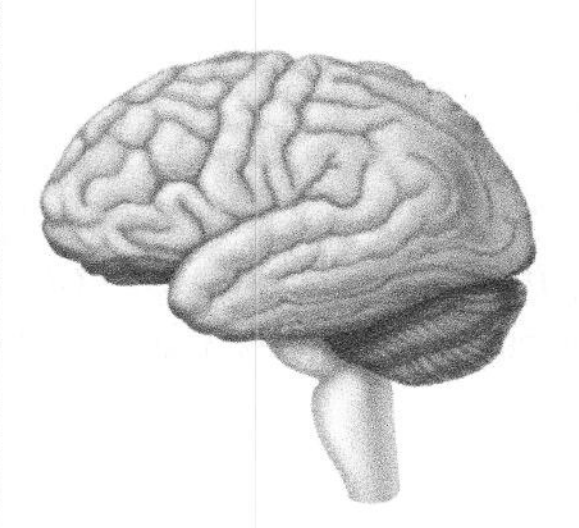

Coordinates body functions

spinal cord, p. 416

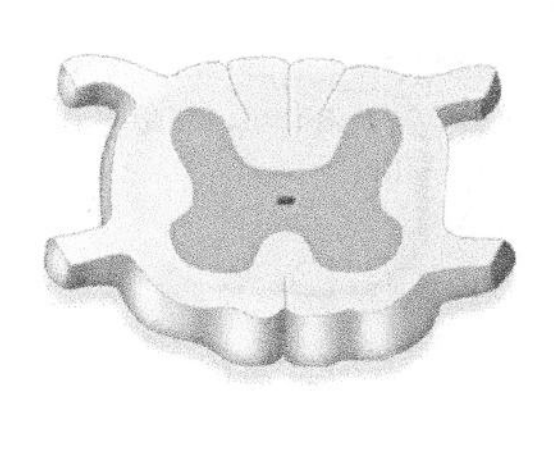

Transmits messages to and from the brain

nerves, p. 418

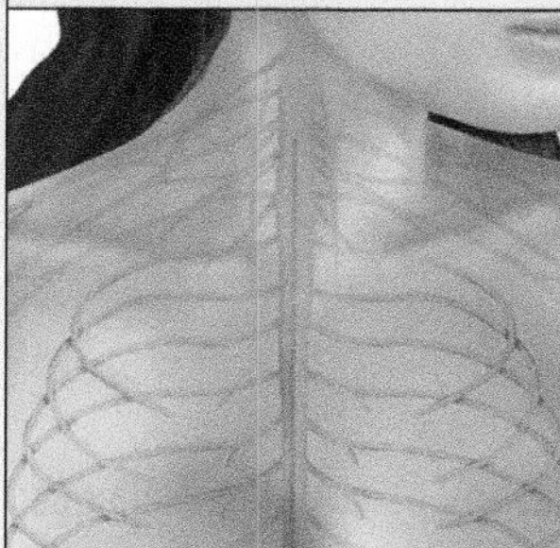

Transmit messages to and from the central nervous system

Anatomy and Physiology of the Nervous System

brain
central nervous system
cranial nerves (KRAY-nee-al)
glands
muscles
nerves
peripheral nervous system (per-IF-er-al)
sensory receptors
spinal cord
spinal nerves

The nervous system is responsible for coordinating all the activity of the body. To do this, it first receives information from both external and internal **sensory receptors** and then uses that information to adjust the activity of **muscles** and **glands** to match the needs of the body.

The nervous system can be subdivided into the **central nervous system** (CNS) and the **peripheral nervous system** (PNS). The central nervous system consists of the **brain** and **spinal cord.** Sensory information comes into the central nervous system, where it is processed. Motor messages then exit the central nervous system carrying commands to muscles and glands. The **nerves** of the peripheral nervous system are **cranial nerves** and **spinal nerves.** Sensory nerves carry information to the central nervous system, and motor nerves carry commands away from the central nervous system. All portions of the nervous system are composed of nervous tissue.

MED TERM TIP

Neuroglial tissue received its name as a result of its function. This tissue holds neurons together. Therefore, it was called *neuroglial*, a term literally meaning "nerve glue."

Nervous Tissue

axon (AK-son)
dendrites (DEN-drights)
myelin (MY-eh-lin)
nerve cell body
neuroglial cells (noo-ROH-glee-all)
neuron (NOO-ron)
neurotransmitter (noo-roh-TRANS-mit-ter)
synapse (sih-NAPSE)
synaptic cleft (sih-NAP-tik)

Nervous tissue consists of two basic types of cells: **neurons** and **neuroglial cells.** Neurons are individual nerve cells. These are the cells that are capable of conducting electrical impulses in response to a stimulus. Neurons have three basic parts: **dendrites,** a **nerve cell body,** and an **axon** (see Figure 12.1A ■). Dendrites are highly branched projections that receive impulses. The nerve cell body contains the nucleus and many of the other organelles of the cell (see Figure 12.1B ■). A neuron has only a single axon, a projection from the nerve cell body that conducts the electrical impulse toward its destination. The point at which the axon of one neuron meets the dendrite of the next neuron is called a **synapse.** Electrical impulses cannot pass directly across the gap between two neurons, called the **synaptic cleft.** They instead require the help of a chemical messenger, called a **neurotransmitter.**

A variety of neuroglial cells are found in nervous tissue. Each has a different support function for the neurons. For example, some neuroglial cells produce **myelin,** a fatty substance that acts as insulation for many axons so that they conduct electrical impulses faster. Neuroglial cells *do not* conduct electrical impulses.

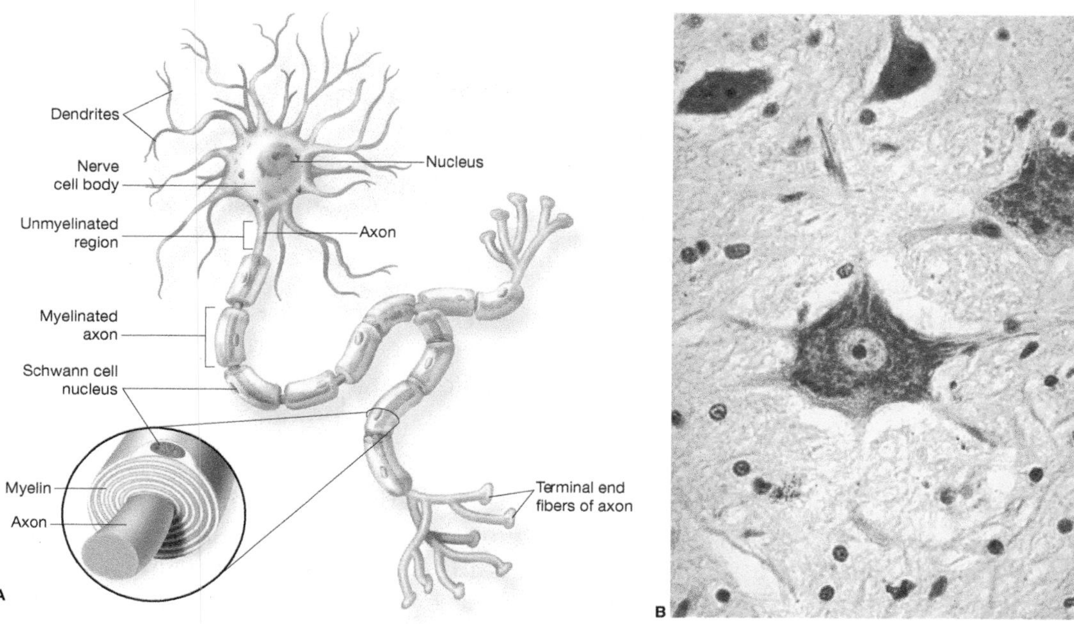

■ **Figure 12.1** (A) The structure of a neuron, showing the dendrites, nerve cell body, and axon. (B) Photomicrograph of typical neuron showing the nerve cell body, nucleus, and dendrites.

Central Nervous System

gray matter
meninges (men-IN-jeez)
myelinated (MY-eh-lih-nayt-ed)
tract
white matter

Because the central nervous system is a combination of the brain and spinal cord, it is able to receive impulses from all over the body, process this information, and then respond with an action. This system consists of both **gray** and **white matter.** Gray matter is comprised of unsheathed or uncovered cell bodies and dendrites. White matter is **myelinated** nerve fibers (see Figure 12.2 ■). The myelin sheath makes the nervous tissue appear white. Bundles of nerve fibers interconnecting different parts of the central nervous system are called **tracts.** The central nervous system is encased and protected by three membranes known as the **meninges.**

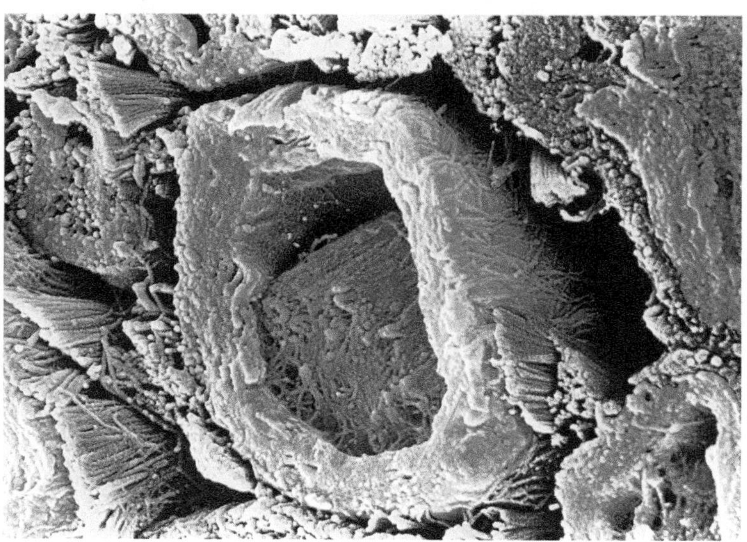

■ **Figure 12.2** Electronmicrograph illustrating an axon (red) wrapped in its myelin sheath (blue). *(Quest/Science Photo Library/Photo Researchers, Inc.)*

MED TERM TIP

Myelin is a lipid and a very white molecule. This is why myelinated neurons are called *white matter.*

The Brain

brain stem
cerebellum (ser-eh-BELL-um)
cerebral cortex (seh-REE-bral / KOR-teks)
cerebral hemisphere
cerebrospinal fluid (ser-eh-broh-SPY-nal)
cerebrum (SER-eh-brum)
diencephalon (dye-en-SEFF-ah-lon)
frontal lobe
gyri (JYE-rye)
hypothalamus (high-poh-THAL-ah-mus)
medulla oblongata (meh-DULL-ah / ob-long-GAH-tah)
midbrain
occipital lobe (ock-SIP-ih-tal)
parietal lobe (pah-RYE-eh-tal)
pons (PONZ)
sulci (SULL-kye)
temporal lobe (TEM-por-al)
thalamus (THAL-ah-mus)
ventricles (VEN-trik-lz)

The brain is one of the largest organs in the body and coordinates most body activities. It is the center for all thought, memory, judgment, and emotion. Each part of the brain is responsible for controlling different body functions, such as temperature regulation, blood pressure, and breathing. There are four sections to the brain: the **cerebrum, cerebellum, diencephalon,** and **brain stem** (see Figure 12.3 ■).

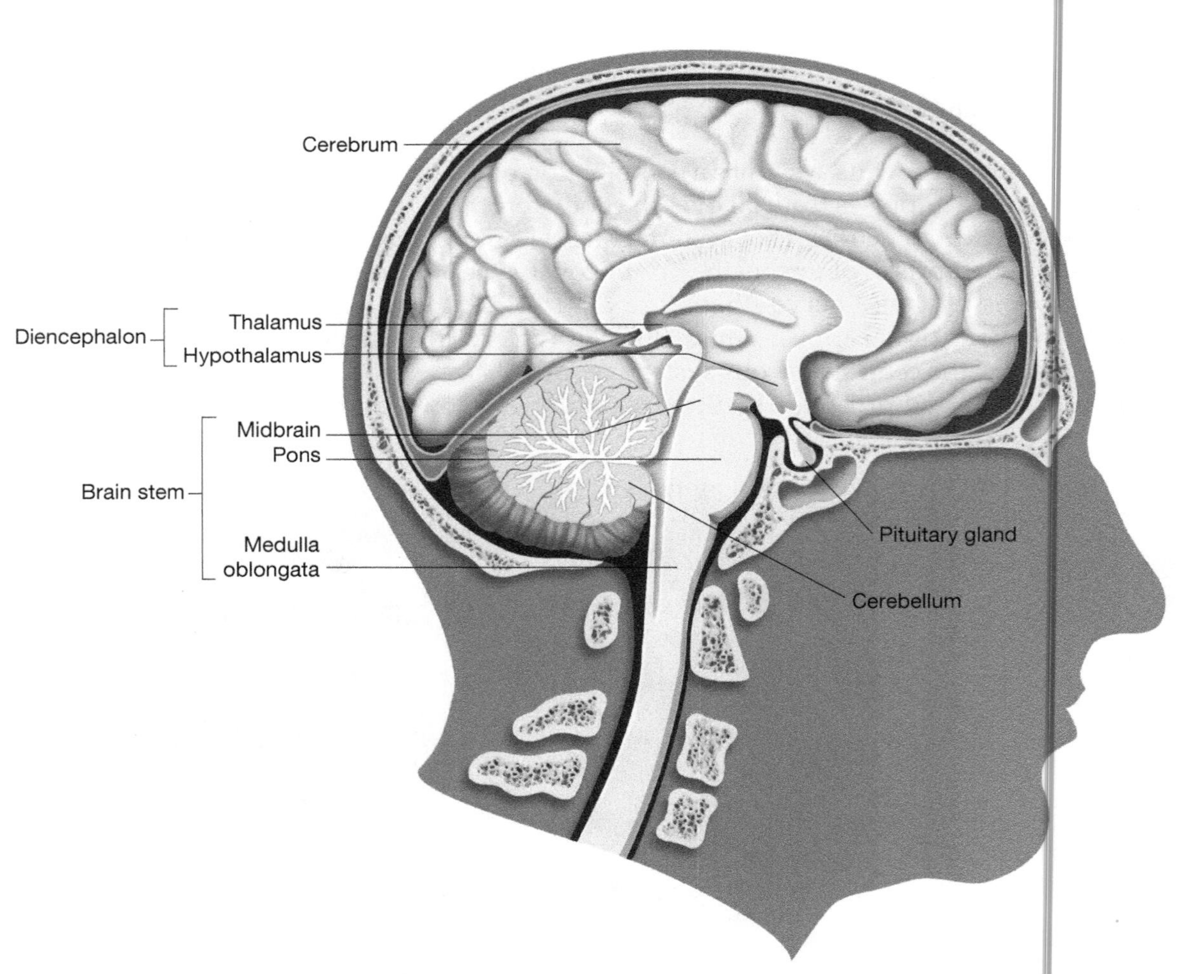

■ **Figure 12.3** The regions of the brain.

The largest section of the brain is the cerebrum. It is located in the upper portion of the brain and is the area that processes thoughts, judgment, memory, problem solving, and language. The outer layer of the cerebrum is the **cerebral cortex,** which is composed of folds of gray matter. The elevated portions of the cerebrum, or convolutions, are called **gyri** and are separated by fissures, or valleys, called **sulci.** The cerebrum is subdivided into left and right halves called **cerebral hemispheres.** Each hemisphere has four lobes. The lobes and their locations and functions are as follows (see Figure 12.4 ■):

1. **Frontal lobe:** Most anterior portion of the cerebrum; controls motor function, personality, and speech
2. **Parietal lobe:** Most superior portion of the cerebrum; receives and interprets nerve impulses from sensory receptors and interprets language
3. **Occipital lobe:** Most posterior portion of the cerebrum; controls vision
4. **Temporal lobe:** Left and right lateral portion of the cerebrum; controls hearing and smell

The diencephalon, located below the cerebrum, contains two of the most critical areas of the brain, the **thalamus** and the **hypothalamus.** The thalamus is composed of gray matter and acts as a center for relaying impulses from the eyes, ears, and skin to the cerebrum. Our pain perception is controlled by the thalamus. The hypothalamus located just below the thalamus controls body temperature, appetite, sleep, sexual desire, and emotions. The hypothalamus is actually responsible for controlling the autonomic nervous system, cardiovascular system, digestive system, and the release of hormones from the pituitary gland.

The cerebellum, the second largest portion of the brain, is located beneath the posterior part of the cerebrum. This part of the brain aids in coordinating voluntary body movements and maintaining balance and equilibrium. The cerebellum refines the muscular movement that is initiated in the cerebrum.

The final portion of the brain is the brain stem. This area has three components: **midbrain, pons,** and **medulla oblongata.** The midbrain acts as a pathway for impulses to

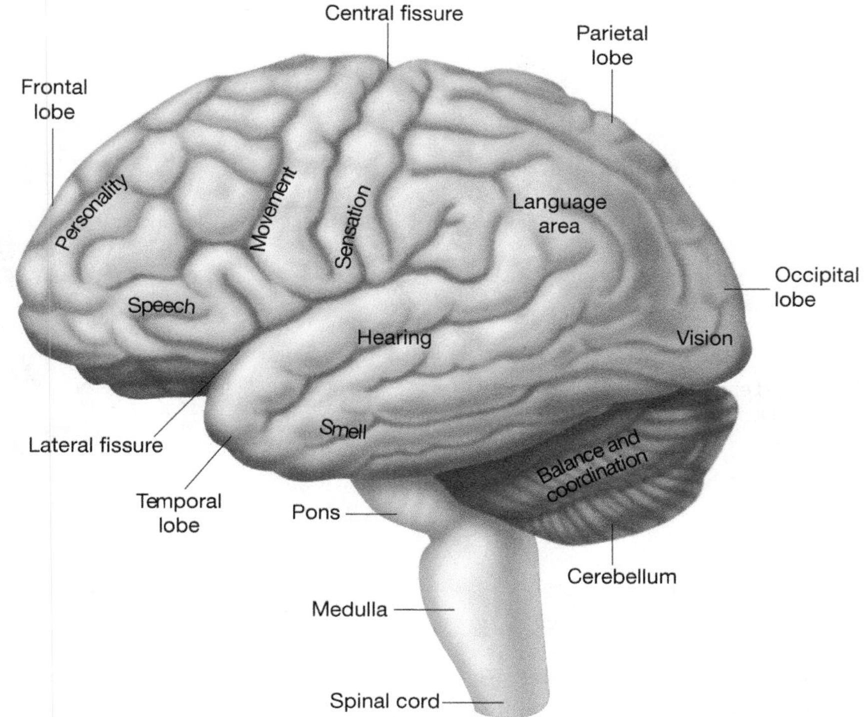

■ **Figure 12.4** The functional regions of the cerebrum.

be conducted between the brain and the spinal cord. The pons—a term meaning bridge—connects the cerebellum to the rest of the brain. The medulla oblongata is the most inferior positioned portion of the brain; it connects the brain to the spinal cord. However, this vital area contains the centers that control respiration, heart rate, temperature, and blood pressure. Additionally, this is the site where nerve tracts cross from one side of the brain to control functions and movement on the other side of the body. In other words, with few exceptions, the left side of the brain controls the right side of the body and vice versa.

The brain has four interconnected cavities called **ventricles:** one in each cerebral hemisphere, one in the thalamus, and one in front of the cerebellum. These contain **cerebrospinal fluid** (CSF), which is the watery, clear fluid that provides protection from shock or sudden motion to the brain and spinal cord.

Spinal Cord

ascending tracts
central canal
descending tracts
spinal cavity
vertebral canal
vertebral column

The function of the spinal cord is to provide a pathway for impulses traveling to and from the brain. The spinal cord is actually a column of nervous tissue extending from the medulla oblongata of the brain down to the level of the second lumbar vertebra within the **vertebral column.** The 33 vertebrae of the backbone line up to form a continuous canal for the spinal cord called the **spinal cavity** or **vertebral canal** (see Figure 12.5 ■).

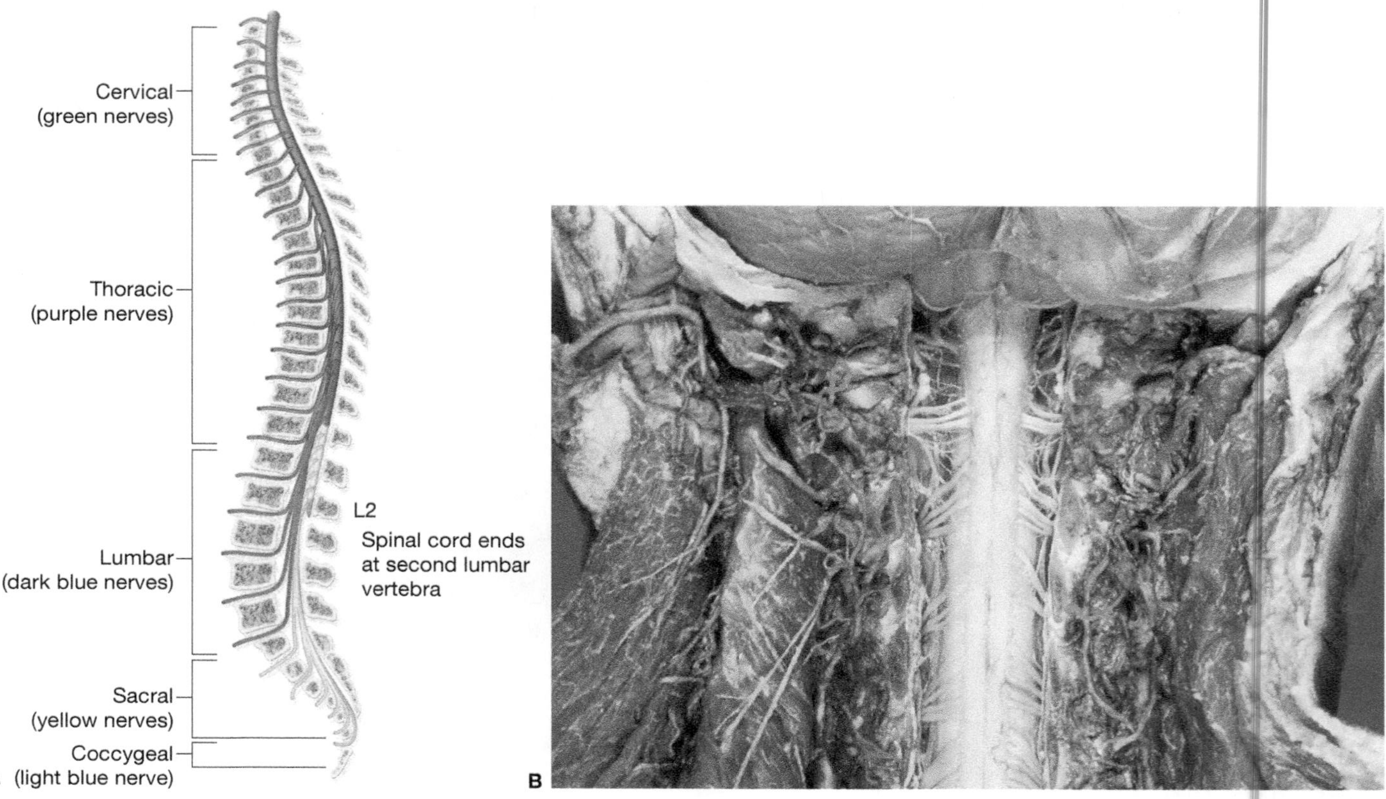

■ **Figure 12.5** (A) The levels of the spinal cord and spinal nerves. (B) Photograph of the spinal cord as it descends from the brain. The spinal nerve roots are clearly visible branching off from the spinal cord. *(Photo Researchers, Inc.)*

Similar to the brain, the spinal cord is also protected by cerebrospinal fluid. It flows down the center of the spinal cord within the **central canal.** The inner core of the spinal cord consists of cell bodies and dendrites of peripheral nerves and therefore is gray matter. The outer portion of the spinal cord is myelinated white matter. The white matter is either **ascending tracts** carrying sensory information up to the brain or **descending tracts** carrying motor commands down from the brain to a peripheral nerve.

Meninges

arachnoid layer (ah-RAK-noyd)
dura mater (DOO-rah / MATE-er)
pia mater (PEE-ah / MATE-er)
subarachnoid space (sub-ah-RAK-noyd)
subdural space (sub-DOO-ral)

The meninges are three layers of connective tissue membranes surrounding the brain and spinal cord (see Figure 12.6 ■). Moving from external to internal, the meninges are:

1. **Dura mater:** Meaning *tough mother;* it forms a tough, fibrous sac around the central nervous system
2. **Subdural space:** Actual space between the dura mater and arachnoid layers
3. **Arachnoid layer:** Meaning *spiderlike;* it is a thin, delicate layer attached to the pia mater by weblike filaments
4. **Subarachnoid space:** Space between the arachnoid layer and the pia mater; it contains cerebrospinal fluid that cushions the brain from the outside
5. **Pia mater:** Meaning *soft mother;* it is the innermost membrane layer and is applied directly to the surface of the brain and spinal cord

MED TERM TIP

Certain disease processes attack the gray matter and the white matter of the central nervous system. For instance, *poliomyelitis* is a viral infection of the gray matter of the spinal cord. The combining term *poli/o* means "gray matter." This disease has almost been eradicated, due to the polio vaccine.

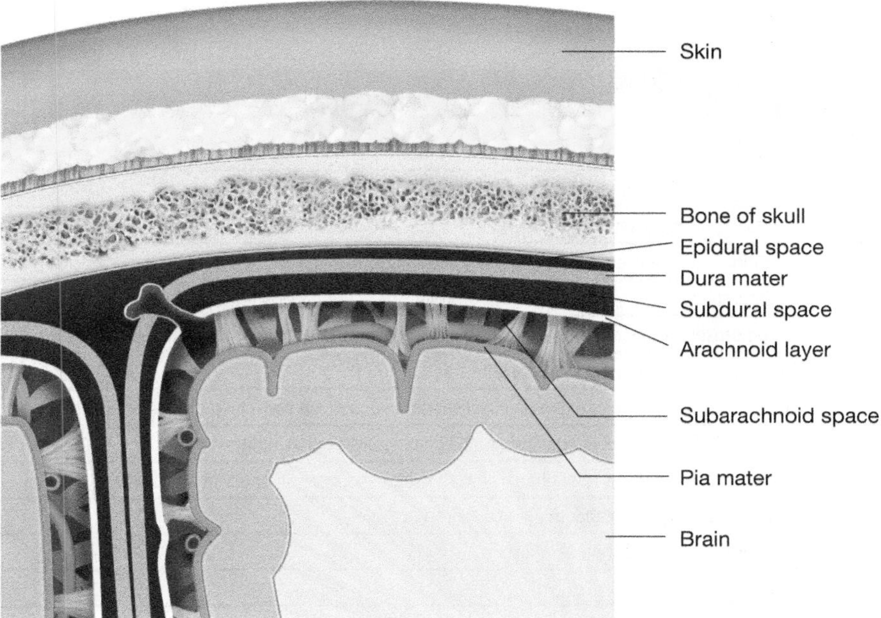

■ **Figure 12.6** The meninges. This figure illustrates the location and structure of each layer of the meninges and their relationship to the skull and brain.

Peripheral Nervous System

afferent neurons (AFF-er-ent)
autonomic nervous system (aw-toh-NOM-ik)
efferent neurons (EFF-er-ent)
ganglion (GANG-lee-on)
motor neurons
nerve root
sensory neurons
somatic nerves

The peripheral nervous system (PNS) includes both the 12 pairs of cranial nerves and the 31 pairs of spinal nerves. A nerve is a group or bundle of axon fibers located outside the central nervous system that carries messages between the central nervous system and the various parts of the body. Whether a nerve is cranial or spinal is determined by where the nerve originates. Cranial nerves arise from the brain, mainly at the medulla oblongata. Spinal nerves split off from the spinal cord, and one pair (a left and a right) exits between each pair of vertebrae. The point where either type of nerve is attached to the central nervous system is called the **nerve root.** The names of most nerves reflect either the organ the nerve serves or the portion of the body the nerve is traveling through. The entire list of cranial nerves is found in Table 12.1 ■. Figure 12.7 ■ illustrates some of the major spinal nerves in the human body.

MED TERM TIP

Because nerve tracts cross from one side of the body to the other side of the brain, damage to one side of the brain results in symptoms appearing on the opposite side of the body. Since nerve cells that control the movement of the right side of the body are located in the left side of the medulla oblongata, a stroke that paralyzed the right side of the body would actually have occurred in the left side of the brain.

Although most nerves carry information to and from the central nervous system, individual neurons carry information in only one direction. **Afferent neurons,** also called **sensory neurons,** carry sensory information from a sensory receptor to the central nervous system. **Efferent neurons,** also called **motor neurons,** carry activity instructions from the central nervous system to muscles or glands out in the body (see Figure 12.8 ■). The nerve cell bodies of the neurons forming the nerve are grouped together in a knot-like mass, called a **ganglion,** located outside the central nervous system.

The nerves of the peripheral nervous system are subdivided into two divisions, the **autonomic nervous system** (ANS) and **somatic nerves,** each serving a different area of the body.

Table 12.1 Cranial Nerves

NUMBER	NAME	FUNCTION
I	Olfactory	Transports impulses for sense of smell
II	Optic	Carries impulses for sense of sight
III	Oculomotor	Motor impulses for eye muscle movement and the pupil of the eye
IV	Trochlear	Controls superior oblique muscle of eye on each side
V	Trigeminal	Carries sensory facial impulses and controls muscles for chewing; branches into eyes, forehead, upper and lower jaw
VI	Abducens	Controls an eyeball muscle to turn eye to side
VII	Facial	Controls facial muscles for expression, salivation, and taste on two-thirds of tongue (anterior)
VIII	Vestibulocochlear	Responsible for impulses of equilibrium and hearing; also called auditory nerve
IX	Glossopharyngeal	Carries sensory impulses from pharynx (swallowing) and taste on one-third of tongue
X	Vagus	Supplies most organs in abdominal and thoracic cavities
XI	Accessory	Controls the neck and shoulder muscles
XII	Hypoglossal	Controls tongue muscles

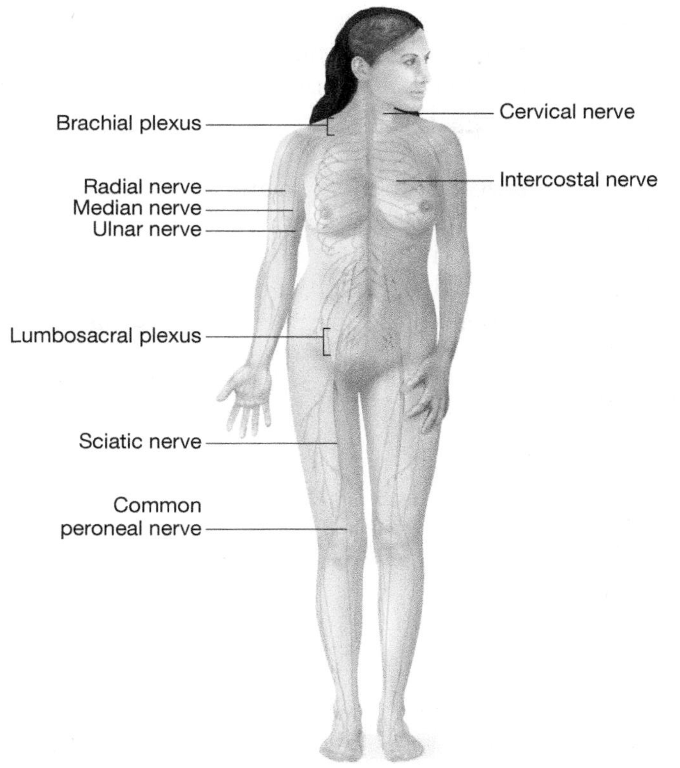

Figure 12.7 The major spinal nerves.

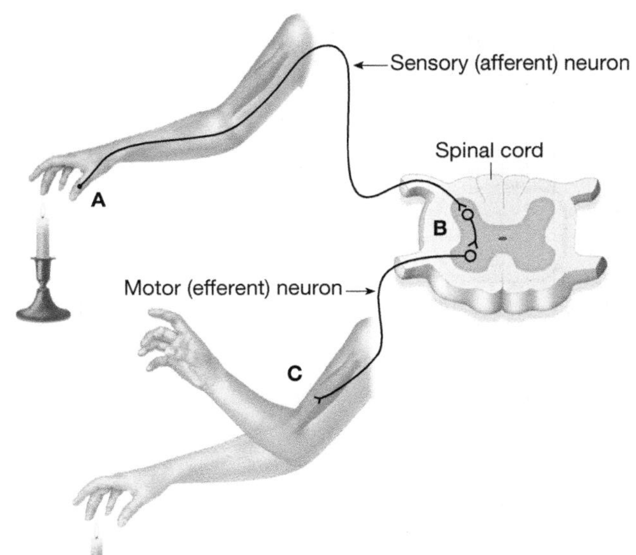

Figure 12.8 The functional structure of the peripheral nervous system. (A) Afferent or sensory neurons carry sensory information to the spinal cord; (B) the spinal cord receives incoming sensory information and delivers motor messages; (C) efferent or motor neurons deliver motor commands to muscles and glands.

Autonomic Nervous System

parasympathetic branch (pair-ah-sim-pah-THET-ik)

sympathetic branch (sim-pah-THET-ik)

The autonomic nervous system is involved with the control of involuntary or unconscious bodily functions. It may increase or decrease the activity of the smooth muscle found in viscera and blood vessels, cardiac muscle, and glands. The autonomic nervous system is divided into two branches: **sympathetic branch** and **parasympathetic branch.** The sympathetic nerves control the "fight or flight" reaction during times of stress and crisis. These nerves increase heart rate, dilate airways, increase blood pressure, inhibit digestion, and stimulate the production of adrenaline during a crisis. The parasympathetic nerves serve as a counterbalance for the sympathetic nerves, the "rest and digest" reaction. Therefore, they cause heart rate to slow down, lower blood pressure, and stimulate digestion.

Somatic Nerves

Somatic nerves serve the skin and skeletal muscles and are mainly involved with the conscious and voluntary activities of the body. The large variety of sensory receptors found in the dermis layer of the skin use somatic nerves to send their information, such as touch, temperature, pressure, and pain, to the brain. These are also the nerves that carry motor commands to skeletal muscles.

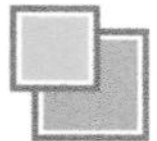

Terminology

Word Parts Used to Build Nervous System Terms

The following lists contain the combining forms, suffixes, and prefixes used to build terms in the remaining sections of this chapter.

Combining Forms

alges/o	sense of pain
angi/o	vessel
arteri/o	artery
astr/o	star
cephal/o	head
cerebell/o	cerebellum
cerebr/o	cerebrum
clon/o	rapid contracting and relaxing
cyt/o	cell
dur/o	dura mater
electr/o	electricity

encephal/o	brain
esthes/o	sensation, feeling
gli/o	glue
hemat/o	blood
isch/o	to hold back
later/o	side
lumb/o	low back
medull/o	medulla oblongata
mening/o	meninges
meningi/o	meninges
my/o	muscle
myel/o	spinal cord

neur/o	nerve
poli/o	gray matter
pont/o	pons
radicul/o	nerve root
scler/o	hard
spin/o	spine
thalam/o	thalamus
thec/o	sheath
tom/o	to cut
ton/o	muscle tone
vascul/o	blood vessel
ventricul/o	ventricle

Suffixes

-al	pertaining to
-algia	pain
-ar	pertaining to
-ary	pertaining to
-asthenia	weakness
-cele	protrusion
-eal	pertaining to
-ectomy	surgical removal
-gram	record
-graphy	process of recording

-ia	condition, state
-ic	pertaining to
-ine	pertaining to
-itis	inflammation
-logy	study of
-nic	pertaining to
-oma	tumor, swelling
-osis	abnormal condition
-otomy	cutting into
-paresis	weakness

-pathy	disease
-phasia	speech
-plasty	surgical repair
-plegia	paralysis
-rrhaphy	suture
-taxia	muscle coordination
-tic	pertaining to
-trophic	pertaining to development

Prefixes

a-	without
an-	without
anti-	against
bi-	two
dys-	abnormal, difficult
endo-	within
epi-	above
hemi-	half
hydro-	water
hyper-	excessive
intra-	within
mono-	one
para-	abnormal, two like parts of a pair
poly-	many
quadri-	four
semi-	partial
sub-	below
un-	not

Anatomical Terms

TERM	WORD PARTS	DEFINITION
cerebellar (ser-eh-BELL-ar)	cerebell/o = cerebellum -ar = pertaining to	Pertaining to the cerebellum.
cerebral (seh-REE-bral)	cerebr/o = cerebrum -al = pertaining to	Pertaining to the cerebrum.
cerebrospinal (ser-eh-broh-SPY-nal)	cerebr/o = cerebrum spin/o = spine -al = pertaining to	Pertaining to the cerebrum and spine.
encephalic (IN-seh-FAL-ik)	encephal/o = brain -ic = pertaining to	Pertaining to the brain.
intrathecal (in-tra-THEE-kal)	intra- = within thec/o = sheath -al = pertaining to	Pertaining to within the meninges, specifically the subdural or subarachnoid space.
medullary (MED-yoo-lair-ee)	medull/o = medulla oblongata -ary = pertaining to	Pertaining to the medulla oblongata.
meningeal (meh-NIN-jee-all)	mening/o = meninges -eal = pertaining to	Pertaining to the meninges.
myelonic (MY-eh-LON-ik)	myel/o = spinal cord -nic = pertaining to	Pertaining to the spinal cord.
neural (NOO-rall)	neur/o = nerve -al = pertaining to	Pertaining to nerves.
neuroglial (noo-RIG-lee-al)	neur/o = nerve gli/o = glue -al = pertaining to	Pertaining to the support cells, glial cells, of nerves.
pontine (pon-TEEN)	pont/o = pons -ine = pertaining to	Pertaining to the pons.
thalamic (tha-LAM-ik)	thalam/o = thalamus -ic = pertaining to	Pertaining to the thalamus.
ventricular (ven-TRIK-yoo-lar)	ventricul/o = ventricle -ar = pertaining to	Pertaining to the ventricles.

Pathology

TERM	WORD PARTS	DEFINITION
Medical Specialties		
anesthesiology (an-es-thee-zee-ol-oh-jee)	an- = without esthes/o = sensation, feeling -logy = study of	Branch of medicine specializing in all aspects of anesthesia, including for surgical procedures, resuscitation measures, and the management of acute and chronic pain. Physician is an *anesthesiologist.*
neurology (noo-rol-oh-jee)	neur/o = nerve -logy = study of	Branch of medicine concerned with diagnosis and treatment of diseases and conditions of the nervous system. Physician is a *neurologist.*
neurosurgery (noo-roh-SIR-jury)	neur/o = nerve	Branch of medicine concerned with treating conditions and diseases of the nervous systems by surgical means. Physician is a *neurosurgeon.*
Signs and Symptoms		
absence seizure		Type of epileptic seizure that lasts only a few seconds to half a minute, characterized by a loss of awareness and an absence of activity. It is formerly known as a *petite mal seizure.*
analgesia (an-al-JEE-zee-ah)	an- = without alges/o = sense of pain -ia = state	Absence of pain.
anesthesia (an-ess-THEE-zee-ah)	an- = without esthes/o = feeling, sensations -ia = condition	Lack of feeling or sensation.
aphasia (ah-FAY-zee-ah)	a- = without -phasia = speech	Inability to communicate verbally or in writing due to damage of the speech or language centers in the brain.
ataxia (ah-TAK-see-ah)	a- = without -taxia = muscle coordination	Lack of muscle coordination.
aura (AW-ruh)		Sensations, such as seeing colors or smelling an unusual odor, that occur just prior to an epileptic seizure or migraine headache.
cephalalgia (seff-al-AL-jee-ah)	cephal/o = head -algia = pain	Headache.
coma (COH-mah)		Profound unconsciousness resulting from an illness or injury.
conscious (KON-shus)		Condition of being awake and aware of surroundings.
convulsion (kon-VULL-shun)		Severe involuntary muscle contractions and relaxations. These have a variety of causes, such as epilepsy, fever, and toxic conditions.

Pathology (continued)

TERM	WORD PARTS	DEFINITION
delirium (dee-LEER-ee-um)		Abnormal mental state characterized by confusion, disorientation, and agitation.
dementia (dee-MEN-she-ah)		Progressive impairment of intellectual function that interferes with performing activities of daily living. Patients have little awareness of their condition. Found in disorders such as Alzheimer's.
dysphasia (dis-FAY-zee-ah)	dys- = abnormal, difficult -phasia = speech	Difficulty communicating verbally or in writing due to damage of the speech or language centers in the brain.
focal seizure (FOE-kal)	-al = pertaining to	Localized seizure often affecting one limb.
hemiparesis (hem-ee-par-EE-sis)	hemi- = half -paresis = weakness	Weakness or loss of motion on one side of the body.
hemiplegia (hem-ee-PLEE-jee-ah)	hemi- = half -plegia = paralysis	Paralysis on only one side of the body.
hyperesthesia (high-per-ess-THEE-zee-ah)	hyper- = excessive esthes/o = feeling, sensations -ia = condition	Abnormally heightened sense of feeling, sense of pain, or sensitivity to touch.
monoparesis (mon-oh-pah-REE-sis)	mono- = one -paresis = weakness	Muscle weakness in one limb.
monoplegia (mon-oh-PLEE-jee-ah)	mono- = one -plegia = paralysis	Paralysis of one limb.
neuralgia (noo-RAL-jee-ah)	neur/o = nerve -algia = pain	Nerve pain.
palsy (PAWL-zee)		Temporary or permanent loss of the ability to control movement.
paralysis (pah-RAL-ih-sis)		Temporary or permanent loss of function or voluntary movement.
paraplegia (pair-ah-PLEE-jee-ah)	para- = two like parts of a pair -plegia = paralysis	Paralysis of the lower portion of the body and both legs.
paresthesia (par-es-THEE-zee-ah)	para- = abnormal esthes/o = sensation, feeling -ia = condition	Abnormal sensation such as burning or tingling.
quadriplegia (kwod-rih-PLEE-jee-ah)	quadri- = four -plegia = paralysis	Paralysis of all four limbs.
seizure (SEE-zyoor)		Sudden, uncontrollable onset of symptoms, such as in an epileptic seizure.
semiconscious (sem-ee-KON-shus)	semi- = partial	State of being aware of surroundings and responding to stimuli only part of the time.

Pathology *(continued)*

TERM	WORD PARTS	DEFINITION
syncope (SIN-koh-pee)		Fainting.
tonic-clonic seizure	ton/o = muscle tone clon/o = rapid contracting and relaxing -ic = pertaining to	Type of severe epileptic seizure characterized by a loss of consciousness and convulsions. The seizure alternates between strong continuous muscle spasms (tonic) and rhythmic muscle contraction and relaxation (clonic). It is also called a *grand mal seizure.*
tremor (TREM-or)		Involuntary repetitive alternating movement of a part of the body.
unconscious (un-KON-shus)	un- = not	State of being unaware of surroundings, with the inability to respond to stimuli.
Brain		
Alzheimer's disease (ALTS-high-merz)		Chronic, organic mental disorder consisting of dementia, which is more prevalent in adults after 65 years of age. Involves progressive disorientation, apathy, speech and gait disturbances, and loss of memory. Named for German neurologist Alois Alzheimer.
astrocytoma (ass-troh-sigh-TOH-mah)	astr/o = star cyt/o = cell -oma = tumor	Tumor of the brain or spinal cord composed of astrocytes, one type of neuroglial cells.
brain tumor		Intracranial mass, either benign or malignant. A benign tumor of the brain can still be fatal since it will grow and cause pressure on normal brain tissue.

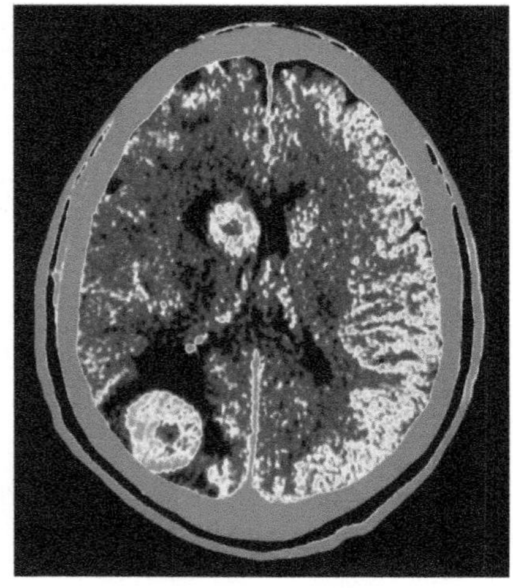

■ **Figure 12.9** Color-enhanced CT scan showing two malignant tumors in the brain. *(Scott Camazine/Photo Researchers, Inc.)*

TERM	WORD PARTS	DEFINITION
cerebellitis (ser-eh-bell-EYE-tis)	cerebell/o = cerebellum -itis = inflammation	Inflammation of the cerebellum.

Pathology *(continued)*

TERM	WORD PARTS	DEFINITION
cerebral aneurysm (AN-yoo-rizm)	cerebr/o = cerebrum -al = pertaining to	Localized abnormal dilation of a blood vessel, usually an artery; the result of a congenital defect or weakness in the wall of the vessel. A ruptured aneurysm is a common cause of a hemorrhagic cerebrovascular accident.

■ **Figure 12.10** Common locations for cerebral artery aneurysms in the Circle of Willis.

TERM	WORD PARTS	DEFINITION
cerebral contusion (kon-TOO-shun)	cerebr/o = cerebrum -al = pertaining to	Bruising of the brain from a blow or impact.
cerebral palsy (CP) (ser-REE-bral / PAWL-zee)	cerebr/o = cerebrum -al = pertaining to	Brain damage resulting from a defect, trauma, infection, or lack of oxygen before, during, or shortly after birth.
cerebrovascular accident (CVA) (ser-eh-broh-VASS-kyoo-lar)	cerebr/o = cerebrum vascul/o = blood vessel -ar = pertaining to	Development of an infarct due to loss in the blood supply to an area of the brain. Blood flow can be interrupted by a ruptured blood vessel (hemorrhage), a floating clot (embolus), a stationary clot (thrombosis), or compression. The extent of damage depends on the size and location of the infarct and often includes dysphasia and hemiplegia. Commonly called a *stroke.*

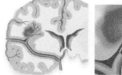

Cerebral hemorrhage: Cerebral artery ruptures and bleeds into brain tissue.

Cerebral embolism: Embolus from another area lodges in cerebral artery and blocks blood flow.

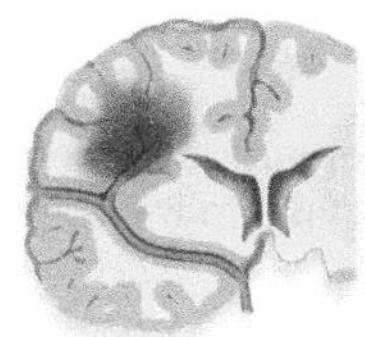

Cerebral thrombosis: Blood clot forms in cerebral artery and blocks blood flow.

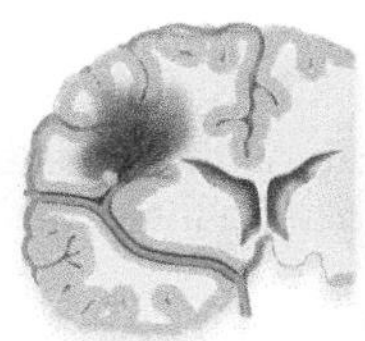

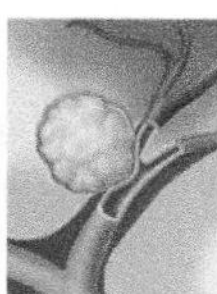

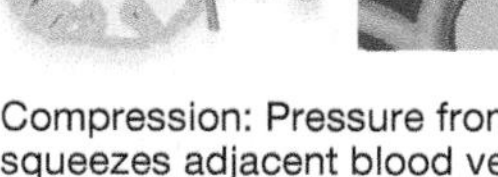

Compression: Pressure from tumor squeezes adjacent blood vessel and blocks blood flow.

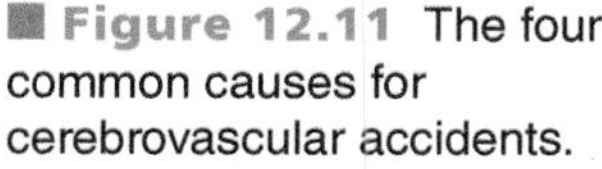

■ **Figure 12.11** The four common causes for cerebrovascular accidents.

Pathology *(continued)*

TERM	WORD PARTS	DEFINITION
concussion (kon-KUSH-un)		Injury to the brain resulting from the brain being shaken inside the skull from a blow or impact. Symptoms vary and may include: headache, blurred vision, nausea or vomiting, dizziness, and balance problems. Also called *mild traumatic brain injury* (TBI).
encephalitis (en-seff-ah-LYE-tis)	encephal/o = brain -itis = inflammation	Inflammation of the brain.
epilepsy (EP-ih-lep-see)		Recurrent disorder of the brain in which seizures and loss of consciousness occur as a result of uncontrolled electrical activity of the neurons in the brain.
hydrocephalus (high-droh-SEFF-ah-lus)	hydro- = water cephal/o = head	Accumulation of cerebrospinal fluid within the ventricles of the brain, causing the head to be enlarged. It is treated by creating an artificial shunt for the fluid to leave the brain. If left untreated, it may lead to seizures and mental retardation.

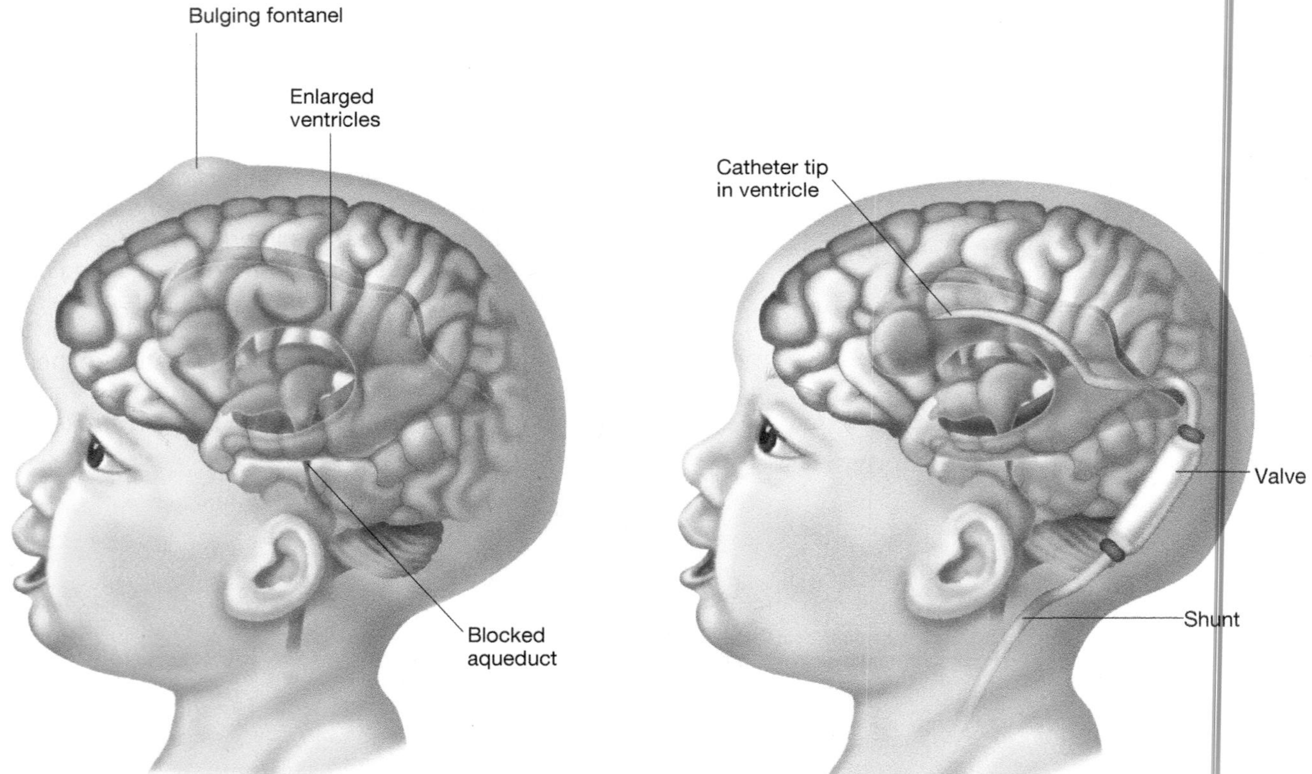

■ **Figure 12.12** Hydrocephalus. The figure on the left is a child with the enlarged ventricles of hydrocephalus. The figure on the right is the same child with a shunt to send the excess cerebrospinal fluid to the abdominal cavity.

Pathology *(continued)*

TERM	WORD PARTS	DEFINITION
migraine (MY-grain)		Specific type of headache characterized by severe head pain, sensitivity to light, dizziness, and nausea.
Parkinson's disease (PARK-in-sons)		Chronic disorder of the nervous system with fine tremors, muscular weakness, rigidity, and a shuffling gait. Named for British physician Sir James Parkinson.
Reye syndrome (RISE / SIN-drohm)		Combination of symptoms first recognized by Australian pathologist R. D. K. Reye that includes acute encephalopathy and damage to various organs, especially the liver. This occurs in children under age 15 who have had a viral infection. It is also associated with taking aspirin. For this reason, it's not recommended for children to use aspirin.
transient ischemic attack (TIA) (TRAN-shent / iss-KEM-ik)	isch/o = to hold back hem/o = blood -ic = pertaining to	Temporary interference with blood supply to the brain, causing neurological symptoms such as dizziness, numbness, and hemiparesis. May eventually lead to a full-blown stroke (cerebrovascular accident).
Spinal Cord		
amyotrophic lateral sclerosis (ALS) (ah-my-oh-TROFF-ik / LAT-er-al / skleh-ROH-sis)	a- = without my/o = muscle -trophic = pertaining to development later/o = side -al = pertaining to scler/o = hard -osis = abnormal condition	Disease with muscular weakness and atrophy due to degeneration of motor neurons of the spinal cord. Also called *Lou Gehrig's disease,* after the New York Yankees baseball player who died from the disease.
meningocele (men-IN-goh-seel)	mening/o = meninges -cele = protrusion	Congenital condition in which the meninges protrude through an opening in the vertebral column (see Figure 12.13B ■). See *spina bifida.*
myelitis (my-eh-LYE-tis)	myel/o = spinal cord -itis = inflammation	Inflammation of the spinal cord.
myelomeningocele (my-eh-loh-meh-NIN-goh-seel)	myel/o = spinal cord mening/o = meninges -cele = protrusion	Congenital condition in which the meninges and spinal cord protrude through an opening in the vertebral column (see Figure 12.13C ■). See *spina bifida.*
poliomyelitis (poh-lee-oh-my-eh-lye-tis)	poli/o = gray matter myel/o = spinal cord -itis = inflammation	Viral inflammation of the gray matter of the spinal cord. Results in varying degrees of paralysis; may be mild and reversible or may be severe and permanent. This disease has been almost eliminated due to the discovery of a vaccine in the 1950s.

Pathology *(continued)*

TERM	WORD PARTS	DEFINITION
spina bifida (SPY-nah / BIFF-ih-dah)	spin/o = spine bi- = two	Congenital defect in the walls of the spinal canal in which the laminae of the vertebra do not meet or close (see Figure 12.13A ■). May result in a meningocele or a myelomeningocele—meninges or the spinal cord being pushed through the opening.

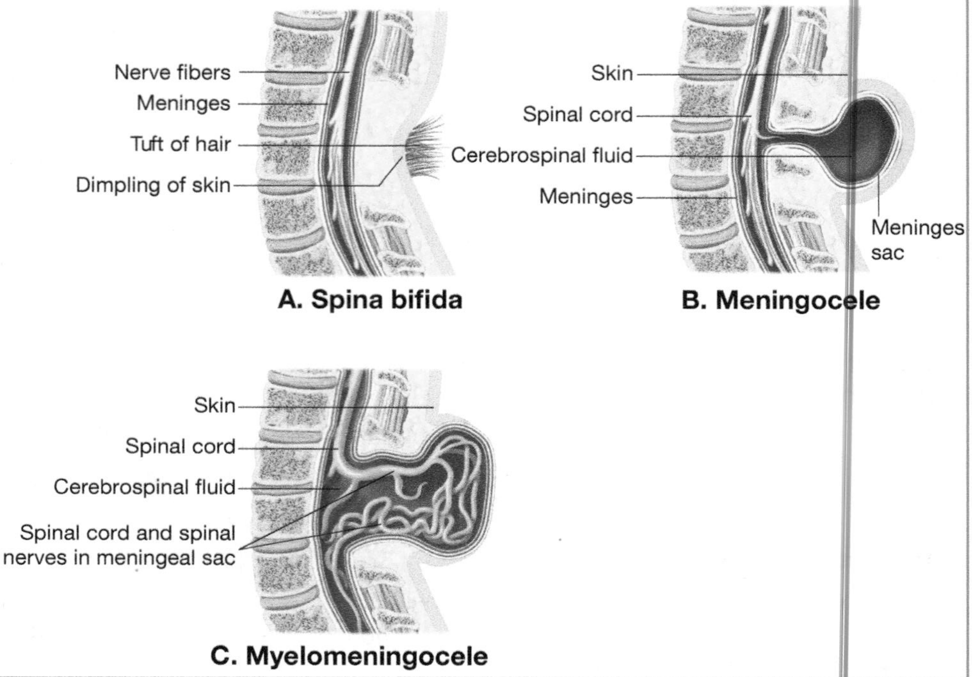

■ **Figure 12.13** Spina bifida. (A) Spina bifica occulta; the vertebra is not complete, but there is no protrusion of nervous system structures. (B) Meningocele; the meninges sac protrudes through the opening in the vertebra. (C) Myelomeningocele; the meninges sac and spinal cord protrude through the opening in the vertebra.

TERM	WORD PARTS	DEFINITION
spinal cord injury (SCI)	spin/o = spine -al = pertaining to	Damage to the spinal cord as a result of trauma. Spinal cord may be bruised or completely severed.
Nerves		
Bell's palsy (BELLZ / PAWL-zee)		One-sided facial paralysis due to inflammation of the facial nerve, probably viral in nature. The patient cannot control salivation, tearing of the eyes, or expression, but most will eventually recover.
Guillain-Barré syndrome (GHEE-yan / bah-RAY)		Disease of the nervous system in which nerves lose their myelin covering. May be caused by an autoimmune reaction. Characterized by loss of sensation and/or muscle control starting in the legs. Symptoms then move toward the trunk and may even result in paralysis of the diaphragm.
multiple sclerosis (MS) (MULL-tih-pl / skleh-ROH-sis)	scler/o = hard -osis = abnormal condition	Inflammatory disease of the central nervous system in which there is extreme weakness and numbness due to loss of myelin insulation from nerves.
myasthenia gravis (my-ass-THEE-nee-ah / GRAV-iss)	my/o = muscle -asthenia = weakness	Disease with severe muscular weakness and fatigue due to insufficient neurotransmitter at a synapse.

Pathology *(continued)*

TERM	WORD PARTS	DEFINITION
neuroma (noo-ROH-mah)	neur/o = nerve -oma = tumor	Nerve tumor or tumor of the connective tissue sheath around a nerve.
neuropathy (noo-ROP-ah-thee)	neur/o = nerve -pathy = disease	General term for disease or damage to a nerve.
polyneuritis (pol-ee-noo-RYE-tis)	poly- = many neur/o = nerve -itis = inflammation	Inflammation of two or more nerves.
radiculitis (rah-dick-yoo-LYE-tis)	radicul/o = nerve root -itis = inflammation	Inflammation of a nerve root; may be caused by a herniated nucleus pulposus.
radiculopathy (rah-dick-yoo-LOP-ah-thee)	radicul/o = nerve root -pathy = disease	Refers to the condition that occurs when a herniated nucleus pulposus puts pressure on a nerve root. Symptoms include pain and numbness along the path of the affected nerve.
shingles (SHING-lz)		Eruption of painful blisters on the body along a nerve path. Thought to be caused by a *Herpes zoster* virus infection of the nerve root.

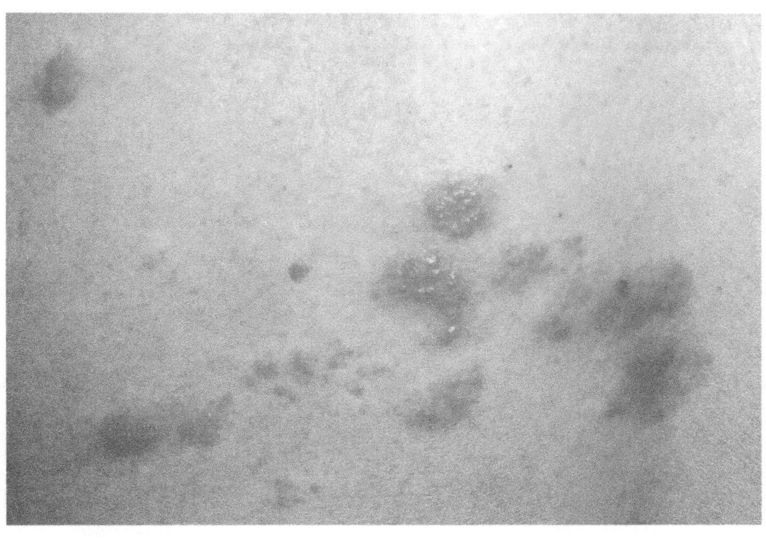

Figure 12.14 Photograph of the skin eruptions associated with shingles. *(Stephen VanHorn/ Shutterstock)*

TERM	WORD PARTS	DEFINITION
Meninges		
epidural hematoma (ep-ih-DOO-ral / hee-mah-TOH-mah)	epi- = above dur/o = dura mater -al = pertaining to hemat/o = blood -oma = swelling	Mass of blood in the space outside the dura mater of the brain and spinal cord.
meningioma (meh-nin-jee-OH-mah)	meningi/o = meninges -oma = tumor	A tumor in the meninges.
meningitis (men-in-JYE-tis)	mening/o = meninges -itis = inflammation	Inflammation of the meninges around the brain or spinal cord caused by bacterial or viral infection. Symptoms include fever, headache, neck stiffness, lethargy, vomiting, irritability, and photophobia.

Pathology (continued)

TERM	WORD PARTS	DEFINITION
subdural hematoma (sub-DOO-ral / hee-mah-TOH-mah)	sub- = below dur/o = dura mater -al = pertaining to hemat/o = blood -oma = swelling	Mass of blood forming beneath the dura mater if the meninges are torn by trauma. May exert fatal pressure on the brain if the hematoma is not drained by surgery.

■ **Figure 12.15** A subdural hematoma. A meningeal vein is ruptured and blood has accumulated in the subdural space, producing pressure on the brain.

Diagnostic Procedures

TERM	WORD PARTS	DEFINITION
Clinical Laboratory Tests		
cerebrospinal fluid analysis (ser-eh-broh-SPY-nal / an-NAL-ih-sis)	cerebr/o = cerebrum spin/o = spine -al = pertaining to	Laboratory examination of the clear, watery, colorless fluid from within the brain and spinal cord. Infections and the abnormal presence of blood can be detected in this test.
Diagnostic Imaging		
brain scan		Image of the brain taken after injection of radioactive isotopes into the circulation.
cerebral angiography (seh-REE-bral / an-jee-OG-rah-fee)	cerebr/o = cerebrum -al = pertaining to angi/o = vessel -graphy = process of recording	X-ray of the blood vessels of the brain after the injection of radiopaque dye.
echoencephalography (ek-oh-en-SEFF-ah-log-rah-fee)	encephal/o = brain -graphy = process of recording	Recording of the ultrasonic echoes of the brain. Useful in determining abnormal patterns of shifting in the brain.
myelogram (MY-eh-loh-gram)	myel/o = spinal cord -gram = record	X-ray record of the spinal cord.

MED TERM TIP

The combining form *myel/o* means "marrow" and is used for both the spinal cord and bone marrow. To the ancient Greek philosophers and physicians, the spinal cord appeared to be much like the marrow found in the medullary cavity of a long bone.

Diagnostic Procedures *(continued)*

TERM	WORD PARTS	DEFINITION
myelography (my-eh-LOG-rah-fee)	myel/o = spinal cord -graphy = process of recording	Injection of radiopaque dye into the spinal canal. An X-ray is then taken to examine the normal and abnormal outlines made by the dye.
positron emission tomography (PET) (PAHZ-ih-tron / ee-MISH-un / toh-MOG-rah-fee)	tom/o = to cut -graphy = process of recording	Image of the brain produced by measuring gamma rays emitted from the brain after injecting glucose tagged with positively charged isotopes. Measurement of glucose uptake by the brain tissue indicates how metabolically active the tissue is.
Additional Diagnostic Tests		
Babinski reflex (bah-BIN-skeez)		Reflex test developed by French neurologist Joseph Babinski to determine lesions and abnormalities in the nervous system. The Babinski reflex is present if the great toe extends instead of flexes when the lateral sole of the foot is stroked. The normal response to this stimulation is flexion of the toe.
electroencephalogram (EEG) (ee-lek-troh-en-SEFF-ah-loh-gram)	electr/o = electricity encephal/o = brain -gram = record	Record of the brain's electrical patterns.
electroencephalography (EEG) (ee-lek-troh-en-SEFF-ah-LOG-rah-fee)	electr/o = electricity encephal/o = brain -graphy = process of recording	Recording the electrical activity of the brain by placing electrodes at various positions on the scalp. Also used in sleep studies to determine if there is a normal pattern of activity during sleep.
lumbar puncture (LP) (LUM-bar / PUNK-chur)	lumb/o = low back -ar = pertaining to	Puncture with a needle into the lumbar area (usually the fourth intervertebral space) to withdraw fluid for examination and for the injection of anesthesia. Also called *spinal puncture* or *spinal tap.*
nerve conduction velocity		Test that measures how fast an impulse travels along a nerve. Can pinpoint an area of nerve damage.

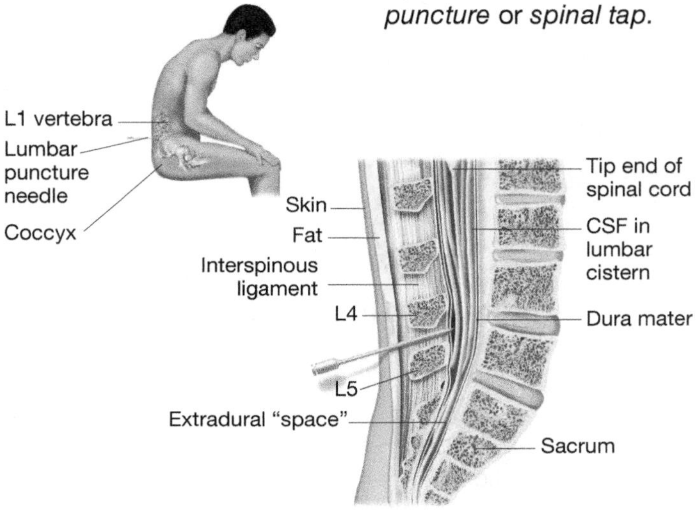

■ **Figure 12.16** A lumbar puncture. The needle is inserted between the lumbar vertebrae and into the spinal canal.

Therapeutic Procedures

TERM	WORD PARTS	DEFINITION
Medical Procedures		
nerve block		Injection of regional anesthetic to stop the passage of sensory or pain impulses along a nerve path.
Surgical Procedures		
carotid endarterectomy (kah-ROT-id / end-ar-ter-EK-toh-mee)	endo- = within arteri/o = artery -ectomy = surgical removal	Surgical procedure for removing an obstruction within the carotid artery, a major artery in the neck that carries oxygenated blood to the brain. Developed to prevent strokes, but is found to be useful only in severe stenosis with transient ischemic attack.
cerebrospinal fluid shunts (ser-eh-bro-SPY-nal)	cerebr/o = cerebrum spin/o = spine -al = pertaining to	Surgical procedure in which a bypass is created to drain cerebrospinal fluid. It is used to treat hydrocephalus by draining the excess cerebrospinal fluid from the brain and diverting it to the abdominal cavity.
laminectomy (lam-ih-NEK-toh-mee)	-ectomy = surgical removal	Removal of a portion of a vertebra, called the lamina, in order to relieve pressure on the spinal nerve.
neurectomy (noo-REK-toh-mee)	neur/o = nerve -ectomy = surgical removal	Surgical removal of a nerve.
neuroplasty (NOOR-oh-plas-tee)	neur/o = nerve -plasty = surgical repair	Surgical repair of a nerve.
neurorrhaphy (noo-ROR-ah-fee)	neur/o = nerve -rrhaphy = suture	To suture a nerve back together. Actually refers to suturing the connective tissue sheath around the nerve.
tractotomy (track-OT-oh-mee)	-otomy = cutting into	Surgical interruption of a nerve tract in the spinal cord. Used to treat intractable pain or muscle spasms.

Pharmacology

CLASSIFICATION	WORD PARTS	ACTION	EXAMPLES
analgesic (an-al-JEE-zik)	an- = without alges/o = sense of pain -ic = pertaining to	Medication to treat minor to moderate pain without loss of consciousness.	aspirin, Bayer, Ecotrin; acetaminophen, Tylenol; ibuprofen, Motrin
anesthetic (an-ess-THET-ik)	an- = without esthes/o = feeling, sensation -tic = pertaining to	Drug that produces a loss of sensation or a loss of consciousness.	lidocaine, Xylocaine; pentobarbital, Nembutal; propofol, Diprivan; procaine, Novocain

Pharmacology *(continued)*

CLASSIFICATION	WORD PARTS	ACTION	EXAMPLES
anticonvulsant (an-tye-kon-VULL-sant)	anti- = against	Substance that reduces the excitability of neurons and therefore prevents the uncontrolled neuron activity associated with seizures.	carbamazepine, Tegretol; phenobarbital, Nembutal
dopaminergic drugs (dope-ah-men-ER-gik)	-ic = pertaining to	Group of medications to treat Parkinson's disease by either replacing the dopamine that is lacking or increasing the strength of the dopamine that is present.	levodopa; L-dopa, Larodopa; levodopa/carbidopa, Sinemet
hypnotic (hip-NOT-tik)	-ic = pertaining to	Drug that promotes sleep.	secobarbital, Seconal; temazepam, Restoril
narcotic analgesic (nar-KOT-tik)	-ic = pertaining to an- = without alges/o = sense of pain -ic = pertaining to	Drug used to treat severe pain; has the potential to be habit forming if taken for a prolonged time. Also called *opiates.*	morphine, MS Contin; oxycodone, OxyContin; meperidine, Demerol
sedative (SED-ah-tiv)		Drug that has a relaxing or calming effect.	amobarbital, Amytal; butabarbital, Butisol

Abbreviations

ALS	amyotrophic lateral sclerosis	**HA**	headache
ANS	autonomic nervous system	**ICP**	intracranial pressure
CNS	central nervous system	**LP**	lumbar puncture
CP	cerebral palsy	**MS**	multiple sclerosis
CSF	cerebrospinal fluid	**PET**	positron emission tomography
CVA	cerebrovascular accident	**PNS**	peripheral nervous system
CVD	cerebrovascular disease	**SCI**	spinal cord injury
EEG	electroencephalogram, electroencephalography	**TBI**	traumatic brain injury
		TIA	transient ischemic attack

Chapter Review

Real-World Applications

Medical Record Analysis

This Discharge Summary contains 12 medical terms. Underline each term and write it in the list below the report. Then define each term.

Discharge Summary

Admitting Diagnosis:	Paraplegia following motorcycle accident.
Final Diagnosis:	Comminuted L2 fracture with epidural hematoma and spinal cord injury resulting in complete paraplegia at the L2 level.
History of Present Illness:	Patient is a 23-year-old male who was involved in a motorcycle accident. He was unconscious for 35 minutes but was fully aware of his surroundings upon regaining consciousness. He was immediately aware of total anesthesia and paralysis below the waist.
Summary of Hospital Course:	CT scan revealed extensive bone destruction at the fracture site and that the spinal cord was severed. Patient was unable to voluntarily contract any lower extremity muscles and was not able to feel touch or pinpricks. Lumbar laminectomy with spinal fusion was performed to stabilize the fracture and remove the epidural hematoma. The immediate postoperative recovery period proceeded normally. Patient began physical therapy and occupational therapy. After 2 months, X-rays indicated full healing of the spinal fusion and patient was transferred to a rehabilitation institute.
Discharge Plans:	Patient was transferred to a rehabilitation institute to continue intensive PT and OT.

	Term	Definition
1	______________	______________________________
2	______________	______________________________
3	______________	______________________________
4	______________	______________________________
5	______________	______________________________
6	______________	______________________________
7	______________	______________________________
8	______________	______________________________
9	______________	______________________________
10	______________	______________________________
11	______________	______________________________
12	______________	______________________________

Chart Note Transcription

The chart note below contains 11 phrases that can be reworded with a medical term that you learned in this chapter. Each phrase is identified with an underline. Determine the medical term and write your answers in the space provided.

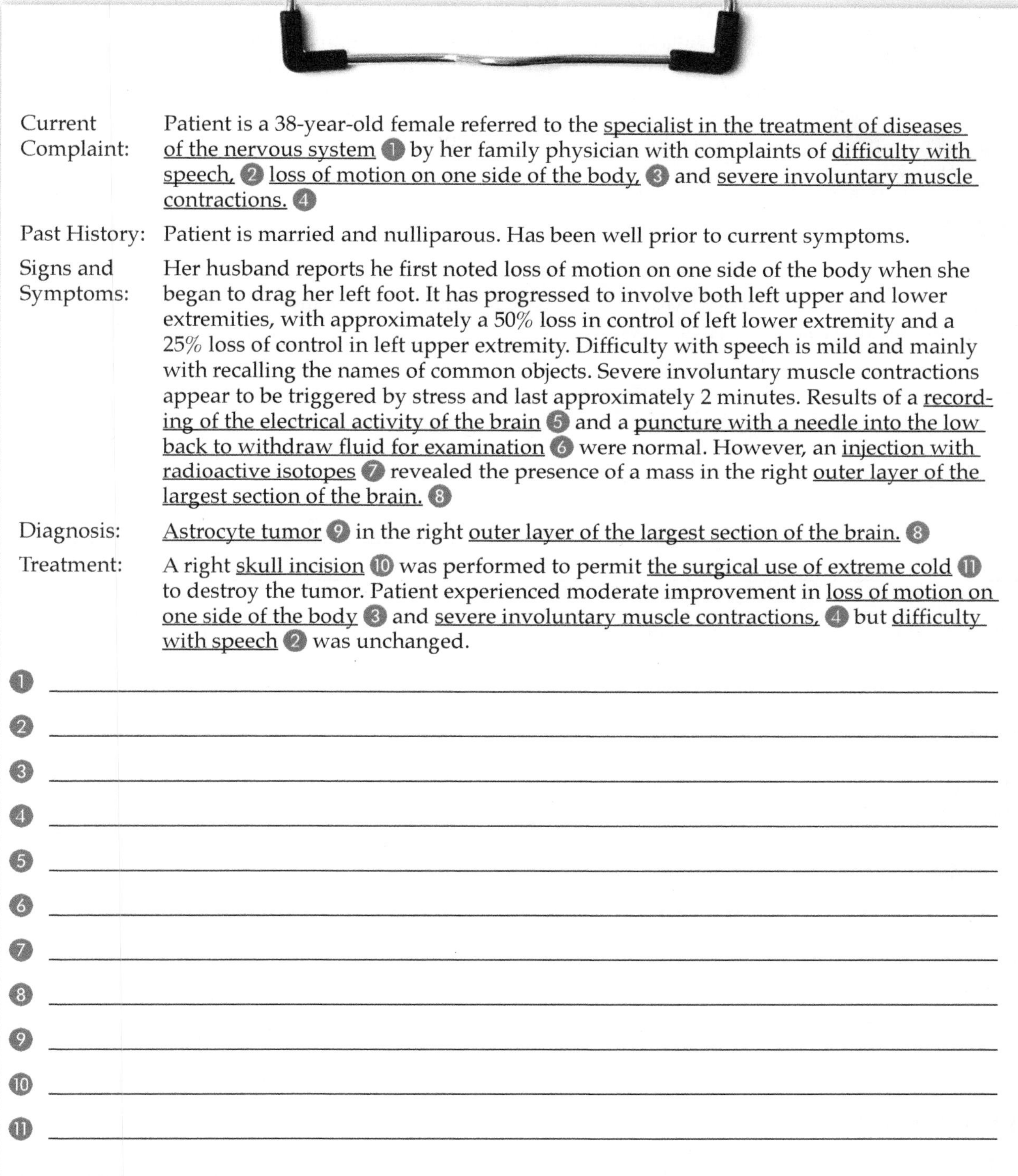

Current Complaint: Patient is a 38-year-old female referred to the specialist in the treatment of diseases of the nervous system (1) by her family physician with complaints of difficulty with speech, (2) loss of motion on one side of the body, (3) and severe involuntary muscle contractions. (4)

Past History: Patient is married and nulliparous. Has been well prior to current symptoms.

Signs and Symptoms: Her husband reports he first noted loss of motion on one side of the body when she began to drag her left foot. It has progressed to involve both left upper and lower extremities, with approximately a 50% loss in control of left lower extremity and a 25% loss of control in left upper extremity. Difficulty with speech is mild and mainly with recalling the names of common objects. Severe involuntary muscle contractions appear to be triggered by stress and last approximately 2 minutes. Results of a recording of the electrical activity of the brain (5) and a puncture with a needle into the low back to withdraw fluid for examination (6) were normal. However, an injection with radioactive isotopes (7) revealed the presence of a mass in the right outer layer of the largest section of the brain. (8)

Diagnosis: Astrocyte tumor (9) in the right outer layer of the largest section of the brain. (8)

Treatment: A right skull incision (10) was performed to permit the surgical use of extreme cold (11) to destroy the tumor. Patient experienced moderate improvement in loss of motion on one side of the body (3) and severe involuntary muscle contractions, (4) but difficulty with speech (2) was unchanged.

(1) ______________________________

(2) ______________________________

(3) ______________________________

(4) ______________________________

(5) ______________________________

(6) ______________________________

(7) ______________________________

(8) ______________________________

(9) ______________________________

(10) ______________________________

(11) ______________________________

Case Study

Below is a case study presentation of a patient with a condition covered in this chapter. Read the case study and answer the questions below. Some questions will ask for information not included within this chapter. Use your text, a medical dictionary, journals, technical materials, multimedia resources, electronic media,, or any other reference material you choose to answer these questions.

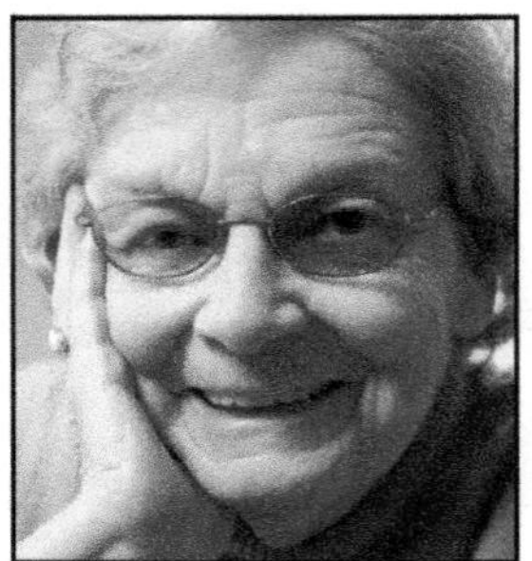
(iofoto/Shutterstock)

Anna Moore, an 83-year-old female, is admitted to the ER with aphasia, hemiparesis on her left side, syncope, and delirium. Her daughter called the ambulance after discovering her mother in this condition at home. Mrs. Moore has a history of hypertension, atherosclerosis, and diabetes mellitus. She was admitted to the hospital after a brain scan revealed an infarct in the right cerebral hemisphere leading to a diagnosis of CVA of the middle cerebral artery.

1. What pathological condition does Ms. Moore have? Look this condition up in a reference source and include a short description of it.

 ____

 ____

2. List and define each of the patient's presenting symptoms in the ER.

 ____

 ____

3. The patient has a history of three significant conditions. Describe each in your own words.

 ____

 ____

4. What diagnostic test did the physician perform? Describe this test and the results in your own words.

 ____

 ____

5. What is an infarct and what causes it?

 ____

 ____

6. List and describe the four common causes of a CVA.

 ____

 ____

Practice Exercises

A. Complete the Statement

1. The study of the nervous system is called ________________________.
2. The organs of the nervous system are the ________________________, ________________________, and ________________________.
3. The two divisions of the nervous system are the ________________________ and ________________________.
4. The neurons that carry impulses away from the brain and spinal cord are called ________________________ neurons.
5. The neurons that carry impulses to the brain and spinal cord are called ________________________ neurons.
6. The largest portion of the brain is the ________________________.
7. The second largest portion of the brain is the ________________________.
8. The occipital lobe controls ________________________.
9. The temporal lobe controls ________________________ and ________________________.
10. The two divisions of the autonomic nervous system are the ________________________ and ________________________.

B. Terminology Matching

Match each term to its definition.

	Term		Definition
1.	_______ olfactory	a.	carries facial sensory impulses
2.	_______ optic	b.	turns eye to side
3.	_______ oculomotor	c.	controls tongue muscles
4.	_______ trochlear	d.	controls eye muscles and pupils
5.	_______ trigeminal	e.	swallowing
6.	_______ abducens	f.	controls facial muscles
7.	_______ facial	g.	controls oblique eye muscles
8.	_______ vestibulocochlear	h.	smell
9.	_______ glossopharyngeal	i.	controls neck and shoulder muscles
10.	_______ vagus	j.	hearing and equilibrium
11.	_______ accessory	k.	vision
12.	_______ hypoglossal	l.	organs in lower body cavities

C. Combining Form Practice

The combining form **neur/o** refers to the nerve. Use it to write a term that means:

1. inflammation of the nerve ______
2. specialist in nerves ______
3. pain in the nerve ______
4. inflammation of many nerves ______
5. removal of a nerve ______
6. surgical repair of a nerve ______
7. nerve tumor ______
8. suture of a nerve ______

The combining form **mening/o** refers to the meninges or membranes. Use it to write a term that means:

9. inflammation of the meninges ______
10. protrusion of the meninges ______
11. protrusion of the spinal cord and the meninges ______

The combining form **encephal/o** refers to the brain. Use it to write a term that means:

12. X-ray record of the brain ______
13. disease of the brain ______
14. inflammation of the brain ______
15. protrusion of the brain ______

The combining form **cerebr/o** refers to the cerebrum. Use it to write a term that means:

16. pertaining to the cerebrum and spinal cord ______
17. pertaining to the cerebrum ______

D. What Does it Stand For?

1. TIA ______
2. MS ______
3. SCI ______
4. CNS ______
5. PNS ______
6. HA ______

7. CP ____________________

8. LP ____________________

9. ALS ____________________

E. Terminology Matching

Match each term to its definition.

1.	_______ aura	a.	loss of ability to control movement
2.	_______ meningitis	b.	sensations before a seizure
3.	_______ coma	c.	seizure with convulsions
4.	_______ shingles	d.	congenital hernia of meninges
5.	_______ syncope	e.	seizure without convulsion
6.	_______ palsy	f.	inflammation of meninges
7.	_______ absence seizure	g.	profound unconsciousness
8.	_______ tonic-clonic seizure	h.	*Herpes zoster* infection
9.	_______ meningocele	i.	fainting

F. What's the Abbreviation?

1. cerebrospinal fluid ____________________
2. cerebrovascular disease ____________________
3. electroencephalogram ____________________
4. intracranial pressure ____________________
5. positron emission tomography ____________________
6. cerebrovascular accident ____________________
7. subarachnoid hemorrhage ____________________
8. autonomic nervous system ____________________

G. Define the Procedures and Tests

1. myelography ______________________________
2. cerebral angiography ______________________________
3. Babinski's reflex ______________________________
4. nerve conduction velocity ______________________________
5. cerebrospinal fluid analysis ______________________________
6. PET scan ______________________________
7. echoencephalography ______________________________
8. lumbar puncture ______________________________

H. Define the Suffix

	Definition	Example from Chapter
1. -plegia		
2. -taxia		
3. -trophic		
4. -paresis		
5. -phasia		

I. Define the Combining Form

	Definition	Example from Chapter Term
1. mening/o		
2. encephal/o		
3. cerebell/o		
4. myel/o		
5. cephal/o		
6. thalam/o		
7. neur/o		
8. radicul/o		
9. cerebr/o		
10. pont/o		

J. Define the Term

1. astrocytoma ______________________________
2. epilepsy ______________________________
3. anesthesia ______________________________
4. hemiparesis ______________________________
5. neurosurgeon ______________________________
6. analgesia ______________________________
7. focal seizure ______________________________
8. quadriplegia ______________________________
9. subdural hematoma ______________________________
10. intrathecal ______________________________

K. Terminology Matching

Match each term to its definition.

1.	_______ neurologist	a.	sudden attack
2.	_______ cerebrovascular accident	b.	a type of severe headache
3.	_______ concussion	c.	loss of intellectual ability
4.	_______ aphasia	d.	physician who treats nervous problem
5.	_______ migraine	e.	stroke
6.	_______ seizure	f.	mild traumatic brain injury
7.	_______ dementia	g.	loss of ability to speak
8.	_______ ataxia	h.	congenital anomaly
9.	_______ spina bifida	i.	state of being unaware
10.	_______ unconscious	j.	lack of muscle coordination

L. Fill in the Blank

Parkinson's disease	transient ischemic attack	cerebral palsy	cerebrospinal fluid shunt
Bell's palsy	subdural hematoma	amyotrophic lateral sclerosis	nerve conduction velocity
delirium	cerebral aneurysm		

1. Dr. Martin noted that the 96-year-old patient suffered from ______________________ when she determined that he was confused, disoriented, and agitated.
2. Lucinda's ______________________ resulted in increasing muscle weakness as the motor neurons in her spinal cord degenerated.
3. The diagnosis of ______________________ was correct because the weakness affected only one side of Charles's face.
4. A cerebral angiogram was ordered because Dr. Larson suspected Mrs. Constantine had a(n) ______________________.
5. Roberta's symptoms included fine tremors, muscular weakness, rigidity, and a shuffling gait, leading to a diagnosis of ______________________.
6. Matthew's hydrocephalus required the placement of a(n) ______________________.
7. Because Mae's hemiparesis was temporary, the final diagnosis was ______________________.
8. Following the car accident, a CT scan showed a(n) ______________________ was putting pressure on the brain, necessitating immediate neurosurgery.
9. Birth trauma resulted in the newborn developing ______________________.
10. A(n) ______________________ test was performed in order to pinpoint the exact position of the nerve damage.

M. Pharmacology Challenge

Fill in the classification for each drug description, then match the brand name.

	Drug Description	Classification	Brand Name
1.	_______ produces loss of sensation	______________________	a. L-Dopa
2.	_______ treats Parkinson's disease	______________________	b. Amytal
3.	_______ promotes sleep	______________________	c. OxyContin
4.	_______ medication for mild pain	______________________	d. Seconal
5.	_______ produces a calming effect	______________________	e. Xylocaine
6.	_______ treats severe pain	______________________	f. Tegretol
7.	_______ treats seizures	______________________	g. Motrin

Labeling Exercise

Image A

Write the labels for this figure on the numbered lines provided.

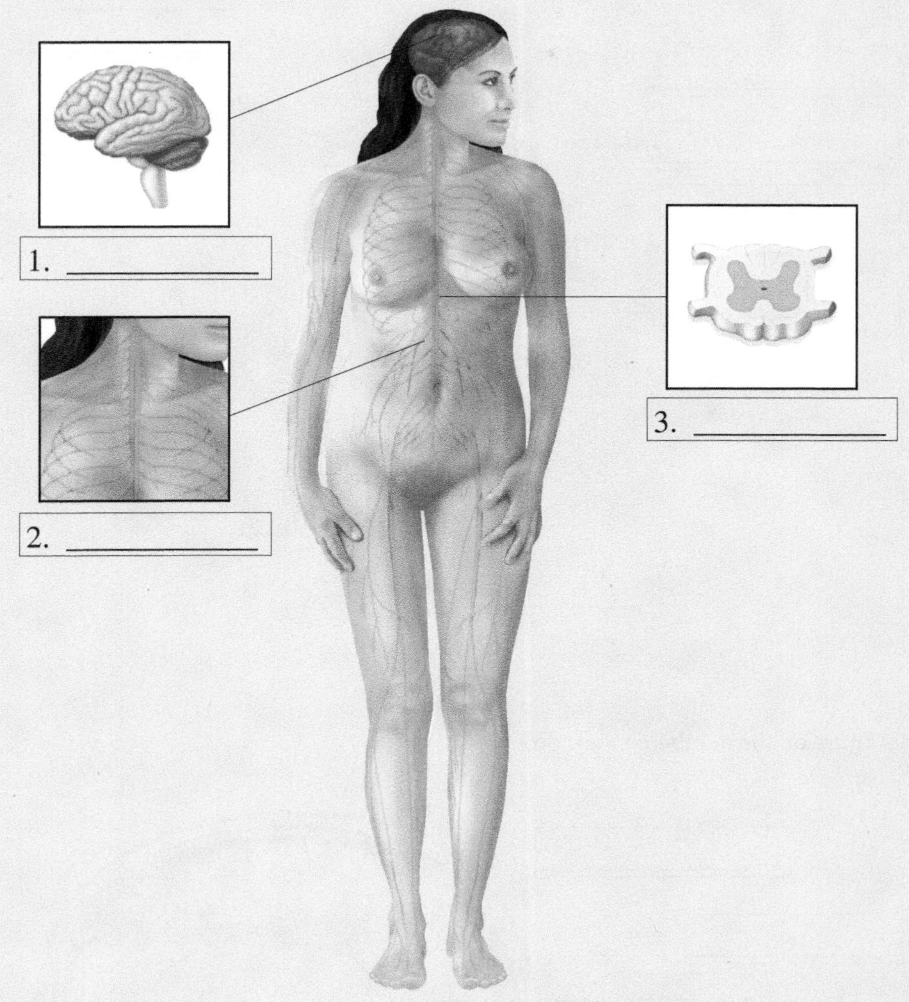

Image B

Write the labels for this figure on the numbered lines provided.

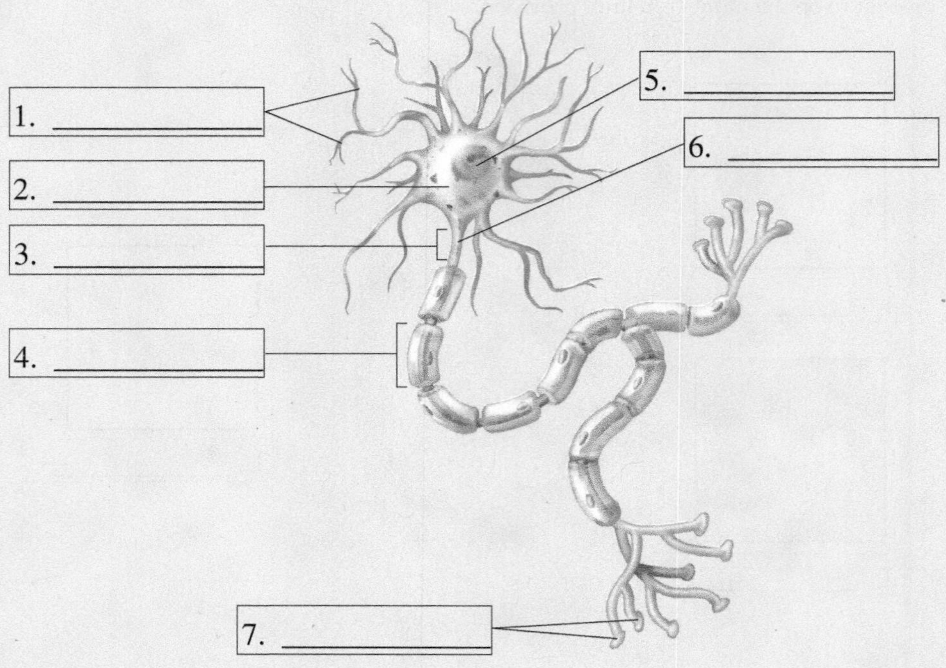

Image C

Write the labels for this figure on the numbered lines provided.

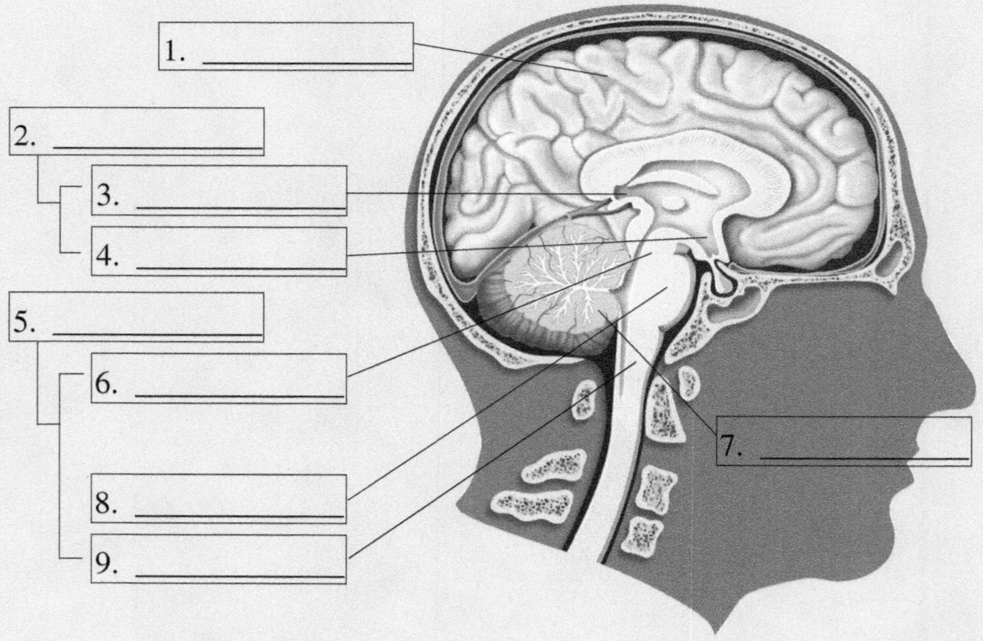

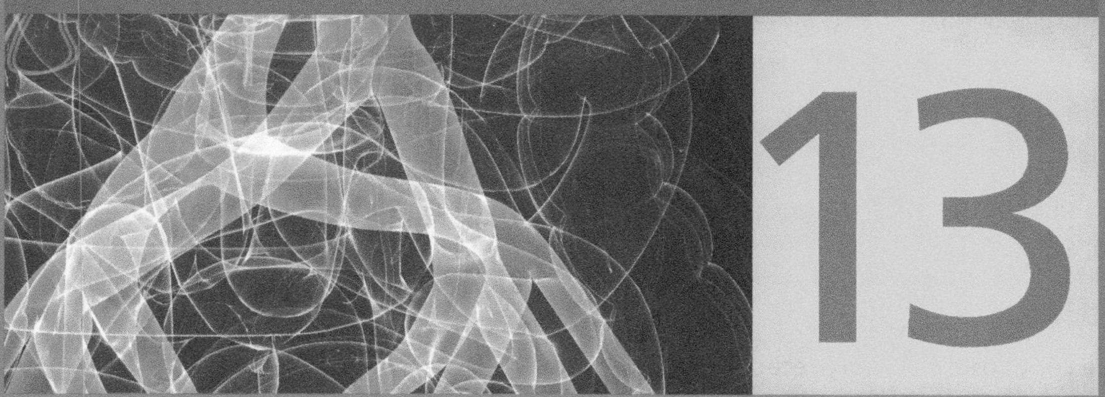

SPECIAL SENSES: THE EYE AND EAR

Learning Objectives

Upon completion of this chapter, you will be able to

- Identify and define the combining forms and suffixes introduced in this chapter.
- Correctly spell and pronounce medical terms and major anatomical structures relating to the eye and ear.
- Locate and describe the major structures of the eye and ear and their functions.
- Describe how we see.
- Describe the path of sound vibration.
- Identify and define eye and ear anatomical terms.
- Identify and define selected eye and ear pathology terms.
- Identify and define selected eye and ear diagnostic procedures.
- Identify and define selected eye and ear therapeutic procedures.
- Identify and define selected medications relating to the eye and ear.
- Define selected abbreviations associated with the eye and ear.

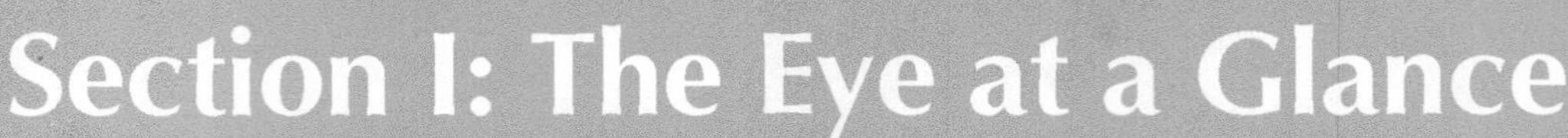

Section I: The Eye at a Glance

Function

The eye contains the sensory receptor cells for vision.

Structures

Here are the primary structures that comprise the eye.

choroid
conjunctiva
eye muscles
eyeball
eyelids
lacrimal apparatus
retina
sclera

Word Parts

Here are the most common word parts (with their meanings) used to build eye terms. For a more comprehensive list, refer to the Terminology section of this chapter.

Combining Forms

ambly/o	dull, dim
aque/o	water
blast/o	immature, embryonic
blephar/o	eyelid
chromat/o	color
conjunctiv/o	conjunctiva
corne/o	cornea
cycl/o	ciliary muscle
dacry/o	tear, tear duct
dipl/o	double
emmetr/o	correct, proper
glauc/o	gray
ir/o	iris
irid/o	iris
kerat/o	cornea
lacrim/o	tears
macul/o	macula lutea
mi/o	lessening
mydr/i	widening
nyctal/o	night
ocul/o	eye
ophthalm/o	eye
opt/o	eye, vision
optic/o	eye, vision
papill/o	optic disk
phac/o	lens
phot/o	light
presby/o	old age
pupill/o	pupil
retin/o	retina
scler/o	sclera
stigmat/o	point
uve/o	choroid
vitre/o	glassy

Suffixes

-ician	specialist
-metrist	specialist in measuring
-opia	vision condition
-opsia	vision condition
-tropia	turned condition

The Eye Illustrated

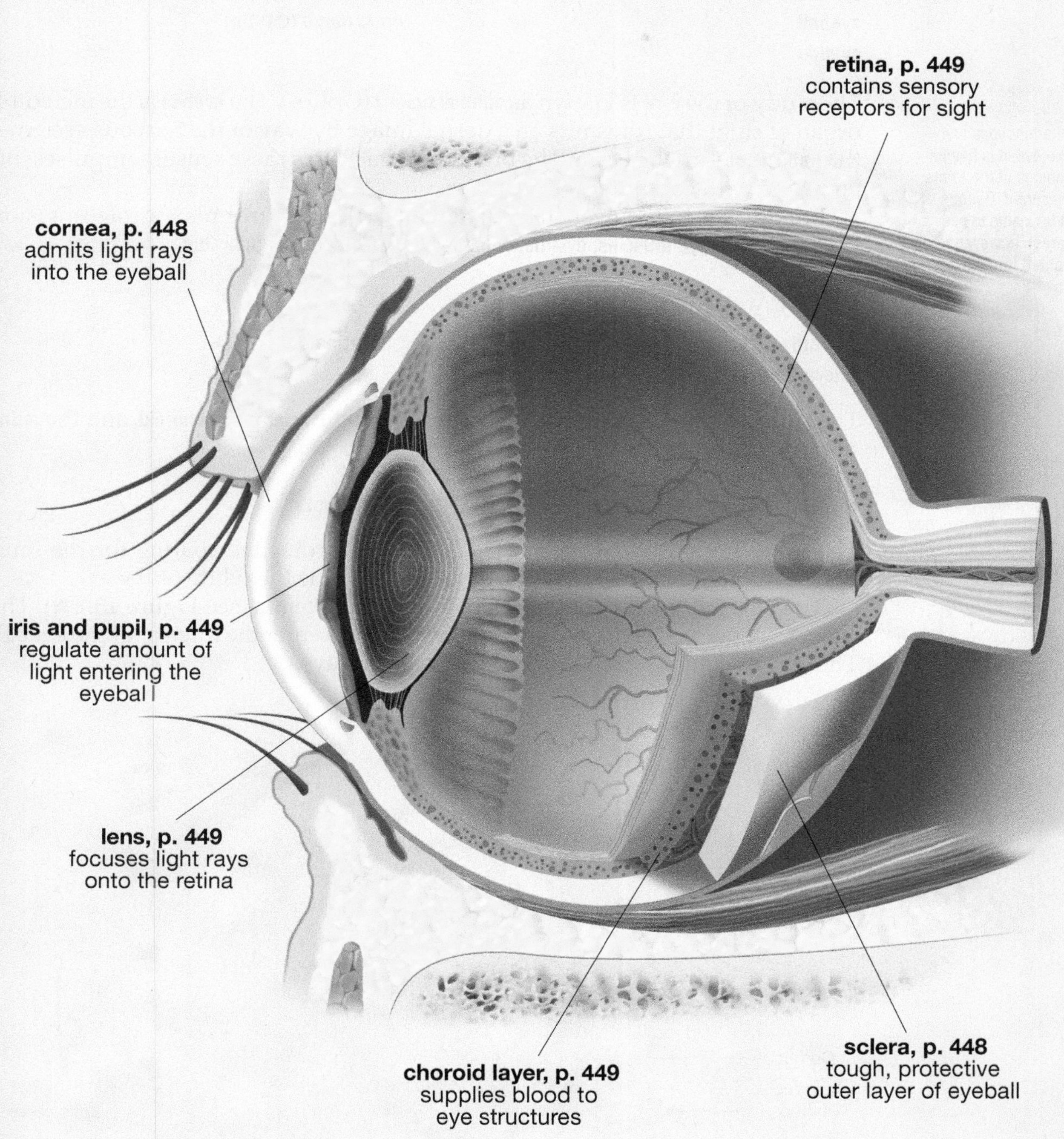

retina, p. 449
contains sensory receptors for sight
cornea, p. 448
admits light rays into the eyeball
iris and pupil, p. 449
regulate amount of light entering the eyeball
lens, p. 449
focuses light rays onto the retina
choroid layer, p. 449
supplies blood to eye structures
sclera, p. 448
tough, protective outer layer of eyeball

Anatomy and Physiology of the Eye

conjunctiva (kon-JUNK-tih-vah)
eye muscles
eyeball
eyelids
lacrimal apparatus (LAK-rim-al)
ophthalmology (off-thal-MALL-oh-gee)
optic nerve (OP-tik)

MED TERM TIP

When studying the functions and terminology of the eye, it is helpful to know the meanings of the terms *opaque* and *transparent.* Opaque means that light is unable to pass through. Transparent, however, means that light is permitted through.

The study of the eye is known as **ophthalmology** (Ophth). The **eyeball** is the incredible organ of sight that transmits an external image by way of the nervous system—the **optic nerve**—to the brain. The brain then translates these sensory impulses into an image with computerlike accuracy.

In addition to the eyeball, several external structures play a role in vision. These are the **eye muscles, eyelids, conjunctiva,** and **lacrimal apparatus.**

The Eyeball

choroid (KOR-oyd)
sclera (SKLAIR-ah)
retina (RET-in-ah)

The actual eyeball is composed of three layers: the **sclera,** the **choroid,** and the **retina.**

MED TERM TIP

The color of the sclera may indicate the presence of disease. For instance, a yellowish cast to the sclera can be present in liver disease and certain anemias.

Sclera

cornea (COR-nee-ah)
refracts

The outer layer, the sclera, provides a tough protective coating for the inner structures of the eye. Another term for the sclera is the white of the eye.

The anterior portion of the sclera is called the **cornea** (see Figure 13.1 ■). This clear, transparent area of the sclera allows light to enter the interior of the eyeball. The cornea actually bends, or **refracts,** the light rays.

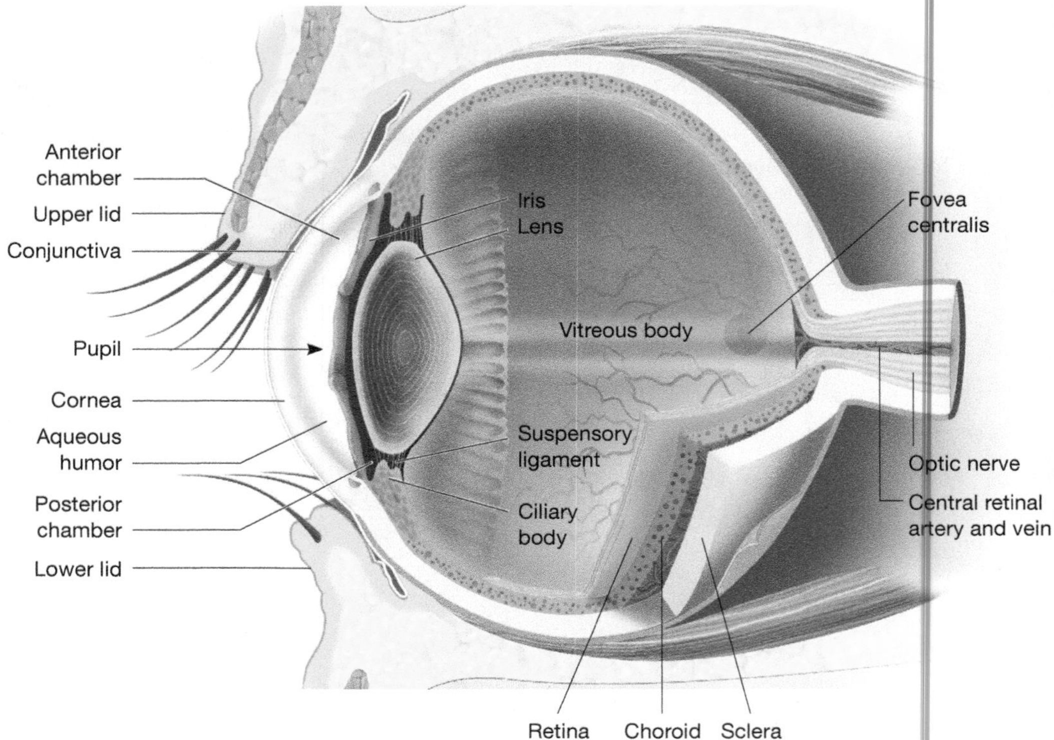

■ **Figure 13.1**
The internal structures of the eye.

Choroid

ciliary body (SIL-ee-ar-ee)
lens
iris
pupil

The second or middle layer of the eyeball is called the choroid. This opaque layer provides the blood supply for the eye.

The anterior portion of the choroid layer consists of the **iris, pupil,** and **ciliary body** (see again Figure 13.1). The iris is the colored portion of the eye and contains smooth muscle. The pupil is the opening in the center of the iris that allows light rays to enter the eyeball. The iris muscle contracts or relaxes to change the size of the pupil, thereby controlling how much light enters the interior of the eyeball. Behind the iris is the **lens.** The lens is not actually part of the choroid layer, but it is attached to the muscular ciliary body. By pulling on the edge of the lens, these muscles change the shape of the lens so it can focus incoming light onto the retina.

MED TERM TIP

The function of the choroid, to provide the rest of the eyeball with blood, is responsible for an alternate name for this layer—*uvea.* The combining form *uve/o* means "vascular."

Retina

aqueous humor (AY-kwee-us)
cones
fovea centralis (FOH-vee-ah / sen-TRAH-lis)
macula lutea (MAK-yoo-lah / loo-TEE-ah)
optic disk
retinal blood vessels (RET-in-al)
rods
vitreous humor (VIT-ree-us)

The third and innermost layer of the eyeball is the retina. It contains the sensory receptor cells (**rods** and **cones**) that respond to light rays. Rods are active in dim light and help us to see in gray tones. Cones are active only in bright light and are responsible for color vision. When one looks directly at an object, the image falls on an area called the **macula lutea,** or yellow spot (see Figure 13.1). In the center of the macula lutea is a depression called the **fovea centralis,** meaning central pit. This pit contains a high concentration of sensory receptor cells and, therefore, is the point of clearest vision. Also visible on the retina is the **optic disk.** This is the point where the **retinal blood vessels** enter and exit the eyeball and where the optic nerve leaves the eyeball (see Figure 13.2 ■). There are no sensory receptor cells in the optic disk and therefore it causes a blind spot in each eye's field of vision. The interior spaces of the eyeball are not empty. The spaces between the cornea and lens are filled with **aqueous humor,** a watery fluid, and the large open area between the lens and retina contains **vitreous humor,** a semisolid gel.

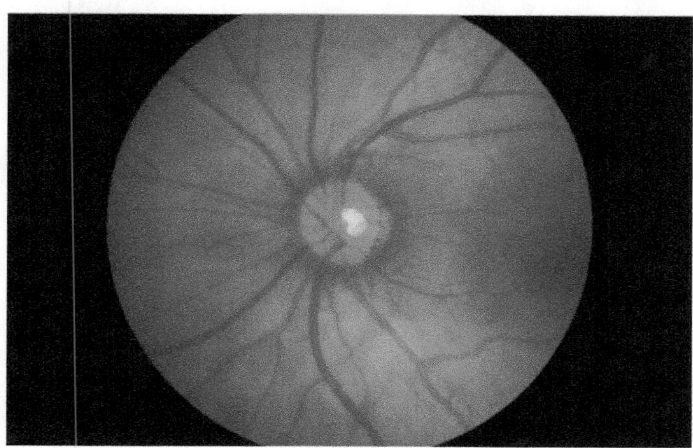

■ **Figure 13.2**
Photograph of the retina of the eye. The optic disk appears yellow and the retinal arteries radiate out from it.

Muscles of the Eye

oblique muscles (oh-BLEEK) **rectus muscles** (REK-tus)

MED TERM TIP

Like many other muscles, the names *rectus* and *oblique* provide clues regarding the direction of their fibers, or their *line of pull.* Rectus means straight and oblique means slanted. Rectus muscles have a straight line of pull. Since the fibers of an oblique muscle are slanted on an angle, they produce rotation.

Six muscles connect the actual eyeball to the skull (see Figure 13.3 ■). These muscles allow for change in the direction of each eye's sightline. In addition, they provide support for the eyeball in the eye socket. Children may be born with a weakness in some of these muscles and may require treatments such as eye exercises or even surgery to correct this problem commonly referred to as crossed eyes or *strabismus* (see Figure 13.4 ■). The muscles involved are the four **rectus** and two **oblique muscles.** Rectus muscles (meaning straight) pull the eye up, down, left, or right in a straight line. Oblique muscles are on an angle and produce diagonal eye movement.

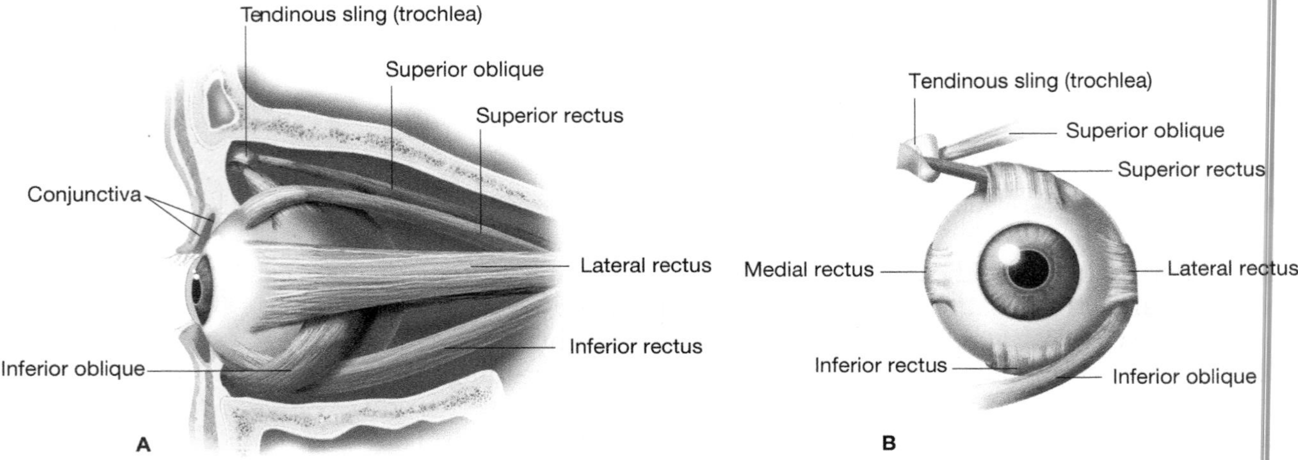

■ **Figure 13.3** The arrangement of the external eye muscles: (A) lateral and (B) anterior views.

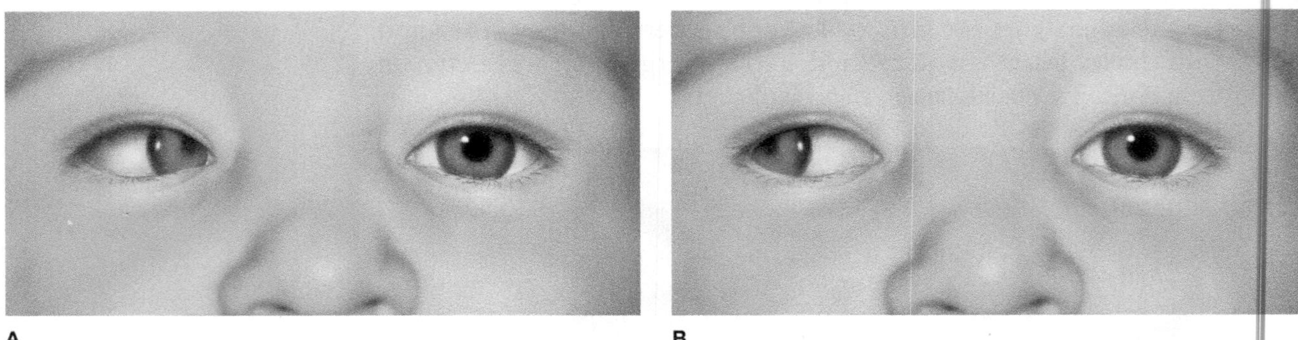

■ **Figure 13.4** Examples of common forms of strabismus: (A) esotropia with the right eye turning inward and (B) exotropia with the right eye turning outward.

The Eyelids

cilia (SIL-ee-ah)
eyelashes
sebaceous glands (see-BAY-shus)

A pair of eyelids over each eyeball provides protection from foreign particles, injury from the sun and intense light, and trauma (see Figure 13.1). Both the upper and lower edges of the eyelids have **eyelashes** or **cilia** that protect the eye from foreign particles. In addition, **sebaceous glands** located in the eyelids secrete lubricating oil onto the eyeball.

Conjunctiva

mucous membrane

The conjunctiva of the eye is a **mucous membrane** lining. It forms a continuous covering on the underside of each eyelid and across the anterior surface of each eyeball (see again Figure 13.1). This serves as protection for the eye by sealing off the eyeball in the socket.

Lacrimal Apparatus

lacrimal ducts
lacrimal gland
nasal cavity
nasolacrimal duct (naz-oh-LAK-rim-al)
tears

The **lacrimal gland** is located under the outer upper corner of each eyelid. These glands produce **tears.** Tears serve the important function of washing and lubricating the anterior surface of the eyeball. **Lacrimal ducts** located in the inner corner of the eye socket then collect the tears and drain them into the **nasolacrimal duct.** This duct ultimately drains the tears into the **nasal cavity** (see Figure 13.5 ■).

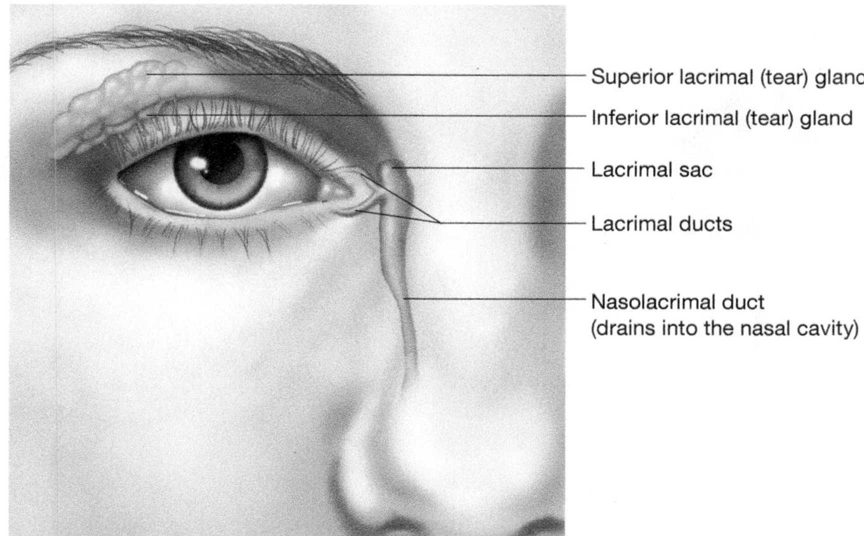

■ **Figure 13.5**
The structure of the lacrimal apparatus.

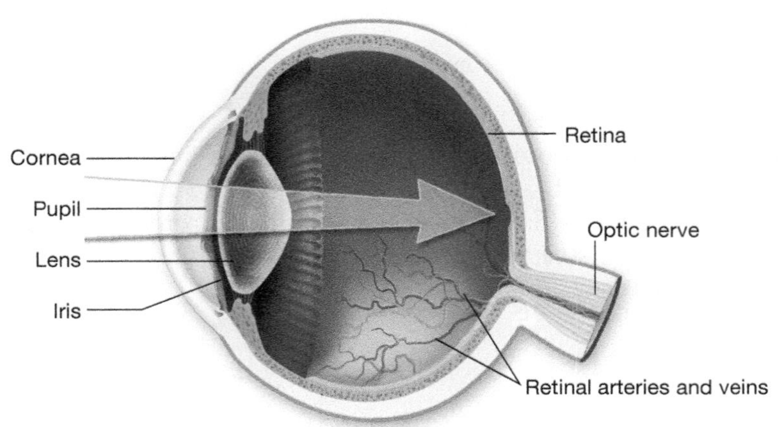

■ **Figure 13.6** The path of light through the cornea, iris, lens, and striking the retina.

How We See

When light rays strike the eye, they first pass through the cornea, pupil, aqueous humor, lens, and vitreous humor (see Figure 13.6 ■). They then strike the retina and stimulate the rods and cones. When the light rays hit the retina, an upside-down image is sent along nerve impulses to the optic nerve (see Figure 13.7 ■). The optic nerve transmits these impulses to the brain, where the upside-down image is translated into the right-side-up image we are looking at.

Vision requires proper functioning of four mechanisms:

1. Coordination of the external eye muscles so that both eyes move together.
2. The correct amount of light admitted by the pupil.
3. The correct focus of light on the retina by the lens.
4. The optic nerve transmitting sensory images to the brain.

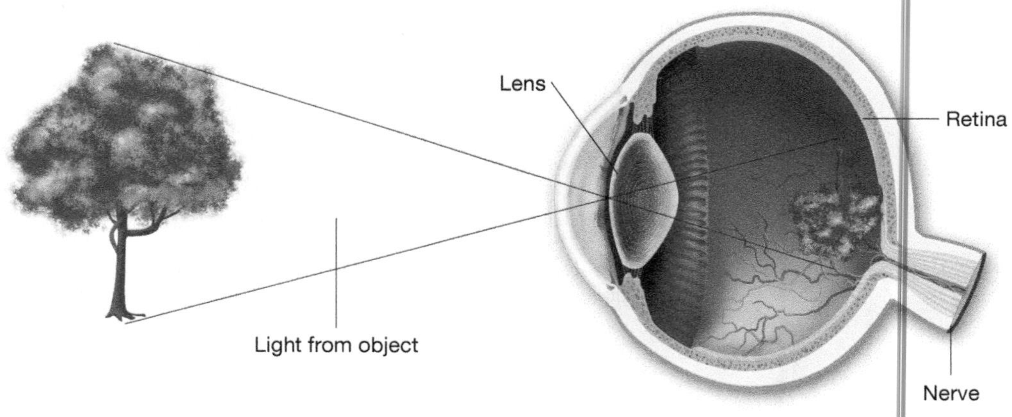

■ **Figure 13.7** The image formed on the retina is inverted. The brain rights the image as part of the interpretation process.

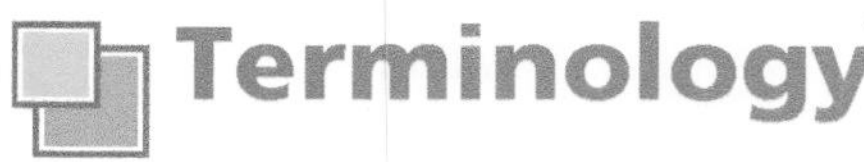

Terminology

Word Parts Used to Build Eye Terms

The following lists contain the combining forms, suffixes, and prefixes used to build terms in the remaining sections of this chapter.

Combining Forms

aden/o	gland
ambly/o	dull, dim
angi/o	vessel
aque/o	water
bi/o	life
blast/o	immature, embryonic
blephar/o	eyelid
chromat/o	color
conjuctiv/o	conjunctiva
corne/o	cornea
cry/o	cold
cycl/o	ciliary body
cyst/o	sac
dacry/o	tears
dipl/o	double
emmetr/o	correct, proper
esthes/o	sensation, feeling
glauc/o	gray
ir/o	iris
irid/o	iris
kerat/o	cornea
lacrim/o	tears
macul/o	macula lutea
mi/o	lessening
myc/o	fungus
mydr/i	widening
nyctal/o	night
ocul/o	eye
ophthalm/o	eye
opt/o	eye, vision
optic/o	eye, vision
papill/o	optic disc
phac/o	lens
phot/o	light
presby/o	old age
pupill/o	pupil
retin/o	retina
scler/o	sclera
stigmat/o	point
ton/o	tone
uve/o	choroid
vitre/o	glassy
xer/o	dry

Suffixes

-al	pertaining to
-algia	pain
-ar	pertaining to
-ary	pertaining to
-atic	pertaining to
-ectomy	surgical removal
-edema	swelling
-graphy	process of recording
-ia	condition
-ic	pertaining to
-ician	specialist
-ism	state of
-itis	inflammation
-logist	one who studies
-logy	study of
-malacia	softening
-meter	instrument to measure
-metrist	specialist in measuring
-metry	process of measuring
-oma	tumor
-opia	vision condition
-opsia	vision condition
-osis	abnormal condition
-otomy	cutting into
-ous	pertaining to
-pathy	disease
-pexy	surgical fixation
-phobia	fear
-plasty	surgical repair
-plegia	paralysis
-ptosis	drooping
-rrhagia	abnormal flow condition
-scope	instrument for viewing
-scopy	process of visually examining
-tic	pertaining to
-tropia	turned condition

Prefixes

a-	without
an-	without
anti-	against
de-	without
eso-	inward

exo-	outward
extra-	outside of
hemi-	half
hyper-	excessive

intra-	within
micro-	small
mono-	one
myo-	to shut

Anatomical Terms

TERM	WORD PARTS	DEFINITION
aqueous (AK-wee-us)	aque/o = water -ous = pertaining to	Pertaining to water or being water-like.
conjunctival (kon-JUNK-tih-vall)	conjuctiv/o = conjunctiva -al = pertaining to	Pertaining to the conjunctiva.
corneal (KOR-nee-all)	corne/o = cornea -al = pertaining to	Pertaining to the cornea. **MED TERM TIP** Word Watch: Be careful using the combining forms *core/o* meaning "pupil" and *corne/o* meaning "cornea."
extraocular (EKS-truh-OK-yoo-lar)	extra- = outside of ocul/o = eye -ar = pertaining to	Pertaining to being outside the eyeball; for example, the extraocular eye muscles.
iridal (ir-id-al)	irid/o = iris -al = pertaining to	Pertaining to the iris.
lacrimal (LAK-rim-al)	lacrim/o = tears -al = pertaining to	Pertaining to tears.
macular (MACK-uoo-lar)	macul/o = macula lutea -ar = pertaining to	Pertaining to the macula lutea.
ocular (OCK-yoo-lar)	ocul/o = eye -ar = pertaining to	Pertaining to the eye.
intraocular (in-trah-OCK-yoo-lar)	intra- = within ocul/o = eye -ar = pertaining to	Pertaining to within the eye.
ophthalmic (off-THAL-mik)	ophthalm/o = eye -ic = pertaining to	Pertaining to the eye.
optic (OP-tik)	opt/o = eye, vision -ic = pertaining to	Pertaining to the eye or vision.
optical (OP-tih-kal)	optic/o = eye, vision -al = pertaining to	Pertaining to the eye or vision.
pupillary (PYOO-pih-lair-ee)	pupill/o = pupil -ary = pertaining to	Pertaining to the pupil.
retinal (RET-in-al)	retin/o = retina -al = pertaining to	Pertaining to the retina.
scleral (SKLAIR-all)	scler/o = sclera -al = pertaining to	Pertaining to the sclera.
uveal (YOO-vee-al)	uve/o = choroid -al = pertaining to	Pertaining to the choroid layer of the eye.
vitreous (VIT-ree-us)	vitre/o = glass -ous = pertaining to	Pertaining to the vitreous humor.

Pathology

TERM	WORD PARTS	DEFINITION
Medical Specialties		
ophthalmologist (opf-thal-MOLL-oh-jist)	ophthalm/o = eye -logist = one who studies	Medical doctor who has specialized in the diagnosis and treatment of eye conditions and diseases.
ophthalmology (opf-thal-MOLL-oh-jee)	ophthalm/o = eye -logy = study of	Branch of medicine involving the diagnosis and treatment of conditions and diseases of the eye and surrounding structures.
optician (op-TISH-an)	opt/o = vision -ician = specialist	Person trained in grinding and fitting corrective lenses.
optometrist (op-TOM-eh-trist)	opt/o = vision -metrist = specialist in measuring	Doctor of optometry.
optometry (op-TOM-eh-tree)	opt/o = vision -metry = process of measuring	Medical profession specializing in examining the eyes, testing visual acuity, and prescribing corrective lenses.
Signs and Symptoms		
blepharoptosis (blef-ah-rop-TOH-sis)	blephar/o = eyelid -ptosis = drooping	Drooping eyelid.
cycloplegia (sigh-kloh-PLEE-jee-ah)	cycl/o = ciliary body -plegia = paralysis	Paralysis of the ciliary body. This affects changing the shape of the lens to bring images into focus.
diplopia (dip-LOH-pee-ah)	dipl/o = double -opia = vision condition	Condition of seeing double.
emmetropia (EM) (em-eh-TROH-pee-ah)	emmetr/o = correct, proper -opia = vision condition	State of normal vision.
iridoplegia (ir-id-oh-PLEE-jee-ah)	irid/o = iris -plegia = paralysis	Paralysis of the iris. This affects changing the size of the pupil to regulate the amount of light entering the eye.
nyctalopia (nik-tah-LOH-pee-ah)	nyctal/o = night -opia = vision condition	Difficulty seeing in dim light; also called *night blindness.* Usually due to damaged rods. **MED TERM TIP** The simple translation of *nyctalopia* is "night vision." However, it is used to mean "night blindness."
ophthalmalgia (off-thal-MAL-jee-ah)	ophthalm/o = eye -algia = pain	Eye pain.
ophthalmoplegia (off-thal-moh-PLEE-jee-ah)	ophthalm/o = eye -plegia = paralysis	Paralysis of one or more of the extraocular eye muscles.
ophthalmorrhagia (off-thal-moh-RAH-jee-ah)	ophthalm/o = eye -rrhagia = abnormal flow condition	Bleeding from the eye.
papilledema (pah-pill-eh-DEEM-ah)	papill/o = optic disc -edema = swelling	Swelling of the optic disk. Often as a result of increased intraocular pressure. Also called *choked disk.*

Pathology *(continued)*

TERM	WORD PARTS	DEFINITION
photophobia (foh-toh-FOH-bee-ah)	phot/o = light -phobia = fear	Although the term translates into *fear of light,* it actually means a strong sensitivity to bright light.
presbyopia (prez-bee-OH-pee-ah)	presby/o = old age -opia = vision condition	Visual loss due to old age, resulting in difficulty in focusing for near vision (such as reading).
scleromalacia (sklair-oh-mah-LAY-she-ah)	scler/o = sclera -malacia = softening	Softening of the sclera.
xerophthalmia (zee-ROP-thal-mee-ah)	xer/o = dry ophthalm/o = eye -ia = condition	Dry eyes.
Eyeball		
achromatopsia (ah-kroh-mah-TOP-see-ah)	a- = without chromat/o = color -opsia = vision condition	Condition of color blindness—unable to perceive one or more colors; more common in males.
amblyopia (am-blee-OH-pee-ah)	ambly/o = dull, dim -opia = vision condition	Loss of vision not as a result of eye pathology. Usually occurs in patients who see two images. In order to see only one image, the brain will no longer recognize the image being sent to it by one of the eyes. May occur if strabismus is not corrected. This condition is not treatable with a prescription lens. Commonly referred to as *lazy eye.*
astigmatism (Astigm) (ah-STIG-mah-tizm)	a- = without stigmat/o = point -ism = state of	Condition in which light rays are focused unevenly on the retina, causing a distorted image, due to an abnormal curvature of the cornea.
cataract (KAT-ah-rakt)		Damage to the lens causing it to become opaque or cloudy, resulting in diminished vision. Treatment is usually surgical removal of the cataract or replacement of the lens.
corneal abrasion	corne/o = cornea -al = pertaining to	Scraping injury to the cornea. If it does not heal, it may develop into an ulcer.
glaucoma (glau-KOH-mah)	glauc/o = gray -oma = mass	Increase in intraocular pressure, which, if untreated, may result in atrophy (wasting away) of the optic nerve and blindness. Glaucoma is treated with medication and surgery. There is an increased risk of developing glaucoma in persons over age 60, of African ancestry, who have sustained a serious eye injury, and in anyone with a family history of diabetes or glaucoma.

MED TERM TIP

The term *cataract* comes from the Latin word meaning "waterfall." This refers to how a person with a cataract sees the world—as if looking through a waterfall.

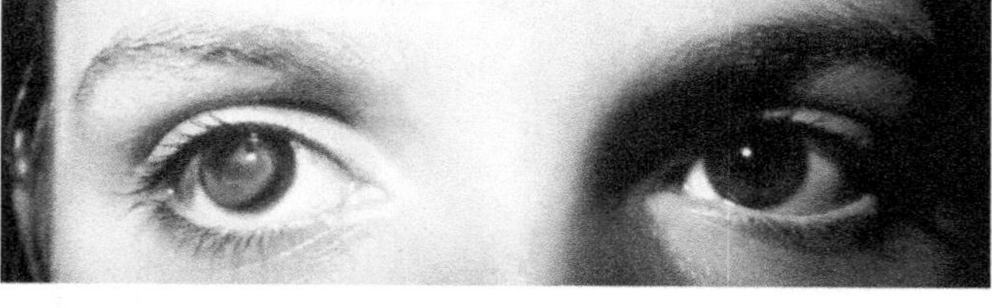

Figure 13.8 Photograph of a person with a cataract in the right eye.

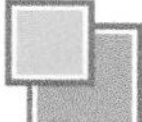

Pathology *(continued)*

TERM	WORD PARTS	DEFINITION
hyperopia (high-per-OH-pee-ah)	hyper- = excessive -opia = vision condition	With this condition a person can see things in the distance but has trouble reading material at close range. Also known as *far-sightedness.* This condition is corrected with converging or biconvex lenses.

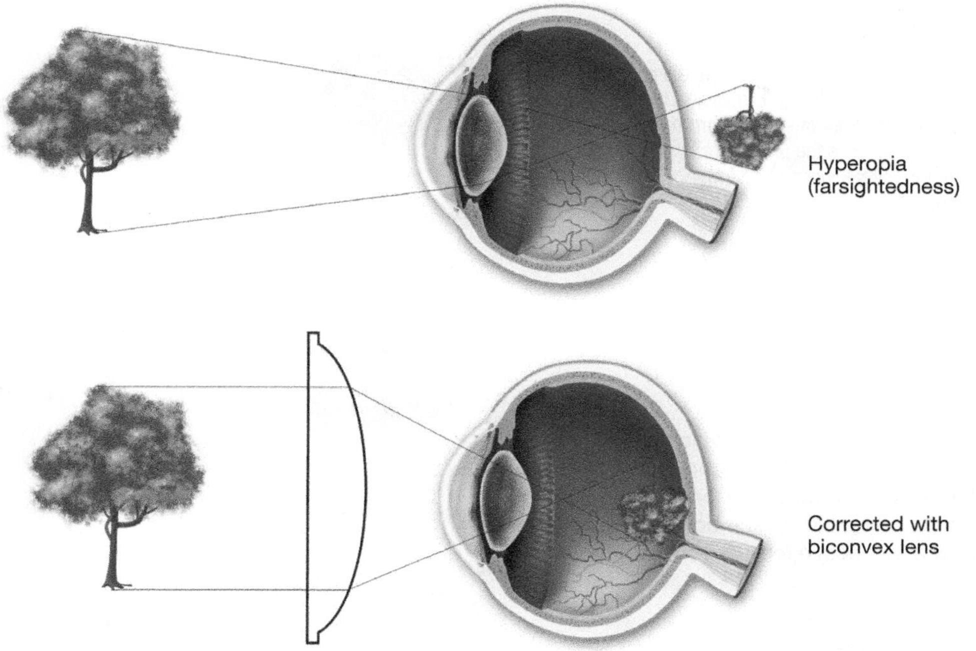

■ **Figure 13.9** Hyperopia (farsightedness). In the uncorrected top figure, the image would come into focus behind the retina, making the image on the retina blurry. The bottom image shows how a biconvex lens corrects this condition.

TERM	WORD PARTS	DEFINITION
iritis (eye-RYE-tis)	ir/o = iris -itis = inflammation	Inflammation of the iris.
keratitis (kair-ah-TYE-tis)	kerat/o = cornea -itis = inflammation	Inflammation of the cornea. **MED TERM TIP** Word Watch: Be careful using the combining form *kerat/o,* which means both "cornea" and "hard protein keratin."
legally blind		Describes a person who has severely impaired vision. Usually defined as having visual acuity of 20/200 that cannot be improved with corrective lenses or having a visual field of less than 20 degrees.
macular degeneration (MAK-yoo-lar)	macul/o = macula lutea -ar = pertaining to	Deterioration of the macular area of the retina of the eye. May be treated with laser surgery to destroy the blood vessels beneath the macula.
monochromatism (mon-oh-KROH-mah-tizm)	mono- = one chromat/o = color -ism = state of	Unable to perceive one color.

Pathology *(continued)*

TERM	WORD PARTS	DEFINITION
myopia (MY) (my-OH-pee-ah)	myo- = to shut -opia = vision condition	With this condition a person can see things close up but distance vision is blurred. Also known as *nearsightedness.* This condition is corrected with diverging or biconcave lenses. Named because persons with myopia often partially shut their eyes, squint, in order to see better.

MED TERM TIP

The term myopia appears to use the combining form, my/o, which means muscle. This combining form comes from the greek word *mys.* But in this case therm uses the prefix myo-, which comes from the Greek word *myo* or *myein,* meaning to shut.

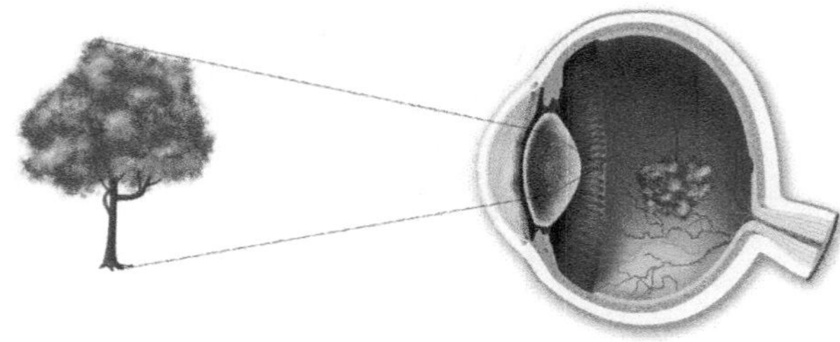

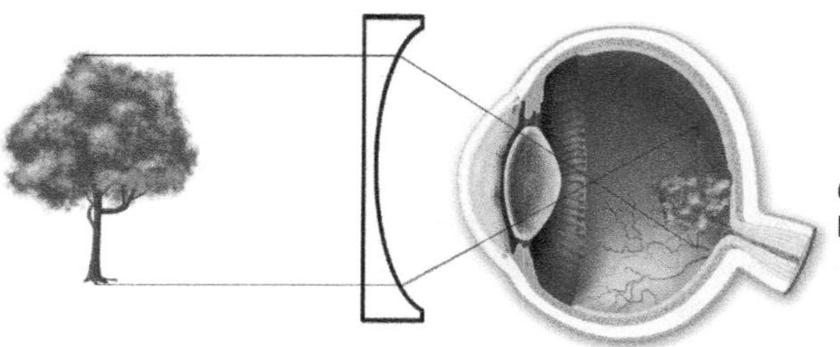

■ **Figure 13.10** Myopia (nearsightedness). In the uncorrected top figure, the image comes into focus in front of the lens, making the image on the retina blurry. The bottom image shows how a biconcave lens corrects this condition.

TERM	WORD PARTS	DEFINITION
oculomycosis (ok-yoo-loh-my-KOH-sis)	ocul/o = eye myc/o = fungus -osis = abnormal condition	Fungus infection of the eye.
retinal detachment (RET-in-al)	retin/o = retina -al = pertaining to	Occurs when the retina becomes separated from the choroid layer. This separation seriously damages blood vessels and nerves, resulting in blindness. May be treated with surgical or medical procedures to stabilize the retina and prevent separation.
retinitis pigmentosa (ret-in-EYE-tis / pig-men-TOH-sah)	retin/o = retina -itis = inflammation	Progressive disease of the eye resulting in the retina becoming hard (sclerosed), pigmented (colored), and atrophying (wasting away). There is no known cure for this condition.
retinoblastoma (RET-in-noh-blast-OH-mah)	retin/o = retina blast/o = immature, embryonic -oma = tumor	Malignant eye tumor occurring in children, usually under the age of 3. Requires enucleation.
retinopathy (ret-in-OP-ah-thee)	retin/o = retina -pathy = disease	General term for disease affecting the retina.
scleritis (skler-EYE-tis)	scler/o = sclera -itis = inflammation	Inflammation of the sclera.

Pathology *(continued)*

TERM	WORD PARTS	DEFINITION
uveitis (yoo-vee-EYE-tis)	uve/o = choroid -itis = inflammation	Inflammation of the choroid layer.
Conjunctiva		
conjunctivitis (kon-junk-tih-VYE-tis)	conjuctiv/o = conjunctiva -itis = inflammation	Inflammation of the conjunctiva usually as the result of a bacterial infection. Commonly called pinkeye.
pterygium (the-RIJ-ee-um)		Hypertrophied conjunctival tissue in the inner corner of the eye.
Eyelids		
blepharitis (blef-ah-RYE-tis)	blephar/o = eyelid -itis = inflammation	Inflammation of the eyelid.
hordeolum (hor-DEE-oh-lum)		Refers to a *stye* (or *sty*), a small purulent inflammatory infection of a sebaceous gland of the eyelid; treated with hot compresses and/or surgical incision.
Lacrimal Apparatus		
dacryoadenitis (dak-ree-oh-ad-eh-NYE-tis)	dacry/o = tears aden/o = gland -itis = inflammation	Inflammation of the lacrimal gland.
dacryocystitis (dak-ree-oh-sis-TYE-tis)	dacry/o = tears cyst/o = sac -itis = inflammation	Inflammation of the lacrimal sac.
Eye Muscles		
esotropia (ST) (ess-oh-TROH-pee-ah)	eso- = inward -tropia = turned condition	Inward turning of the eye; also called *cross-eyed.* An example of a form of strabismus (muscle weakness of the eye).
exotropia (XT) (eks-oh-TROH-pee-ah)	exo- = outward -tropia = turned condition	Outward turning of the eye; also called *wall-eyed.* Also an example of strabismus (muscle weakness of the eye).
strabismus (strah-BIZ-mus)		Eye muscle weakness commonly seen in children resulting in the eyes looking in different directions at the same time. May be corrected with glasses, eye exercises, and/or surgery.
Brain-Related Vision Pathologies		
hemianopia (hem-ee-ah-NOP-ee-ah)	hemi- = half a- = without -opia = vision condition	Loss of vision in half of the visual field. A stroke patient may suffer from this disorder.
nystagmus (niss-TAG-mus)		Jerky-appearing involuntary eye movements, usually left and right. Often an indication of brain injury.

Diagnostic Procedures

TERM	WORD PARTS	DEFINITION
Eye Examination Tests		
color vision tests		Use of polychromic (multicolored) charts to determine the ability of the patient to recognize color.
■ Figure 13.11 An example of color blindness test. A person with red-green color blindness would not be able to distinguish the green 27 from the surrounding red circles.		
fluorescein angiography (floo-oh-RESS-ee-in / an-jee-OG-rah-fee)	angi/o = vessel -graphy = process of recording	Process of injecting a dye (fluorescein) to observe the movement of blood and detect lesions in the macular area of the retina. Used to determine if there is a detachment of the retina.
fluorescein staining (floo-oh-RESS-ee-in)		Applying dye eye drops that are a bright green fluorescent color. Used to look for corneal abrasions or ulcers.
keratometer (KAIR-ah-toh-mee-ter)	kerat/o = cornea -meter = instrument to measure	An instrument used to measure the curvature of the cornea.
keratometry (kair-ah-TOM-eh-tree)	kerat/o = cornea -metry = process of measuring	Measurement of the curvature of the cornea using an instrument called a *keratometer.*
ophthalmoscope (off-THAL-moh-scope)	ophthalm/o = eye -scope = instrument for viewing	Instrument used to examine the inside of the eye through the pupil.
ophthalmoscopy (off-thal-MOSS-koh-pee)	ophthalm/o = eye -scopy = process of visually examining	Examination of the interior of the eyes using an instrument called an *ophthalmoscope* (see Figure 13.12 ■). The physician dilates the pupil in order to see the cornea, lens, and retina. Used to identify abnormalities in the blood vessels of the eye and some systemic diseases.

Diagnostic Procedures *(continued)*

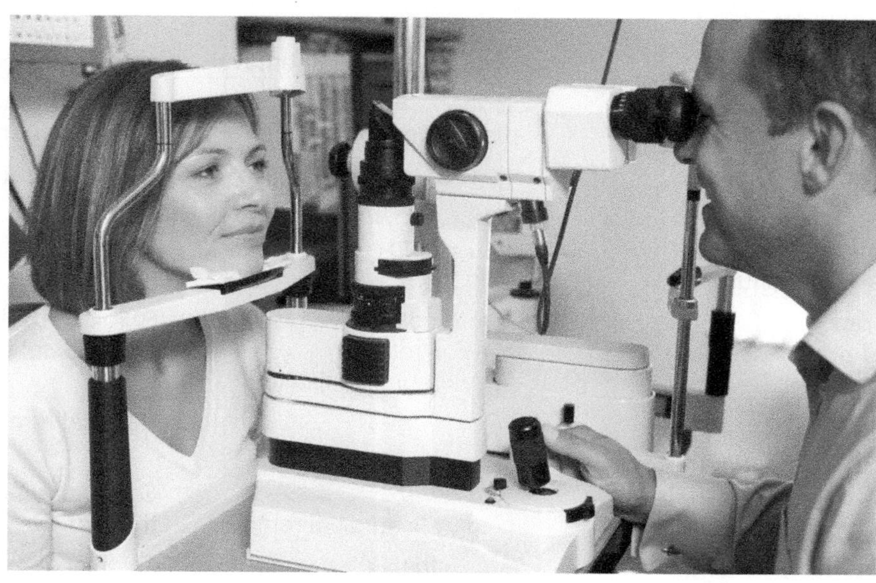

■ **Figure 13.12** Examination of the interior of the eye using an ophthalmoscope. *(Monkey Business Images/Shutterstock)*

TERM	WORD PARTS	DEFINITION
optometer (op-TOM-eh-ter)	opt/o = vision -meter = instrument to measure	Instrument used to measure how well the eye is able to focus images clearly on the retina.
refractive error test (ree-FRAK-tiv)		Vision test for a defect in the ability of the eye to accurately focus the image that is hitting it. Refractive errors result in myopia and hyperopia.
slit lamp microscopy	micro- = small -scopy = process of visually examining	Examining the conjunctiva, cornea, iris and lens of the eye.
Snellen chart (SNEL-enz)		Chart used for testing distance vision named for Dutch ophthalmologist Hermann Snellen. It contains letters of varying size and is administered from a distance of 20 feet. A person who can read at 20 feet what the average person can read at this distance is said to have 20/20 vision.
tonometry (tohn-OM-eh-tree)	ton/o = tone -metry = process of measuring	Measurement of the intraocular pressure of the eye using a *tonometer* to check for the condition of glaucoma. Generally part of a normal eye exam for adults.
visual acuity (VA) **test** (VIZH-oo-al / ah-KYOO-ih-tee)	-al = pertaining to	Measurement of the sharpness of a patient's vision. Usually, a Snellen chart is used for this test in which the patient identifies letters from a distance of 20 feet.

Therapeutic Procedures

TERMS	WORD PARTS	DEFINITION
Surgical Procedures		
blepharectomy (blef-ah-REK-toh-mee)	blephar/o = eyelid -ectomy = surgical removal	Surgical removal of all or part of the eyelid.
blepharoplasty (BLEF-ah-roh-plass-tee)	blephar/o = eyelid -plasty = surgical repair	Surgical repair of the eyelid. A common plastic surgery to correct blepharoptosis.
conjunctivoplasty (kon-junk-tih-VOH-plas-tee)	conjuctiv/o = conjunctiva -plasty = surgical repair	Surgical repair of the conjunctiva.
cryoextraction (cry-oh-eks-TRAK-shun)	cry/o = cold	Procedure in which cataract is lifted from the lens with an extremely cold probe.
cryoretinopexy (cry-oh-RET-ih-noh-pek-see)	cry/o = cold retin/o = retina -pexy = surgical fixation	Surgical fixation of the retina by using extreme cold.
enucleation (ee-new-klee-AH-shun)		Surgical removal of an eyeball.
iridectomy (ir-id-EK-toh-mee)	irid/o = iris -ectomy = surgical removal	Surgical removal of a small portion of the iris.
iridosclerotomy (ir-ih-doh-skleh-ROT-oh-mee)	irid/o = iris scler/o = sclera -otomy = cutting into	To cut into the iris and sclera.
keratoplasty (KAIR-ah-toh-plass-tee)	kerat/o = cornea -plasty = surgical repair	Surgical repair of the cornea is the simple translation of this term that is utilized to mean corneal transplant.
laser-assisted insitu keratomileusis (LASIK) (in-SIH-tyoo / kair-ah-toh-mih-LOO-sis) ■ **Figure 13.13** LASIK surgery uses a laser to reshape the cornea. *(mehmetcan/Shutterstock)*	kerat/o = cornea	Correction of myopia using laser surgery to remove corneal tissue.
laser photocoagulation (LAY-zer / foh-toh-koh-ag-yoo-LAY-shun)	phot/o = light	Use of a laser beam to destroy very small precise areas of the retina. May be used to treat retinal detachment or macular degeneration.
phacoemulsification (fak-oh-ee-mull-sih-fih-KAY-shun)	phac/o = lens	Use of high-frequency sound waves to emulsify (liquefy) a lens with a cataract, which is then aspirated (removed by suction) with a needle.
photorefractive keratectomy (PRK) (foh-toh-ree-FRAK-tiv / kair-ah-TEK-toh-mee)	phot/o = light kerat/o = cornea -ectomy = surgical removal	Use of a laser to reshape the cornea and correct errors of refraction.
prosthetic lens implant (pros-THET-ik)		Use of an artificial lens to replace the lens removed during cataract surgery.

Therapeutic Procedures *(continued)*

TERMS	WORD PARTS	DEFINITION
radial keratotomy (RK) (RAY-dee-all / kair-ah-TOT-oh-mee)	-al = pertaining to kerat/o = cornea -otomy = cutting into	Spokelike incisions around the cornea that result in it becoming flatter. A surgical treatment for myopia.
retinopexy (ret-ih-noh-PEX-ee)	retin/o = retina -pexy = surgical fixation	Surgical fixation of the retina. One treatment for a detaching retina.
scleral buckling (SKLAIR-al)	scler/o = sclera -al = pertaining to	Placing a band of silicone around the outside of the sclera that stabilizes a detaching retina.
sclerotomy (skleh-ROT-oh-mee)	scler/o = sclera -otomy = cutting into	To cut into the sclera.
strabotomy (strah-BOT-oh-mee)	-otomy = cutting into	Incision into the eye muscles in order to correct strabismus.

Pharmacology

CLASSIFICATION	WORD PARTS	ACTION	EXAMPLES
anesthetic ophthalmic solution (off-THAL-mik)	an- = without esthes/o = sensation, feeling -ic = pertaining to ophthalm/o = eye -ic = pertaining to	Eye drops for pain relief associated with eye infections, corneal abrasions, or surgery.	proparacain, Ak-Taine, Ocu-Caine; tetracaine, Opticaine, Pontocaine
antibiotic ophthalmic solution (off-THAL-mik)	anti- = against bi/o = life -ic = pertaining to ophthalm/o = eye -ic = pertaining to	Eye drops for the treatment of bacterial eye infections.	erythromycin, Del-Mycin, Ilotycin Ophthalmic
antiglaucoma medications (an-tye-glau-KOH-mah)	anti- = against glauc/o = gray -oma = mass	Group of drugs that reduce intraocular pressure by lowering the amount of aqueous humor in the eyeball. May achieve this by either reducing the production of aqueous humor or increasing its outflow.	timolol, Betimol, Timoptic; acetazolamide, Ak-Zol, Dazamide; prostaglandin analogs, Lumigan, Xalatan
artificial tears		Medications, many of them over the counter, to treat dry eyes.	buffered isotonic solutions, Akwa Tears, Refresh Plus, Moisture Eyes
miotic drops (my-OT-ik)	mi/o = lessening -tic = pertaining to	Any substance that causes the pupil to constrict. These medications may also be used to treat glaucoma.	physostigmine, Eserine Sulfate, Isopto Eserine; carbachol, Carbastat, Miostat
mydriatic drops (mid-ree-AT-ik)	mydr/i = widening -atic = pertaining to	Any substance that causes the pupil to dilate by paralyzing the iris and/or ciliary body muscles. Particularly useful during eye examinations and eye surgery.	atropine sulfate, Atropine-Care Ophthalmic, Atropisol Ophthalmic
ophthalmic decongestants	ophthalm/o = eye -ic = pertaining to de- = without	Over-the-counter medications that constrict the arterioles of the eye and reduce redness and itching of the conjunctiva.	tetrahydrozoline, Visine, Murine

Abbreviations

ARMD	age-related macular degeneration
Astigm	astigmatism
c.gl.	correction with glasses
D	diopter (lens strength)
DVA	distance visual acuity
ECCE	extracapsular cataract extraction
EENT	eye, ear, nose, and throat
EM	emmetropia
EOM	extraocular movement
ICCE	intracapsular cataract extraction
IOP	intraocular pressure
LASIK	laser-assisted insitu keratomileusis
OD	right eye
Ophth.	ophthalmology
OS	left eye
OU	each eye/both eyes
PERRLA	pupils equal, round, react to light and accommodation
PRK	photorefractive keratectomy
REM	rapid eye movement
s.gl.	without correction or glasses
SMD	senile macular degeneration
ST	esotropia
VA	visual acuity
VF	visual field
XT	exotropia

MED TERM TIP

The abbreviations for right eye (OD) and left eye (OS) are easy to remember when we know their origins. OD stands for *oculus* (eye) *dexter* (right). OS has its origin in *oculus* (eye) *sinister* (left). At one time in history it was considered to be sinister if a person looked at another from only the left side. Hence the term *oculus sinister* (OS) means left eye.

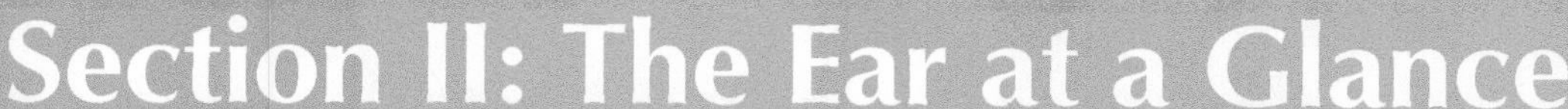

Section II: The Ear at a Glance

Function

The ear contains the sensory receptors for hearing and equilibrium (balance).

Structures

Here are the primary structures that comprise the ear.

auricle
external ear
inner ear
middle ear

Word Parts

Here are the most common word parts (with their meanings) used to build ear terms. For a more comprehensive list, refer to the Terminology section of this chapter.

Combining Forms

acous/o	hearing
audi/o	hearing
audit/o	hearing
aur/o	ear
auricul/o	ear
cerumin/o	cerumen
cochle/o	cochlea
labyrinth/o	labyrinth (inner ear)
myring/o	tympanic membrane (eardrum)
ot/o	ear
salping/o	auditory tube (eustachian tube)
staped/o	stapes
tympan/o	tympanic membrane (eardrum)

Suffixes

-cusis	hearing
-otia	ear condition

The Ear Illustrated

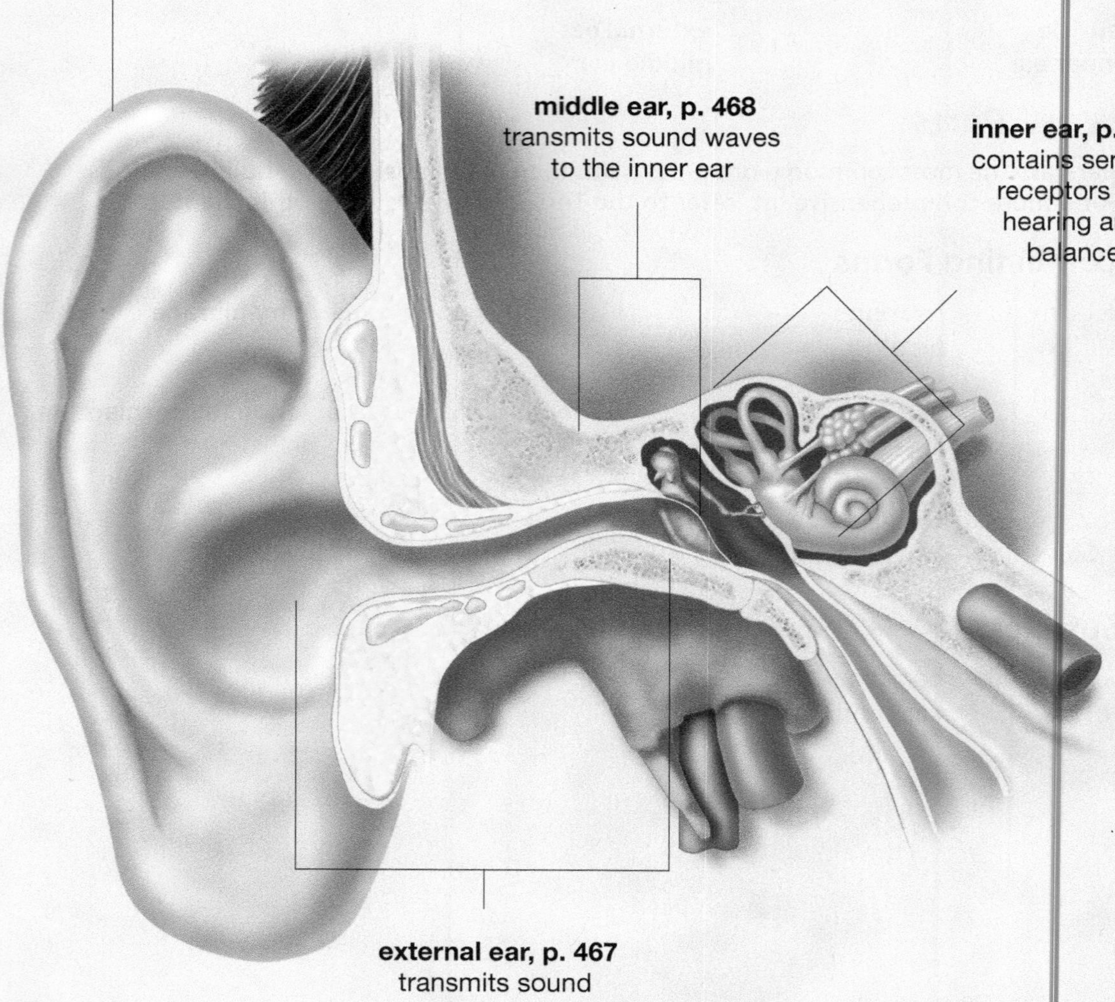

auricle, p. 467
directs sound waves into the ear canal
middle ear, p. 468
transmits sound waves to the inner ear
inner ear, p. 468
contains sensory receptors for hearing and balance
external ear, p. 467
transmits sound waves to the middle ear

Anatomy and Physiology of the Ear

audiology (aw-dee-OL-oh-jee)
cochlear nerve (KOK-lee-ar)
equilibrium (ee-kwih-LIB-ree-um)
external ear
hearing
inner ear
middle ear
otology (oh-TOL-oh-jee)
vestibular nerve (ves-TIB-yoo-lar)
vestibulocochlear nerve (ves-tib-yoo-loh-KOK-lee-ar)

The study of the ear is referred to as **otology** (Oto), and the study of hearing disorders is called **audiology.** While there is a large amount of overlap between these two areas, there are also examples of ear problems that do not affect hearing. The ear is responsible for two senses: **hearing** and **equilibrium,** or our sense of balance. Hearing and equilibrium sensory information is carried to the brain by cranial nerve VIII, the **vestibulocochlear nerve.** This nerve is divided into two major branches. The **cochlear nerve** carries hearing information, and the **vestibular nerve** carries equilibrium information.

The ear is subdivided into three areas: **external ear, middle ear,** and **inner ear.**

External Ear

auditory canal (AW-dih-tor-ee)
auricle (AW-rih-k'l)
cerumen (seh-ROO-men)
external auditory meatus (AW-dih-tor-ee / me-A-tus)
pinna (PIN-ah)
tympanic membrane (tim-PAN-ik)

The external ear consists of three parts: the **auricle,** the **auditory canal,** and the **tympanic membrane** (see Figure 13.14 ■). The auricle or **pinna** is what is commonly referred to as the *ear* because this is the only visible portion. The auricle with its earlobe

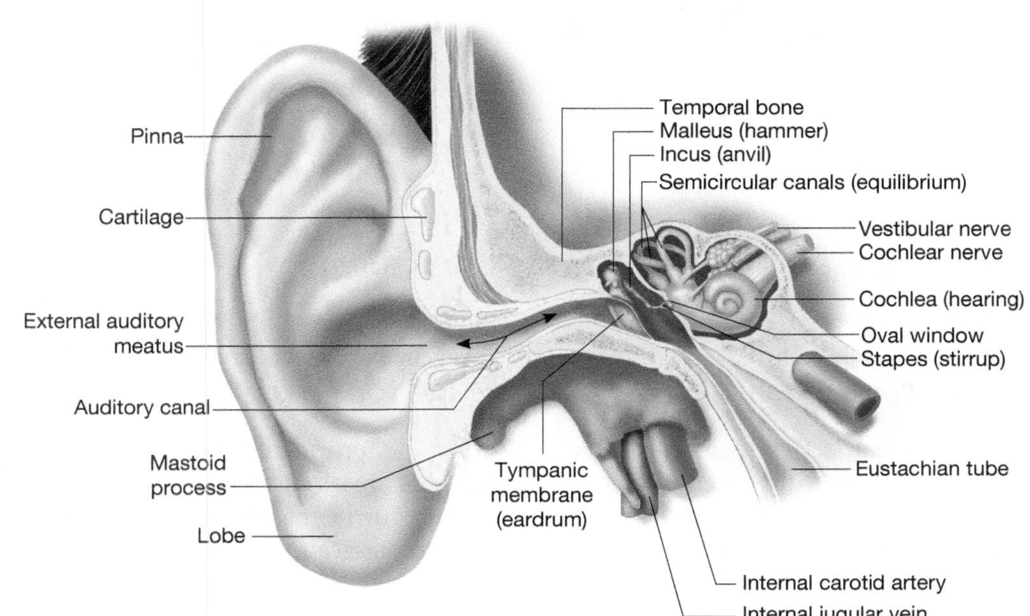

■ **Figure 13.14** The internal structures of the outer, middle, and inner ear.

has a unique shape in each person and functions like a funnel to capture sound waves as they go past the outer ear and channel them through the **external auditory meatus.** The sound then moves along the auditory canal and causes the tympanic membrane (eardrum) to vibrate. The tympanic membrane actually separates the external ear from the middle ear. Earwax or **cerumen** is produced in oil glands in the auditory canal. This wax helps to protect and lubricate the ear. It is also just barely liquid at body temperature. This causes cerumen to slowly flow out of the auditory canal, carrying dirt and dust with it. Therefore, the auditory canal is self-cleaning.

MED TERM TIP

The term *tympanic membrane* comes from the Greek word for "drumhead." The tympanic membrane or eardrum vibrates to sound waves like a drum head.

Middle Ear

auditory tube (AW-dih-tor-ee)
eustachian tube (yoo-STAY-she-en)
incus (ING-kus)
malleus (MAL-ee-us)
ossicles (OSS-ih-kls)
oval window
stapes (STAY-peez)

MED TERM TIP

The three bones in the middle ear are referred to by terms that are similar to their shape. Thus, the malleus is called the hammer, the incus is the anvil, and the stapes is the stirrup (see Figure 13.15).

The middle ear is located in a small cavity in the temporal bone of the skull. This air-filled cavity contains three tiny bones called **ossicles** (see Figure 13.15 ■). These three bones, the **malleus, incus,** and **stapes,** are vital to the hearing process. They amplify the vibrations in the middle ear and transmit them to the inner ear from the malleus to the incus and finally to the stapes. The stapes, the last of the three ossicles, is attached to a very thin membrane that covers the opening to the inner ear called the **oval window.**

The **eustachian tube** or **auditory tube** connects the nasopharynx with the middle ear (see Figure 13.14). Each time you swallow the eustachian tube opens. This connection allows pressure to equalize between the middle ear cavity and the atmospheric pressure.

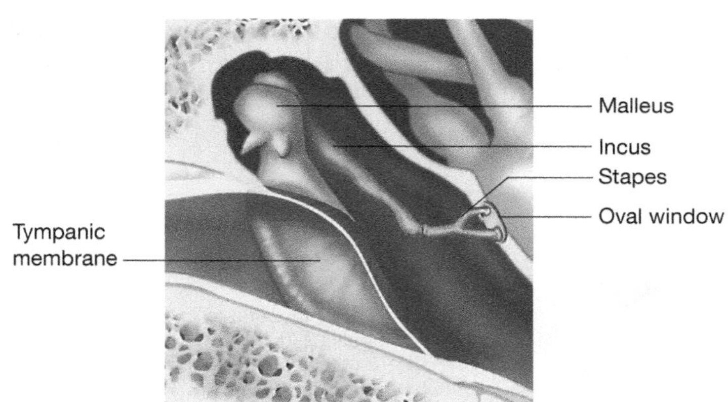

■ **Figure 13.15** Closeup view of the ossicles within the middle ear. These three bones extend from the tympanic membrane to the oval window.

Inner Ear

cochlea (KOK-lee-ah)
labyrinth (LAB-ih-rinth)
organs of Corti (KOR-tee)
saccule (SAK-yool)
semicircular canals
utricle (YOO-trih-k'l)

MED TERM TIP

Frequently, children will twirl in circles and fall or stumble from dizziness when they stop. This is caused from a temporary imbalance in the inner ear.

The inner ear is also located in a cavity within the temporal bone (see again Figure 13.14). This fluid-filled cavity is referred to as the **labyrinth** because of its shape. The labyrinth contains the hearing and equilibrium sensory organs: the **cochlea** for hearing and the **semicircular canals, utricle,** and **saccule** for equilibrium. Each of these organs contains hair cells, which are the actual sensory receptor cells. In the cochlea, the hair cells are referred to as **organs of Corti.**

How We Hear

conductive hearing loss (kon-DUK-tiv)
sensorineural hearing loss (sen-soh-ree-NOO-ral)

Figure 13.16 ■ outlines the path of sound through the outer ear and middle ear and into the cochlea of the inner ear. Sound waves traveling down the external auditory canal strike the eardrum, causing it to vibrate. The ossicles conduct these vibrations across the middle ear from the eardrum to the oval window. Oval window movements initiate vibrations in the fluid that fills the cochlea. As the fluid vibrations strike a hair cell, they bend the small hairs and stimulate the nerve ending. The nerve ending then sends an electrical impulse to the brain on the cochlear portion of the vestibulocochlear nerve.

Hearing loss can be divided into two main categories: **conductive hearing loss** and **sensorineural hearing loss.** Conductive refers to disease or malformation of the outer or middle ear. All sound is weaker and muffled in conductive hearing loss since it is not conducted correctly to the inner ear. Sensorineural hearing loss is the result of damage or malformation of the inner ear (cochlea) or the cochlear nerve. In this hearing loss, some sounds are distorted and heard incorrectly. There can also be a combination of both conductive and sensorineural hearing loss.

MED TERM TIP

Hearing impairment is becoming a greater problem for the general population for several reasons. First, people are living longer. Hearing loss can accompany old age, and there are a greater number of people over 50 years of age requiring hearing assistance. In addition, sound technology has produced music quality that was never available before. However, listening to loud music either naturally or through earphones can cause gradual damage to the hearing mechanism.

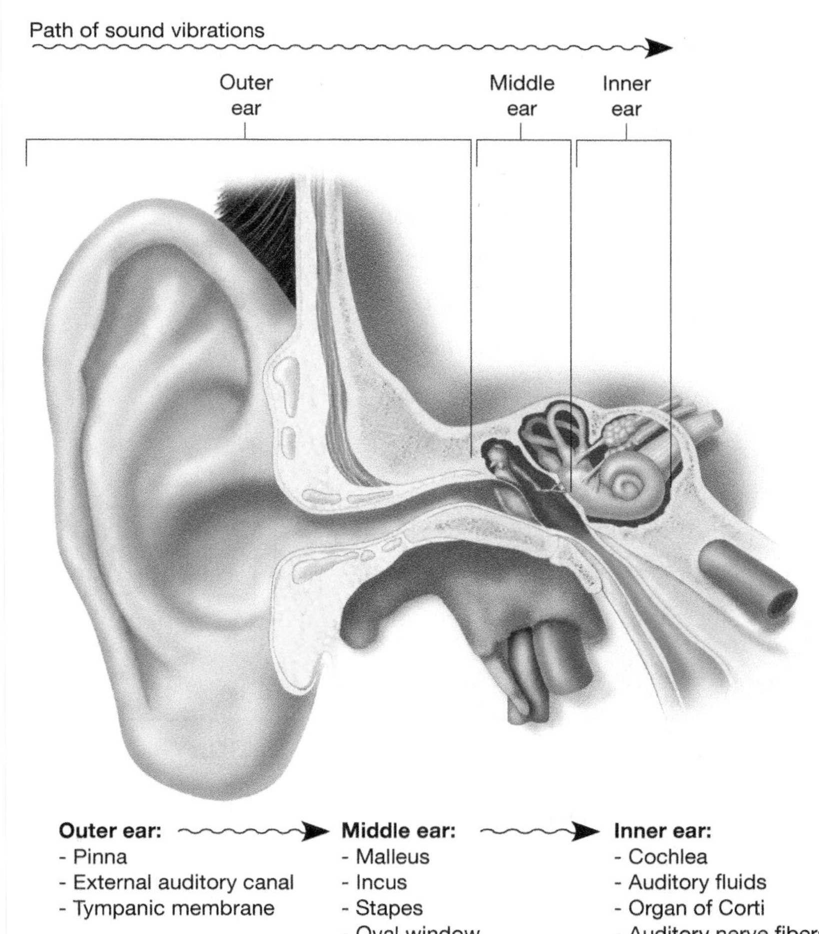

■ **Figure 13.16** The path of sound waves through the outer, middle, and inner ear.

Terminology

Word Parts Used to Build Ear Terms

The following lists contain the combining forms, suffixes, and prefixes used to build terms in the remaining sections of this chapter.

Combining Forms

acous/o	hearing
audi/o	hearing
audit/o	hearing
aur/o	ear
auricul/o	ear
bi/o	life
cerumin/o	cerumen
cochle/o	cochlea
labyrinth/o	labyrinth
laryng/o	larynx
myc/o	fungus
myring/o	tympanic membrane
neur/o	nerve
ot/o	ear
presby/o	old age
py/o	pus
rhin/o	nose
salping/o	auditory tube
staped/o	stapes
tympan/o	tympanic membrane

Suffixes

-al	pertaining to
-algia	pain
-ar	pertaining to
-cusis	hearing
-ectomy	pertaining to
-emesis	vomiting
-gram	record
-ic	pertaining to
-itis	inflammation
-logy	study of
-meter	instrument to measure
-metry	process of measuring
-oma	mass, tumor
-ory	pertaining to
-osis	abnormal condition
-otia	ear condition
-otomy	cutting into
-plasty	surgical repair
-rrhagia	abnormal flow
-rrhea	discharge
-rrhexis	rupture
-sclerosis	hardening
-scope	instrument to visually examine
-scopy	process of visually examining
-tic	pertaining to

Prefixes

an- = without
anti- = against
bi- = two
macro- = large
micro- = small
mono- = one

Anatomical Terms

TERM	WORD PARTS	DEFINITION
acoustic (ah-KOOS-tik)	acous/o = hearing -tic = pertaining to	Pertaining to hearing.
auditory (AW-dih-tor-ee)	audit/o = hearing -ory = pertaining to	Pertaining to hearing.

Anatomical Terms *(continued)*

TERM	WORD PARTS	DEFINITION
aural (AW-ral)	aur/o = ear -al = pertaining to	Pertaining to the ear. **MED TERM TIP** Word Watch: Be careful when using two terms that sound the same—*aural* meaning "pertaining to the ear" and *oral* meaning "pertaining to the mouth."
auricular (aw-RIK-cu-lar)	auricul/o = ear -ar = pertaining to	Pertaining to the ear.
binaural (bin-AW-rall)	bi- = two aur/o = ear -al = pertaining to	Pertaining to both ears.
cochlear (KOK-lee-ar)	cochle/o = cochlea -ar = pertaining to	Pertaining to the cochlea.
monaural (mon-AW-rall)	mono- = one aur/o = ear -al = pertaining to	Pertaining to one ear.
otic (OH-tik)	ot/o = ear -ic = pertaining to	Pertaining to the ear.
tympanic (tim-PAN-ik)	tympan/o = tympanic membrane -ic = pertaining to	Pertaining to the tympanic membrane.

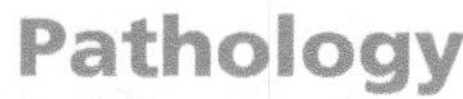

Pathology

TERM	WORD PARTS	DEFINITION
Medical Specialties		
audiology (aw-dee-OL-oh-jee)	audi/o = hearing -logy = study of	Medical specialty involved with measuring hearing function and identifying hearing loss. Specialist is an *audiologist.*
otorhinolaryngology (ENT) (oh-toh-rye-noh-lair-in-GOL-oh-jee)	ot/o = ear rhin/o = nose laryng/o = larynx -logy = study of	Branch of medicine involving the diagnosis and treatment of conditions and diseases of the ear, nose, and throat. Also referred to as *ENT.* Physician is an *otorhinolaryngologist.*
Signs and Symptoms		
macrotia (mah-KROH-she-ah)	macro- = large -otia = ear condition	Condition of having abnormally large ears.
microtia (my-KROH-she-ah)	micro- = small -otia = ear condition	Condition of having abnormally small ears.
otalgia (oh-TAL-jee-ah)	ot/o = ear -algia = pain	Ear pain.
otopyorrhea (oh-toh-pye-oh-REE-ah)	ot/o = ear py/o = pus -rrhea = discharge	Discharge of pus from the ear.
otorrhagia (oh-toh-RAH-jee-ah)	ot/o = ear -rrhagia = abnormal flow	Bleeding from the ear.

Pathology *(continued)*

TERM	WORD PARTS	DEFINITION
presbycusis (pres-bih-KOO-sis)	presby/o = old age -cusis = hearing condition	Normal loss of hearing that can accompany the aging process.
residual hearing (rih-ZID-yoo-al)	-al = pertaining to	Amount of hearing that is still present after damage has occurred to the auditory mechanism.
tinnitus (tin-EYE-tus)		Ringing in the ears.
tympanorrhexis (tim-pan-oh-REK-sis)	tympan/o = tympanic membrane -rrhexis = rupture	Rupture of the tympanic membrane.
vertigo (VER-tih-goh)		Dizziness caused by the sensation that the room is spinning.
Hearing Loss		
anacusis (an-ah-KOO-sis)	an- = without -cusis = hearing	Total absence of hearing; inability to perceive sound. Also called *deafness.*
deafness		Inability to hear or having some degree of hearing impairment.
External Ear		
ceruminoma (seh-roo-men-oh-ma)	cerumin/o = cerumen -oma = mass	Excessive accumulation of earwax resulting in a hard wax plug. Sound becomes muffled.
otitis externa (OE) (oh-TYE-tis / ex-TERN-ah)	ot/o = ear -itis = inflammation	External ear infection. May be caused by bacteria or fungus. Also called *otomycosis* and commonly referred to as *swimmer's ear.*
otomycosis (oh-toh-my-KOH-sis)	ot/o = ear myc/o = fungus -osis = abnormal condition	Fungal infection of the ear. One type of otitis externa.
Middle Ear		
myringitis (mir-ing-JYE-tis)	myring/o = tympanic membrane -itis = inflammation	Inflammation of the tympanic membrane.
otitis media (OM) (oh-TYE-tis / MEE-dee-ah)	ot/o = ear -itis = inflammation	Seen frequently in children; commonly referred to as a *middle ear infection.* Often preceded by an upper respiratory infection during which pathogens move from the pharynx to the middle ear via the eustachian tube. Fluid accumulates in the middle ear cavity. The fluid may be watery, *serous otitis media,* or full of pus, *purulent otitis media.*
otosclerosis (oh-toh-sklair-OH-sis)	ot/o = ear -sclerosis = hardening	Loss of mobility of the stapes bone, leading to progressive hearing loss.
salpingitis (sal-pin-JIH-tis)	salping/o = auditory tube -itis = inflammation	Inflammation of the auditory tube. **MED TERM TIP** Word Watch: Be careful using the combining form *salping/o,* which can mean either "Eustachian tube" or "fallopian tube."
tympanitis (tim-pan-EYE-tis)	tympan/o = tympanic membrane -itis = inflammation	Inflammation of the tympanic membrane.

Pathology *(continued)*

TERM	WORD PARTS	DEFINITION
Inner Ear		
acoustic neuroma (ah-KOOS-tik / noor-OH-mah)	acous/o = hearing -tic = pertaining to neur/o = nerve -oma = tumor	Benign tumor of the eighth cranial nerve sheath. The pressure causes symptoms such as tinnitus, headache, dizziness, and progressive hearing loss.
labyrinthitis (lab-ih-rin-THIGH-tis)	labyrinth/o = labyrinth -itis = inflammation	May affect both the hearing and equilibrium portions of the inner ear. Also referred to as an *inner ear infection.*
Ménière's disease (may-nee-ARZ)		Abnormal condition within the labyrinth of the inner ear that can lead to a progressive loss of hearing. The symptoms are dizziness or vertigo, hearing loss, and tinnitus (ringing in the ears). Named for French physician Prosper Ménière.

Diagnostic Procedures

TERM	WORD PARTS	DEFINITION
Audiology Tests		
audiogram (AW-dee-oh-gram)	audi/o = hearing -gram = record	Graphic record that illustrates the results of audiometry.
audiometer (aw-dee-OM-eh-ter)	audi/o = hearing -meter = instrument to measure	Instrument to measure hearing.
audiometry (aw-dee-OM-eh-tree)	audi/o = hearing -metry = process of measuring	Test of hearing ability by determining the lowest and highest intensity (decibels) and frequencies (hertz) that a person can distinguish. The patient may sit in a sound-proof booth and receive sounds through earphones as the technician decreases the sound or lowers the tones.

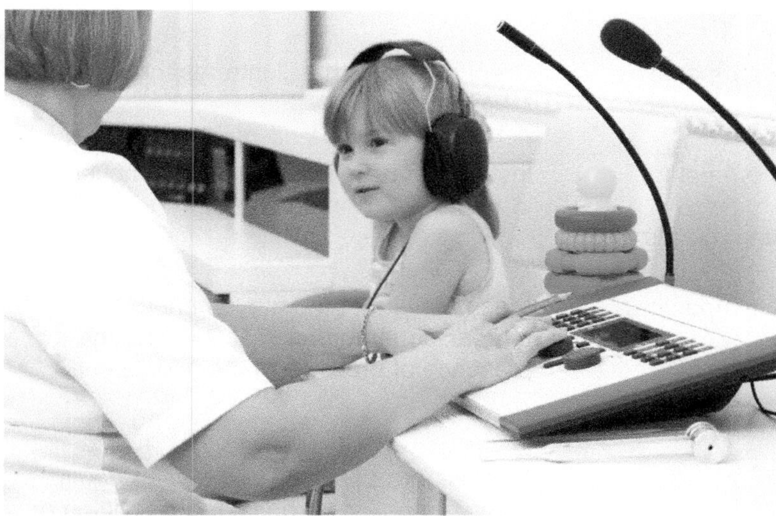

■ **Figure 13.17** Audiometry exam being administered to a young child who is wearing the ear phones through which sounds are given. *(Capifrutta/Shutterstock)*

TERM	WORD PARTS	DEFINITION
decibel (dB) (DES-ih-bel)		Measures the intensity or loudness of a sound. Zero decibels is the quietest sound measured and 120 dB is the loudest sound commonly measured.

Diagnostic Procedures *(continued)*

TERM	WORD PARTS	DEFINITION
hertz (Hz)		Measurement of the frequency or pitch of sound. The lowest pitch on an audiogram is 250 Hz. The measurement can go as high as 8000 Hz, which is the highest pitch measured.
Rinne and Weber tuning-fork tests (RIN-eh)		Tests that assess both nerve and bone conduction of sound. The physician holds a tuning fork, an instrument that produces a constant pitch when it is struck, against or near the bones on the side of the head.
Otology Tests		
otoscope (OH-toh-scope)	ot/o = ear -scope = instrument to visually examine	Instrument to view inside the ear canal.
otoscopy (oh-TOSS-koh-pee)	ot/o = ear -scopy = process of visually examining	Examination of the ear canal, eardrum, and outer ear using an *otoscope.*

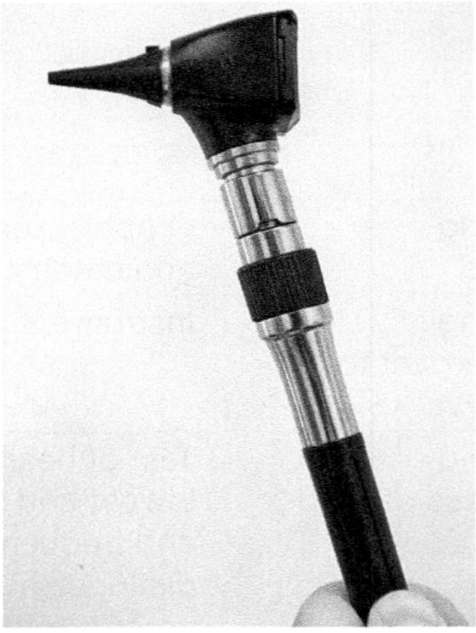

MED TERM TIP

Small children are prone to placing objects in their ears. In some cases, as with peas and beans, these become moist in the ear canal and swell, which makes removal difficult. *Otoscopy,* or the examination of the ear using an *otoscope,* can aid in identifying and removing the cause of hearing loss if it is due to foreign bodies.

Figure 13.18 An otoscope, used to visually examine the external auditory ear canal and tympanic membrane.

TERM	WORD PARTS	DEFINITION
tympanogram (TIM-pah-no-gram)	tympan/o = tympanic membrane -gram = record	Graphic record that illustrates the results of tympanometry.
tympanometer (tim-pah-NOM-eh-ter)	tympan/o = tympanic membrane -meter = instrument to measure	Instrument used to measure the movement of the tympanic membrane.
tympanometry (tim-pah-NOM-eh-tree)	tympan/o = tympanic membrane -metry = process of measuring	Measurement of the movement of the tympanic membrane. Can indicate the presence of pressure in the middle ear.
Balance Tests		
falling test		Test used to observe balance and equilibrium. The patient is observed balancing on one foot, then with one foot in front of the other, and then walking forward with eyes open. The same test is conducted with the the patient's eyes closed. Swaying and falling with the eyes closed can indicate an ear and equilibrium malfunction.

Therapeutic Procedures

TERM	WORD PARTS	DEFINITION
Audiology Procedures		
American Sign Language (ASL) 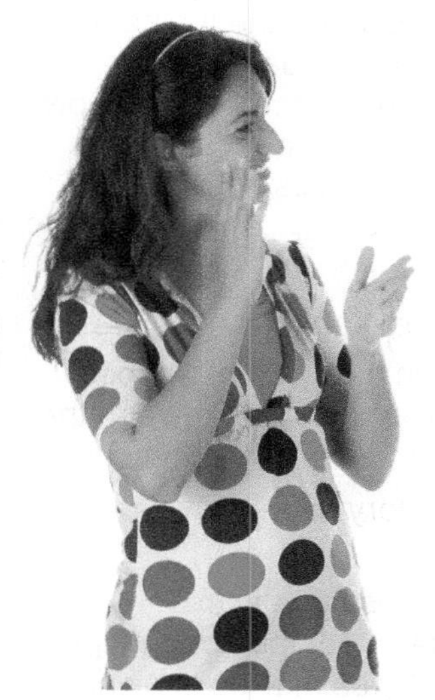 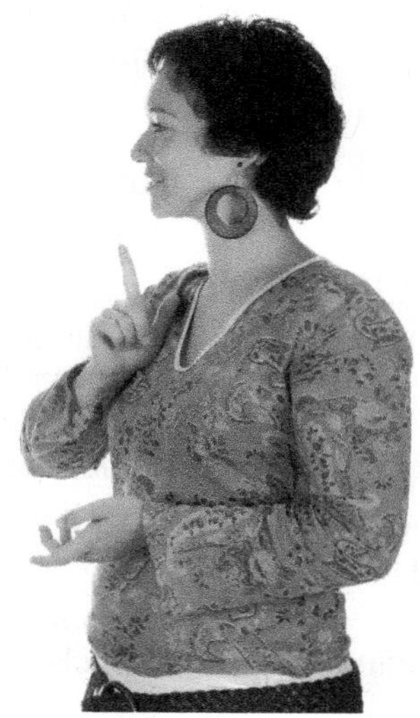		Nonverbal method of communicating in which the hands and fingers are used to indicate words and concepts. Used by both persons who are deaf and persons with speech impairments. ■ **Figure 13.19** Two women having a conversation using American Sign Language. *(Vladimir Mucibabic/ Shutterstock)*
hearing aid		Apparatus or mechanical device used by persons with impaired hearing to amplify sound. Also called an *amplification device.*
Surgical Procedures		
cochlear implant (KOK-lee-ar) 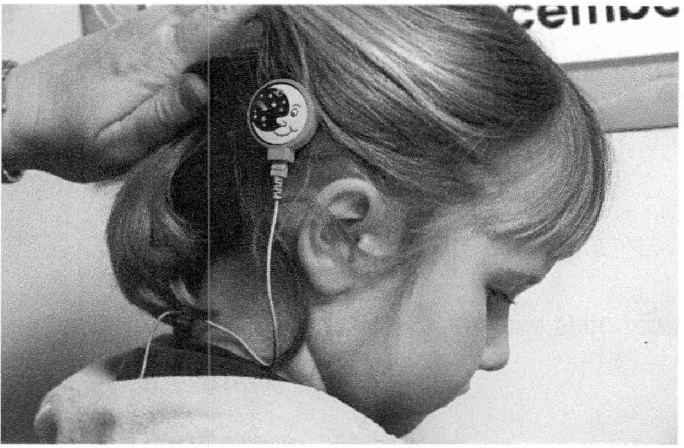	cochle/o = cochlea -ar = pertaining to	Mechanical device surgically placed under the skin behind the outer ear (pinna) that converts sound signals into magnetic impulses to stimulate the auditory nerve. Can be beneficial for those with profound sensorineural hearing loss. ■ **Figure 13.20** Photograph of a child with a cochlear implant. This device sends electrical impulses directly to the brain.
labyrinthectomy (lab-ih-rin-THEK-toh-mee)	labyrinth/o = labyrinth -ectomy = surgical removal	Surgical removal of the labyrinth.
labyrinthotomy (lab-ih-rinth-OT-oh-mee)	labyrinth/o = labyrinth -otomy = cutting into	To cut into the labyrinth.
myringectomy (mir-in-GEK-toh-mee)	myring/o = tympanic membrane -ectomy = surgical removal	Surgical removal of the tympanic membrane.
myringoplasty (mir-IN-goh-plass-tee)	myring/o = tympanic membrane -plasty = surgical repair	Surgical repair of the tympanic membrane.

Therapeutic Procedures *(continued)*

TERM	WORD PARTS	DEFINITION
myringotomy (mir-in-GOT-oh-mee)	myring/o = tympanic membrane -otomy = cutting into	Surgical puncture of the eardrum with removal of fluid and pus from the middle ear to eliminate a persistent ear infection and excessive pressure on the tympanic membrane. A pressure equalizing tube is placed in the tympanic membrane to allow for drainage of the middle ear cavity; this tube typically falls out on its own.
otoplasty (OH-toh-plas-tee)	ot/o = ear -plasty = surgical repair	Surgical repair of the external ear.
pressure equalizing tube (PE tube)		Small tube surgically placed in a child's eardrum to assist in drainage of trapped fluid and to equalize pressure between the middle ear cavity and the atmosphere.
salpingotomy (sal-pin-GOT-oh-mee)	salping/o = auditory tube -otomy = cutting into	To cut into the auditory tube.
stapedectomy (stay-pee-DEK-toh-mee)	staped/o = stapes -ectomy = pertaining to	Removal of the stapes bone to treat otosclerosis (hardening of the bone). A prosthesis or artificial stapes may be implanted.
tympanectomy (tim-pan-EK-toh-mee)	tympan/o = tympanic membrane -ectomy = surgical removal	Surgical removal of the tympanic membrane.
tympanoplasty (tim-pan-oh-PLASS-tee)	tympan/o = tympanic membrane -plasty = surgical repair	Surgical repair of the tympanic membrane.
tympanotomy (tim-pan-OT-oh-mee)	tympan/o = tympanic membrane -otomy = cutting into	To cut into the tympanic membrane.

Pharmacology

CLASSIFICATION	WORD PARTS	ACTION	EXAMPLES
antibiotic otic solution (OH-tik)	anti- = against bi/o = life -tic = pertaining to ot/o = ear -ic = pertaining to	Eardrops to treat otitis externa.	Neomycin, polymyxin B and hydrocortisone solution, Otocort, Cortisporin, Otic Care
antiemetics (an-tye-ee-mit-tiks)	anti- = against -emesis = vomiting -tic = pertaining to	Medications effective in treating the nausea associated with vertigo.	meclizine, Antivert, Meni-D; prochlorperazine, Compazine
anti-inflammatory otic solution (OH-tik)	anti- = against -ory = pertaining to ot/o = ear -ic = pertaining to	Reduces inflammation, itching, and edema associated with otitis externa.	antipyrine and benzoaine, Allergan Ear Drops, A/B Otic
wax emulsifiers		Substances used to soften earwax to prevent buildup within the external ear canal.	carbamide peroxide, Debrox Drops, Murine Ear Drops

Abbreviations

AD	right ear	**HEENT**	head, ears, eyes, nose, throat
AS	left ear	**Hz**	hertz
ASL	American Sign Language	**OM**	otitis media
AU	both ears	**Oto**	otology
BC	bone conduction	**PE tube**	pressure equalizing tube
dB	decibel	**PORP**	partial ossicular replacement prosthesis
EENT	eyes, ears, nose, throat	**SOM**	serous otitis media
ENT	ear, nose, and throat	**TORP**	total ossicular replacement prosthesis

Chapter Review

Real-World Applications

Medical Record Analysis

This Ophthalmology Consultation Report contains 11 medical terms. Underline each term and write it in the list below the report. Then define each term.

Ophthalmology Consultation Report

Reason for Consultation:	Evaluation of progressive loss of vision in right eye.
History of Present Illness:	Patient is a 79-year-old female who has noted gradual deterioration of vision and increasing photophobia during the past year, particularly in the right eye. She states that it feels like there is a film over her right eye. She denies any change in vision in her left eye. Patient has used corrective lenses her entire adult life for hyperopia.
Results of Physical Examination:	Visual acuity test showed no change in this patient's long-standing hyperopia. The pupils react properly to light. Intraocular pressure is normal. Ophthalmoscopy after application of mydriatic drops revealed presence of large opaque cataract in lens of right eye. There is a very small cataract forming in the left eye. There is no evidence of retinopathy, macular degeneration, or keratitis.
Assessment:	Diminished vision in right eye secondary to cataract.
Recommendations:	Phacoemulsification of cataract followed by prosthetic lens implant.

	Term	Definition
1	______________	______________
2	______________	______________
3	______________	______________
4	______________	______________
5	______________	______________
6	______________	______________
6	______________	______________
7	______________	______________
8	______________	______________
9	______________	______________
10	______________	______________

Chart Note Transcription

The chart note below contains 10 phrases that can be reworded with a medical term that you learned in this chapter. Each phrase is identified with an underline. Determine the medical term and write your answers in the space provided.

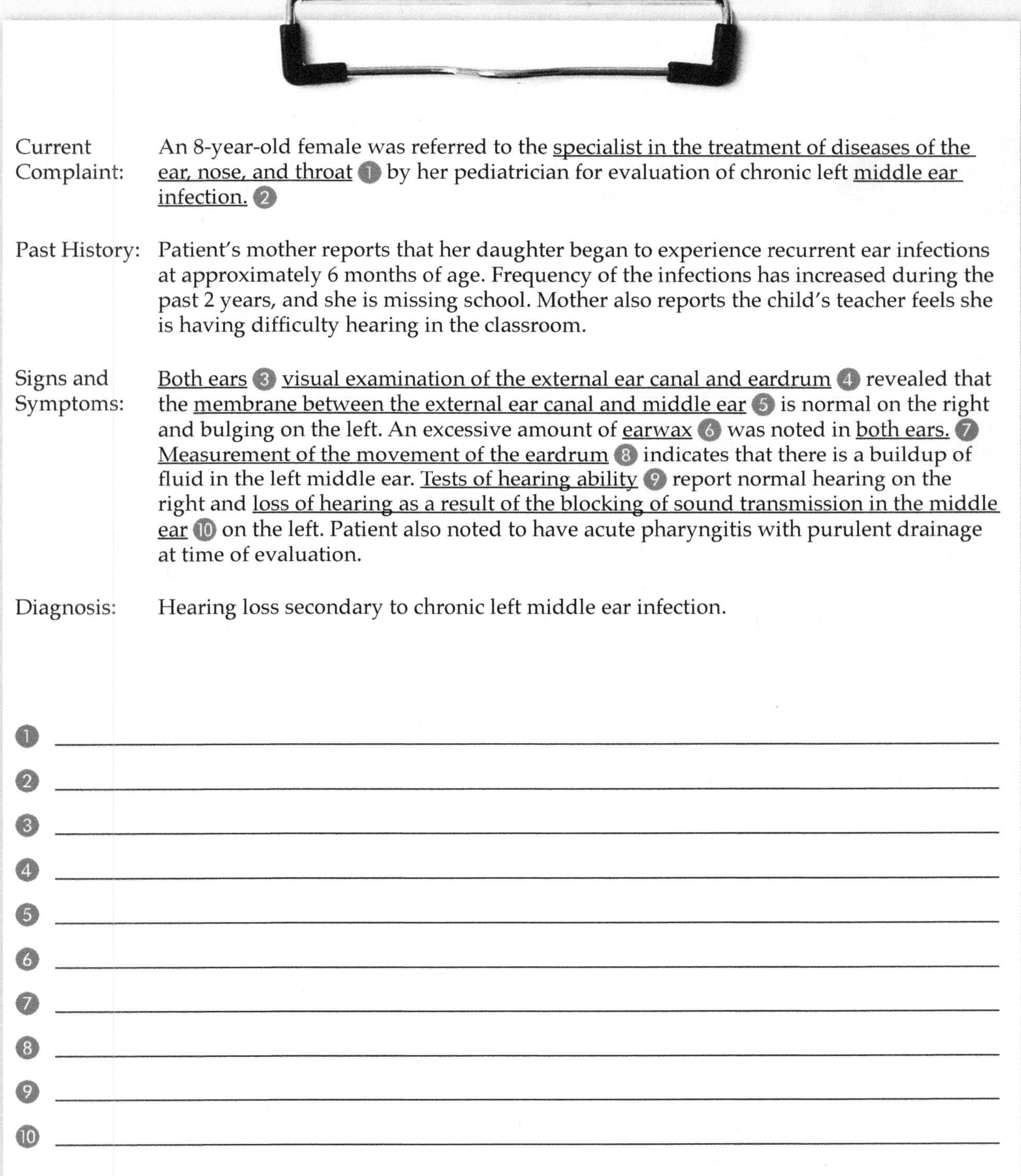

Current Complaint: An 8-year-old female was referred to the specialist in the treatment of diseases of the ear, nose, and throat (1) by her pediatrician for evaluation of chronic left middle ear infection. (2)

Past History: Patient's mother reports that her daughter began to experience recurrent ear infections at approximately 6 months of age. Frequency of the infections has increased during the past 2 years, and she is missing school. Mother also reports the child's teacher feels she is having difficulty hearing in the classroom.

Signs and Symptoms: Both ears (3) visual examination of the external ear canal and eardrum (4) revealed that the membrane between the external ear canal and middle ear (5) is normal on the right and bulging on the left. An excessive amount of earwax (6) was noted in both ears. (7) Measurement of the movement of the eardrum (8) indicates that there is a buildup of fluid in the left middle ear. Tests of hearing ability (9) report normal hearing on the right and loss of hearing as a result of the blocking of sound transmission in the middle ear (10) on the left. Patient also noted to have acute pharyngitis with purulent drainage at time of evaluation.

Diagnosis: Hearing loss secondary to chronic left middle ear infection.

(1) ______________________

(2) ______________________

(3) ______________________

(4) ______________________

(5) ______________________

(6) ______________________

(7) ______________________

(8) ______________________

(9) ______________________

(10) ______________________

Case Study

Below is a case study presentation of a patient with a condition covered in this chapter. Read the case study and answer the questions below. Some questions will ask for information not included within this chapter. Use your text, a medical dictionary, journals, technical materials, multimedia resources, electronic media, or any other reference material you choose to answer these questions.

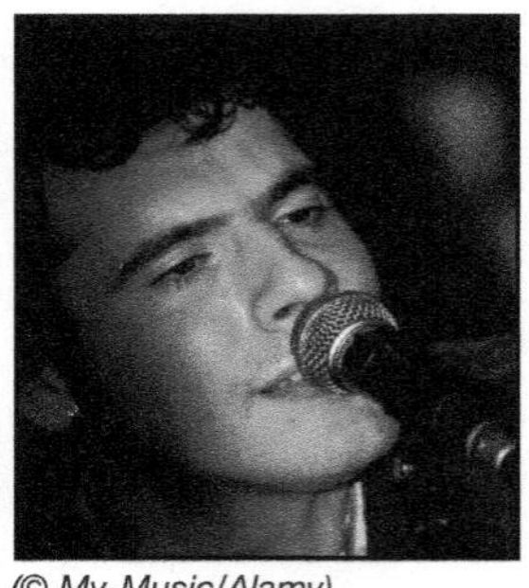

(© My-Music/Alamy)

This 35-year-old male musician was seen in the EENT clinic complaining of a progressive hearing loss over the past 15 years. He is now unable to hear what is being said if there is any environmental noise present. He states that he has played with a group of musicians using amplified instruments and no earplugs for the past 20 years. External ear structures appear normal bilaterally with otoscopy. Tympanometry is normal bilaterally. Audiometry reveals diminished hearing bilaterally. Rinne and Weber tuning-fork tests indicate that the patient has a moderate amount of conductive hearing loss but rule out sensorineural hearing loss. Diagnosis is moderate bilateral conductive hearing loss as a result of prolonged exposure to loud noise. Patient is referred for evaluation for a hearing aid.

1. Which type of hearing loss does this patient appear to have? Look this condition up in a reference source and include a short description of it.

____

____

2. Explain how the other type of hearing loss (the type ruled out by the Rinne and Weber tuning-fork tests) is different from what this patient has.

____

____

3. What diagnostic tests did the physician perform? Describe them in your own words.

____

____

4. Explain the difference between a hearing aid and a cochlear implant.

____

____

5. How do you think this patient could have avoided this hearing loss?

____

____

Practice Exercises

A. Complete the Statement

1. The study of the eye is ____________________.
2. Another term for eyelashes is ____________________.
3. The glands responsible for tears are called ____________________ glands.
4. The clear, transparent portion of the sclera is called the ____________________.
5. The innermost layer of the eye, which is composed of sensory receptors, is the ____________________.
6. The pupil of the eye is actually a hole in the ____________________.
7. The three bones in the middle ear are the ____________________, ____________________, and ____________________.
8. The study of the ear is called ____________________.
9. Another term for the eardrum is ____________________.
10. ____________________ is produced in the oil glands in the auditory canal.
11. The ____________________ tube connects the nasopharynx with the middle ear.
12. The ____________________ is responsible for conducting impulses from the ear to the brain.

B. Pharmacology Challenge

Fill in the classification for each drug description, then match the brand name.

	Drug Description	Classification		Brand Name
1.	________ treats dry eyes	____________________	a.	Atropine-Care
2.	________ reduces intraocular pressure	____________________	b.	Allergan Ear Drops
3.	________ ear drops for ear infection	____________________	c.	Timoptic
4.	________ dilates pupil	____________________	d.	Opticaine
5.	________ treats nausea from vertigo	____________________	e.	Debrox Drops
6.	________ eye drops for bacterial infection	____________________	f.	Eserine Sulfate
7.	________ treats ear itching	____________________	g.	Antivert
8.	________ constricts pupil	____________________	h.	Refresh Plus
9.	________ softens cerumen	____________________	i.	Otocort
10.	________ eye drops for pain	____________________	j.	Del-Mycin

C. Combining Form Practice

The combining form **blephar/o** refers to the eyelid. Use it to write a term that means:

1. inflammation of the eyelid ______
2. surgical repair of the eyelid ______
3. drooping of the upper eyelid ______

The combining form **retin/o** refers to the retina. Use it to write a term that means:

4. a disease of the retina ______
5. surgical fixation of the retina ______

The combining form **ophthalm/o** refers to the eye. Use it to write a term that means:

6. the study of the eye ______
7. pertaining to the eye ______
8. an eye examination using a scope ______

The combining form **irid/o** refers to the iris. Use it to write a term that means:

9. iris paralysis ______
10. removal of the iris ______

The combining form **ot/o** refers to the ear. Write a word that means:

11. ear surgical repair ______
12. pus flow from the ear ______
13. pain in the ear ______
14. inflammation of the ear ______

The combining form **tympan/o** refers to the eardrum. Write a word that means:

15. eardrum rupture ______
16. eardrum incision ______
17. eardrum inflammation ______

The combining form **audi/o** refers to hearing. Write a word that means:

18. record of hearing ______
19. instrument to measure hearing ______
20. study of hearing ______

D. Name That Suffix

	Suffix	Example from Chapter
1. to turn		
2. vision		
3. inflammation of		
4. the study of		
5. cutting into		
6. surgical repair		
7. surgical fixation		
8. pain		
9. ear condition		
10. hearing		

E. Define the Combining Form

	Definition	Example from Chapter
1. **dacry/o**		
2. **uve/o**		
3. **aque/o**		
4. **phot/o**		
5. **kerat/o**		
6. **vitre/o**		
7. **dipl/o**		
8. **glauc/o**		
9. **presby/o**		
10. **ambly/o**		
11. **aur/o**		
12. **staped/o**		
13. **acous/o**		
14. **salping/o**		
15. **myring/o**		

F. Answer the Question

1. Describe the difference between conductive hearing loss and sensorineural hearing loss. ______________________________

____

2. List in order the eyeball structures light rays pass through: ______________, ______________, ______________, ______________

3. Describe the role of the conjunctiva. ______________________________

____

4. List the ossicles and what they do. ______________________________

____

G. Terminology Matching

Match each term to its definition.

1.	_______ emmetropia	a.	opacity of the lens
2.	_______ sclera	b.	muscle regulating size of pupil
3.	_______ cataract	c.	nearsightedness
4.	_______ conjunctiva	d.	protective membrane of eye
5.	_______ iris	e.	blind spot
6.	_______ xerophthalmia	f.	involuntary movements of eye
7.	_______ myopia	g.	white of eye
8.	_______ nystagmus	h.	normal vision
9.	_______ optic disk	i.	dry eyes
10.	_______ vitreous humor	j.	material filling eyeball

H. What Does it Stand For?

1. Oto ______________________________
2. OU ______________________________
3. REM ______________________________
4. Hz ______________________________
5. SMD ______________________________
6. PERRLA ______________________________

7. IOP ______________________________

8. dB ______________________________

9. OD ______________________________

10. VF ______________________________

I. Terminology Matching

Match each term to its definition.

1.	________ myringotomy	a.	removal of stapes bone
2.	________ tympanoplasty	b.	reconstruction of eardrum
3.	________ otoplasty	c.	surgical puncture of eardrum
4.	________ stapedectomy	d.	change size of pinna
5.	________ anacusis	e.	absence of hearing
6.	________ falling test	f.	treats sensorineural hearing loss
7.	________ PE tube	g.	tuning fork tests
8.	________ cochlear implant	h.	swimmer's ear
9.	________ otitis externa	i.	drains off fluid
10.	________ Rinne & Weber	j.	balance test

J. What's the Abbreviation?

1. pressure equalizing tube ______________________________
2. eye, ear, nose, and throat ______________________________
3. bone conduction ______________________________
4. both ears ______________________________
5. otitis media ______________________________
6. emmetropia ______________________________
7. exotropia ______________________________
8. left eye ______________________________
9. extraocular movement ______________________________
10. visual acuity ______________________________

K. Fill in the Blank

emmetropia	tonometry	Ménière's disease
hyperopia	cataract	hordeolum
acoustic neuroma	strabismus	myopia
otorhinolaryngologist	presbycusis	
conjunctivitis	inner ear	

1. Cheri is having a regular eye checkup. The pressure reading test that the physician will do to detect glaucoma is ____________________.
2. Carlos's ophthalmologist tells him that he has normal vision. This is called ____________________.
3. Ana has been given an antibiotic eye ointment for pinkeye. The medical term for this condition is ____________________.
4. Adrian is nearsighted and cannot read signs in the distance. This is called ____________________.
5. Ivan is scheduled to have surgery to have the opaque lens of his right eye removed. This condition is a(n) ____________________.
6. Roberto has developed a stye on the corner of his left eye. He has been told to treat it with hot compresses. This condition is called a(n) ____________________.
7. Judith has twin boys with crossed eyes that will require surgical correction. The medical term for this condition is ____________________.
8. Beth is farsighted and has difficulty reading textbooks. Her eyeglass correction will be for ____________________.
9. Grace was told by her physician that her hearing loss was a part of the aging process. The term for this is ____________________.
10. Stacey is having frequent middle ear infections and wishes to be treated by a specialist. She would go to a(n) ____________________.
11. Warren was told that his dizziness may be caused by a problem in the ____________________ area.
12. Shantel is suffering from an abnormal condition of the inner ear, vertigo, and tinnitus. She may have ____________________.
13. Keisha was told that her tumor of the eighth cranial nerve was benign, but she still experienced a hearing loss as a result of the tumor. This tumor is called a(n) ____________________.

L. Define the Term

1. amblyopia ______________________________

2. diplopia ______________________________

3. mydriatic ______________________________

4. miotic ______________________________

5. presbyopia ______________________________

6. tinnitus ______________________________

7. stapes ______________________________

8. tympanometry ______________________________

9. eustachian tube ______________________________

10. labyrinth ______________________________

11. audiogram ______________________________

12. otitis media ______________________________

Labeling Exercise

Image A

Write the labels for this figure on the numbered lines provided.

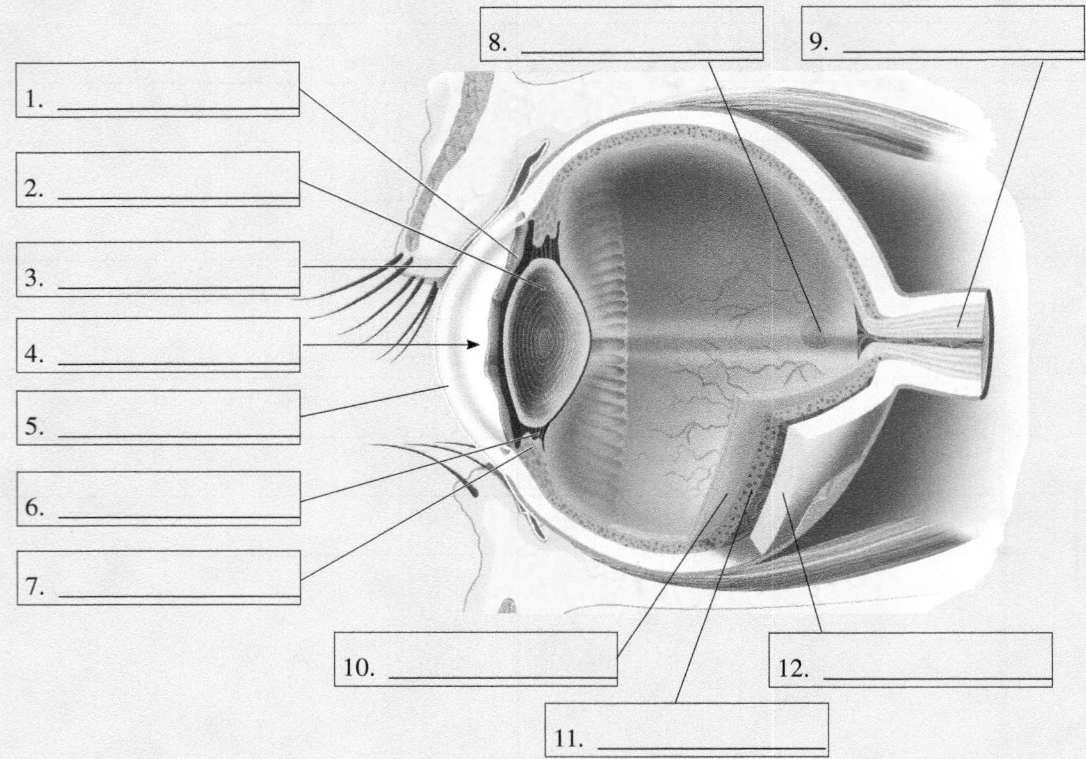

Image B

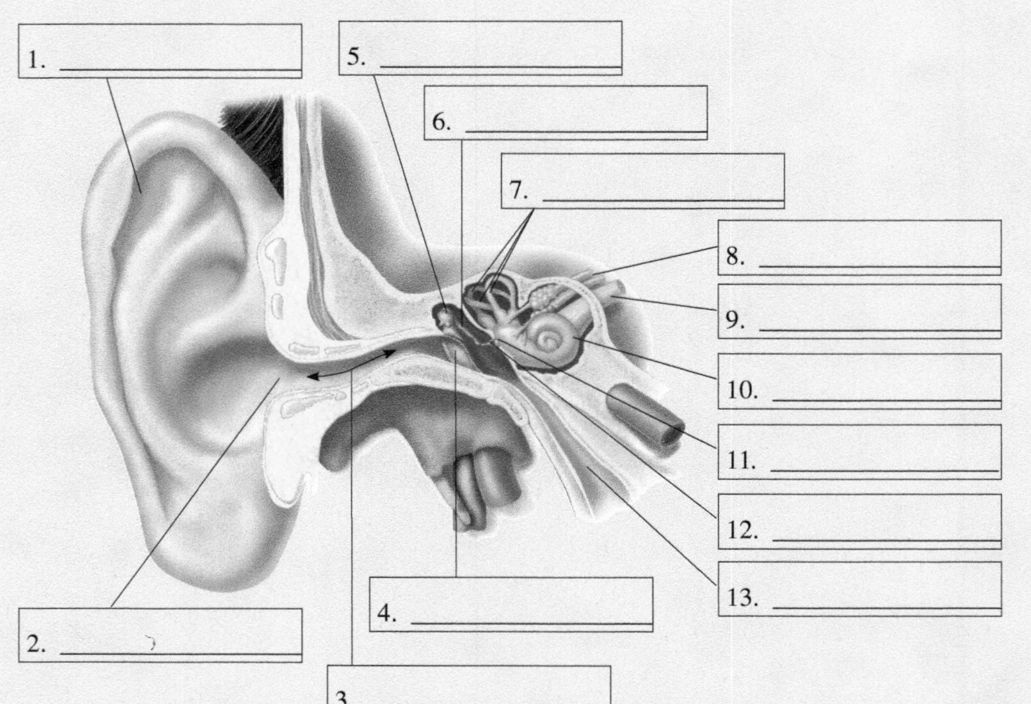

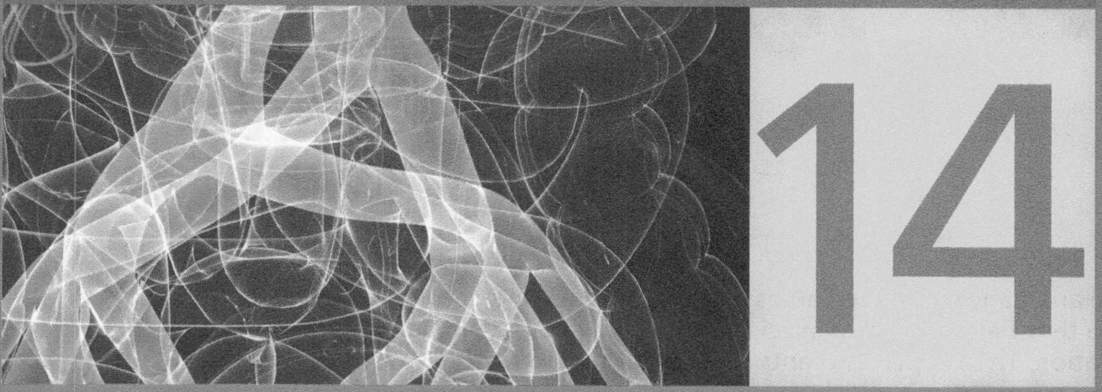

SPECIAL TOPICS

Learning Objectives

Upon completion of this chapter, you will be able to

- Identify and define the combining forms and suffixes introduced in this chapter.
- Correctly spell and pronounce medical terms relating to the medical fields introduced in this chapter.
- Describe pertinent information relating to pharmacology.
- Describe pertinent information relating to mental health.
- Describe pertinent information relating to diagnostic imaging.
- Describe pertinent information relating to rehabilitation services.
- Describe pertinent information relating to surgery.
- Describe pertinent information relating to oncology.
- Identify and define vocabulary terms relating to the topics.
- Identify and define selected pathology terms relating to the topics.
- Identify and define selected diagnostic procedures relating to the topics.
- Identify and define selected therapeutic procedures relating to the topics.
- Define selected abbreviations associated with the topics.

Introduction

There are many specialized areas within medicine, and each has medical terms relating to that field, as well as specialists that provide patient support within each specialization. This chapter presents medical terminology from six of these fields.

In addition many health care processes, procedures, and diseases are identified by naming them for the person that made the discovery. These are referred to as *eponyms.* A medical eponym is therefore any word related to medicine, whose name is derived from a person. Several examples of eponyms are found in this chapter.

1. Pharmacology
2. Mental Health
3. Diagnostic Imaging
4. Rehabilitation Services
5. Surgery
6. Oncology

Section I: Pharmacology at a Glance

Word Parts

Here are the most common word parts (with their meanings) used to build pharmacy terms.

Combining Forms

aer/o	air
bucc/o	cheek
chem/o	drug
cutane/o	skin
derm/o	skin
enter/o	intestine
hal/o	to breathe
iatr/o	physician, medicine, treatment
idi/o	distinctive
lingu/o	tongue
muscul/o	muscle
or/o	mouth
pharmac/o	drug
rect/o	rectum
thec/o	sheath (meninges)
topic/o	a specific area
toxic/o	poison
vagin/o	vagina
ven/o	vein

Suffixes

-al	pertaining to
-ary	pertaining to
-genic	produced by
-ic	pertaining to
-ical	pertaining to
-ist	specialist
-logy	study of
-phylaxis	protection

Prefixes

anti-	against
contra-	against
in-	inward
intra-	within
para-	near, beside
pro-	before
sub-	under
trans-	through

Pharmacology

pharmacology (far-ma-KALL-oh-jee)

Pharmacology is the study of the origin, characteristics, and effects of drugs. Drugs are obtained from many different sources. Some drugs, such as vitamins, are found naturally in the foods we eat. Others, such as hormones, are obtained from animals. Penicillin and some of the other antibiotics are developed from mold, which is a fungus. Plants have been the source of many of today's drugs. Many drugs, such as those used in chemotherapy, are synthetic, meaning they are developed by artificial means in a laboratory.

Drug Names

brand name
chemical name
generic name
nonproprietary name (non-prah-PRYE-ah-tair-ee)
pharmaceutical (far-mih-SOO-tih-kal)
pharmacist (FAR-mah-sist)
proprietary name (proh-PRYE-ah-tair-ee)
trademark

MED TERM TIP

The terms *drug* and *medication* have the same meaning. However, the general public often uses the term *drug* to refer to a narcotic type of medication. The term can also mean illegal chemical substances. For purposes of medical terminology, use of the word *drug* means medication.

All drugs are chemicals. The **chemical name** describes the chemical formula or molecular structure of a particular drug. For example, the chemical name for ibuprofen, an over-the-counter pain medication, is 2-*p*-isobutylphenyl propionic acid. Just as in this case, chemical names are usually very long, so a shorter name is given to the drug. This name is the **generic** or **nonproprietary name,** and it is recognized and accepted as the official name for a drug.

Each drug has only one generic name, such as ibuprofen, and this name is not subject to copyright protection, so any **pharmaceutical** manufacturer may use it. However, the pharmaceutical company that originally developed the drug has exclusive rights to produce it for 17 years. After that time, any manufacturer may produce and sell the drug. When a company manufactures a drug for sale, it must choose a **brand name,** or **proprietary name** for its product. This is the company's **trademark** for the drug. For example, ibuprofen is known by several brand names, including Motrin™, Advil™, and Nuprin™. All three contain the same ibuprofen; they are just marketed by different pharmaceutical companies. (See Table 14.1 ■ for examples of different drug names.)

Generic drugs are usually priced lower than brand name drugs. A physician can indicate on the prescription if the **pharmacist** may substitute a generic drug for a brand name. The physician may prefer that a particular brand name drug be used if he or she believes it to be more effective than the generic drug.

MED TERM TIP

Look for these word parts:

chem/o = drug
pharmac/o = drug
-al = pertaining to
-ary = pertaining to
-ic = pertaining to
-ical = pertaining to
-ist = specialist
-logy = study of

Table 14.1 Examples of Different Drug Names

CHEMICAL NAME	GENERIC NAME	BRAND NAMES
2-***p***-isobutylphenyl propionic acid	Ibuprofen	Motrin™
		Advil™
		Nuprin™
Acetylsalicylic acid	Aspirin	Anacin™
		Bufferin™
		Excedrin™
S-2-[1-(methylamino) ethyl] benzenemethanol hydrochloride	Pseudoephedrine hydrochloride	Sudafed™
		Actifed™
		Nucofed™

Legal Classification of Drugs

controlled substances
Drug Enforcement Agency
over-the-counter drug
prescription (prih-SKRIP-shun)
prescription drug (prih-SKRIP-shun)

A **prescription drug** can only be ordered by licensed healthcare practitioners such as physicians, dentists, or physician assistants. These drugs must include the words "Caution: Federal law prohibits dispensing without prescription" on their labels. Antibiotics, such as penicillin, and heart medications, such as digoxin, are available only by prescription. A **prescription** is the written explanation to the pharmacist regarding the name of the medication, the dosage, and the times of administration. A licensed practitioner can also give a prescription order orally to a pharmacist.

A drug that does not require a prescription is referred to as an **over-the-counter** (OTC) **drug.** Many medications or drugs can be purchased without a prescription, for example, aspirin, antacids, and antidiarrheal medications. However, taking aspirin along with an anticoagulant, such as coumadin, can cause internal bleeding in some people, and OTC antacids interfere with the absorption of the prescription drug tetracycline into the body. It is better for the physician or pharmacist to advise the patient on the proper OTC drugs to use with prescription drugs.

MED TERM TIP

It is critical that patients receive the correct drug, but it is not possible to list or remember all the drug names. You must acquire the habit of looking up any drug name you do not recognize in the *Physician's Desk Reference (PDR)*. Every medical office or medical facility should have a copy of this book.

Certain drugs are **controlled substances** if they have a potential for being addictive (habit forming) or can be abused. The **Drug Enforcement Agency** (DEA) enforces the control of these drugs. Some of the more commonly prescribed controlled substances are:

- butabarbital
- chloral hydrate
- codeine
- diazepam
- oxycontin
- morphine
- phenobarbital
- secobarbital

Controlled drugs are classified as Schedule I through Schedule V, indicating their potential for abuse. The differences between each schedule are listed in Table 14.2 ■.

Table 14.2 Schedule for Controlled Substances

CLASSIFICATION	MEANING
Schedule I	Drugs with the highest potential for addiction and abuse. They are not accepted for medical use. Examples are heroin and LSD.
Schedule II	Drugs with a high potential for addiction and abuse accepted for medical use in the United States. Examples are codeine, cocaine, morphine, opium, and secobarbital.
Schedule III	Drugs with a moderate to low potential for addiction and abuse. Examples are butabarbital, anabolic steroids, and acetaminophen with codeine.
Schedule IV	Drugs with a lower potential for addiction and abuse than Schedule III drugs. Examples are chloral hydrate, phenobarbital, and diazepam.
Schedule V	Drugs with a low potential for addiction and abuse. An example is low-strength codeine combined with other drugs to suppress coughing.

How to Read a Prescription

A prescription is not difficult to read once you understand the symbols that are used. Symbols and abbreviations based on Latin and Greek words are used to save time for the physician. For example, the abbreviation po, meaning to be taken by mouth, comes from the Latin term *per os,* which means "by mouth."

See Figure 14.1 ■ for an example of a prescription. In this example, the prescribed medication (Rx) is Tagamet (a medication to reduce stomach acid) in the 800 milligram (mg) size. The instructions on the label are to say (Sig) to take 1 (ī) by mouth (po) every (q) bedtime (hs). The pharmacist is to dispense (disp) 30 tablets (#30). The prescription concludes by informing the pharmacist to refill the prescription two times, and he or she may substitute with another medication. Each prescription must contain the date, physician's name, address, and Drug Enforcement Agency number as well as the patient's name and date of birth. The physician must also sign his or her name at the bottom of the prescription. A blank prescription cannot be handed to a patient.

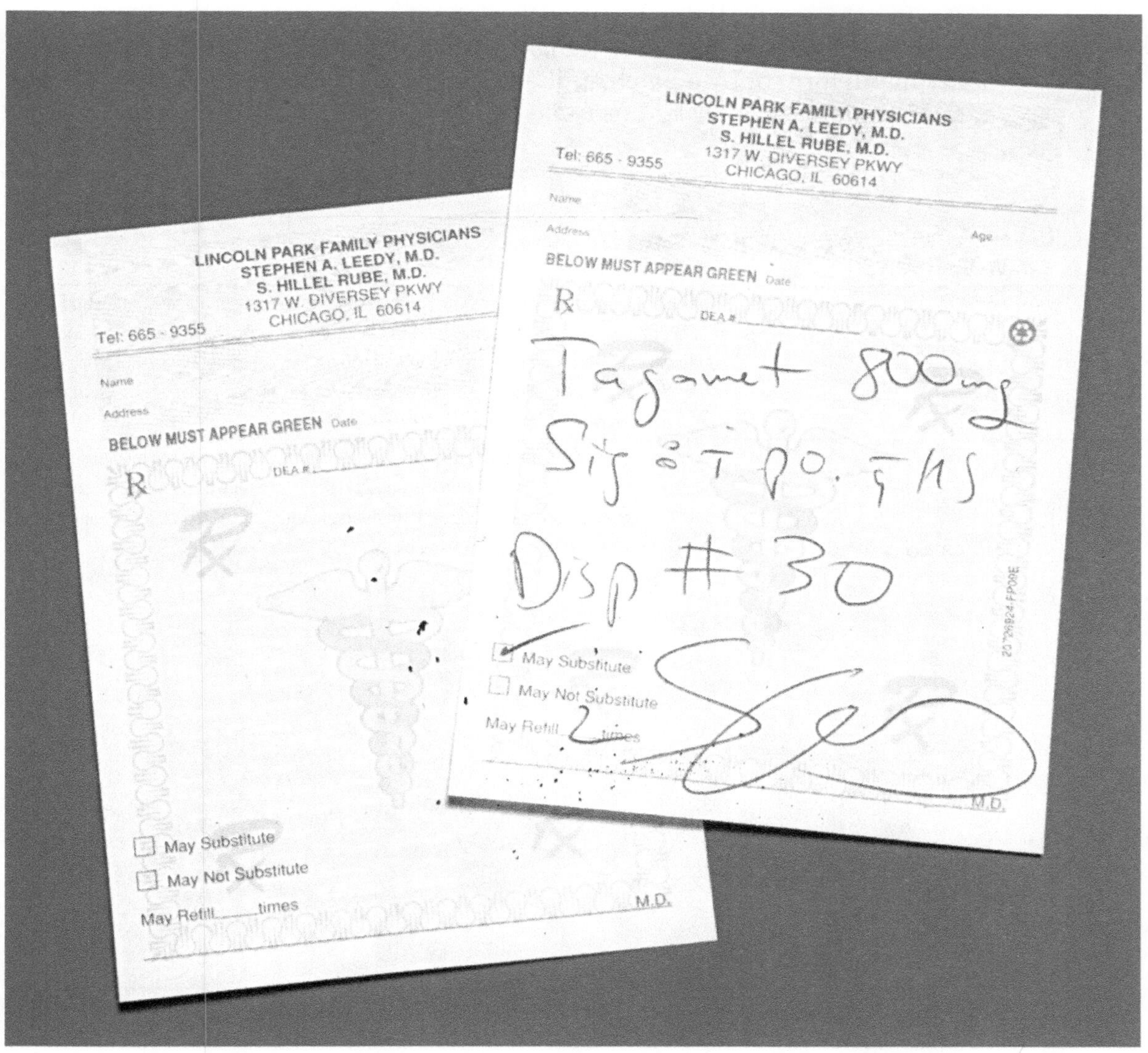

■ **Figure 14.1** A sample prescription written by a physician.

The physician's instruction to the patient will be placed on the label. The pharmacist will also include instructions about the medication and alert the patient to side effects that may need to be reported to the physician. In addition, any special instructions regarding the medication (i.e., take with meals, do not take along with dairy products) will also be supplied by the pharmacist.

Routes and Methods of Drug Administration

aerosol (AIR-oh-sol)
buccal (BUCK-al)
eardrops
eyedrops
inhalation (in-hah-LAY-shun)
oral (OR-al)
parenteral (par-EN-ter-al)
rectal (REK-tal)
sublingual (sub-LING-gwal)
suppositories (suh-POZ-ih-tor-ees)
topical (TOP-ih-kal)
transdermal (tranz-DER-mal)
vaginal (VAJ-in-al)

MED TERM TIP

Many abbreviations have multiple meanings, such as od, which can mean overdose (od) or right eye (OD), depending on whether the letters are lowercase or uppercase. Care must be taken when reading abbreviations since some may be written too quickly, making them difficult to decipher. Never create your own abbreviations.

The method by which a drug is introduced into the body is referred to as the *route of administration*. To be effective, drugs must be administered by a particular route. In some cases, there may be a variety of routes by which a drug can be administered. For instance, the female hormone estrogen can be administered orally in pill form or by a patch applied to the skin. The most common routes of administration are described in Table 14.3 ■.

Table 14.3 Common Routes of Drug Administration

METHOD	WORD PARTS	DESCRIPTION
oral	or/o = mouth -al = pertaining to	Includes all drugs given by mouth. The advantages are ease of administration and a slow rate of absorption via the stomach and intestinal wall. The disadvantages include slowness of absorption and destruction of some chemical compounds by gastric juices. In addition, some medications, such as aspirin, can have a corrosive action on the stomach lining.
sublingual	sub- = under lingu/o = tongue -al = pertaining to	Includes drugs that are held under the tongue and not swallowed. The medication is absorbed by the blood vessels on the underside of the tongue as the saliva dissolves it. The rate of absorption is quicker than the oral route. Nitroglycerin to treat angina pectoris (chest pain) is administered by this route.
inhalation	in- = inward hal/o = to breathe	Includes drugs inhaled directly into the nose and mouth. **Aerosol** sprays are administered by this route (see Figure 14.3). ■

■ **Figure 14.2** Sublingual medication administration. Photograph of a male patient placing a nitroglycerine tablet under his tongue.

Table 14.3 Common Routes of Drug Administration (continued)

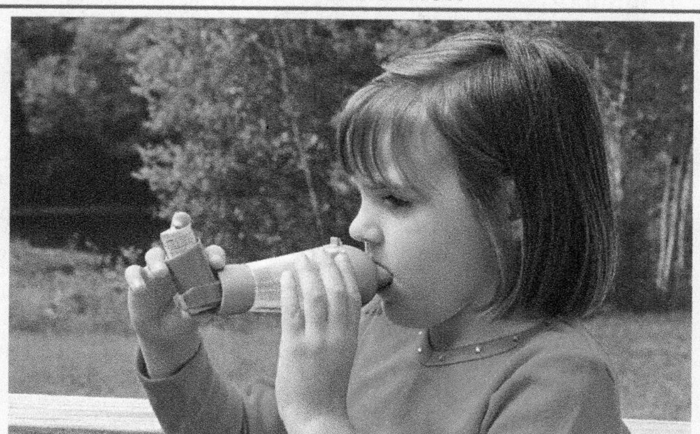

■ **Figure 14.3** Inhalation medication administration. Photograph of a young girl using a metered-dose inhaler.

METHOD	WORD PARTS	DESCRIPTION
parenteral	para- = near, beside enter/o = intestine -al = pertaining to	An invasive method of administering drugs as it requires the skin to be punctured by a needle. The needle with syringe attached is introduced either under the skin or into a muscle, vein, or body cavity.
intracavitary (in-trah-KAV-ih-tair-ee)	intra- = within -ary = pertaining to	Injection into a body cavity such as the peritoneal and chest cavity.
intradermal (ID) (in-trah-DER-mal)	intra- = within derm/o = skin -al = pertaining to	Very shallow injection just under the top layer of skin. Commonly used in skin testing for allergies and tuberculosis testing.

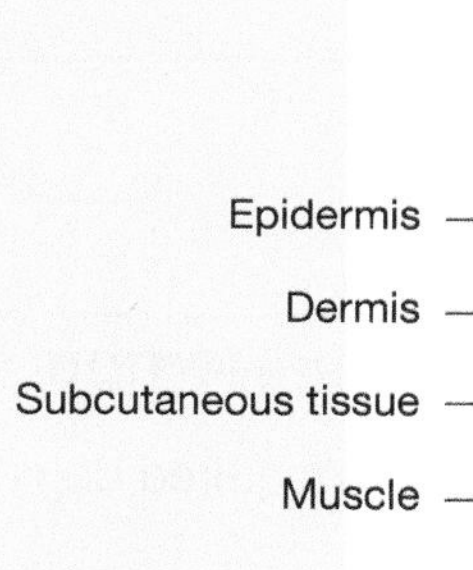
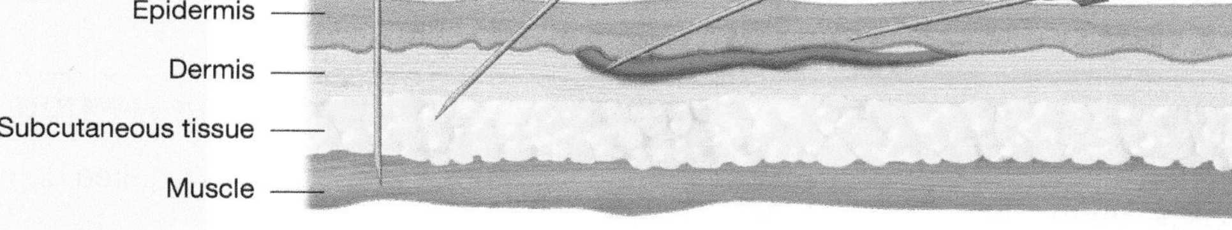

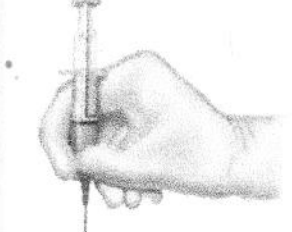

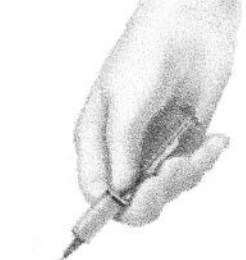

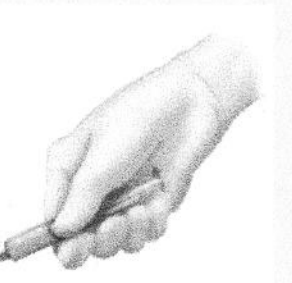

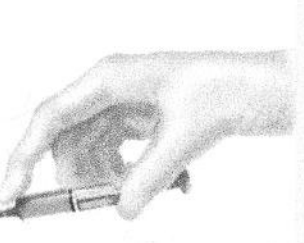

■ **Figure 14.4** Parenteral medication administration. The angle of needle insertion for four different types of parenteral injections.

METHOD	WORD PARTS	DESCRIPTION
intramuscular (IM) (in-trah-MUSS-kyoo-lar)	intra- = within muscul/o = muscle -ar = pertaining to	Injection directly into the muscle of the buttocks, thigh, or upper arm. Used when there is a large amount of medication or it is irritating (see again Figure 14.4).
intrathecal (in-trah-THEE-kal)	intra- = within thec/o = sheath (meninges) -al = pertaining to	Injection into the meningeal space surrounding the brain and spinal cord.

Table 14.3 Common Routes of Drug Administration (continued)

METHOD	WORD PARTS	DESCRIPTION
intravenous (IV) (in-trah-VEE-nus)	intra- = within ven/o = vein -ous = pertaining to	Injection into the veins. This route may be set up to deliver medication very quickly or to deliver a continuous drip of medication (see again Figure 14.4).
subcutaneous (Subc, SubQ) (sub-kyoo-TAY-nee-us)	sub- = under cutane/o = skin -ous = pertaining to	Injection into the subcutaneous layer of the skin, usually the upper, outer arm or abdomen (see again Figure 14.4); for example, insulin injection.
transdermal	trans- = through derm/o = skin -al = pertaining to	Includes medications that coat the underside of a patch, which is applied to the skin where it is then absorbed. Examples include birth control patches, nicotine patches, and sea sickness patches.
rectal	rect/o = rectum -al = pertaining to	Includes medications introduced directly into the rectal cavity in the form of **suppositories** or solution. Drugs may have to be administered by this route if the patient is unable to take them by mouth due to nausea, vomiting, or surgery.
topical	topic/o = a specific area -al = pertaining to	Includes medications applied directly to the skin or mucous membranes. They are distributed in ointment, cream, or lotion form, and are used to treat skin infections and eruptions.
vaginal	vagin/o = vagina -al = pertaining to	Includes tablets and suppositories that may be inserted vaginally to treat vaginal yeast infections and other irritations.
eyedrops		Includes drops used during eye examinations to dilate the pupil of the eye for better examination of the interior of the eye. They are also placed into the eye to control eye pressure in glaucoma and treat infections.
eardrops		Includes drops placed directly into the ear canal for the purpose of relieving pain or treating infection.
buccal	bucc/o = cheek -al = pertaining to	Includes drugs that are placed under the lip or between the cheek and gum.

Pharmacology Terms

TERM	WORD PARTS	DEFINITION
addiction (ah-DICK-shun)		Acquired dependence on a drug.
additive		Sum of the action of two (or more) drugs given. In this case, the total strength of the medications is equal to the sum of the strength of each individual drug.
antidote (AN-tih-doht)	anti- = against	Substance that will neutralize poisons or their side effects.
broad spectrum		Ability of a drug to be effective against a wide range of microorganisms.
contraindication (kon-trah-in-dih-KAY-shun)	contra- = against	Condition in which a particular drug should not be used.
cumulative action		Action that occurs in the body when a drug is allowed to accumulate or stay in the body.

Pharmacology Terms *(continued)*

TERM	WORD PARTS	DEFINITION
drug interaction		Occurs when the effect of one drug is altered because it was taken at the same time as another drug.
drug tolerance		Decrease in susceptibility to a drug after continued use of the drug.
habituation (hah-bich-yoo-AY-shun)		Development of an emotional dependence on a drug due to repeated use.
iatrogenic (eye-ah-troh-JEN-ik)	iatr/o = medicine -genic = produced by	Usually an unfavorable response resulting from taking a medication.
idiosyncrasy (id-ee-oh-SIN-krah-see)	idi/o = distinctive	Unusual or abnormal response to a drug or food.
placebo (plah-SEE-boh)		Inactive, harmless substance used to satisfy a patient's desire for medication. This is also used in research when given to a control group of patients in a study in which another group receives a drug. The effect of the placebo versus the drug is then observed.
potentiation (poe-ten-chee-A-shun)		Giving a patient a second drug to boost (potentiate) the effect of another drug. The total strength of the drugs is greater than the sum of the strength of the individual drugs.
prophylaxis (proh-fih-LAK-sis)	pro- = before -phylaxis = protection	Prevention of disease. For example, an antibiotic can be used to prevent the occurrence of a disease.
side effect		Response to a drug other than the effect desired. Also called an *adverse reaction.*
tolerance (TAHL-er-ans)		Development of a capacity for withstanding a large amount of a substance, such as foods, drugs, or poison, without any adverse effect. A decreased sensitivity to further doses will develop.
toxicity (tok-SISS-ih-tee)	toxic/o = poison	Extent or degree to which a substance is poisonous.
unit dose		Drug dosage system that provides prepackaged, prelabeled, individual medications that are ready for immediate use by the patient.

Abbreviations

@	at
ā	before
ac	before meals
ad lib	as desired
ante	before
APAP	acetaminophen (Tylenol™)
aq	aqueous (water)
ASA	aspirin
bid	twice a day
c̄	with
cap(s)	capsule(s)
d	day
d/c, DISC	discontinue
DC, disc	discontinue
DEA	Drug Enforcement Agency
dil	dilute
disp	dispense
dtd	give of such a dose
Dx	diagnosis
et	and
FDA	Federal Drug Administration
gm	gram
gr	grain
gt	drop
gtt	drops
hs	at bedtime
i̇	one
ID	intradermal
i̇i̇	two
i̇i̇i̇	three
IM	intramuscular
inj	injection
IV	intravenous
kg	kilogram
L	liter
mcg	microgram
mEq	milliequivalent
mg	milligram
mL	milliliter
no sub	no substitute
noc	night
non rep	do not repeat
NPO	nothing by mouth
NS	normal saline
od	overdose
oint	ointment
OTC	over the counter
oz	ounce
p̄	after
pc	after meals
PCA	patient-controlled administration
PDR	*Physician's Desk Reference*
per	with
po	by mouth
prn	as needed
pt	patient
q	every
qam	every morning
qh	every hour
qhs	at bedtime
qid	four times a day
qs	quantity sufficient
Rx	take
s̄	without
Sig	label as follows/directions
sl	under the tongue
sol	solution
s̄s̄	one-half
stat	at once/immediately
Subc, SubQ	subcutaneous
suppos, supp	suppository
susp	suspension
syr	syrup
T, tbsp	tablespoon
t, tsp	teaspoon
tab	tablet
tid	three times a day
TO	telephone order
top	apply topically
VO	verbal order
wt	weight
x	times

Section II: Mental Health at a Glance

Word Parts

Here are the most common word parts (with their meanings) used to build mental health terms.

Combining Forms

amnes/o	forgetfulness	path/o	disease
anxi/o	fear, worry	ped/o	child
chondr/o	cartilage	pharmac/o	drug
compuls/o	drive, compel	phob/o	irrational fear
deluss/o	false belief	phren/o	mind
depress/o	to press down	psych/o	mind
electr/o	electricity	pyr/o	fire
factiti/o	artificial, contrived	schiz/o	split
hallucin/o	imagined perception	soci/o	society
klept/o	to steal	somat/o	body
ment/o	mind	somn/o	sleep
obsess/o	besieged by thoughts		

Suffixes

-al	pertaining to	-logist	one who studies
-ar	pertaining to	-logy	study of
-ia	state, condition	-mania	frenzy
-iatrist	physician	-orexia	appetite
-iatry	medical treatment	-ous	pertaining to
-ic	pertaining to	-philia	attracted to
-ism	state of	-therapy	treatment
-logical	pertaining to the study of	-tic	pertaining to

Prefixes

an-	without	dis-	apart
anti-	against	ex-	outward
auto-	self	hyper-	excessive
bi-	two	hypo-	below
de-	without	in-	not

 Mental Health Disciplines

Psychology

abnormal psychology
clinical psychologist (sigh-KALL-oh-jist)
normal psychology
psychology (sigh-KALL-oh-jee)

Psychology is the study of human behavior and thought processes. This behavioral science is primarily concerned with understanding how human beings interact with their physical environment and with each other. Behavior can be divided into two categories: normal and abnormal. The study of **normal psychology** includes how the personality develops, how people handle stress, and the stages of mental development. In contrast, **abnormal psychology** studies and treats behaviors that are outside of normal and that are detrimental to the person or society. These maladaptive behaviors range from occasional difficulty coping with stress, to bizarre actions and beliefs, to total withdrawal. A **clinical psychologist,** though not a physician, is a specialist in evaluating and treating persons with mental and emotional disorders.

> **MED TERM TIP**
> All social interactions pose some problems for some people. These problems are not necessarily abnormal. One means of judging if behavior is abnormal is to compare one person's behavior with others in the community. Also, if a person's behavior interferes with the activities of daily living, it is often considered abnormal.

Psychiatry

psychiatric nurse (sigh-kee-AT-rik)
psychiatric social worker
psychiatrist (sigh-KIGH-ah-trist)
psychiatry (sigh-KIGH-ah-tree)

Psychiatry is the branch of medicine that deals with the diagnosis, treatment, and prevention of mental disorders. A **psychiatrist** is a medical physician specializing in the care of patients with mental, emotional, and behavioral disorders. Other health professions also have specialty areas in caring for clients with mental illness. Good examples are **psychiatric nurses** and **psychiatric social workers.**

> **MED TERM TIP**
> Look for these word parts:
> psych/o = mind
> -iatrist = physician
> -iatry = medical treatment
> -logist = one who studies
> -logy = study of

Genetics

Medical genetics seeks to understand how genetic variation relates to human health and disease, hence much of the research into the causes of mental disease, such as Alzheimer's, includes the study of genetics. This research is done by a **geneticist**. A **geneticist** is a biologist who studies genetics, the science of genes, heredity, and variation of organisms. Medical terminology associated with a geneticist will focus on these areas of study. To help treat mental health disease, and perhaps find a cure, continued research and discovery is essential.

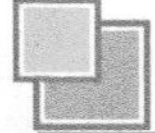 Pathology

The legal definition of mental disorder is "impaired judgment and lack of self-control." The guide for terminology and classifications relating to psychiatric disorders is the *Diagnostic and Statistical Manual of Mental Disorders, Fourth Edition* (Text Revision) (DSM-IV-TR™), which is published by the American Psychiatric Association (2004). The DSM organizes mental disorders into 14 major diagnostic categories of mental disorders.

> **MED TERM TIP**
> Mental disorders are sometimes more simply characterized by whether they are a *neurosis* or a *psychosis.* Neuroses are inappropriate coping mechanisms to handle stress, such as phobias and panic attacks. Psychoses involve extreme distortions of reality and disorganization of a person's thinking, including bizarre behaviors, hallucinations, and delusions. Schizophrenia is an example of a psychosis.

TERM	WORD PARTS	DEFINITION
Anxiety disorders	anxi/o = fear, worry	Characterized by persistent worry and apprehension.
panic attacks	-ic = pertaining to	Feeling of intense apprehension, terror, or sense of impending danger.
anxiety (ang-ZY-eh-tee)	anxi/o = fear, worry	Feeling of dread in the absence of a clearly identifiable stress trigger.
phobias (FOH-bee-ahs)	phob/o = irrational fear -ia = state, condition	Irrational fear, such as *arachnophobia,* or fear of spiders.

Pathology (continued)

TERM	WORD PARTS	DEFINITION
obsessive–compulsive disorder (OCD) (ob-SESS-iv / kom-PUHL-siv)	obsess/o = besieged by thoughts compuls/o = drive, compel	Performing repetitive rituals to reduce anxiety.
Cognitive disorders		Deterioration of mental functions due to temporary brain or permanent brain dysfunction.
dementia (dee-MEN-she-ah)	de- = without ment/o = mind -ia = state, condition	Progressive confusion and disorientation.
Alzheimer's disease (ALTS-high-merz)		Degenerative brain disorder with gradual loss of cognitive abilities.
Disorders diagnosed in infancy and childhood		Mental disorders associated with childhood; include:
mental retardation	ment/o = mind -al = pertaining to	Subaverage intellectual functioning.
attention-deficit/hyperactivity disorder (ADHD)	hyper- = excessive	Inattention and impulsive behavior.
autism (AW-tizm)	auto- = self -ism = state of	Condition involving deficits in social interaction, communication skills, and restricted patterns of behavior.
Dissociative disorders	dis- = apart soci/o = society	Disorders in which severe emotional conflict is so repressed that a split in the personality may occur or the person may lose memory.
amnesia (am-NEE-zee-ah)	amnes/o = forgetfulness -ia = state, condition	Loss of memory.
dissociative identity disorder		Having two or more distinct personalities.
Eating disorders		Abnormal behaviors related to eating; include:
anorexia nervosa (an-oh-REK-see-ah / ner-VOH-sah)	an- = without -orexia = appetite	Refusal to eat.

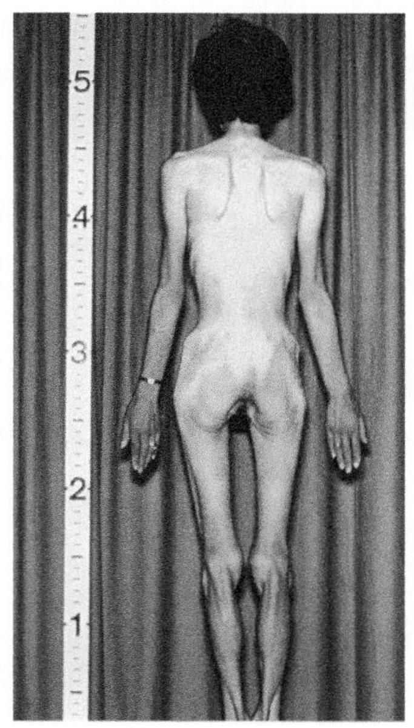

■ **Figure 14.5** Photograph of a young woman suffering from anorexia nervosa, posterior view. *(Custom Medical Stock Photo, Inc.)*

Pathology *(continued)*

TERM	WORD PARTS	DEFINITION
bulimia (boo-LIM-ee-ah)	-ia = state, condition	Binge eating and intentional vomiting.
Factitious disorders	factiti/o = artificial, contrived -ous = pertaining to	Intentionally feigning illness symptoms in order to gain attention.
malingering		Pretending to be ill or injured.
Impulse control disorders		Inability to resist an impulse to perform some act that is harmful to the individual or others; include:
kleptomania (klep-toh-MAY-nee-ah)	klept/o = to steal -mania = frenzy	Stealing.
pyromania (pie-roh-MAY-nee-ah)	pyr/o = fire -mania = frenzy	Setting fires.
explosive disorder	ex- = outward	Violent rages.
pathological gambling (path-ah-LOJ-ih-kal)	path/o = disease -logical = pertaining to the study of	Inability to stop gambling.
Mood disorders		Characterized by instability in mood; include:
major depression	depress/o = to press down	Feelings of hopelessness, helplessness, worthlessness; lack of pleasure in any activity; potential for suicide.
mania (MAY-nee-ah)	-mania = frenzy	Extreme elation.
bipolar disorder (BPD)	bi- = two -ar = pertaining to	Alternation between periods of deep depression and mania.

MED TERM TIP

The healthcare professional must take all threats of suicide from patients seriously. Psychologists tell us that there is no clear suicide type, which means that we cannot predict who will actually take his or her own life. Always tell the physician about any discussion a patient has concerning suicide. If you believe a patient is in danger of suicide, do not be afraid to ask, "Are you thinking about suicide?"

TERM	WORD PARTS	DEFINITION
Personality disorders		Inflexible or maladaptive behavior patterns that affect a person's ability to function in society; include:
paranoid personality disorder		Exaggerated feelings of persecution.
narcissistic personality disorder (nar-sis-SIST-ik)		Abnormal sense of self-importance.
antisocial personality disorder	anti- = against soci/o = society -al = pertaining to	Behaviors that are against legal or social norms.

Pathology *(continued)*

TERM	WORD PARTS	DEFINITION
passive aggressive personality		Indirect expression of hostility or anger.
Schizophrenia	schiz/o = split phren/o = mind -ia = state, condition	Mental disorders characterized by distortions of reality such as:
delusion (dee-LOO-zhun)	deluss/o = false belief	A false belief held even in the face of contrary evidence.
hallucination (hah-loo-sih-NAY-shun)	hallucin/o = imagined perception	Perceiving something that is not there.
Sexual disorders		Disorders include aberrant sexual activity and sexual dysfunction; include:
pedophilia (pee-doh-FILL-ee-ah)	ped/o = child -philia = attracted to	Sexual interest in children.
masochism (MAS-oh-kizm)	-ism = state of	Gratification derived from being hurt or abused.
voyeurism (VOY-er-izm)	-ism = state of	Gratification derived from observing others engaged in sexual acts.
Sleeping disorders		Disorders relating to sleeping; include:
insomnia (in-SOM-nee-ah)	in- = not somn/o = sleep -ia = state, condition	Inability to sleep.
sleepwalking		Getting up and walking around unaware while sleeping.
Somatoform disorders	somat/o = body	Patient has physical symptoms for which no physical disease can be determined; include:
hypochondria (high-poh-KON-dree-ah)	hypo- = below chondr/o = cartilage -ia = state, condition	A preoccupation with health concerns. Named for the location of the liver and spleen, below the rib cartilage. The ancient Greeks thought these organs controlled mood.
conversion reaction		Anxiety is transformed into physical symptoms such as heart palpitations, paralysis, or blindness.
Substance-related disorders		Overindulgence or dependence on chemical substances including alcohol, illegal drugs, and prescription drugs.

Therapeutic Procedures

TERM	WORD PARTS	DEFINITION
Electroconvulsive therapy (ECT) (ee-lek-troh-kon-VULL-siv)	electr/o = electricity	Procedure occasionally used for cases of prolonged major depression. This controversial treatment involves placement of an electrode on one or both sides of the patient's head and a current is turned on briefly causing a convulsive seizure. A low level of voltage is used in modern electroconvulsive therapy, and the patient is administered a muscle relaxant and anesthesia. Advocates of this treatment state that it is a more effective way to treat severe depression than using drugs. It is not effective with disorders other than depression, such as schizophrenia and alcoholism.
Psychopharmacology (sigh-koh-far-mah-KALL-oh-jee)	psych/o = mind pharmac/o = drug -logy = study of	Study of the effects of drugs on the mind and particularly the use of drugs in treating mental disorders. The main classes of drugs for the treatment of mental disorders are:
antipsychotic drugs	anti- = against psych/o = mind -tic = pertaining to	Major tranquilizers include chlorpromazine (Thorazine™), haloperidol (Haldol™), clozapine (Clozaril™), and risperidone. These drugs have transformed the treatment of patients with psychoses and schizophrenia by reducing patient agitation and panic and shortening schizophrenic episodes. One of the side effects of these drugs is involuntary muscle movements, which approximately one-fourth of all adults who take the drugs develop.
antidepressant drugs	anti- = against depress/o = to press down	Classified as stimulants and alter the patient's mood by affecting levels of neurotransmitters in the brain. Antidepressants, such as serotonin norepinephrine reuptake inhibitors, are nonaddictive but they can produce unpleasant side effects such as dry mouth, weight gain, blurred vision, and nausea.
minor tranquilizers		Include Valium™ and Xanax™. These are also classified as central nervous system depressants and are prescribed for anxiety.
lithium		Special category of drug used successfully to calm patients who suffer from bipolar disorder (depression alternating with manic excitement).

Therapeutic Procedures *(continued)*

TERM	WORD PARTS	DEFINITION
Psychotherapy (sigh-koh-THAIR-ah-pee)	psych/o = mind -therapy = treatment	A method of treating mental disorders by mental rather than chemical or physical means. It includes:
psychoanalysis	psych/o = mind	Method of obtaining a detailed account of the past and present emotional and mental experiences from the patient to determine the source of the problem and eliminate the effects. It is a system developed by Sigmund Freud that encourages the patient to discuss repressed, painful, or hidden experiences with the hope of eliminating or minimizing the problem.
humanistic psychotherapy	-tic = pertaining to psych/o = mind -therapy = treatment	Therapist does not delve into the patients' past when using these methods. Instead, it is believed that patients can learn how to use their own internal resources to deal with their problems. The therapist creates a therapeutic atmosphere, which builds patient self-esteem and encourages discussion of problems, thereby gaining insight in how to handle them. Also called *client-centered* or *nondirective psychotherapy.*
family and group psychotherapy	psych/o = mind -therapy = treatment	Often described as solution focused, the therapist places minimal emphasis on patient past history and strong emphasis on having patient state and discuss goals and then find a way to achieve them.

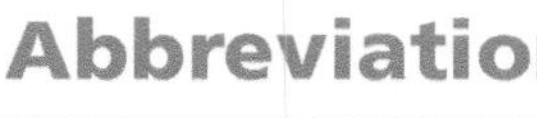

Abbreviations

AD	Alzheimer's disease	**ECT**	electroconvulsive therapy
ADD	attention-deficit disorder	**MA**	mental age
ADHD	attention-deficit/hyperactivity disorder	**MMPI**	Minnesota Multiphasic Personality Inventory
BPD	bipolar disorder	**OCD**	obsessive–compulsive disorder
CA	chronological age	**SAD**	seasonal affective disorder
DSM	*Diagnostic and Statistical Manual of Mental Disorders*		

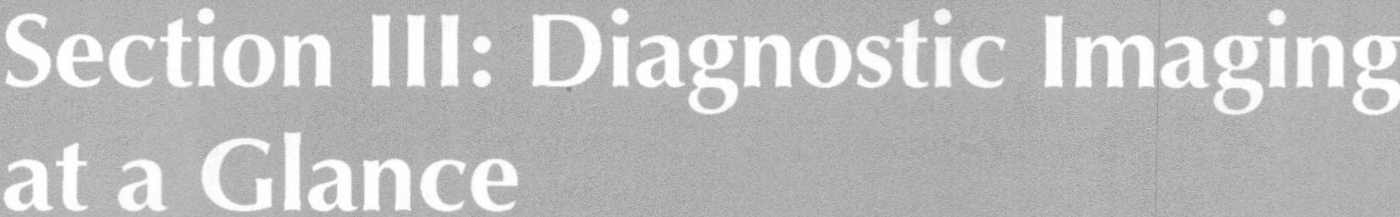

Section III: Diagnostic Imaging at a Glance

Word Parts

Here are the most common word parts (with their meanings) used to build diagnostic imaging terms.

Combining Forms

anter/o	front
fluor/o	fluorescence, luminous
later/o	side
nucle/o	nucleus
poster/o	back
radi/o	ray (X-ray)
roentgen/o	X-ray
son/o	sound
tom/o	to cut

Suffixes

-al	pertaining to
-ar	pertaining to
-graphy	process of recording
-ic	pertaining to
-ior	pertaining to
-logist	one who studies
-logy	study of
-lucent	to shine through
-opaque	nontransparent
-scopy	process of visually examining

Prefix

ultra-	beyond

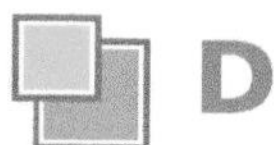

Diagnostic Imaging

roentgenology (rent-gen-ALL-oh-jee) **X-rays**

Diagnostic imaging is the medical specialty that uses a variety of methods to produce images of the internal structures of the body. These images are then used to diagnose disease. This area of medicine began as **roentgenology** (roentgen/o = X-ray; -logy = study of), named after German physicist Wilhelm Roentgen who discovered roentgen rays in 1895. This discovery, now commonly known as **X-rays,** revolutionized the diagnosis of disease.

Diagnostic Imaging is one of the more technical fields of medical and dental care. To improve understanding of the many processes specific to this field you may need to consult and interpret technical materials to expand your knowledge for the various procedures included in this chapter.

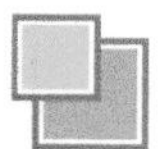

Diagnostic Imaging Terms

TERM	WORD PARTS	DEFINITION
anteroposterior view (AP view)	anter/o = front poster/o = back -ior = pertaining to	Positioning the patient so that the X-rays pass through the body from the anterior side to the posterior side.
barium (Ba) (BAH-ree-um)		Soft metallic element from the earth used as a radiopaque X-ray dye.
film		Thin sheet of cellulose material coated with a light-sensitive substance that is used in taking photographs. There is a special photographic film that is sensitive to X-rays.
film badge		Badge containing film that is sensitive to X-rays. This is worn by all personnel in radiology to measure the amount of X-rays to which they are exposed.
lateral view	later/o = side -al = pertaining to	Positioning of the patient so that the side of the body faces the X-ray machine.
oblique view (oh-BLEEK)		Positioning of the patient so that the X-rays pass through the body on an angle.
posteroanterior view (PA view)	poster/o = back anter/o = front -ior = pertaining to	Positioning of the patient so that the X-rays pass through the body from the posterior side to the anterior side.
radiography (ray-dee-OG-rah-fee)	radi/o = X-ray -graphy = process of recording	Making of X-ray pictures.
radioisotope (ray-dee-oh-EYE-soh-tohp)	radi/o = X-ray	Radioactive form of an element.
radiologist (ray-dee-ALL-oh-jist)	radi/o = X-ray -logist = one who studies	Physician who uses images to diagnose abnormalities and radiant energy to treat various conditions such as cancer.
radiolucent (ray-dee-oh-LOO-cent)	radi/o = X-ray -lucent = to shine through	Structures that allow X-rays to pass through; expose the photographic plate and appear as black areas on the X-ray.
radiopaque (ray-dee-oh-PAYK)	radi/o = X-ray -opaque = nontransparent	Structures that are impenetrable to X-rays, appearing as a light area on the radiograph (X-ray).

Diagnostic Imaging Terms *(continued)*

TERM	WORD PARTS	DEFINITION
roentgen (RENT-gen)	roentgen/o = X-ray	Unit for describing an exposure dose of radiation.
scan		Recording on a photographic plate the emission of radioactive waves after a substance has been injected into the body.
shield		Device used to protect against radiation.
tagging		Attaching a radioactive material to a chemical, and tracing it as it moves through the body.
uptake		Absorption of radioactive material and medicines into an organ or tissue.
X-ray		High-energy wave that can penetrate most solid matter and present the image on photographic film.

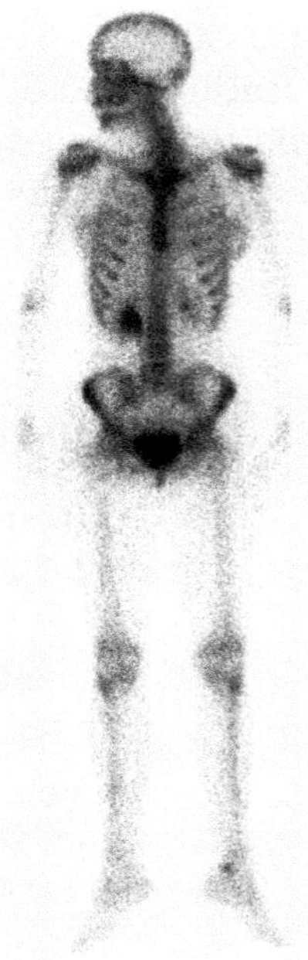

■ **Figure 14.6** Nuclear medicine. Bone scan produced after injection of a radioactive substance into the body. *(Getty Images, Inc/Photodisc)*

Diagnostic Imaging Procedures

TERM	WORD PARTS	DEFINITION
computed tomography scan (CT scan) (toh-MOG-rah-fee)	tom/o = to cut -graphy = process of recording	Imaging technique that is able to produce a cross-sectional view of the body. X-ray pictures are taken at multiple angles through the body. A computer then uses all these images to construct a composite cross-section.

Diagnostic Imaging Procedures *(continued)*

TERM	WORD PARTS	DEFINITION
contrast studies 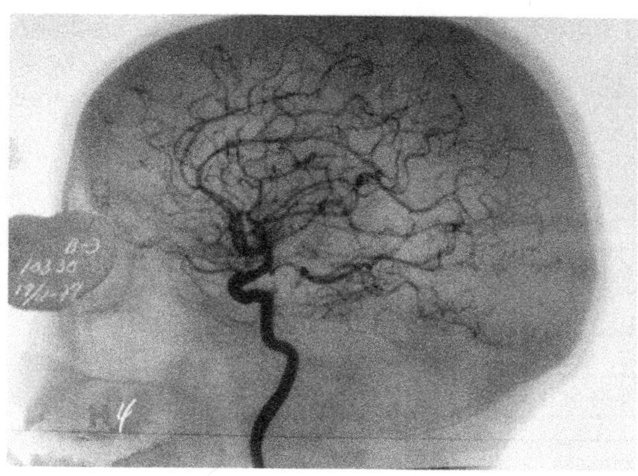 ■ **Figure 14.7** Contrast study. X-ray of cerebral blood vessels taken after injection of a radiopaque substance into the bloodstream.		Radiopaque substance is injected or swallowed. X-rays are then taken that will outline the body structure containing the radiopaque substance. For example, angiograms and myelograms.
Doppler ultrasonography	ultra- = beyond son/o = sound -graphy = process of recording	Use of ultrasound to record the velocity of blood flowing through blood vessels. Used to detect blood clots and blood vessel obstructions.
fluoroscopy (floo-or-OS-koh-pee)	fluor/o = luminous -scopy = process of visually examining	X-rays strike a fluorescing screen rather than a photographic plate, causing it to glow. The glowing screen changes from minute to minute; therefore movement, such as the heart beating or the digestive tract moving, can be seen.
magnetic resonance imaging (MRI) (REZ-oh-nence) 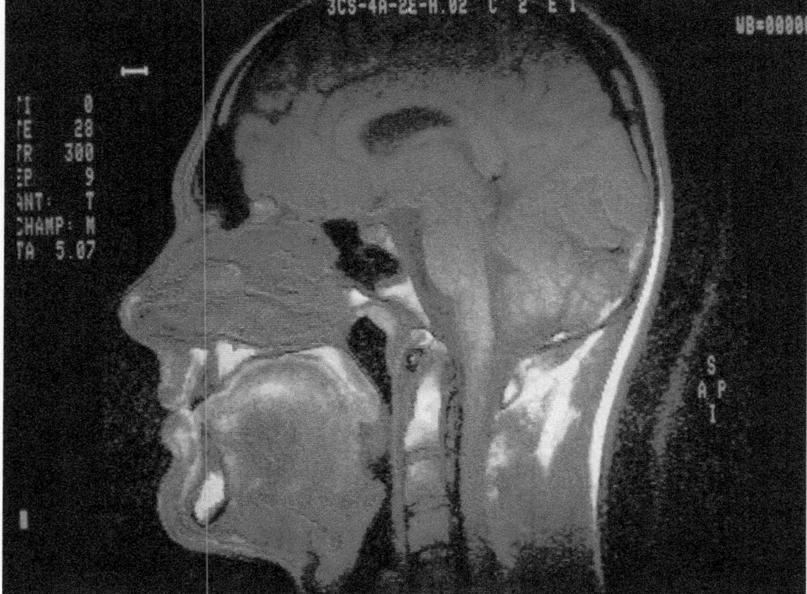 	-ic = pertaining to	Use of electromagnetic energy to produce an image of soft tissues in any plane of the body. Atoms behave differently when placed in a strong magnetic field. When the body is exposed to this magnetic field the nuclei of the body's atoms emit radio-frequency signals that can be used to create an image. ■ **Figure 14.8** Color-enhanced magnetic resonance image (MRI) showing a sagittal view of the head. *(Photo Researchers, Inc.)*

Diagnostic Imaging Procedures *(continued)*

TERM	WORD PARTS	DEFINITION
nuclear medicine	nucle/o = nucleus -ar = pertaining to	Use of radioactive substances to diagnose diseases. A radioactive substance known to accumulate in certain body tissues is injected or inhaled. After waiting for the substance to travel to the body area of interest, the radioactivity level is recorded. Commonly referred to as a *scan* (see again Figure 14.6). See Table 14.4 ■ for examples of the radioactive substances used in nuclear medicine.

Table 14.4 Substances Used to Visualize Various Body Organs in Nuclear Medicine

ORGAN	SUBSTANCE
bone	technetium (^{99m}Tc)–labeled phosphate
tumors	gallium (^{67}Ga)
lungs	xenon (^{133}Xe)
liver	technetium (^{99m}Tc)–labeled sulfur
heart	thallium (^{201}Tl)
thyroid	iodine (^{131}I)

TERM	WORD PARTS	DEFINITION
positron emission tomography (PET) (POS-ih-tron / eh-MIS-shun / toh-MOG-rah-fee)	tom/o = to cut -graphy = process of recording	Image is produced following the injection of radioactive glucose. The glucose will accumulate in areas of high metabolic activity. Therefore, this process will highlight areas that are consuming a large quantity of glucose. This may show an active area of the brain or a tumor.

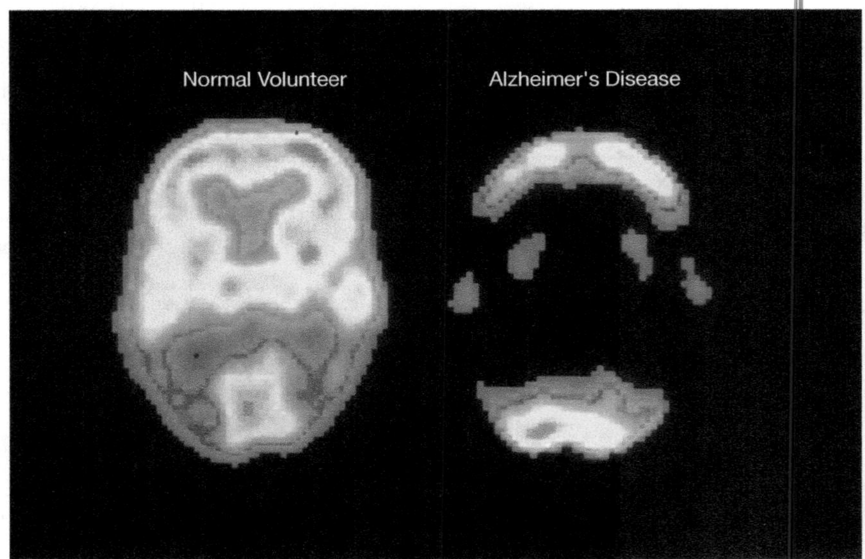

■ **Figure 14.9** Positron emission tomography (PET) image showing the difference in the metabolic activity of the brain of a person with Alzheimer's disease and that of a normal person. *(Science Source/Photo Researchers Inc.)*

TERM	WORD PARTS	DEFINITION
radiology (ray-dee-ALL-oh-jee)	radi/o = X-ray -logy = study of	Use of high-energy radiation, X-rays, to expose a photographic plate. The image is a black-and-white picture with radiopaque structures such as bone appearing white and radiolucent tissue such as muscles appearing dark.

Diagnostic Imaging Procedures *(continued)*

TERM	WORD PARTS	DEFINITION
ultrasound (US) (ULL-trah-sound)	ultra- = beyond	Use of high-frequency sound waves to produce an image. Sound waves directed into the body from a transducer will bounce off internal structures and echo back to the transducer. The speed of the echo is dependent on the density of the tissue. A computer is able to correlate speed of echo with density and produce an image. Used to visualize internal organs, heart valves, and fetuses.

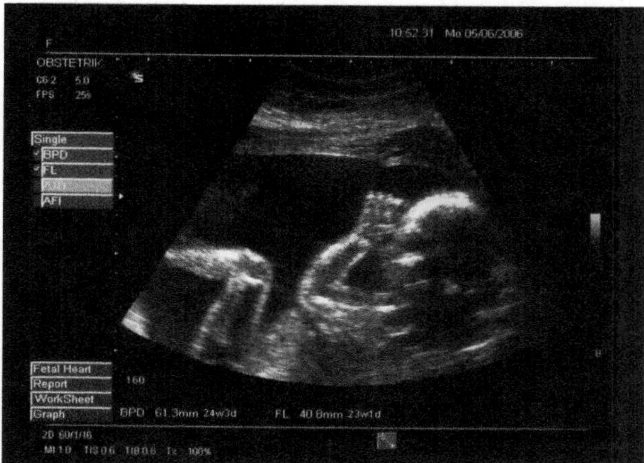

■ **Figure 14.10** Ultrasound showing the outline of a fetus.

Abbreviations

^{67}Ga	radioactive gallium	**DI**	diagnostic imaging
^{99m}Tc	radioactive technetium	**DSA**	digital subtraction angiography
^{131}I	radioactive iodine	**ERCP**	endoscopic retrograde cholangiopancreatography
^{201}Tl	radioactive thallium	**Fx**	fracture
^{133}Xe	radioactive xenon	**GB**	gallbladder X-ray
Angio	angiography	**IVC**	intravenous cholangiogram
AP	anteroposterior	**IVP**	intravenous pyelogram
Ba	barium	**KUB**	kidneys, ureters, bladder
BaE	barium enema	**LAT**	lateral
CAT	computerized axial tomography	**LGI**	lower gastrointestinal series
Ci	curie	**LL**	left lateral
CT	computerized tomography	**mA**	milliampere
CXR	chest X-ray	**mCi**	millicurie
decub	lying down		

Abbreviations *(continued)*

MRA	magnetic resonance angiography
MRI	magnetic resonance imaging
NMR	nuclear magnetic resonance
PA	posteroanterior
PET	positron emission tomography
PTC	percutaneous transhepatic cholangiography
R	roentgen
Ra	radium
rad	radiation-absorbed dose
RL	right lateral
RRT	registered radiologic technologist
UGI	upper gastrointestinal series
US	ultrasound

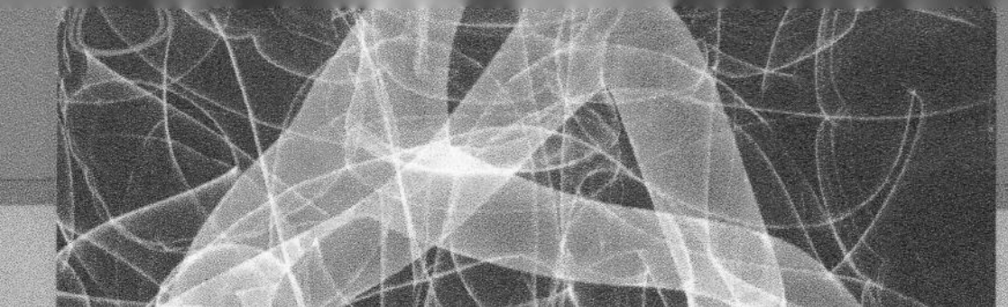

Section IV: Rehabilitation Services at a Glance

Word Parts

Here are the most common word parts (with their meanings) used to build rehabilitation services terms.

Combining Forms

cry/o	cold
cutane/o	skin
electr/o	electric current
erg/o	work
habilitat/o	ability
hydr/o	water
my/o	muscle
orth/o	straight, correct
phon/o	sound
physic/o	body
prosthet/o	addition
therm/o	heat

Suffixes

-al	pertaining to
-graphy	process of recording
-ic	pertaining to
-nomics	pertaining to laws
-ous	pertaining to
-phoresis	carrying
-therapy	treatment
-tic	pertaining to

Prefixes

re-	again
trans-	across
ultra-	beyond

Rehabilitation Services

occupational therapy **physical therapy**

The goal of rehabilitation is to prevent disability and restore as much function as possible following disease, illness, or injury. Rehabilitation services include the healthcare specialties of **physical therapy** (PT) and **occupational therapy** (OT).

Physical Therapy

Physical therapy (PT) involves treating disorders using physical means and methods. Physical therapy personnel assess joint motion, muscle strength and endurance, function of heart and lungs, performance of activities required in daily living, and the ability to carry out other responsibilities. Physical therapy treatment includes gait training, therapeutic exercise, massage, joint and soft tissue mobilization, thermotherapy, cryotherapy, electrical stimulation, ultrasound, and hydrotherapy. These methods strengthen muscles, improve motion and circulation, reduce pain, and increase function.

Occupational Therapy

Occupational therapy (OT) assists patients to regain, develop, and improve skills that are important for independent functioning (activities of daily living). Occupational therapy personnel work with people who, because of illness, injury, or developmental or psychological impairments, require specialized training in skills that will enable them to lead independent, productive, and satisfying lives in regard to personal care, work, and leisure. Occupational therapists instruct patients in the use of adaptive equipment and techniques, body mechanics, and energy conservation. They also employ modalities such as heat, cold, and therapeutic exercise.

Rehabilitation Services Terms

TERM	WORD PARTS	DEFINITION
activities of daily living (ADL)		Activities usually performed in the course of a normal day, such as eating, dressing, and washing.

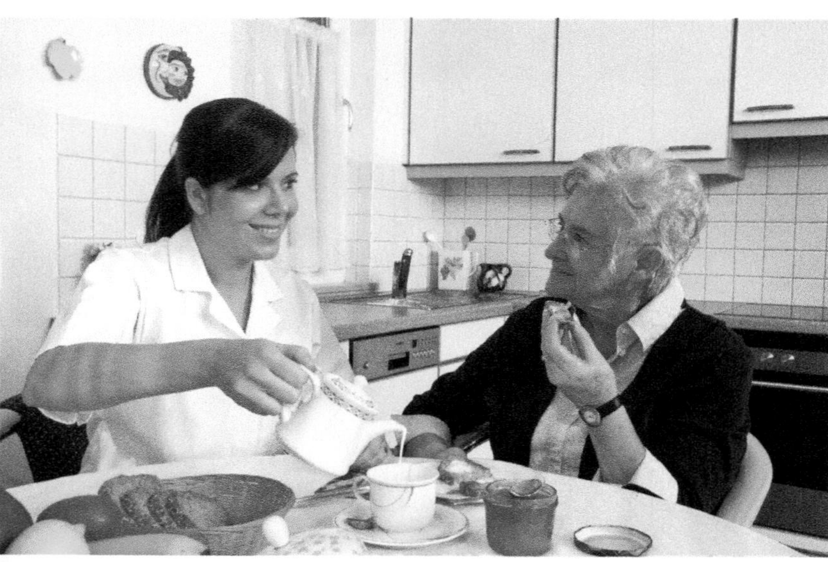

■ **Figure 14.11** Photograph of an occupational therapist assisting a patient with learning independence in activities of daily living (ADLs). *(Gina Sanders/ Shutterstock)*

Rehabilitation Services Terms *(continued)*

TERM	WORD PARTS	DEFINITION
adaptive equipment		Modification of equipment or devices to improve the function and independence of a person with a disability.
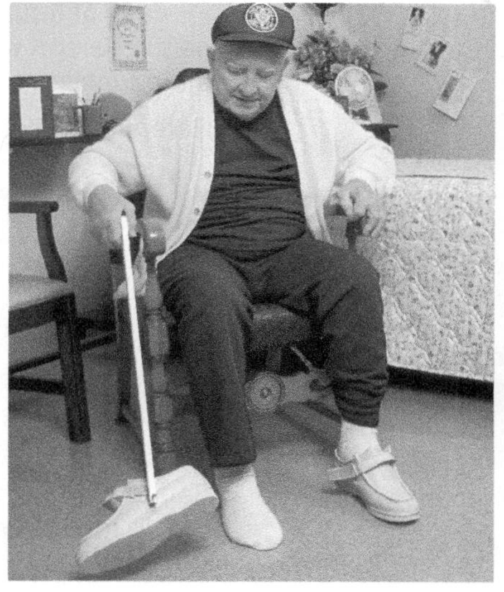 A	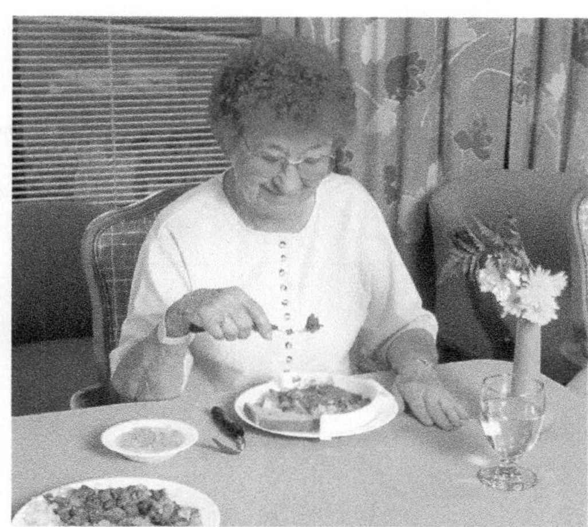 B	■ Figure 14.12 Using adaptive equipment: (A) male putting on shoe; (B) female eating one handed.
body mechanics	-ic = pertaining to	Use of good posture and position while performing activities of daily living to prevent injury and stress on body parts.
ergonomics (er-goh-NOM-iks)	erg/o = work -nomics = pertaining to laws	Study of human work including how the requirements for performing work and the work environment affect the musculoskeletal and nervous systems.
fine motor skills		Use of precise and coordinated movements in such activities such as writing, buttoning, and cutting.
gait (GAYT)		Manner of walking.
gross motor skills		Use of large muscle groups that coordinate body movements such as walking, running, jumping, and balance.
lower extremity (LE)		Refers to one of the legs.
mobility		State of having normal movement of all body parts.
orthotics (or-THOT-iks)	orth/o = straight -tic = pertaining to	Use of equipment, such as splints and braces, to support a paralyzed muscle, promote a specific motion, or correct musculoskeletal deformities.
physical medicine	physic/o = body -al = pertaining to	Branch of medicine focused on restoring function. Primarily cares for patients with musculoskeletal and nervous system disorders. Physician is a *physiatrist.*
prosthetics (pros-THET-iks)	prosthet/o = addition -ic = pertaining to	Artificial devices, such as limbs and joints, that replace a missing body part.

Rehabilitation Services Terms *(continued)*

TERM	WORD PARTS	DEFINITION
range of motion (ROM)		Range of movement of a joint, from maximum flexion through maximum extension. It is measured as degrees of a circle.
rehabilitation	re- = again habilitat/o = ability	Process of treatment and exercise that can help a person with a disability attain maximum function and well-being.
upper extremity (UE)		Refers to one of the arms.

Therapeutic Procedures

TERM	WORD PARTS	DEFINITION
active exercises		Exercises that a patient performs without assistance.
active range of motion (AROM)		Range of motion for joints that a patient is able to perform without assistance from someone else.
active-resistive exercises		Exercises in which the patient works against resistance applied to a muscle, such as a weight. Used to increase strength.
cryotherapy (cry-oh-THAIR-ah-pee)	cry/o = cold -therapy = treatment	Using cold for therapeutic purposes.
debridement (day-breed-MON)		Removal of dead or damaged tissue from a wound. Commonly performed for burn therapy.
electromyography (EMG) (ee-LEK-troh-my-OG-rah-fee)	electr/o = electricity my/o = muscle -graphy = process of recording	The recording of a muscle's response to electrical stimulation. The graphic record produced is an *electromyogram.*
gait training		Assisting a patient to learn to walk again or how to use an assistive device to walk.

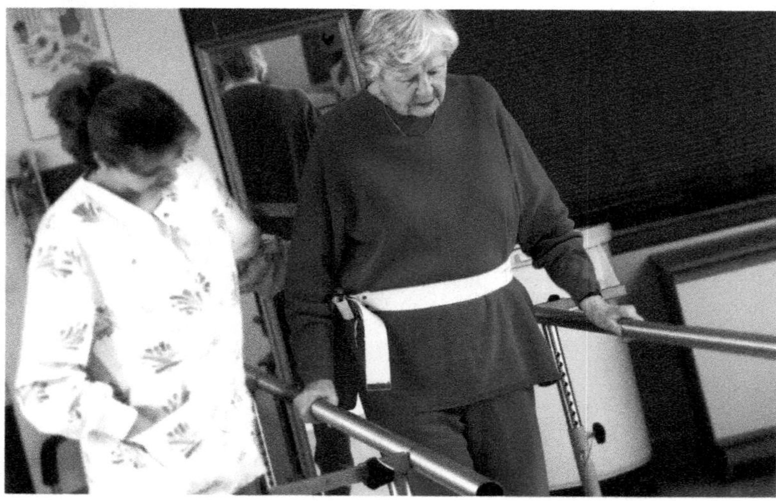

Figure 14.13 Physical therapist assisting a patient to walk in the parallel bars. *(auremar/Shutterstock)*

Therapeutic Procedures *(continued)*

TERM	WORD PARTS	DEFINITION
hydrotherapy (high-droh-THAIR-ah-pee)	hydr/o = water -therapy = treatment	Application of warm water as a therapeutic treatment. Can be done in baths, swimming pools, and whirlpools.
massage		Kneading or applying pressure by hands to a part of the patient's body to promote muscle relaxation and reduce tension.
mobilization		Treatments such as exercise and massage to restore movement to joints and soft tissue.
moist hot packs		Applying moist warmth to a body part to produce the slight dilation of blood vessels in the skin. Causes muscle relaxation in the deeper regions of the body and increases circulation, which aids healing.
nerve conduction velocity		Test to determine if nerves have been damaged by recording the rate at which an electrical impulse travels along a nerve. If the nerve is damaged, the velocity will be decreased.
pain control		Managing pain through a variety of means, including medications, biofeedback, and mechanical devices.
passive range of motion (PROM)		Therapist putting a patient's joints through available range of motion without assistance from the patient.
phonophoresis (foh-noh-foh-REE-sis)	phon/o = sound -phoresis = carrying	Use of ultrasound waves to introduce medication across the skin and into the subcutaneous tissues.
postural drainage with clapping	-al = pertaining to	Draining secretions from the bronchi or a lung cavity by having the patient lie so that gravity allows drainage to occur. Clapping is using the hand in a cupped position to perform percussion on the chest. Assists in loosening secretions and mucus.
therapeutic exercise (thair-ah-PEW-tik)	-ic = pertaining to	Exercise planned and carried out to achieve a specific physical benefit, such as improved range of motion, muscle strength, or cardiovascular function.
thermotherapy (ther-moh-THAIR-ah-pee)	therm/o = heat -therapy = treatment	Applying heat to the body for therapeutic purposes.
traction		Process of pulling or drawing, usually with a mechanical device. Used in treating orthopedic (bone and joint) problems and injuries.
transcutaneous electrical nerve stimulation (TENS) (tranz-kyoo-TAY-nee-us)	trans- = across cutane/o = skin -ous = pertaining to electr/o = electricity -al = pertaining to	Application of an electric current to a peripheral nerve to relieve pain.

Therapeutic Procedures *(continued)*

TERM	WORD PARTS	DEFINITION
ultrasound (US)	ultra- = beyond	Use of high-frequency sound waves to create heat in soft tissues under the skin. It is particularly useful for treating injuries to muscles, tendons, and ligaments, as well as muscle spasms.
whirlpool		Bath in which there are continuous jets of hot water reaching the body surfaces.

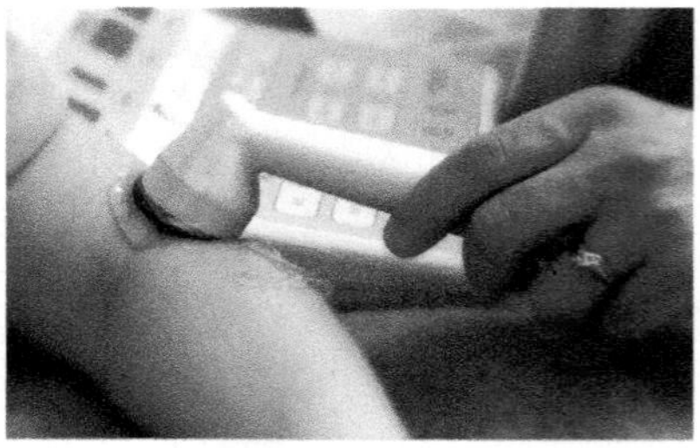

■ **Figure 14.14** Patient receiving ultrasound treatment to the left elbow. *(GWImages/Shutterstock)*

Abbreviations

AAROM	active assistive range of motion	**PROM**	passive range of motion
ADL	activities of daily living	**PT**	physical therapy
AROM	active range of motion	**ROM**	range of motion
EMG	electromyogram	**TENS**	transcutaneous electrical stimulation
e-stim	electrical stimulation	**UE**	upper extremity
LE	lower extremity	**US**	ultrasound
OT	occupational therapy		

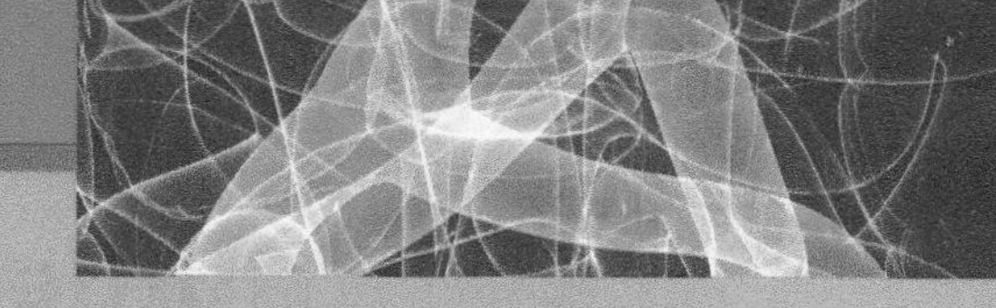

Section V: Surgery at a Glance

Word Parts

Here are the most common word parts (with their meanings) used to build surgery terms.

Combining Forms

alges/o	pain	hem/o	blood
aspir/o	to breathe in	later/o	side
cis/o	to cut	lith/o	stone
cry/o	cold	recumb/o	to lie back
cutane/o	skin	sect/o	to cut
dilat/o	to widen	specul/o	to look at
electr/o	electricity	tenacul/o	to hold
esthes/o	sensation, feeling	topic/o	a specific area
hal/o	to breathe	ven/o	vein

Suffixes

-al	pertaining to	-otomy	to cut into
-ia	state, condition	-ous	pertaining to
-ic	pertaining to	-scopic	pertaining to visually examining
-ist	specialist	-stasis	standing still
-logist	one who studies	-stat	standing still
-logy	study of		

Prefixes

an-	without	peri-	around
dis-	apart	post-	after
endo-	within	pre-	before
in-	inward	re-	again
intra-	within	sub-	under

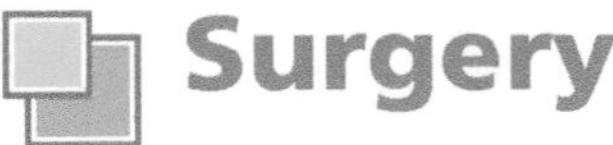

Surgery

operative report
surgeon
surgery

Surgery is the branch of medicine dealing with operative procedures to correct deformities and defects, repair injuries, and diagnose and cure diseases. A **surgeon** is a physician who has completed additional training of 5 years or more in a surgical specialty area. These specialty areas include orthopedics; neurosurgery; gynecology; ophthalmology; urology; and thoracic, vascular, cardiac, plastic, and general surgery. The surgeon must complete an **operative report** for every procedure that he or she performs. This is a detailed description that includes:

- preoperative diagnosis
- indication for the procedure
- name of the procedure
- surgical techniques employed
- findings during surgery
- postoperative diagnosis
- name of the surgeon

This report also includes information pertaining to the patient such as name, address, age, patient number, and date of the procedure.

Surgical terminology includes terms related to anesthesiology, surgical instruments, surgical procedures, incisions, and suture materials. Specific surgical procedures are frequently named by using the combining form for the body part being operated on and adding a suffix that describes the procedure. For example, an incision into the chest is a *thoracotomy,* removal of the stomach is *gastrectomy,* and surgical repair of the skin is *dermatoplasty.*

Anesthesia

anesthesia (an-ess-THEE-zee-ah)
anesthesiologist (an-es-thee-zee-OL-jist)
general anesthesia
inhalation (in-hah-LAY-shun)
intravenous (in-trah-VEE-nus)
local anesthesia
nurse anesthetist (ah-NES-the-tist)
regional anesthesia
subcutaneous (sub-kyoo-TAY-nee-us)
topical anesthesia

An **anesthesiologist** is a physician who specializes in the practice of administering anesthetics. A **nurse anesthetist** is a registered nurse who has received additional training and education in the administration of anesthetic medications. **Anesthesia** results in the loss of feeling or sensation. The most common types of anesthesia are general, regional, local, and topical anesthesia (see Table 14.5 ■).

MED TERM TIP

Look for these word parts:

an- = without
esthesi/o = sensation, feeling
-ist = specialist
-logist = one who studies

Surgical Instruments

Physicians have developed surgical instruments since the time of the early Egyptians. Instruments include surgical knives, saws, clamps, drills, and needles. Some of the more commonly used surgical instruments are listed in Table 14.6 ■ and are shown in Figure 14.15 ■.

Table 14.5 Types of Anesthesia

TYPE	WORD PARTS	DESCRIPTION
general anesthesia (GA)	an- = without esthes/o = sensation, feeling -ia = state, condition	Produces a loss of consciousness including an absence of pain sensation. The patient's vital signs (VS)—heart rate, breathing rate, pulse, and blood pressure—are carefully monitored when using a general anesthetic.
intravenous (IV)	intra- = within ven/o = vein -ous = pertaining to	Route for administering general anesthesia via injection into a vein.
inhalation	in- = inward hal/o = to breath	Route for administering general anesthesia by breathing it in.
regional anesthesia	-al = pertaining to an- = without esthes/o = sensation, feeling -ia = state, condition	Also referred to as a nerve block. This anesthetic interrupts a patient's pain sensation in a particular region of the body, such as the arm. The anesthetic is injected near the nerve that will be blocked from sensation. The patient usually remains conscious.
local anesthesia	-al = pertaining to an- = without esthes/o = sensation, feeling -ia = state, condition	Produces a loss of sensation in one localized part of the body. The patient remains conscious.
subcutaneous	sub- = under cutane/o = skin -ous = pertaining to	Method of applying local anesthesia involving injecting the anesthetic under the skin. This type of anesthetic is used to deaden the skin prior to suturing a laceration.
topical	topic/o = a specific area -al = pertaining to	Method of applying local anesthesia involving placing a liquid or gel directly onto a specific area of skin. This type of anesthetic is used on the skin, the cornea, and the mucous membranes in dental work.

Table 14.6 Common Surgical Instruments

INSTRUMENT	WORD PARTS	USE
aspirator (AS-pih-ray-tor)	aspir/o = to breathe in	Suctions fluid
clamp		Grasps tissue; controls bleeding
curette (kyoo-RET)		Scrapes and removes tissue
dilator (dye-LAY-tor)	dilat/o = to widen	Enlarges an opening by stretching
forceps (FOR-seps)		Grasps tissue
hemostat (HEE-moh-stat)	hem/o = blood -stat = standing still	Forceps to grasp blood vessel to control bleeding
probe		Explores tissue
scalpel		Cuts and separates tissue
speculum (SPEK-yoo-lum)	specul/o = to look at	Spreads apart walls of a cavity
tenaculum (the-NAK-yoo-lum)	tenacul/o = to hold	Long-handled clamp
trephine (treh-FINE)		Saw that removes disk-shaped piece of tissue or bone

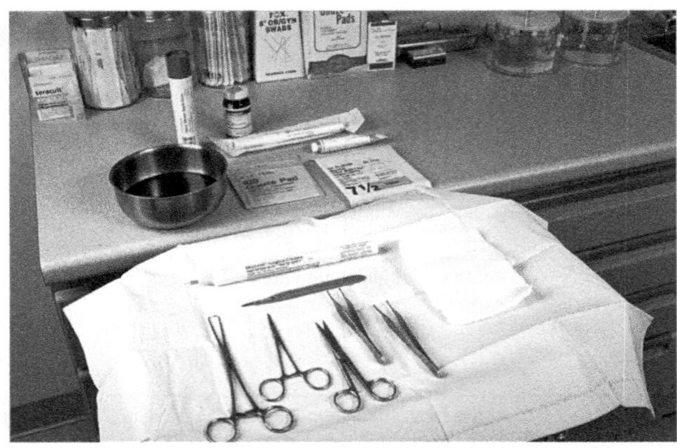

■ **Figure 14.15** Surgical instruments prepared for a procedure.

Surgical Positions

Patients are placed in specific positions so the surgeon is able to reach the area that is to be operated on. Table 14.7 ■ describes and Figure 14.16 ■ illustrates some common surgical positions.

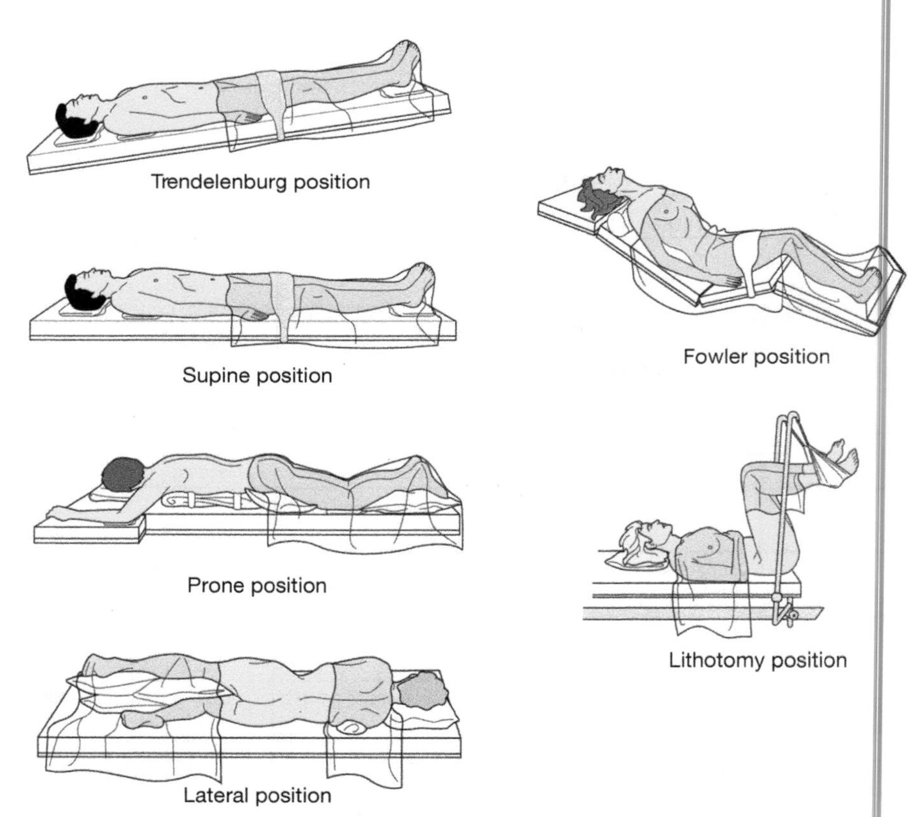

■ **Figure 14.16** Examples of common surgical positions.

Table 14.7 Common Surgical Positions		
POSITION	**WORD PARTS**	**DESCRIPTION**
Fowler		Sitting with back positioned at a 45° angle
lateral recumbent (ree-KUM-bent)	later/o = side -al = pertaining to recumb/o = to lie back	Lying on either the left or right side
lithotomy (lith-OT-oh-mee)	lith/o = tone -otomy = to cut into	Lying face up with hips and knees bent at 90° angles
prone (PROHN)		Lying horizontal and face down
supine (soo-PINE)		Lying horizontal and face up; also called dorsal recumbent
Trendelenburg (TREN-dee-len-berg)		Lying face up and on an incline with head lower than legs

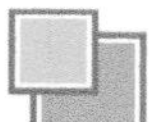

Surgery Terms

TERM	WORD PARTS	DEFINITION
analgesic (an-al-JEE-zik)	an- = without alges/o = pain -ic = pertaining to	Medication to relieve pain.
anesthetic (an-ess-THET-ik)	an- = without esthes/o = sensation, feeling -ic = pertaining to	Medication to produce partial to complete loss of sensation.
cauterization (kaw-ter-ih-ZAY-shun)		Use of heat, cold, electricity, or chemicals to scar, burn, or cut tissues.
circulating nurse		Nurse who assists the surgeon and scrub nurse by providing needed materials during the procedure and by handling the surgical specimen. This person does not wear sterile clothing and may enter and leave the operating room during the procedure.
cryosurgery (cry-oh-SER-jer-ee)	cry/o = cold	Technique of exposing tissues to extreme cold to produce cell injury and destruction. Used in the treatment of malignant tumors or to control pain and bleeding.
day surgery		Type of outpatient surgery in which the patient is discharged on the same day he or she is admitted; also called *ambulatory surgery.*
dissection (dih-SEK-shun)	dis- = apart sect/o = to cut	Surgical cutting of parts for separation and study.
draping		Process of covering the patient with sterile cloths that allow only the operative site to be exposed to the surgeon.

Surgery Terms *(continued)*

TERM	WORD PARTS	DEFINITION
electrocautery (ee-lek-troh-KAW-ter-ee)	electr/o = electricity	Use of an electric current to stop bleeding by coagulating blood vessels.
endoscopic surgery (en-doh-SKOP-ik)	endo- = within -scopic = pertaining to visually examining	Use of a lighted instrument to examine the interior of a cavity.
hemostasis (hee-moh-STAY-sis)	hem/o = blood -stasis = standing still	Stopping the flow of blood using instruments, pressure, and/or medication.
intraoperative (in-trah-OP-er-ah-tiv)	intra- = within	Period of time during surgery.
laser surgery		Use of a controlled beam of light for cutting, hemostasis, or tissue destruction.
perioperative (per-ee-OP-er-ah-tiv)	peri- = around	Period of time that includes before, during, and after a surgical procedure.
postoperative (post-op) (post-OP-er-ah-tiv)	post- = after	Period of time immediately following the surgery.
preoperative (preop, pre-op) (pree-OP-er-ah-tiv)	pre- = before	Period of time preceding surgery.
resection (ree-SEK-shun)	re- = again sect/o = to cut	To surgically cut out or remove; excision.
scrub nurse		Surgical assistant who hands instruments to the surgeon. This person wears sterile clothing and maintains the sterile operative field.
suture material (SOO-cher)		Used to close a wound or incision. Examples are catgut, silk thread, or staples. They may or may not be removed when the wound heals, depending on the type of material that is used.

Abbreviations

D & C	dilation and curettage	**PARR**	postanesthetic recovery room
Endo	endoscopy	**preop, pre-op**	preoperative
EUA	exam under anesthesia	**prep**	preparation, prepared
GA	general anesthesia	**T & A**	tonsillectomy and adenoidectomy
I & D	incision and drainage	**TAH**	total abdominal hysterectomy
MUA	manipulation under anesthesia	**TURP**	transurethral resection of prostate
OR	operating room		

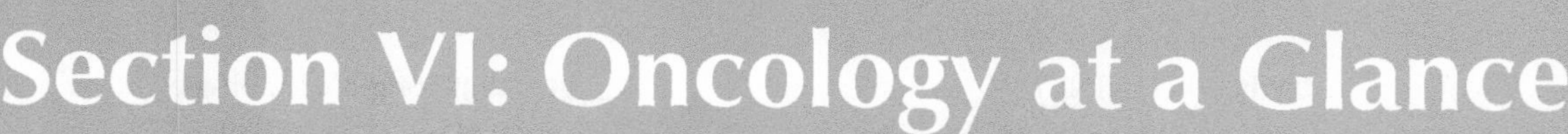

Section VI: Oncology at a Glance

Word Parts

Here are the most common word parts (with their meanings) used to build oncology terms.

Combining Forms

bi/o	life	miss/o	to send back
blast/o	primitive cell	morbid/o	ill
capsul/o	to box	mort/o	death
carcin/o	cancerous	mutat/o	to change
chem/o	drug	onc/o	tumor
cyt/o	cell	path/o	disease
immun/o	protection	radic/o	root
lapar/o	abdomen	radi/o	rays (X-rays)
laps/o	to slide back	tox/o	poison

Suffixes

-al	pertaining to	-oma	tumor
-gen	that which produces	-opsy	to view
-genic	producing	-otomy	to cut into
-logic	pertaining to studying	-plasia	growth, formation
-logist	one who studies	-plasm	growth, formation
-logy	study of	-therapy	treatment

Prefixes

en-	inward	neo-	new
hyper-	excessive	re-	again
in-	within		

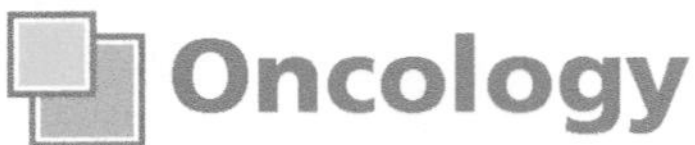

Oncology

benign (bee-NINE)
carcinoma (kar-sin-NOH-mah)
malignant (mah-LIG-nant)
oncology (ong-KALL-oh-jee)
protocol (PROH-toh-kall)
tumors

Oncology is the branch of medicine dealing with **tumors.** A tumor can be classified as **benign** or **malignant.** A benign tumor is one that is generally not progressive or recurring. Generally, a benign tumor will have the suffix *-oma* at the end of the term. However, a malignant tumor indicates that there is a cancerous growth present (see Figure 14.17 ■). These terms will usually have the word *carcinoma* added. The medical specialty of oncology primarily treats patients who have cancer.

The treatment for cancer can consist of a variety or a combination of treatments. The **protocol** (prot) for a particular patient will consist of the actual plan of care, including the medications, surgeries, and treatments such as chemotherapy and radiation therapy. Often, the entire healthcare team, including the physician, oncologist, radiologist, geneticist, nurse, patient, and family, will assist in designing the treatment plan.

MED TERM TIP

Carcinoma or cancer (Ca) can affect almost every organ in the body. The medical term reflects the area of the body affected as well as the type of tumor cell. For example, there can be an esophageal carcinoma, gastric adenocarcinoma, or adenocarcinoma of the uterus.

Staging Tumors

grade
metastases (meh-TASS-tah-seez)
pathologist (path-ALL-oh-jist)
staging

The process of classifying tumors based on their degree of tissue invasion and the potential response to therapy is referred to as **staging.** The TNM staging system is frequently used, with the *T* referring to the tumor's size and invasion, the *N* referring to lymph node involvement, and the *M* referring to the presence of **metastases** (mets) of the tumor cells (see Figure 14.18 ■).

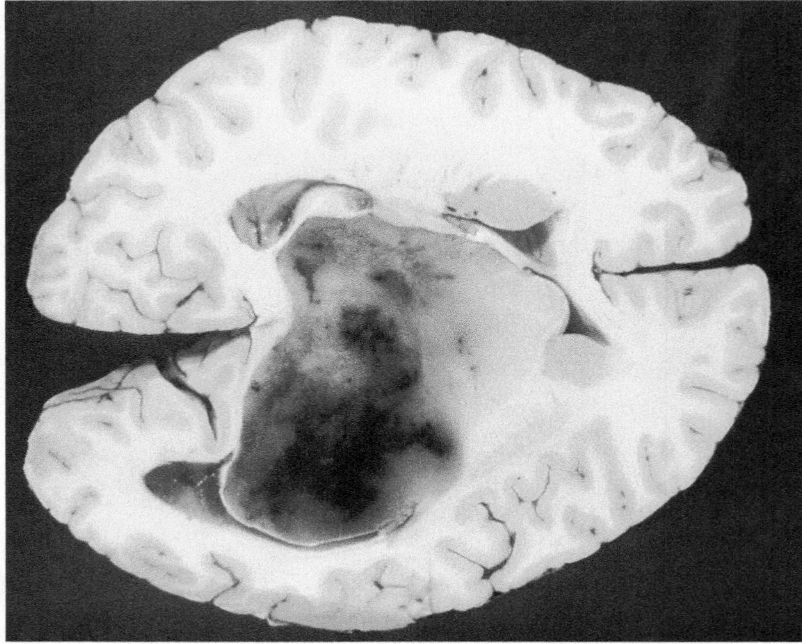

■ **Figure 14.17** Photograph of a brain specimen with a large malignant tumor. *(Biophoto Associates/Photo Researchers, Inc.)*

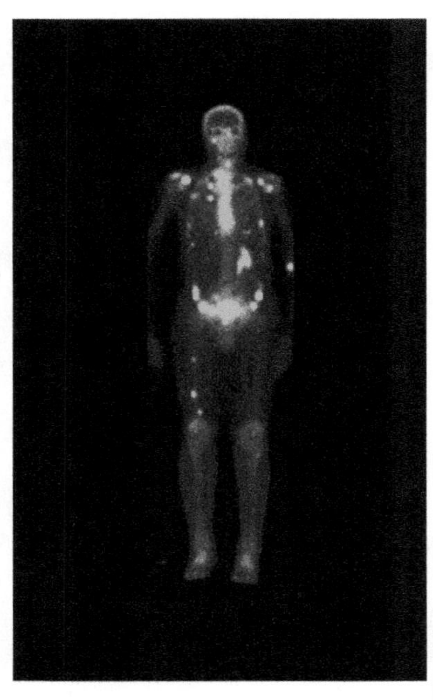

■ **Figure 14.18** Nuclear medicine bone scan showing metastatic tumors in the skeleton. *(Medical Body Scans/Photo Researchers, Inc.)*

In addition, a tumor can be graded from grade I through grade IV. The **grade** is based on the microscopic appearance of the tumor cells. The **pathologist** rates or grades the cells based on whether the tumor resembles the normal tissue. The classification system is illustrated in Table 14.8 ■. The cells in a grade I tumor are well differentiated, which makes it easier to treat than the more advanced grades.

MED TERM TIP

Look for these word parts:

carcin/o = cancer
onc/o = tumor
path/o = disease
-logist = one who studies
-logy = study of
-oma = tumor

Table 14.8 Tumor Grade Classification

GRADE	MEANING
GX	Grade cannot be determined
GI	Cells are well differentiated
GII	Cells are moderately differentiated
GIII	Cells are poorly differentiated
GIV	Cells are undifferentiated

Oncology Terms

TERM	WORD PARTS	DEFINITION
carcinogen (kar-SIN-oh-jen)	carcin/o = cancer -gen = that which produces	Substance or chemical agent that produces or increases the risk of developing cancer. For example, cigarette smoke and insecticides are considered to be carcinogens.
carcinoma in situ (CIS) (kar-sin-NOH-mah)	carcin/o = cancer -oma = tumor	Malignant tumor whose cells have not spread beyond the original site.
encapsulated (en-CAP-soo-lay-ted)	en- = inward capsul/o = to box	Growth enclosed in a sheath of tissue that prevents tumor cells from invading surrounding tissue.
hyperplasia (high-per-PLAY-zee-ah)	hyper- = excessive -plasia = growth	Excessive development of normal cells within an organ.
invasive disease (in-VAY-siv)	in- = within	Tendency of a malignant tumor to spread to immediately surrounding tissue and organs.

MED TERM TIP

The term *benign* comes from the Latin term *bene,* which means "kind or good." On the other hand, the term *malignant* comes from the Latin term *mal,* meaning "bad or malicious."

Oncology Terms *(continued)*

TERM	WORD PARTS	DEFINITION
metastasis (mets) (meh-TASS-tah-sis)		Movement and spread of cancer cells from one part of the body to another. Metastases is plural.

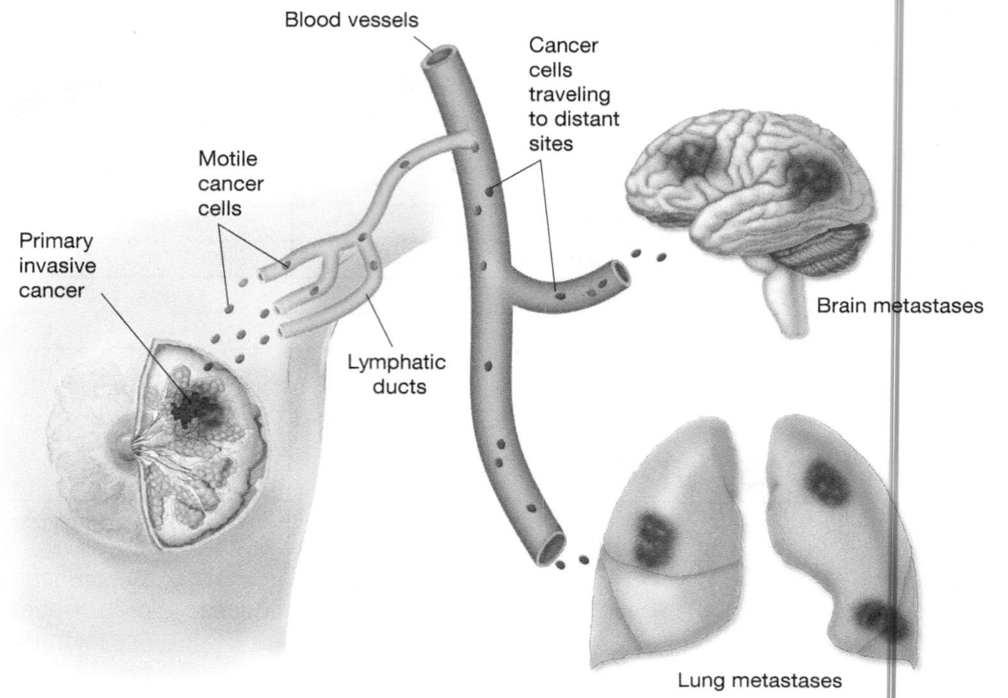

■ **Figure 14.19** Illustration showing how the primary breast tumor metastasized through the lymphatic and blood vessels to secondary sites in the brain and lungs.

TERM	WORD PARTS	DEFINITION
morbidity (mor-BID-ih-tee)	morbid/o = ill	Number representing the sick persons in a particular population.
mortality (mor-TAL-ih-tee)	mort/o = death	Number representing the deaths in a particular population.
mutation (mew-TAY-shun)	mutat/o = to change	Change or transformation from the original.
neoplasm (NEE-oh-plazm)	neo- = new -plasm = growth	New and abnormal growth or tumor. These can be benign or malignant.
oncogenic (ong-koh-JEN-ik)	onc/o = tumor -genic = producing	Cancer causing.
primary site		Term used to designate where a malignant tumor first appeared.
relapse (REE-laps)	re- = again laps/o = to slide back	Return of disease symptoms after a period of improvement.
remission (rih-MISH-un)	re- = again miss/o = to send back	Period during which the symptoms of a disease or disorder leave. Can be temporary.

Diagnostic Procedures

TERM	WORD PARTS	DEFINITION
biopsy (bx) (BYE-op-see)	bi/o = life -opsy = to view	Excision of a small piece of tissue for microscopic examination to assist in determining a diagnosis.
cytologic testing (sigh-toh-LAH-jik)	cyt/o = cell -logic = pertaining to studying	Examination of cells to determine their structure and origin. Pap smears are considered a form of cytologic testing.
exploratory surgery		Surgery performed for the purpose of determining if cancer is present or if a known cancer has spread. Biopsies are generally performed.
staging laparotomy (lap-ah-ROT-oh-mee)	lapar/o = abdomen -otomy = to cut into	Surgical procedure in which the abdomen is entered to determine the extent and staging of a tumor.

Therapeutic Procedures

TERM	WORD PARTS	DEFINITION
chemotherapy (chemo) (kee-moh-THAIR-ah-pee)	chem/o = drug -therapy = treatment	Treating disease by using chemicals that have a toxic effect on the body, especially cancerous tissue.
hormone therapy		Treatment of cancer with natural hormones or with chemicals that produce hormone-like effects.
immunotherapy (im-yoo-noh-THAIR-ah-pee)	immun/o = protection -therapy = treatment	Strengthening the immune system to attack cancerous cells.
palliative therapy (PAL-ee-ah-tiv)		Treatment designed to reduce the intensity of painful symptoms, but does not produce a cure.
radiation therapy	radi/o = X-rays	Exposing tumors and surrounding tissues to X-rays, gamma rays, neutrons, protons, and other sources to kill cancer cells and shrink tumors.
radical surgery	radic/o = root -al = pertaining to	Extensive surgery to remove as much tissue associated with a tumor as possible.
radioactive implant (ray-dee-oh-AK-tiv)	radi/o = rays	Embedding a radioactive source directly into tissue to provide a highly localized radiation dosage to damage nearby cancerous cells. Also called *brachytherapy.*

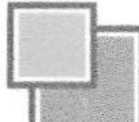

Abbreviations

bx	biopsy	**mets**	metastases
Ca	cancer	**MTX**	methotrexate
chemo	chemotherapy	**prot**	protocol
CIS	carcinoma in situ	**st**	stage
5-FU	5-fluorouracil	**TNM**	tumor, nodes, metastases
GA	gallium		

Chapter Review

Real-World Applications

Chart Note Transcription

The chart note below contains 11 phrases that can be reworded with a medical term that you learned in this chapter. Each phrase is identified with an underline. Determine the medical term and write your answers in the space provided.

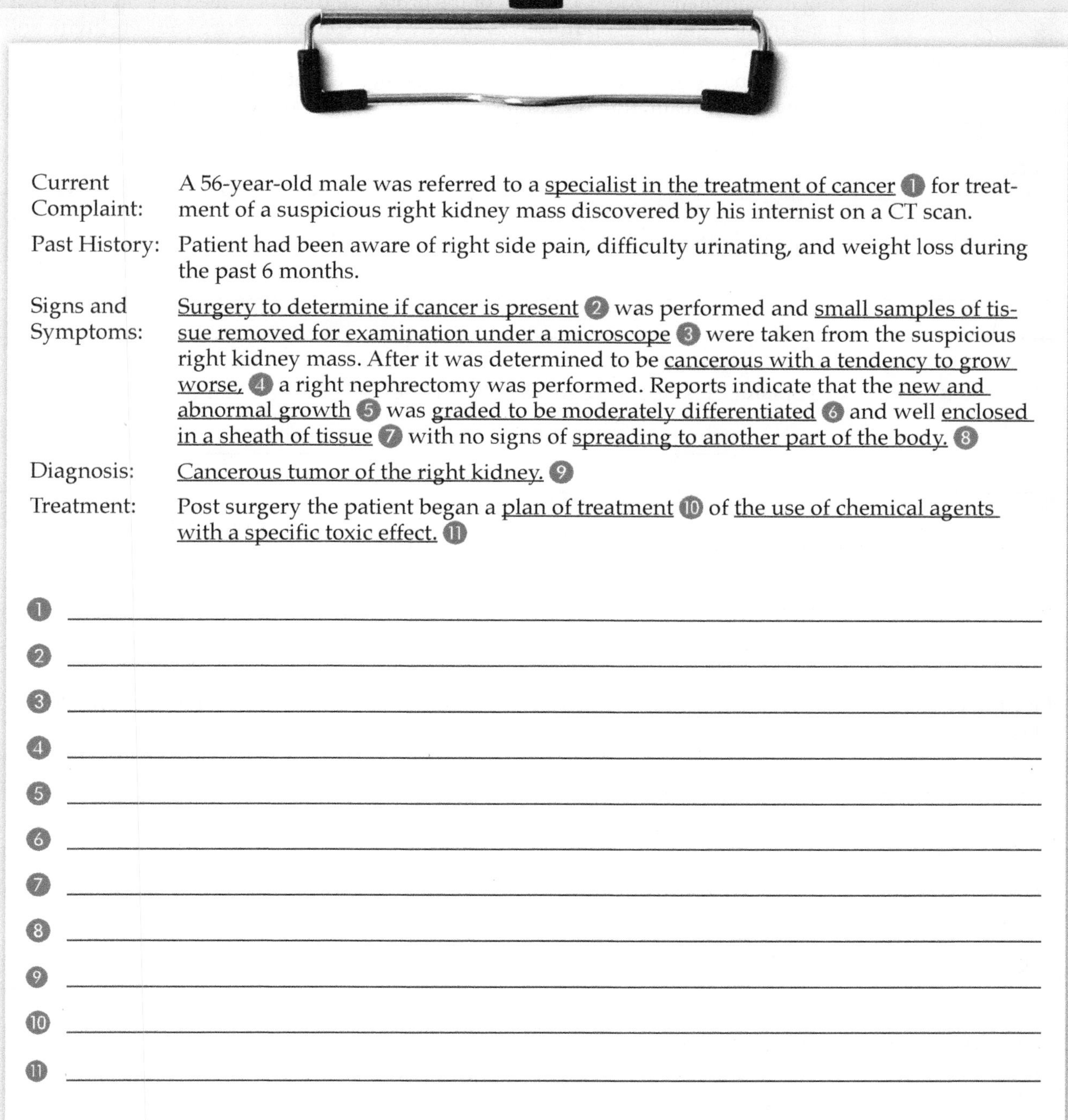

Current Complaint:	A 56-year-old male was referred to a specialist in the treatment of cancer (1) for treatment of a suspicious right kidney mass discovered by his internist on a CT scan.
Past History:	Patient had been aware of right side pain, difficulty urinating, and weight loss during the past 6 months.
Signs and Symptoms:	Surgery to determine if cancer is present (2) was performed and small samples of tissue removed for examination under a microscope (3) were taken from the suspicious right kidney mass. After it was determined to be cancerous with a tendency to grow worse, (4) a right nephrectomy was performed. Reports indicate that the new and abnormal growth (5) was graded to be moderately differentiated (6) and well enclosed in a sheath of tissue (7) with no signs of spreading to another part of the body. (8)
Diagnosis:	Cancerous tumor of the right kidney. (9)
Treatment:	Post surgery the patient began a plan of treatment (10) of the use of chemical agents with a specific toxic effect. (11)

(1) ______________________

(2) ______________________

(3) ______________________

(4) ______________________

(5) ______________________

(6) ______________________

(7) ______________________

(8) ______________________

(9) ______________________

(10) ______________________

(11) ______________________

Case Study

Below is a case study presentation of a patient with a condition covered by this chapter. Read the case study and answer the questions below. Some questions will ask for information not included within this chapter. Use your text, a medical dictionary, journals, technical materials, multimedia resources, electronic media, or any other reference material you choose to answer these questions.

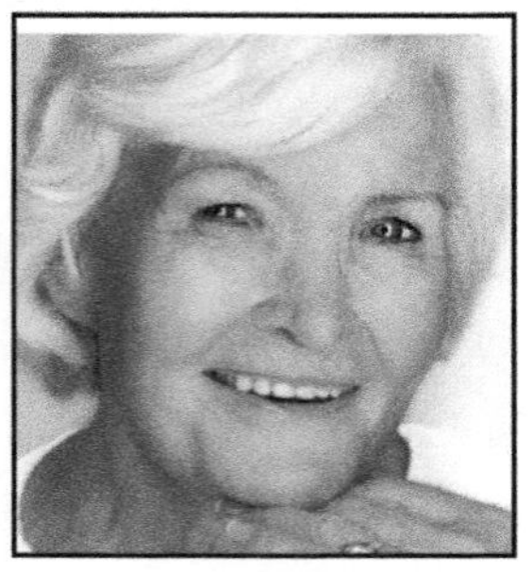

(Martina Ebel/Shuterstock)

Patient is a 72-year-old female complaining of increasing dyspnea with activity during the past 6 months. She now has a frequent harsh cough producing thick sputum and occasional hemoptysis. Patient is thin and short of stature. She is not SOB sitting in examination room. CT scan of the bronchial tree confirmed the presence of a mass in the right lung. Sputum was collected for sputum culture and sensitivity and sputum cytology. Sputum specimen was negative for the presence of bacteria. Sputum cytology revealed bronchogenic carcinoma. Patient will be referred to thoracic surgeon for consultation regarding lobectomy. Following recovery from this surgery she is to return to oncology clinic for chemotherapy and to determine if the tumor has metastasized.

1. What is this patient's diagnosis? Look it up and write a short description.

2. The patient had three complaints. List the three complaints and describe each in your own words.

3. Describe in your own words the diagnostic imaging procedure used on this patient and the results.

4. List and describe in your own words the clinical laboratory diagnostic test run on this patient and the results of each test.

5. What surgical procedure will this patient undergo? Describe it in your own words.

6. What does the term *metastasized* mean?

Practice Exercises

A. Complete the Statement

1. The reference book containing important information regarding medications is the ____________________.
2. A person specializing in the dispensing of medications is a ____________________.
3. The accepted official name for a drug is the ____________________ name.
4. The trade name for a drug is the ____________________ name.
5. What does the chemical name represent? ____________________
6. What federal agency enforces controls over the use of drugs causing dependency? ____________________

B. Drug Administration Practice

Name the route of drug administration for the following descriptions.

1. under the tongue ____________________
2. into the anus or rectum ____________________
3. applied to the skin ____________________
4. injected under the first layer of skin ____________________
5. injected into a muscle ____________________
6. injected into a vein ____________________
7. by mouth ____________________

C. Define the Term

1. idiosyncrasy ____________________
2. parenteral ____________________
3. placebo ____________________
4. toxicity ____________________
5. side effect ____________________
6. unit dose ____________________
7. habituation ____________________
8. antidote ____________________
9. contraindication ____________________
10. prophylaxis ____________________

D. What Does it Stand For?

1. gr ______________________________
2. bid ______________________________
3. tid ______________________________
4. ad lib ______________________________
5. prn ______________________________
6. ante ______________________________
7. OTC ______________________________
8. gt ______________________________
9. Sig ______________________________
10. stat ______________________________
11. mg ______________________________
12. aq ______________________________
13. noc ______________________________
14. NPO ______________________________
15. hs ______________________________
16. IV ______________________________
17. TO ______________________________
18. gtt ______________________________
19. pc ______________________________
20. d/c ______________________________

E. Prescription Practice

Write out the following prescription instructions in the space provided.

1. Pravachol, 20 mg, Sig. ī daily hs, 30, refill 3x, no sub. ______________________________
2. Lanoxin, 0.125 mg, Sig. īīī stat, then īī q AM, 100, refills prn. ______________________________
3. Synthroid, 0.075 mg, Sig. ī daily, 100, refill x4. ______________________________
4. Norvasc, 5 mg, ī q am, 60, refillable. ______________________________

F. Terminology Matching

Match each term to its definition.

1.	_______ cognitive disorder	a.	hypochondria
2.	_______ factitious disorder	b.	kleptomania
3.	_______ dissociative disorder	c.	masochism
4.	_______ eating disorder	d.	narcissistic personality
5.	_______ sleeping disorder	e.	insomnia
6.	_______ mood disorder	f.	bipolar disease
7.	_______ impulse control disorder	g.	panic attacks
8.	_______ somatoform disorder	h.	amnesia
9.	_______ personality disorder	i.	dementia
10.	_______ sexual disorder	j.	anorexia nervosa
11.	_______ anxiety disorder	k.	malingering

G. Name the Treatment

Identify each mental health treatment from its description.

1. depressant drugs prescribed for anxiety ______________________________
2. client-centered psychotherapy ______________________________
3. drug used to calm patients with bipolar disorder ______________________________
4. reduces patient agitation and panic and shortens schizophrenic episodes ______________________________
5. obtains a detailed account of the past and present emotional and mental experiences ______________________________
6. stimulants that alter the patient's mood by affecting neurotransmitter levels ______________________________

H. Name the Anesthesia

Identify the type of anesthesia for each description.

1. produces loss of consciousness and absence of pain ______________________________
2. produces loss of sensation in one localized part of the body ______________________________
3. anesthetic applied directly onto a specific skin area ______________________________
4. also referred to as a nerve block ______________________________

I. Terminology Matching

Match thet term to its definition.

1. _______ ultrasound
2. _______ MRI
3. _______ Doppler US
4. _______ nuclear medicine scan
5. _______ CT scan
6. _______ contrast study
7. _______ fluoroscopy
8. _______ radiography
9. _______ PET scan

a. radiopaque substances used to outline hollow structures
b. records velocity of blood flowing through vessels
c. image created by electromagnetic energy
d. glowing screen shows movement
e. making an X-ray
f. multiple-angle X-rays compiled into a cross-section
g. uses radioactive substances
h. image of internal organs using sound waves
i. indicates metabolic activity

J. What Does it Stand For?

1. ROM _______________
2. OT _______________
3. ADL _______________
4. LE _______________
5. EMG _______________
6. TENS _______________
7. PT _______________
8. PROM _______________
9. e-stim _______________
10. US _______________

K. Name the Procedure Described

Identify the rehabilitation procedure described by each phrase.

1. kneading or applying pressure by hands _______________
2. removal of dead and damaged tissue from a wound _______________
3. using water for treatment purposes _______________

4. drainage of secretions from the bronchi ______________________________

5. exercises performed by a patient without resistance ______________________________

6. medication introduced by ultrasound waves ______________________________

7. use of cold for therapeutic purposes ______________________________

8. pulling with a mechanical device ______________________________

L. Terminology Matching

Match each term to its definition.

1. _______ forceps
2. _______ tenaculum
3. _______ Trendelenburg
4. _______ lithotomy
5. _______ curette
6. _______ aspirator
7. _______ supine
8. _______ probe
9. _______ scalpel
10. _______ lateral recumbent

a. scrapes and removes tissue
b. cuts and separates tissue
c. lying horizontal and face up
d. lying on either the left or right side
e. long-handled clamp
f. explores tissue
g. lying face up with hips and knees bent at 90° angle
h. grasps tissue
i. suctions fluid
j. lying face up on an incline, head lower than legs

M. What Does it Stand For?

1. MRI ______________________________

2. Ba ______________________________

3. AP ______________________________

4. CT ______________________________

5. RL ______________________________

6. PA ______________________________

7. LL ______________________________

8. PET ______________________________

9. UGI ______________________________

10. KUB ______________________________

N. Terminology Matching

Match each term to its definition.

1. _______ oncogenic
2. _______ benign
3. _______ encapsulated
4. _______ relapse
5. _______ primary site
6. _______ protocol
7. _______ staging laparotomy
8. _______ cytologic testing
9. _______ radioactive implant
10. _______ bx

a. examine cells to determine their structure and origin
b. the plan for care for any individual patient
c. biopsy
d. growth that is not recurrent or progressive
e. placing a radioactive substance directly into the tissue
f. where the malignant tumor first appeared
g. growth is enclosed in a tissue sheath
h. cancer causing
i. abdominal surgery to determine extent of tumor

O. Matching

Match the name to the process or procedure.

1. _______ German psychiatrist Alois Alzheimer
2. _______ German surgeon Friedrich Trendelenburg
3. _______ American physician/surgeon George Ryerson Fowler
4. _______ German physicist Wilhelm Roentgen
5. _______ Austrian physicist Christian Johann Doppler

a. x-rays
b. brain disorder
c. ultrasonography
d. sitting position
e. lying face up position

Select two of those listed and research and describe the origins for the eponym.

____

____

P. Practices and Procedures

List and accurately spell one specialty practice and one surgical, diagnostic procedure, or treatment for each health science field.

1. Pharmacology____
2. Mental Health____
3. Diagnostic Imaging____
4. Rehabilitation Services____

5. Surgery____________________

6. Oncology____________________

Q. Interpret Technical Materials

Interpret technical materials to describe the process for creating a new imaging technology.

Technical Materials name____________________

Process____________________

R. Research

Research and report on how genetics influence cancer. Be sure to use associated medical terminology. Cite the source of your research. Present your findings to the class.

S. Scenario

Interpret the contents of the scenario and summarize your observations using medical terminology.
Robby Johnson is 17 years old and has been in a serious motorcycle accident. He is unconscious and there is fear from his vital sign measures that he may be going into shock. The paramedics have arrived and have applied a neck brace and placed him on a gurney. He is being transported by ambulance to City University Hospital. His parents were immediately called and have arrived at the emergency department where he is to be admitted. His injuries seem to be very severe and it appears he will need surgery. The hospital does not have any record of his blood type as he has not needed to have blood work done previously. His parents say that he is in good health and is current with his vaccinations.

Since he will need surgery, the hospital must have his blood typed. There is also the chance he may have a head injury and some internal injuries. In addition to blood typing, he will also need to have x-rays to determine if there are broken bones and an MRI to check his head wound. He is scheduled for surgery within the next couple of hours as soon as all of the testing can be completed.

The tests show he does not have a head injury, just some cuts and bruises on his face and several of his teeth are out of alignment. He does however, have several cracked ribs, a punctured lung, a severe cut on his left arm, and a broken thigh bone on his left leg. Summarize your observations below:

List four specialists that will help with his diagnosis and treatment:

1.____________________

2.____________________

3.____________________

4.____________________

T. Matching

Match the practice for each health care team member.

1. _______ Surgeon	a. corrects malocclusion
2. _______ Radiation Technologist	b. records information on patient charts
3. _______ Oncologist	c. treats mental conditions
4. _______ Pharmacy Technician	d. assists with filling and dispensing prescriptions
5. _______ Psychiatrist	e. performs surgical procedures
6. _______ Physical Therapist	f. completes blood testing and other diagnostics
5. _______ EMR Specialist	g. administers radiology testing procedures
8. _______ Nurse Anesthetist	h. helps patients regain motion and strength
9. _______ Orthodontist	i. a biologist who studies genetics
10. _______ Clinical Lab Technologist	j. administers medications during surgery
11. _______ Geneticist	k. treats patients with cancer

Identify the health care specialists from the list above that will cooperate, contribute, and collaborate as a part of the team that will help care for Robby, as described in the previous activity.

Appendices

Appendix I

Word Parts Arranged Alphabetically and Defined

The word parts that have been presented in this textbook are summarized with their definitions for quick reference. Prefixes are listed first, followed by combining forms and suffixes.

Prefix	Definition
a-	without, away from
ab-	away from
ad-	toward
allo-	other, different from usual
an-	without
ante-	before, in front of
anti-	against
auto-	self
bi-	two
brady-	slow
circum-	around
contra-	against
de-	without
dis-	apart
dys-	abnormal, difficult, painful
e-	outward, without
en-	inward
endo-	inner, within
epi-	upon, over, above
eso-	inward
eu-	normal, good
ex-	external, outward
exo-	outward
extra-	outside of
hemi-	half
hetero-	different
homo-	same
hydro-	water
hyper-	excessive, over, above
hypo-	below, under, insufficient
in-	inward, without, not, within
inter-	among, between
intra-	inside, within
macro-	large
micro-	small
mono-	one
multi-	many
myo-	to shut
neo-	new
nulli-	none
pan-	all
para-	abnormal, two like parts of a pair, beside, near
per-	through
peri-	around
poly-	many
post-	after
pre-	before, in front of
primi-	first
pro-	before
pseudo-	false
quadri-	four
re-	again
retro-	backward, behind
semi-	partial, half
sub-	below, under
supra-	above
tachy-	fast, rapid
tetra-	four
trans-	across, through
tri-	three
ultra-	beyond, excess
un-	not
xeno-	strange, foreign

Combining Form	Definition
abdomin/o	abdomen
acous/o	hearing
acr/o	extremities
aden/o	gland
adenoid/o	adenoids
adip/o	fat
adren/o	adrenal glands

Combining Form	Definition
adrenal/o	adrenal glands
aer/o	air
agglutin/o	clumping
albin/o	white
alges/o	sense of pain
alveol/o	alveolus; air sac
ambly/o	dull, dim
amnes/o	forgetfulness
amni/o	amnion
an/o	anus
andr/o	male
angi/o	vessel
ankyl/o	stiff joint
anter/o	front
anthrac/o	coal
anxi/o	fear, worry
aort/o	aorta
append/o	appendix
appendic/o	appendix
aque/o	water
arteri/o	artery
arthr/o	joint
articul/o	joint
aspir/o	to breathe in
astr/o	star
atel/o	incomplete
ather/o	fatty substance
atri/o	atrium
audi/o	hearing
audit/o	hearing
aur/o	ear
auricul/o	ear
axill/o	axilla, underarm
azot/o	nitrogenous waste
bacteri/o	bacteria
balan/o	glans penis
bar/o	weight
bas/o	base
bi/o	life
blast/o	immature, embryonic
blephar/o	eyelid
brachi/o	arm
bronch/o	bronchus
bronchi/o	bronchus
bronchiol/o	bronchiole
bucc/o	cheek
burs/o	bursa, sac
calc/o	calcium
capsul/o	to box
carcin/o	cancer
cardi/o	heart
carp/o	carpus, wrist
caud/o	tail
cec/o	cecum
cephal/o	head

Combining Form	Definition
cerebell/o	cerebellum
cerebr/o	cerebrum
cerumin/o	cerumen
cervic/o	neck, cervix
chem/o	chemical, drug
chol/e	bile, gall
cholangi/o	bile duct
cholecyst/o	gallbladder
choledoch/o	common bile duct
chondr/o	cartilage
chori/o	chorion
chrom/o	color
chromat/o	color
cirrh/o	yellow
cis/o	to cut
clavicul/o	clavicle
clon/o	rapid contracting and relaxing
coagul/o	clotting
coccyg/o	coccyx
cochle/o	cochlea
col/o	colon
colon/o	colon
colp/o	vagina
compuls/o	drive, compel
coni/o	dust
conjunctiv/o	conjunctiva
corne/o	cornea
coron/o	heart
corpor/o	body
cortic/o	outer portion, cortex
cost/o	rib
crani/o	skull
crin/o	to secrete
crur/o	leg
cry/o	cold
crypt/o	hidden
culd/o	cul-de-sac
cutane/o	skin
cyan/o	blue
cycl/o	ciliary body, ciliary muscle
cyst/o	bladder, pouch, sac
cyt/o	cell
dacry/o	tear duct, tears
deluss/o	false belief
dent/o	tooth
depress/o	to press down
derm/o	skin
dermat/o	skin
diaphor/o	profuse sweating
diaphragmat/o	diaphragm
dilat/o	to widen
dipl/o	double
dist/o	away from
diverticul/o	pouch
dors/o	back of body

Combining Form	Definition
duct/o	to bring
duoden/o	duodenum
dur/o	dura mater
electr/o	electricity
embol/o	plug
embry/o	embryo
emmetr/o	correct, proper
encephal/o	brain
enter/o	small intestine
eosin/o	rosy red
epididym/o	epididymis
epiglott/o	epiglottis
episi/o	vulva
epitheli/o	epithelium
erg/o	work
erythr/o	red
esophag/o	esophagus
esthes/o	sensation, feeling
estr/o	female
extens/o	to stretch out
factiti/o	artificial, contrived
fasci/o	fibrous band
femor/o	femur
fet/o	fetus
fibr/o	fibers
fibrin/o	fibers, fibrous
fibul/o	fibula
flex/o	to bend
fluor/o	fluorescence, luminous
fus/o	pouring
gastr/o	stomach
genit/o	genitals
gingiv/o	gums
glauc/o	gray
gli/o	glue
glomerul/o	glomerulus
gloss/o	tongue
gluc/o	glucose
glute/o	buttock
glyc/o	sugar
glycos/o	sugar, glucose
gonad/o	sex glands
granul/o	granules
gynec/o	female, woman
habilitat/o	ability
hal/o	to breathe
hallucin/o	imagined perception
hem/o	blood
hemat/o	blood
hepat/o	liver
hidr/o	sweat
hist/o	tissue
home/o	sameness
humer/o	humerus
hydr/o	water

Combining Form	Definition
hymen/o	hymen
hyster/o	uterus
iatr/o	physician, medicine, treatment
ichthy/o	scaly, dry
idi/o	distinctive
ile/o	ileum
ili/o	ilium
immun/o	immunity, protection
infer/o	below
inguin/o	groin region
iod/o	iodine
ir/o	iris
irid/o	iris
isch/o	to hold back
ischi/o	ischium
jejun/o	jejunum
kal/i	potassium
kerat/o	cornea, hard, horny
ket/o	ketones
keton/o	ketones
kinesi/o	movement
klept/o	to steal
kyph/o	hump
labi/o	lip
labyrinth/o	labyrinth (inner ear)
lacrim/o	tears
lact/o	milk
lamin/o	lamina, part of vertebra
lapar/o	abdomen
laps/o	to slide back
laryng/o	larynx, voice box
later/o	side
leuk/o	white
lingu/o	tongue
lip/o	fat
lith/o	stone
lob/o	lobe
lord/o	bent backwards
lumb/o	loin, low back
lymph/o	lymph
lymphaden/o	lymph node
lymphangi/o	lymph vessel
macul/o	macula lutea
mamm/o	breast
mandibul/o	mandible
mast/o	breast
maxill/o	maxilla
meat/o	meatus
medi/o	middle
medull/o	inner portion, medulla, oblongata
melan/o	black
men/o	menses, menstruation
mening/o	meninges
meningi/o	meninges

Combining Form	Definition
ment/o	mind
metacarp/o	metacarpals
metatars/o	metatarsals
metr/o	uterus
mi/o	lessening
mineral/o	minerals, electrolytes
miss/o	to send back
morbid/o	ill
morph/o	shape
mort/o	death
muc/o	mucus
muscul/o	muscles
mutat/o	to change
my/o	muscle
myc/o	fungus
mydr/i	widening
myel/o	bone marrow, spinal cord
myocardi/o	heart muscle
myos/o	muscle
myring/o	tympanic membrane (eardrum)
nas/o	nose
nat/o	birth
natr/o	sodium
necr/o	death
nephr/o	kidney
neur/o	nerve
neutr/o	neutral
noct/i	night
nucle/o	nucleus
nyctal/o	night
o/o	egg
obsess/o	besieged by thoughts
ocul/o	eye
odont/o	tooth
olig/o	scanty
onc/o	tumor
onych/o	nail
oophor/o	ovary
ophthalm/o	eye
opt/o	eye, vision
optic/o	eye, vision
or/o	mouth
orch/o	testes
orchi/o	testes
orchid/o	testes
orth/o	straight, correct, upright
oste/o	bone
ot/o	ear
ovari/o	ovary
ox/o, ox/i	oxygen
palat/o	palate
pancreat/o	pancreas
papill/o	optic disc
parathyroid/o	parathyroid gland

Combining Form	Definition
patell/o	patella
path/o	disease
pector/o	chest
ped/o	child, foot
pedicul/o	lice
pelv/o	pelvis
pen/o	penis
perine/o	perineum
peritone/o	peritoneum
phac/o	lens
phag/o	eat, swallow
phalang/o	phalanges
pharmac/o	drug
pharyng/o	pharynx (throat)
phleb/o	vein
phob/o	irrational fear
phon/o	sound
phot/o	light
phren/o	mind
physic/o	body
pineal/o	pineal gland
pituitar/o	pituitary gland
plant/o	sole of foot
pleur/o	pleura
pneum/o	lung, air
pneumon/o	lung, air
pod/o	foot
poli/o	gray matter
polyp/o	polyp
pont/o	pons
poster/o	back
presby/o	old age
proct/o	rectum and anus
prostat/o	prostate gland
prosthet/o	addition
protein/o	protein
proxim/o	near to
psych/o	mind
pub/o	genital region, pubis
pulmon/o	lung
pupill/o	pupil
py/o	pus
pyel/o	renal pelvis
pylor/o	pylorus
pyr/o	fire
radi/o	radius, ray (X-ray)
radic/o	root
radicul/o	nerve root
rect/o	rectum
recumb/o	to lie back
ren/o	kidney
retin/o	retina
rhin/o	nose
rhytid/o	wrinkle
roentgen/o	X-ray

Combining Form	Definition
rotat/o	to revolve
sacr/o	sacrum
salping/o	auditory tube (eustachian tube), uterine tubes, fallopian tubes
sanguin/o	blood
sarc/o	flesh (muscular substance)
scapul/o	scapula
schiz/o	split
scler/o	hard, sclera
scoli/o	crooked, bent
seb/o	oil
sect/o	to cut
sept/o	a wall
septic/o	infection
sialaden/o	salivary gland
sigmoid/o	sigmoid colon
sinus/o	sinus
soci/o	society
somat/o	body
somn/o	sleep
son/o	sound
specul/o	to look at
spermat/o	sperm
sphygm/o	pulse
spin/o	spine
spir/o	breathing
splen/o	spleen
spondyl/o	vertebrae
staped/o	stapes
stern/o	sternum
steth/o	chest
stigmat/o	point
super/o	above
synov/o	synovial membrane
synovi/o	synovial membrane
system/o	systems
tars/o	ankle, tarsus
ten/o	tendon
tenacul/o	to hold
tend/o	tendon
tendin/o	tendon
testicul/o	testes, testicle
thalam/o	thalamus

Combining Form	Definition
thec/o	sheath (meninges)
therm/o	heat
thorac/o	chest, thorax
thromb/o	clot
thym/o	thymus gland
thyr/o	thyroid gland
thyroid/o	thyroid gland
tibi/o	tibia
tom/o	to cut
ton/o	tone
tonsill/o	tonsils
topic/o	a specific area
tox/o	poison
toxic/o	poison
trache/o	trachea, windpipe
trich/o	hair
tuss/o	cough
tympan/o	tympanic membrane (eardrum)
uln/o	ulna
ungu/o	nail
ur/o	urine
ureter/o	ureter
urethr/o	urethra
urin/o	urine
uter/o	uterus
uve/o	choroid
vagin/o	vagina
valv/o	valve
valvul/o	valve
varic/o	dilated vein
vas/o	vas deferens, vessel, duct
vascul/o	blood vessel
ven/o	vein
ventr/o	belly
ventricul/o	brain ventricle, ventricle
vers/o	to turn
vertebr/o	vertebra
vesic/o	bladder
vesicul/o	seminal vesicle
viscer/o	internal organ
vitre/o	glassy
vulv/o	vulva
xer/o	dry

Suffix	Definition
-ac	pertaining to
-al	pertaining to
-algia	pain
-an	pertaining to
-apheresis	removal, carry away
-ar	pertaining to
-arche	beginning
-ary	pertaining to

Suffix	Definition
-asthenia	weakness
-atic	pertaining to
-blast	immature, embryonic
-capnia	carbon dioxide
-cele	hernia, protrusion
-centesis	puncture to withdraw fluid
-cide	to kill
-clasia	to surgically break

Suffix	Definition
-crit	separation of
-cusis	hearing
-cyesis	state of pregnancy
-cyte	cell
-cytosis	more than the normal number of cells
-derma	skin condition
-desis	fuse, stabilize
-dipsia	thirst
-dynia	pain
-eal	pertaining to
-ectasis	dilation
-ectomy	surgical removal
-edema	swelling
-emesis	vomit
-emia	blood condition
-gen	that which produces
-genesis	produces, generates
-genic	producing, produced by
-globin	protein
-globulin	protein
-gram	record or picture
-graph	instrument for recording
-graphy	process of recording
-gravida	pregnancy
-ia	condition, state
-iac	pertaining to
-iasis	abnormal condition
-iatrist	physician
-iatry	medical treatment
-ic	pertaining to
-ical	pertaining to
-ician	specialist
-ile	pertaining to
-ine	pertaining to
-ion	action, condition
-ior	pertaining to
-ism	state of
-ist	specialist
-istry	specialty of
-itis	inflammation
-kinesia	movement
-listhesis	slipping
-lith	stone
-lithiasis	condition of stones
-logic	pertaining to studying
-logical	pertaining to the study of
-logist	one who studies
-logy	study of
-lucent	to shine through
-lysis	destruction
-lytic	destruction
-malacia	abnormal softening
-mania	frenzy

Suffix	Definition
-manometer	instrument to measure pressure
-megaly	enlargement, large
-meter	instrument for measuring
-metrist	specialist in measuring
-metry	process of measuring
-nic	pertaining to
-nomics	pertaining to laws
-oid	resembling
-ole	small
-oma	mass, tumor, swelling
-opaque	nontransparent
-opia	vision condition
-opsia	vision condition
-opsy	view of
-orexia	appetite
-ory	pertaining to
-ose	pertaining to
-osis	abnormal condition
-osmia	smell
-ostomy	surgically create an opening,
-otia	ear condition
-otomy	cutting into
-ous	pertaining to
-para	to bear (offspring)
-paresis	weakness
-partum	childbirth
-pathy	disease
-penia	abnormal decrease, too few
-pepsia	digestion
-pexy	surgical fixation
-phagia	eat, swallow
-phasia	speech
-phil	attracted to
-philia	attracted to
-phobia	fear
-phonia	voice
-phoresis	carrying
-phylaxis	protection
-plasia	development, growth, formation
-plasm	formation, development, growth
-plastic	pertaining to development
-plasty	surgical repair
-plegia	paralysis
-pnea	breathing
-poiesis	formation
-porosis	porous
-prandial	pertaining to a meal
-pressin	to press down
-ptosis	drooping
-ptysis	spitting
-rrhage	abnormal flow, excessive

Suffix	Definition
-rrhagia	abnormal flow condition
-rrhagic	pertaining to abnormal flow
-rrhaphy	suture
-rrhea	discharge, flow
-rrhexis	rupture
-salpinx	uterine tube
-sclerosis	hardening
-scope	instrument for viewing
-scopic	pertaining to visually examining
-scopy	process of visually examining
-spasm	involuntary muscle contraction
-spermia	condition of sperm
-stasis	standing still
-stat	standing still
-stenosis	narrowing

Suffix	Definition
-taxia	muscle coordination
-tension	pressure
-therapy	treatment
-thorax	chest
-tic	pertaining to
-tocia	labor, childbirth
-tome	instrument to cut
-tonia	tone
-tonic	pertaining to tone
-tripsy	surgical crushing
-trophic	pertaining to development
-trophy	nourishment, development
-tropia	turned condition
-tropin	to stimulate
-ule	small
-uria	condition of the urine

Appendix II

Word Parts Arranged Alphabetically by Definition

The definitions of the word parts that have been presented in this textbook are presented here and are arranged alphabetically. Prefixes are listed first, followed by combining forms and suffixes.

Definition	Prefix
abnormal	dys-, para-
above	hyper-, epi-, supra-
across	trans-
after	post-
again	re-
against	anti-, contra-
all	pan-
among	inter-
apart	dis-
around	circum-, peri-
away from	a-, ab-
backward	retro-
before	ante-, pre-, pro-
behind	retro-
below	hypo-, sub-
beside	para-
between	inter-
beyond	ultra-
different from usual	allo-
different	hetero-
difficult	dys-
excess	ultra-
excessive	hyper-
external	ex-
false	pseudo-
fast	tachy-
first	primi-
foreign	xeno-
four	quadri-, tetra-
good	eu-
half	semi-, hemi-
in front of	ante-, pre-
inner	endo-
inside	intra-
inward	en-, eso-, in-
large	macro-
many	multi-, poly-
near	para-
new	neo-
none	nulli-
normal	eu-
not	in-, un-
one	mono-
other	allo-
outside of	extra-
outward	ex-, exo-, e-
over	epi-, hyper-
painful	dys-
partial	semi-
same	homo-
self	auto-
to shut	myo-
slow	brady-
small	micro-
strange	xeno-
three	tri-
through	trans-, per-
toward	ad-
two	bi-
two like parts of a pair	para-
under	hypo-, sub-
upon	epi-
water	hydro-
within	endo-, in-, intra-
without	e-, a-, an-, de-, in-

Definition	Combining Form
abdomen	abdomin/o, lapar/o
ability	habilitat/o
above	super/o
addition	prosthet/o
adenoids	adenoid/o
adrenal glands	adren/o, adrenal/o
air	aer/o, pneum/o, pneumon/o
air sac	alveol/o
alveolus	alveol/o
amnion	amni/o
ankle	tars/o

Definition	Combining Form
anus	an/o
aorta	aort/o
appendix	append/o, appendic/o
arm	brachi/o
artery	arteri/o
artificial	factiti/o
atrium	atri/o
auditory tube	salping/o
away from	dist/o
axilla	axill/o
back	poster/o
back of body	dors/o
bacteria	bacteri/o
base	bas/o
belly	ventr/o
below	infer/o
to bend	flex/o
bent	scoli/o
bent backwards	lord/o
besieged by thoughts	obsess/o
bile duct	cholangi/o
bile	chol/e
birth	nat/o
black	melan/o
bladder	vesic/o, cyst/o
blood	hem/o, hemat/o, sanguin/o
blood vessel	vascul/o
blue	cyan/o
body	corpor/o, physic/o, somat/o
bone	oste/o
bone marrow	myel/o
to box	capsul/o
brain	encephal/o
brain ventricle	ventricul/o
breast	mamm/o, mast/o
to breathe	hal/o
to breathe in	aspir/o
breathing	spir/o
to bring	duct/o
bronchiole	bronchiol/o
bronchus	bronch/o, bronchi/o
bursa	burs/o
buttock	glute/o
calcium	calc/o
cancer	carcin/o
carpus	carp/o

Definition	Combining Form
cartilage	chondr/o
cavity	sinus/o
cecum	cec/o
cell	cyt/o
cerebellum	cerebell/o
cerebrum	cerebr/o
cerumen	cerumin/o
cervix	cervic/o
to change	mutat/o
cheek	bucc/o
chemical	chem/o
chest	pect/o, steth/o, thorac/o
child	ped/o
chorion	chori/o
choroid	uve/o
ciliary body	cycl/o
ciliary muscle	cycl/o
clavicle	clavicul/o
clot	thromb/o
clotting	coagul/o
clumping	agglutin/o
coal	anthrac/o
coccyx	coccyg/o
cochlea	cochle/o
cold	cry/o
colon	col/o, colon/o
color	chrom/o, chromat/o
common bile duct	choledoch/o
compel	compuls/o
conjunctiva	conjunctiv/o
contrived	factiti/o
cornea	corne/o, kerat/o
correct	emmetr/o, orth/o
cortex	cortic/o
cough	tuss/o
crooked	scoli/o
cul-de-sac	culd/o
to cut	cis/o, sect/o, tom/o
death	mort/o, necr/o
diaphragm	diaphragmat/o
dilated vein	varic/o
dim	ambly/o
disease	path/o
distinctive	idi/o
double	dipl/o
drive	compuls/o
drug	chem/o, pharmac/o
dry	ichthy/o, xer/o

Definition	Combining Form	Definition	Combining Form
duct	vas/o	**glassy**	vitre/o
dull	ambly/o	**glomerulus**	glomerul/o
duodenum	duoden/o	**glucose**	glycos/o, gluc/o
dura mater	dur/o	**glue**	gli/o
dust	coni/o	**granules**	granul/o
ear	aur/o, auricul/o, ot/o	**gray**	glauc/o
		gray matter	poli/o
eardrum	myring/o, tympan/o	**groin region**	inguin/o
eat	phag/o	**gums**	gingiv/o
egg	o/o	**hair**	trich/o
electricity	electr/o	**hard**	kerat/o, scler/o
electrolytes	mineral/o	**head**	cephal/o
embryo	embry/o	**hearing**	audi/o, audit/o, acous/o
embryonic	blast/o		
epididymis	epididym/o	**heart**	cardi/o, coron/o
epiglottis	epiglott/o	**heart muscle**	myocardi/o
epithelium	epitheli/o	**heat**	therm/o
esophagus	esophag/o	**hidden**	crypt/o
eustachian tube	salping/o	**to hold**	tenacul/o
extremities	acr/o	**to hold back**	isch/o
eye	ocul/o, ophthalm/o, opt/o, optic/o	**horny**	kerat/o
		humerus	humer/o
eyelid	blephar/o	**hump**	kyph/o
fallopian tubes	salping/o	**hymen**	hymen/o
false belief	deluss/o	**ileum**	ile/o
fat	adip/o, lip/o	**ilium**	ili/o
fatty substance	ather/o	**ill**	morbid/o
fear	anxi/o	**imagined perception**	hallucin/o
feeling	esthes/o	**immature**	blast/o
female	estr/o, gynec/o	**immunity**	immun/o
femur	femor/o	**incomplete**	atel/o
fetus	fet/o	**infection**	septic/o
fibers	fibr/o, fibrin/o	**inner portion**	medull/o
fibrous	fibrin/o	**internal organ**	viscer/o
fibrous band	fasci/o	**iodine**	iod/o
fibula	fibul/o	**iris**	ir/o, irid/o
fire	pyr/o	**irrational fear**	phob/o
flesh (muscular substance)	sarc/o	**ischium**	ischi/o
fluorescence	fluor/o	**jejunum**	jejun/o
foot	ped/o, pod/o	**joint**	arthr/o, articul/o
forgetfulness	amnes/o	**ketones**	ket/o, keton/o
front	anter/o	**kidney**	nephr/o, ren/o
fungus	myc/o	**labyrinth**	labyrinth/o
gall	chol/e	**inner ear**	labyrinth/o
gallbladder	cholecyst/o	**lamina**	lamin/o
genital region	pub/o	**larynx**	laryng/o
genitals	genit/o	**leg**	crur/o
gland	aden/o	**lens**	phac/o
glans penis	balan/o	**lessening**	mi/o

Definition	Combining Form	Definition	Combining Form
lice	pedicul/o	nucleus	nucle/o
to lie back	recumb/o	oil	seb/o
life	bi/o	old age	presby/o
light	phot/o	outer portion	cortic/o
lip	labi/o	ovary	oophor/o, ovari/o
liver	hepat/o	oxygen	ox/o, ox/i
lobe	lob/o	palate	palat/o
loin	lumb/o	pancreas	pancreat/o
to look at	specul/o	parathyroid gland	parathyroid/o
low back	lumb/o	part of vertebra	lamin/o
luminous	fluor/o	patella	patell/o
lung	pulmon/o, pneum/o, pneumon/o	pelvis	pelv/o
lymph	lymph/o	penis	pen/o
lymph node	lymphaden/o	perineum	perine/o
lymph vessel	lymphangi/o	peritoneum	peritone/o
macula lutea	macul/o	phalanges	phalang/o
male	andr/o	pharynx	pharyng/o
mandible	mandibul/o	physician	iatr/o
maxilla	maxill/o	pineal gland	pineal/o
meatus	meat/o	pituitary gland	pituitar/o
medicine	iatr/o	pleura	pleur/o
medulla oblongata	medull/o	plug	embol/o
meninges	mening/o, meningi/o, thec/o	point	stigmat/o
menses	men/o	poison	tox/o, toxic/o
menstruation	men/o	polyp	polyp/o
metacarpals	metacarp/o	pons	pont/o
metatarsals	metatars/o	potassium	kal/i
middle	medi/o	pouch	diverticul/o, cyst/o
milk	lact/o	pouring	fus/o
mind	ment/o, phren/o, psych/o	to press down	depress/o
minerals	mineral/o	profuse sweating	diaphor/o
mouth	or/o	proper	emmetr/o
movement	kinesi/o	prostate gland	prostat/o
mucus	muc/o	protection	immun/o
muscle	my/o, myos/o, muscul/o	protein	protein/o
nail	onych/o, ungu/o	pubis	pub/o
near to	proxim/o	pulse	sphygm/o
neck	cervic/o	pupil	pupill/o
nerve	neur/o	pus	py/o
nerve root	radicul/o	pylorus	pylor/o
neutral	neutr/o	radius	radi/o
night	noct/l, nyctal/o	rapid contracting and relaxing	clon/o
nitrogenous waste	azot/o	ray (X-ray)	radi/o
nose	nas/o, rhin/o	rectum	rect/o
		rectum and anus	proct/o
		red	erythr/o
		renal pelvis	pyel/o
		retina	retin/o

Definition	Combining Form
to revolve	rotat/o
rib	cost/o
root	radic/o
rosy red	eosin/o
sac	burs/o, cyst/o
sacrum	sacr/o
salivary gland	sialaden/o
sameness	home/o
scaly	ichthy/o
scanty	olig/o
scapula	scapul/o
sclera	scler/o
to secrete	crin/o
seminal vesicle	vesicul/o
to send back	miss/o
sensation	esthes/o
sense of pain	alges/o
sex glands	gonad/o
shape	morph/o
sheath (meninges)	thec/o
side	later/o
sigmoid colon	sigmoid/o
sinus	sinus/o
skin	cutane/o, derm/o, dermat/o
skull	crani/o
sleep	somn/o
to slide back	laps/o
small intestine	enter/o
society	soci/o
sodium	natr/o
sole of foot	plant/o
sound	phon/o, son/o
specific area	topic/o
sperm	spermat/o
spinal cord	myel/o
spine	spin/o
spleen	splen/o
split	schiz/o
stapes	staped/o
star	astr/o
to steal	klept/o
sternum	stern/o
stiff joint	ankyl/o
stomach	gastr/o
stone	lith/o
straight	orth/o
to stretch out	extens/o
sugar	glyc/o, glycos/o

Definition	Combining Form
swallow	phag/o
sweat	hidr/o
synovial membrane	synov/o, synovi/o
systems	system/o
tail	caud/o
tarsus	tars/o
tear duct	dacry/o
tears	dacry/o, lacrim/o
tendon	ten/o, tend/o, tendin/o
testes	orch/o, orchi/o, orchid/o, testicul/o
thalamus	thalam/o
thorax	thorac/o
throat	pharyng/o
thymus gland	thym/o
thyroid gland	thyr/o, thyroid/o
tibia	tibi/o
tissue	hist/o
tone	ton/o
tongue	gloss/o, lingu/o
tonsils	tonsill/o
tooth	dent/o, odont/o
trachea	trache/o
treatment	iatr/o
tumor	onc/o
to turn	vers/o
tympanic membrane	myring/o, tympan/o
ulna	uln/o
underarm	axill/o
upright	orth/o
ureter	ureter/o
urethra	urethr/o
urine	ur/o, urin/o
uterine tubes	salping/o
uterus	hyster/o, metr/o, uter/o
vagina	colp/o, vagin/o
valve	valv/o, valvul/o
vas deferens	vas/o
vein	phleb/o, ven/o
ventricle	ventricul/o
vertebra	vertebr/o, spondyl/o
vessel	angi/o, vas/o
vision	opt/o, optic/o
voice box	laryng/o
vulva	episi/o, vulv/o
wall	sept/o
water	aque/o, hydr/o

Definition	Combining Form
weight	bar/o
white	albin/o, leuk/o
to widen	dilat/o
widening	mydr/i
windpipe	trache/o
woman	gynec/o
work	erg/o
worry	anxi/o
wrinkle	rhytid/o
wrist	carp/o
X-ray	roentgen/o
yellow	cirrh/o

Definition	Suffix
abnormal condition	-iasis, -osis
abnormal decrease	-penia
abnormal flow condition	-rrhagia
abnormal flow	-rrhage
abnormal flow (pertaining to)	-rrhagic
abnormal softening	-malacia
action	-ion
appetite	-orexia
attracted to	-phil, -philia
to bear (offspring)	-para
beginning	-arche
blood condition	-emia
breathing	-pnea
carbon dioxide	-capnia
carry away	-apheresis
carrying	-phoresis
cell	-cyte
chest	-thorax
childbirth	-partum, -tocia
condition	-ion, -ia
condition of sperm	-spermia
condition of stones	-lithiasis
condition of the urine	-uria
cut (instrument to)	-tome
cutting into	-otomy
destruction	-lytic, -lysis
development	-plasia, -trophy, -plasm
development (pertaining to)	-plastic, -trophic
digestion	-pepsia
dilation	-ectasis
discharge	-rrhea
disease	-pathy
drooping	-ptosis
ear condition	-otia
eat	-phagia
embryonic	-blast
enlargement	-megaly
excessive flow	-rrhage
fallopian tube	-salpinx
fear	-phobia
flow	-rrhea
formation	-poiesis, -plasia, -plasm
frenzy	-mania
fuse	-desis
generates	-genesis
growth	-plasia, -plasm
hardening	-sclerosis
hearing	-cusis
hernia	-cele
immature	-blast
inflammation	-itis
pressure (instrument to measure)	-manometer
involuntary muscle contraction	-spasm
to kill	-cide
labor	-tocia
large	-megaly
laws (pertaining to)	-nomics
mass	-oma
meal (pertaining to a)	-prandial
measuring (instrument for)	-meter
measuring (process of)	-metry
medical treatment	-iatry
more than the normal number of cells	-cytosis
movement	-kinesia
muscle coordination	-taxia
narrowing	-stenosis
nontransparent	-opaque
nourishment	-trophy
one who studies	-logist
pain	-algia, -dynia
paralysis	-plegia
pertaining to	-ac, -al, -an, -ar, -ary, -atic, -eal, -ia, -iac, -ic, -ical, -ile, -ine, -ior, -nic, -ory, -ose, -ous, -tic
physician	-iatrist

Definition	Suffix
porous	-porosis
pregnancy	-gravida
pregnancy (state of)	-cyesis
pressure	-tension
to press down	-pressin
produced by	-genic
produces	-genesis
producing	-genic
protection	-phylaxis
protein	-globin, -globulin
protrusion	-cele
puncture to withdraw fluid	-centesis
record or picture	-gram
recording (instrument for)	-graph
recording (process of)	-graphy
removal	-apheresis
resembling	-oid
rupture	-rrhexis
separation of	-crit
to shine through	-lucent
skin condition	-derma
slipping	-listhesis
small	-ole, -ule
smell	-osmia
specialist	-ician, -ist
specialist in measuring	-metrist
specialty of	-istry
speech	-phasia
spitting	-ptysis
stabilize	-desis
standing still	-stasis, -stat
state	-ia
state of	-ism

Definition	Suffix
to stimulate	-tropin
stone	-lith
studying (pertaining to)	-logic
study of	-logy
study of (pertaining to the)	-logical
surgical fixation	-pexy
surgical removal	-ectomy
surgical repair	-plasty
to surgically break	-clasia
surgically create an opening	-ostomy
suture	-rrhaphy
swallow	-phagia
swelling	-edema, -oma
that which produces	-gen
thirst	-dipsia
tone	-tonia
tone (pertaining to)	-tonic
too few	-penia
treatment	-therapy
tumor	-oma
turned condition	-tropia
uterine tube	-salpinx
viewing (instrument for)	-scope
view of	-opsy
vision condition	-opia, -opsia
visually examining (pertaining to)	-scopic
visually examining (process of)	-scopy
voice	-phonia
vomit	-emesis
weakness	-asthenia, -paresis

Appendix III
Abbreviations

Abbreviation	Meaning
@	at
5-FU	5-fluorouracil
^{67}Ga	radioactive gallium
^{99m}Tc	radioactive technetium
^{131}I	radioactive iodine
^{133}Xe	radioactive xenon
^{201}Tl	radioactive thallium
α	alpha
$\bar{a}$	before
AAROM	active assistive range of motion
AB	abortion
ABGs	arterial blood gases
ac	before meals
ACTH	adrenocorticotropic hormone
ad lib	as desired
AD	Alzheimer's disease, right ear
ADD	attention-deficit disorder
ADH	antidiuretic hormone
ADHD	attention-deficit/hyperactivity disorder
ADL	activities of daily living
AE	above elbow
AF	atrial fibrillation
AGN	acute glomerulonephritis
AI	artificial insemination
AIDS	acquired immunodeficiency syndrome
AK	above knee
ALL	acute lymphocytic leukemia
ALS	amyotrophic lateral sclerosis
ALT	alanine transaminase
AMI	acute myocardial infarction
AML	acute myelogenous leukemia
Angio	angiography
ANS	autonomic nervous system
ante	before
AP	anteroposterior
APAP	acetaminophen (Tylenol™)
aq	aqueous (water)
ARC	AIDS-related complex
ARDS	adult (or acute) respiratory distress syndrome
ARF	acute renal failure
ARMD	age-related macular degeneration
AROM	active range of motion
AS	arteriosclerosis, left ear
ASA	aspirin
ASD	atrial septal defect
ASHD	arteriosclerotic heart disease
ASL	American Sign Language
AST	aspartate transaminase
Astigm	astigmatism
ATN	acute tubular necrosis
AU	both ears
AV, A-V	atrioventricular
β	beta
Ba	barium
BaE	barium enema
basos	basophils
BBB	bundle branch block (L for left; R for right)
BC	bone conduction
BCC	basal cell carcinoma
BDT	bone density testing
BE	barium enema, below elbow
bid	twice a day
BK	below knee
BM	bowel movement
BMD	bone mineral density
BMR	basal metabolic rate
BMT	bone marrow transplant
BNO	bladder neck obstruction
BP	blood pressure
BPD	bipolar disorder
BPH	benign prostatic hyperplasia
bpm	beats per minute
Bronch	bronchoscopy
BS	bowel sounds
BSE	breast self-examination
BUN	blood urea nitrogen
BX, bx	biopsy
$\bar{c}$	with
C1, C2, etc.	first cervical vertebra, second cervical vertebra, etc.
Ca	calcium, cancer
CA	chronological age
CABG	coronary artery bypass graft
CAD	coronary artery disease
cap(s)	capsule(s)
CAPD	continuous ambulatory peritoneal dialysis
CAT	computerized axial tomography
cath	catheterization
CBC	complete blood count
CBD	common bile duct
CC	cardiac catheterization, chief complaint, clean catch urine specimen
CCU	coronary care unit

Abbreviation	Meaning
c.gl.	correction with glasses
chemo	chemotherapy
CHF	congestive heart failure
Ci	curie
CIS	carcinoma in situ
Cl^-	chloride
CLL	chronic lymphocytic leukemia
CML	chronic myelogenous leukemia
CNS	central nervous system
CO_2	carbon dioxide
CoA	coarctation of the aorta
COPD	chronic obstructive pulmonary disease
CP	cerebral palsy, chest pain
CPK	creatine phosphokinase
CPR	cardiopulmonary resuscitation
CRF	chronic renal failure
C&S	culture and sensitivity
CS, C-section	cesarean section
CSD	congenital septal defect
CSF	cerebrospinal fluid
CT	calcitonin, computerized tomography
CTA	clear to auscultation
CTS	carpal tunnel syndrome
CV	cardiovascular
CVA	cerebrovascular accident
CVD	cerebrovascular disease
CVS	chorionic villus sampling
Cx	cervix
CXR	chest X-ray
cysto	cystoscopy
d	day
D	diopter (lens strength)
dB	decibel
D & C	dilation and curettage
d/c, DISC	discontinue
DC, disc	discontinue
DEA	Drug Enforcement Agency
decub	decubitus ulcer, lying down
Derm, derm	dermatology
DI	diabetes insipidus, diagnostic imaging
diff	differential
dil	dilute
disp	dispense
DJD	degenerative joint disease
DM	diabetes mellitus
DOE	dyspnea on exertion
DPT	diphtheria, pertussis, tetanus injection
DRE	digital rectal exam
DSA	digital subtraction angiography
DSM	*Diagnostic and Statistical Manual of Mental Disorders*
dtd	give of such a dose
DTR	deep tendon reflex
DVA	distance visual acuity
DVT	deep vein thrombosis
Dx	diagnosis
DXA	dual-energy absorptiometry
e-stim	electrical stimulation
ECC	extracorporeal circulation
ECCE	extracapsular cataract extraction
ECG, EKG	electrocardiogram
ECHO	echocardiogram
ECT	electroconvulsive therapy
ED	erectile dysfunction
EDC	estimated date of confinement
EEG	electroencephalogram, electroencephalography
EENT	eye, ear, nose, and throat
EGD	esophagogastroduodenoscopy
ELISA	enzyme-linked immunosorbent assay
EM	emmetropia
EMB	endometrial biopsy
EMG	electromyogram
Endo	endoscopy
ENT	ear, nose, and throat
EOM	extraocular movement
eosins, eos	eosinophils
ERCP	endoscopic retrograde cholangiopancreatography
ERT	estrogen replacement therapy
ERV	expiratory reserve volume
ESR, SR, sed rate	erythrocyte sedimentation rate
ESRD	end-stage renal disease
ESWL	extracorporeal shockwave lithotripsy
et	and
EU	excretory urography
EUA	exam under anesthesia
FBS	fasting blood sugar
FDA	Federal Drug Administration
FEKG	fetal electrocardiogram
FHR	fetal heart rate
FHT	fetal heart tone
FOBT	fecal occult blood test
FRC	functional residual capacity
FS	frozen section
FSH	follicle-stimulating hormone
FTND	full-term normal delivery
FX, Fx	fracture
GA	gallium, general anesthesia

Abbreviation	Meaning
GB	gallbladder, gallbladder X-ray
GC	gonorrhea
GERD	gastroesophageal reflux disease
GH	growth hormone
GI, grav I	first pregnancy
GI	gastrointestinal
gm	gram
GOT	glutamic oxaloacetic transaminase
gr	grain
gt	drop
gtt	drops
GTT	glucose tolerance test
GU	genitourinary
GVHD	graft versus host disease
GYN, gyn	gynecology
H_2O	water
HA	headache
HAV	hepatitis A virus
HBV	hepatitis B virus
HCG, hCG	human chorionic gonadotropin
HCl	hydrochloric acid
HCO_3^-	bicarbonate
HCT, Hct, crit	hematocrit
HCV	hepatitis C virus
HD	Hodgkin's disease, hemodialysis
HDN	hemolytic disease of the newborn
HDV	hepatitis D virus
HEENT	head, ears, eyes, nose, throat
HEV	hepatitis E virus
Hgb, Hb, HGB	hemoglobin
HIV	human immunodeficiency virus
HMD	hyaline membrane disease
HNP	herniated nucleus pulposus
HPV	human papilloma virus
HRT	hormone replacement therapy
hs	at bedtime
HSG	hysterosalpingography
HSV-1	herpes simplex virus type 1
HSV	herpes simplex virus
HTN	hypertension
Hz	hertz
$\hat{\text{i}}$	one
$\hat{\text{ii}}$	two
$\hat{\text{iii}}$	three
IBD	inflammatory bowel disease
IBS	irritable bowel syndrome
IC	inspiratory capacity
ICCE	intracapsular cataract extraction
ICP	intracranial pressure
ICU	intensive care unit
I&D	incision and drainage
ID	intradermal
IDDM	insulin-dependent diabetes mellitus
Ig	immunoglobulins (IgA, IgD, IgE, IgG, IgM)
IM	intramuscular
inj	injection
I&O	intake and output
IOP	intraocular pressure
IPD	intermittent peritoneal dialysis
IPPB	intermittent positive pressure breathing
IRDS	infant respiratory distress syndrome
IRV	inspiratory reserve volume
IU	international unit
IUD	intrauterine device
IV	intravenous
IVC	intravenous cholangiogram, intravenous cholangiography
IVF	*in vitro* fertilization
IVP	intravenous pyelogram
JRA	juvenile rheumatoid arthritis
K^+	potassium
kg	kilogram
KS	Kaposi's sarcoma
KUB	kidney, ureter, bladder
L1, L2, etc.	first lumbar vertebra, second lumbar vertebra, etc.
L	liter
LASIK	laser-assisted in-situ keratomileusis
LAT, lat	lateral
LBW	low birth weight
LE	lower extremity
LGI	lower gastrointestinal series
LH	luteinizing hormone
LL	left lateral
LLE	left lower extremity
LLL	left lower lobe
LLQ	left lower quadrant
LMP	last menstrual period
LP	lumbar puncture
LUE	left upper extremity
LUL	left upper lobe
LUQ	left upper quadrant
LVAD	left ventricular assist device
LVH	left ventricular hypertrophy
lymphs	lymphocytes
MA	mental age
mA	milliampere
MAO	monoamine oxidase

Abbreviation	Meaning
mcg	microgram
mCi	millicurie
MD	muscular dystrophy
MDI	metered-dose inhaler
mEq	milliequivalent
mets	metastases
mg	milligram
MI	myocardial infarction, mitral insufficiency
mL	milliliter
mm Hg	millimeters of mercury
MM	malignant melanoma
MMPI	Minnesota Multiphasic Personality Inventory
mono	mononucleosis
monos	monocytes
MR	mitral regurgitation
MRA	magnetic resonance angiography
MRI	magnetic resonance imaging
MS	mitral stenosis, multiple sclerosis, musculoskeletal
MSH	melanocyte-stimulating hormone
MTX	methotrexate
MUA	manipulation under anesthesia
MVP	mitral valve prolapse
Na^+	sodium
NB	newborn
NG	nasogastric (tube)
NHL	non-Hodgkin's lymphoma
NIDDM	non-insulin-dependent diabetes mellitus
NK	natural killer cells
NMR	nuclear magnetic resonance
no sub	no substitute
noc	night
non rep	do not repeat
NPH	neutral protamine Hagedorn (insulin)
NPO	nothing by mouth
NS	nephrotic syndrome, normal saline
NSAID	nonsteroidal anti-inflammatory drug
n&v	nausea and vomiting
O_2	oxygen
OA	osteoarthritis
OB	obstetrics
OCD	obsessive–compulsive disorder
OCPs	oral contraceptive pills
od	overdose
OD	right eye
oint	ointment
OM	otitis media
O&P	ova and parasites
Ophth.	ophthalmology
OR	operating room
ORIF	open reduction–internal fixation
Orth, ortho	orthopedics
OS	left eye
OT	occupational therapy
OTC	over the counter
Oto	otology
OU	each eye/both eyes
oz	ounce
$\bar{p}$	after
P	pulse
PA	pernicious anemia, posteroanterior
PAC	premature atrial contraction
Pap	Papanicolaou test
PARR	postanesthetic recovery room
PBI	protein-bound iodine
pc	after meals
PCA	patient-controlled administration
PCP	pneumocystis pneumonia
PCV	packed cell volume
PDA	patent ductus arteriosus
PDR	*Physician's Desk Reference*
PE tube	pressure equalizing tube
per	with
PERRLA	pupils equal, round, react to light and accommodation
PET	positron emission tomography
PFT	pulmonary function test
pH	acidity or alkalinity of urine
PI, para I	first delivery
PID	pelvic inflammatory disease
PMN, polys	polymorphonuclear neutrophil
PMS	premenstrual syndrome
PNS	peripheral nervous system
PO, po	by mouth
PORP	partial ossicular replacement prosthesis
pp	postprandial
PPD	purified protein derivative
preop, pre-op	preoperative
prep	preparation, prepared
PRK	photorefractive keratectomy
PRL	prolactin
prn	as needed
PROM	passive range of motion
prot	protocol
PSA	prostate-specific antigen
PT, pro-time	prothrombin time
pt	patient

Abbreviation	Meaning
PT	physical therapy
PTC	percutaneous transhepatic cholangiography
PTCA	percutaneous transluminal coronary angioplasty
PTH	parathyroid hormone
PUD	peptic ulcer disease
PVC	premature ventricular contraction
q	every
qam	every morning
qh	every hour
qhs	at bedtime
qid	four times a day
qs	quantity sufficient
R	respiration, roentgen
Ra	radium
RA	rheumatoid arthritis, room air
rad	radiation-absorbed dose
RAI	radioactive iodine
RBC	red blood cell
RDS	respiratory distress syndrome
REM	rapid eye movement
Rh+	Rh-positive
Rh–	Rh-negative
RIA	radioimmunoassay
RL	right lateral
RLE	right lower extremity
RLL	right lower lobe
RLQ	right lower quadrant
RML	right middle lobe
ROM	range of motion
RP	retrograde pyelogram
RPR	rapid plasma reagin (test for syphilis)
RRT	registered radiologic technologist, registered respiratory therapist
RUE	right upper extremity
RUL	right upper lobe
RUQ	right upper quadrant
RV	reserve volume
Rx	take
$\bar{s}$	without
$\overline{ss}$	one-half
S1	first heart sound
S2	second heart sound
SA, S-A	sinoatrial
SAD	seasonal affective disorder
SARS	severe acute respiratory syndrome
SC	subcutaneous
SCC	squamous cell carcinoma
SCI	spinal cord injury

Abbreviation	Meaning
SCIDS	severe combined immunodeficiency syndrome
segs	segmented neutrophils
s.gl.	without correction or glasses
SG, sp. gr.	specific gravity
SG	skin graft
SIDS	sudden infant death syndrome
Sig	label as follows/directions
SK	streptokinase
sl	under the tongue
SLE	systemic lupus erythematosus
SMAC	sequential multiple analyzer computer
SMD	senile macular degeneration
SOB	shortness of breath
sol	solution
SOM	serous otitis media
SPP	suprapubic prostatectomy
ST	esotropia
st	stage
stat	at once/immediately
STD	sexually transmitted disease
STSG	split-thickness skin graft
Subc, SubQi subcu, SC, sc, subq	subcutaneous
suppos, supp	suppository
susp	suspension
syr	syrup
T & A	tonsillectomy and adenoidectomy
T, tbsp	tablespoon
t, tsp	teaspoon
T1, T2, etc.	first thoracic vertebra, second thoracic vertebra, etc.
T_3	triiodothyronine
T_4	thyroxine
tab	tablet
TAH-BSO	total abdominal hysterectomy–bilateral salpingo-oophorectomy
TAH	total abdominal hysterectomy
TB	tuberculosis
TENS	transcutaneous electrical stimulation
TFT	thyroid function test
THA	total hip arthroplasty
THR	total hip replacement
TIA	transient ischemic attack
tid	three times a day
TKA	total knee arthroplasty
TKR	total knee replacement
TLC	total lung capacity
TNM	tumor, nodes, metastases

Abbreviation	Meaning
TO	telephone order
top	apply topically
TORP	total ossicular replacement prosthesis
tPA	tissue-type plasminogen activator
TPN	total parenteral nutrition
TPR	temperature, pulse, and respiration
TSH	thyroid-stimulating hormone
TSS	toxic shock syndrome
TUR	transurethral resection
TURP	transurethral resection of the prostate
TV	tidal volume
u	unit
U/A, UA	urinalysis
UC	urine culture, uterine contractions
UE	upper extremity
UGI	upper gastrointestinal series
URI	upper respiratory infection
US	ultrasound
UTI	urinary tract infection
UV	ultraviolet
VA	visual acuity
VC	vital capacity
VCUG	voiding cystourethrography
VD	venereal disease
VF	visual field
Vfib	ventricular fibrillation
VO	verbal order
VSD	ventricular septal defect
VT	ventricular tachycardia
WBC	white blood cell
wt	weight
x	times
XT	exotropia

Glossary/Index

A

Abbreviations, 11. ***See also*** individual subject headings
Abdomen
anatomical divisions of, 36***t***
clinical divisions of, 36***t***
abdominal, pertaining to abdomen, 33, 39
Abdominal aorta, 382***f***
Abdominal cavity, superior portion of abdominopelvic cavity, 34, 34***f***, 35***t***
Abdominal region, 33, 33***f***
Abdominopelvic cavity, ventral cavity consisting of abdominal and pelvic cavities; contains digestive, urinary, and reproductive organs, 34, 35, 36***t***
Abducens nerve, 418***t***
Abduction, directional term meaning to move away from median or middle line of body, 9, 116***t***, 116***f***
Abnormal psychology, study and treatment of behaviors outside of normal and detrimental to person or society; these maladaptive behaviors range from occasional difficulty coping with stress, to bizarre actions and beliefs, to total withdrawal, 500
ABO system, major system of blood typing, 182
Abortifacient, medication that terminates a pregnancy, 351
Abortion (AB), 336
Abrasion, scraping away a portion of skin surface; performed to remove acne scars, tattoos, and scar tissue, 58
Abruptio placentae, emergency condition in which placenta tears away from uterine wall before twentieth week of pregnancy; requires immediate delivery of baby, 345
Abscess, a collection of pus in skin, 63
Absence seizure, type of epileptic seizure that lasts only a few seconds to half a minute, characterized by loss of awareness and absence of activity; also called ***petit mal seizure,*** 422
Accessory nerve, 418***t***
Accessory organs, accessory organs to digestive system consist of organs that are part of system, but not part of continuous tube from mouth to anus; accessory organs are liver, pancreas, gallbladder, and salivary glands, 258, 264–65
ACE inhibitor drugs, medication that produces vasodilation and decreases blood pressure, 163
Achromatopsia, condition of color blindness; more common in males, 456
Acidosis, excessive acidity of body fluids due to accumulation of acids, as in diabetic acidosis, 392
Acne, inflammatory disease of sebaceous glands and hair follicles resulting in papules and pustules, 63
Acne rosacea, hypertrophy of sebaceous glands causing thickened skin generally on nose, forehead, and cheeks, 63
Acne vulgaris, common form of acne occurring in adolescence from oversecretion of oil glands; characterized by papules, pustules, blackheads, and whiteheads, 63
Acoustic, pertaining to hearing, 470
Acoustic neuroma, benign tumor of eighth cranial nerve sheath, which can cause symptoms from pressure being exerted on tissues, 473
Acquired immunity, protective response of body to a specific pathogen, 197
Acquired immunodeficiency syndrome (AIDS), disease involving a defect in cell-mediated immunity system; syndrome of opportunistic infections occurring in final stages of infection with human immunodeficiency virus (HIV); virus attacks T_4 lymphocytes and destroys them, which reduces person's ability to fight infection, 66, 202
Acromegaly, chronic disease of adults resulting in elongation and enlargement of bones of head and extremities, 393, 393***f***
Action, type of movement a muscle produces, 115
Active acquired immunity, immunity developing after direct exposure to a pathogen, 196, 197
Active exercises, exercises that a patient performs without assistance, 516

Active range of motion (AROM), range of motion for joints that a patient is able to perform without assistance of someone else, 516
Active-resistive exercises, exercises in which patient will work against artificial resistance applied to a muscle, such as a weight; used to increase strength, 516
Activities of daily living (ADL), activities usually performed in course of a normal day, such as eating, dressing, and washing, 514, 514***f***
Acute care hospitals, hospitals that typically provide services to diagnose (laboratory, diagnostic imaging) and treat (surgery, medications, therapy) diseases for a short period of time; in addition, they usually provide emergency and obstetrical care; also called general hospital, 13
Acute respiratory distress syndrome, 234
Acute tubular necrosis (ATN), damage to renal tubules due to presence of toxins in urine or to ischemia; results in oliguria, 308
Adam's apple, 222, 388***f***
Adaptive equipment, equipment that has been structured to aid in mobility, eating, and managing other activities of daily living; equipment includes special walkers and spoons for stroke patient, 514, 515***f***
Addiction, acquired dependence on a drug, 496
Addison's disease, disease resulting from a deficiency in adrenocortical hormones; there may be an increased pigmentation of skin, generalized weakness, and weight loss, 391
Additive, sum of action of two (or more) drugs given; in this case, total strength of medications is equal to sum of strength of each individual drug, 496
Adduction, directional term meaning to move toward median or middle line of body, 9, 116***t***, 116***f***
Adenocarcinoma, malignant adenoma in a glandular organ, 395
Adenoidectomy, excision of adenoids, 205
Adenoiditis, inflammation of adenoid tissue, 201
Adenoids, another term for pharyngeal tonsils; tonsils are a collection of lymphatic tissue found in nasopharynx to combat microorganisms entering body through nose or mouth, 196, 222
Adhesion, scar tissue forming in fascia surrounding a muscle making it difficult to stretch muscle, 120
Adipose, type of connective tissue; also called fat; it stores energy and provides protective padding for underlying structures, 25
Adjective suffixes, 8
Adrenal, pertaining to adrenal gland, 389
Adrenal cortex, outer portion of adrenal glands; secretes several families of hormones: mineralocorticoids, glucocorticoids, and steroid sex hormones, 380***t,*** 382, 382***f***
Adrenal feminization, development of female secondary sexual characteristics (such as breasts) in a male; often as a result of increased estrogen secretion by adrenal cortex, 391
Adrenal glands, pair of glands in endocrine system located just above each kidney; glands are composed of two sections, cortex and medulla, that function independently of each other; cortex secretes steroids, such as aldosterone, cortisol, androgens, estrogens, and progestins; medulla secretes epinephrine and norepinephrine; adrenal glands are regulated by adrenocorticotropin hormone, which is secreted by pituitary gland, 30***t,*** 380**,** 382, 382***f,*** 391
Adrenal medulla, inner portion of adrenal gland; secretes epinephrine and norepinephrine, 380***t,*** 382, 382***f***
Adrenal virilism, development of male secondary sexual characteristics (such as deeper voice and facial hair) in a female; often as a result of increased androgen secretion by adrenal cortex, 391
Adrenalectomy, excision of adrenal gland, 396
Adrenaline, hormone produced by adrenal medulla; also known as epinephrine; some of its actions include increasing heart rate and force of contraction, bronchodilation, and relaxation of intestinal muscles, 380***t,*** 382
Adrenalitis, inflammation of adrenal gland, 391
Adrenocorticotropic hormone (ACTH), hormone secreted by anterior pituitary; regulates function of adrenal gland cortex, 381***t,*** 384, 385
Adrenomegaly, enlarged adrenal gland, 390
Adrenopathy, adrenal gland disease, 390
Adult respiratory distress syndrome (ARDS), acute respiratory failure in adults characterized by tachypnea, dyspnea, cyanosis, tachycardia, and hypoxemia, 234
Adverse reaction, 497
Aerosol, drugs inhaled directly into nose and mouth, 494, 494***t***
Aerosol therapy, medication suspended in mist intended to be inhaled; delivered by a ***nebulizer***, which delivers mist for period of time while patient breathes, or a ***metered dose inhaler*** (MDI), which delivers a single puff of mist, 240
Afferent, 299
Afferent arteriole, arteriole that carries blood into glomerulus, 299, 300***f,*** 302***f***

Afferent neurons, nerve that carries impulses to brain and spinal cord from skin and sense organs; also called sensory neurons, 418
Agglutinate, clumping together to form small clusters; platelets agglutinate to start clotting process, 182
Agranulocytes, nongranular leukocyte; this is one of two types of leukocytes found in plasma that are classified as either monocytes or lymphocytes, 181, 181***t***
AIDS-related complex (ARC), early stage of AIDS; there is a positive test for virus but only mild symptoms of weight loss, fatigue, skin rash, and anorexia, 202
Alanine transaminase (ALT), enzyme normally present in blood; blood levels are increased in persons with liver disease, 276
Albinism, condition in which person is not able to produce melanin; albino person has white hair and skin and pupils of eye are red, 63
Albumin, protein normally found circulating in bloodstream; it is abnormal for albumin to be in urine, 180, 303
Aldosterone, hormone produced by adrenal cortex; regulates levels of sodium and potassium in body and as a side effect volume of water lost in urine, 380***t*,** 382
Alimentary canal, also known as gastrointestinal system or digestive system; system covers area between mouth and anus and includes 30 feet of intestinal tubing; has a wide range of functions; system serves to store and digest food, absorb nutrients, and eliminate waste; major organs of system are mouth, pharynx, esophagus, stomach, small intestine, colon, rectum, and anus, 258
Allergen, antigen capable of causing a hypersensitivity or allergy in body, 201
Allergist, physician who specializes in testing for and treating allergies, 200
Allergy, hypersensitivity to a substance in environment or medication, 201
Allograft, skin graft from one person to another; donor is usually a cadaver, 70
Alopecia, absence or loss of hair, especially of head, 69
Alveolar, pertaining to alveoli,
Alveoli, tiny air sacs at end of each bronchiole; alveoli are surrounded by capillary network; gas exchange takes place as oxygen and carbon dioxide diffuse across alveolar and capillary walls, 223, 224***f***
Alzheimer's disease (AD), chronic, organic mental disorder consisting of dementia that is more prevalent in adults between 40 and 60; involves progressive disorientation, apathy, speech and gait disturbances, and loss of memory, 424, 501
Amblyopia, loss of vision not as a result of eye pathology; usually occurs in patients who see two images; in order to see only one image, brain will no longer recognize image being sent to it by one of eyes; may occur if strabismus is not corrected; commonly referred to as lazy eye, 456
Ambulatory care center, facility that provides services that do not require overnight hospitalization; services range from simple surgeries, to diagnostic testing, to therapy; also called a surgical center or outpatient clinic, 13
Amenorrhea, absence of menstruation, which can be result of many factors, including pregnancy, menopause, and dieting, 342
American Sign Language (ASL), nonverbal method of communicating in which hands and fingers are used to indicate words and concepts; used by people who are deaf and speech impaired, 475, 475***f***
Amino acids, organic substances found in plasma, used by cells to build proteins, 180
Amnesia, loss of memory in which people forget their identity as a result of head injury or disorder, such as epilepsy, senility, and alcoholism; can be either temporary or permanent, 501
Amniocentesis, puncturing of amniotic sac using a needle and syringe for purpose of withdrawing amniotic fluid for testing; can assist in determining fetal maturity, development, and genetic disorders, 348
Amnion, inner of two membranous sacs surrouding fetus; amniotic sac contains amniotic fluid in which baby floats, 338, 340
Amniorrhea, discharge of amniotic fluid, 342
Amniotic, pertaining to amnion, 340
Amniotic fluid, fluid inside amniotic sac, 336, 337***f*,** 338
Amniotomy, incision into amniotic sac, 349
Amplification device, 475
Amputation, partial or complete removal of a limb for a variety of reasons, including tumors, gangrene, intractable pain, crushing injury, or uncontrollable infection, 107
Amylase, digestive enzyme found in saliva that begins digestion of carbohydrates, 264
Amyotrophic lateral sclerosis (ALS), disease with muscular weakness and atrophy due to degeneration of motor neurons of spinal cord; also called ***Lou Gehrig's disease,*** after New York Yankees' baseball player who died from disease, 427

Anacusis, total absence of hearing; unable to perceive sound; also called ***deafness,*** 472

Anal, pertaining to anus, 267

Anal fistula, abnormal tubelike passage from surface around anal opening directly into rectum, 272

Anal sphincter, ring of muscle that controls anal opening, 263

Analgesia, reduction in perception of pain or sensation due to neurological condition or medication, 422

Analgesic, substance that relieves pain without loss of consciousness; may be either narcotic or non-narcotic; narcotic drugs are derived from opium poppy and act on brain to cause pain relief and drowsiness, 432, 523

Anaphylactic shock, life-threatening condition resulting from ingestion of food or medications that produce severe allergic response; circulatory and respiratory problems occur, including respiratory distress, hypotension, edema, tachycardia, and convulsions, 201

Anaphylaxis, severe reaction to antigen, 201

Anastomosis, creating a passageway or opening between two organs or vessels, 279

Anatomical position, used to describe positions and relationships of a structure in human body; for descriptive purposes assumption is always that person is in anatomical position; body is standing erect with arms at side of body, palms of hands facing forward, and eyes looking straight ahead; legs are parallel with feet and toes pointing forward, 31, 32***f***

Ancillary reports, report in patient's medical record from various treatments and therapies patient has received, such as rehabilitation, social services, respiratory therapy, or from dietician, 12

Androgen, class of steroid hormones secreted by adrenal cortex; these hormones, such as testosterone, produce a masculinizing effect, 380***t***, 382

Androgen therapy, replacement male hormones to treat patients who produce insufficient hormone naturally, 362

Anemia, reduction in number of red blood cells (RBCs) or amount of hemoglobin in blood; results in less oxygen reaching tissues, 186

Anesthesia, partial or complete loss of sensation with or without loss of consciousness as a result of drug, disease, or injury, 422, 520, 521***t***

Anesthesiologist, physician who has specialization in practice of administering anesthetics, 422, 520

Anesthesiologist's report, medical record document that relates details regarding drugs given to patient and patient's response to anesthesia and vital signs during surgery, 12

Anesthesiology, branch of medicine specializing in all aspects of anesthesia, including for surgical procedures, resuscitation measures, and management of acute and chronic pain; physician is ***anesthesiologist***, 422

Anesthetic, substance that produces a lack of feeling that may be of local or general effect, depending on type of administration, 72, 432, 523

Anesthetic ophthalmic solution, eyedrops for pain relief associated with eye infections and corneal abrasions, 463

Aneurysm, weakness in wall of artery that results in localized widening of artery, 157, 157***f***

Aneurysmectomy, surgical removal of aneurysm, 162

Angiitis, inflammation of vessels, 153

Angina pectoris, severe chest pain with sensation of constriction around heart; caused by a deficiency of oxygen to heart muscle, 154, 155***f***

Angiogram, record of a vessel, 159

Angiography, process of taking X-ray of blood or lymphatic vessels after injection of a radiopaque substance, 159

Angioplasty, surgical repair of blood vessels, 163, 163***f***

Angiospasm, involuntary muscle contraction of a vessel, 153

Angiostenosis, narrowing of a vessel, 153

Anhidrosis, abnormal condition of no sweat, 58

Ankylosing spondylitis, inflammatory spinal condition that resembles rheumatoid arthritis; results in gradual stiffening and fusion of vertebrae; more common in men than women, 103

Anorchism, congenital absence of one or both testes, 358

Anorexia, loss of appetite that can accompany other conditions such as gastrointestinal (GI) upset, 269

Anorexia nervosa, type of eating disorder characterized by severe disturbance in body image and marked refusal to eat, 501, 501***f***

Anorexiant, substance that treats obesity by suppressing appetite, 281

Anosmia, loss of sense of smell, 230

Anoxia, lack of oxygen, 230

Antacid, substance that neutralizes acid in stomach, 281

Antagonistic pairs, pair of muscles arranged around a joint that produce opposite actions, 115, 116–18***t***

Anteflexion, while uterus is normally in this position, exaggeration of forward bend of uterus is abnormal; forward bend is near neck of uterus; position of cervix, or opening of uterus, remains normal, 334

Antepartum, before birth, 341

Anterior, directional term meaning near or on front or belly side of body, 34***f,*** 37***t***

Anterior lobe, anterior portion of pituitary gland; secretes adrenocorticotropin hormone, follicle-stimulating hormone, growth hormone, luteinizing hormone, melanocyte-stimulating hormone, prolactin, and thyroid-stimulating hormone, 385

Anterior pituitary gland, 385***f,*** 386***f***

Anterior tibial artery, 148***f***

Anterior tibial vein, 150***f***

Anteroposterior view (AP), positioning patient so that X-rays pass through body from anterior side to posterior side, 507

Anthracosis, type of pneumoconiosis that develops from collection of coal dust in lung; also called black lung or miner's lung, 234

Anti-inflammatory otic solution, reduces inflammation, itching, and edema associated with otitis externa, 476

Anti-virals, substance that weakens viral infection in body, often by interfering with virus's ability to replicate, 281

Antiarrhythmic, controls cardiac arrhythmias by altering nerve impulses within heart, 163

Antibiotic, substance that destroys or prohibits growth of microorganisms; used to treat bacterial infections; not found effective in treating viral infections; to be effective, it must be taken regularly for specified period, 72, 242, 315

Antibiotic ophthalmic solution, eyedrops for treatment of bacterial eye infections, 463

Antibiotic otic solution, eardrops to treat otitis externa, 476

Antibody, protein material produced in body as a response to invasion of foreign substance, 198

Antibody-mediated immunity, production of antibodies by B cells in response to an antigen; also called ***humoral immunity,*** 197

Anticoagulant, substance that prevents or delays clotting or coagulation of blood, 163, 189

Anticonvulsant, prevents or relieves convulsions; drugs such as phenobarbital reduce excessive stimulation in brain to control seizures and other symptoms of epilepsy, 433

Antidepressant drugs, medications classified as stimulants that alter patient's mood by affecting levels of neurotransmitters in brain, 504

Antidiarrheal, prevents or relieves diarrhea, 281

Antidiuretic hormone (ADH), hormone secreted by posterior pituitary; promotes water reabsorption by kidney tubules, 381***t,*** 385

Antidote, substance that will neutralize poisons or their side effects, 496

Antiemetic, substance that controls nausea and vomiting, 281, 476

Antifungal, substance that kills fungi infecting skin, 72

Antigen, substance capable of inducing formation of antibody; antibody then intereacts with antigen in antigen–antibody reaction, 197

Antigen-antibody complex, combination of antigen with its specific antibody; increases susceptibility to phagocytosis and immunity, 198

Antiglaucoma medications, group of drugs that reduce intraocular pressure by lowering amount of aqueous humor in eyeball; may achieve this by either reducing production of aqueous humor or increasing its outflow, 463

Antihemorrhagic, substance that prevents or stops hemorrhaging, 189

Antihistamine, substance that acts to control allergic symptoms by counteracting histamine, which exists naturally in body, and which is released in allergic reactions, 205, 242

Antilipidemic, substance that reduces amount of cholesterol and lipids in bloodstream; treats hyperlipidemia, 163

Antiparasitic, substance that kills mites or lice, 72

Antiplatelet agent, substance that interferes with action of platelets; prolongs bleeding time; commonly referred to as blood thinner; used to prevent heart attacks and strokes, 163, 189

Antiprostatic agents, medications to treat early cases of benign prostatic hypertrophy; may prevent surgery for mild cases, 362

Antipruritic, substance that reduces severe itching, 72

Antipsychotic drugs, major tranquilizer drugs that have transformed treatment of patients with psychoses and schizophrenia by reducing patient agitation and panic and shortening schizophrenic episodes, 504

Antiseptic, substance used to kill bacteria in skin cuts and wounds or at a surgical site, 72

Antisocial personality disorder, personality disorder in which patient engages in behaviors that are illegal or outside of social norms, 502

Antispasmodic, medication to prevent or reduce bladder muscle spasms, 315
Antithyroid agents, medication given to block production of thyroid hormones in patients with hypersecretion disorders, 397
Antitussive, substance that controls or relieves coughing; codeine is an ingredient in many prescription cough medicines that acts upon the brain to control coughing, 243
Antrum, tapered distal end of the stomach, 262, 262***f***
Anuria, complete suppression of urine formed by kidneys and complete lack of urine excretion, 305
Anus, terminal opening of digestive tube, 263, 264***f***
Anvil, 467***f,*** 468
Anxiety, feeling of apprehension or worry, 500
Anxiety disorders, characterized by persistent worry and apprehension; includes panic attacks, anxiety, phobias, and obsessive-compulsive disorder, 500
Aorta, largest artery in body; located in mediastinum and carries oxygenated blood away from left side of heart, 35***t,*** 140***f,*** 141***f,*** 142***f,*** 144, 145***f,*** 146***f,*** 195***f***, 384***f***
Aortic, pertaining to aorta, 152
Aortic arch, 148***f***
Aortic semilunar valve, 144***f***
Aortic valve, semilunar valve between left ventricle of heart and aorta in heart; prevents blood from flowing backwards into ventricle, 142***f,*** 143, 144***f,*** 145***f***
Apex, directional term meaning tip or summit; an area of lungs and heart, 37***t,*** 141, 141***f,*** 145***f,*** 224, 225***f***
Apgar score, evaluation of neonate's adjustment to outside world; observes color, heart rate, muscle tone, respiratory rate, and response to stimulus, 348
Aphagia, not eating, 269
Aphasia, inability to communicate through speech; often after effect of stroke (CVA), 422
Aphonia, no voice, 230
Aphthous ulcers, painful ulcers in mouth of unknown cause; commonly called ***canker sores***, 270
Aplastic anemia, severe form of anemia that develops as consequence of loss of functioning red bone marrow; results in decrease in number of all formed elements; treatment may eventually require bone marrow transplant, 186
Apnea, condition of not breathing, 230
Apocrine gland, type of sweat gland that opens into hair follicles located in pubic, anal, and mammary areas; glands secrete substance that can produce odor when it comes into contact with bacteria on skin causing what is commonly referred to as body odor, 56
Appendectomy, surgical removal of appendix, 279
Appendicitis, inflammation of appendix, 272
Appendicular skeleton, appendicular skeleton consists of bones of upper and lower extremities, shoulder, and pelvis, 89, 92, 93***f***
Appendix, 36***t,*** 263***f,*** 264***f***
Aqueous, pertaining to water or being water-like, 454
Aqueous humor, watery fluid filling spaces between cornea and lens, 448***f,*** 449
Arachnoid layer, delicate middle layer of meninges, 417, 417***f***
Areola, pigmented area around nipple of breast, 336, 336***f***
Arrector pili, small slip of smooth muscle attached to hairs; when this muscle contracts hair shaft stands up and results in "goose bumps," 53***f,*** 55, 55***f***
Arrhythmia, irregularity in heartbeat or action, 154
Arterial, pertaining to artery, 152
Arterial anastomosis, surgical joining together of two arteries; performed if artery is severed or if damaged section of artery is removed, 162
Arterial blood gases (ABG), lab test that measures amount of oxygen, carbon dioxide, and nitrogen in blood, and pH, 238
Arteries, blood vessels that carry blood away from heart, 28***t,*** 87***f,*** 140, 147, 147***f,*** 148***f***
Arteriole, smallest branch of arteries; carries blood to capillaries, 147, 152, 193***f***
Arteriorrhexis, ruptured artery, 157
Arteriosclerosis (AS), condition with thickening, hardening, and loss of elasticity of walls of arteries, 157
Arthralgia, pain in a joint, 100
Arthrocentesis, removal of synovial fluid with needle from joint space, such as in knee, for examination, 107
Arthroclasia, surgically breaking loose a stiffened joint, 107
Arthrodesis, surgical fusion or stiffening of a joint to provide stability; sometimes done to relieve pain of arthritis, 107
Arthrogram, record of a joint, 106
Arthrography, visualization of joint by radiographic study after injection of contrast medium into joint space, 106
Arthroscope, instrument to view inside joint, 3, 106
Arthroscopic surgery, use of arthroscope to facilitate performing surgery on joint, 107
Arthroscopy, examination of interior of joint by entering joint with arthroscope; arthroscope contains small television camera allowing

Autism, type of mental disorder diagnosed in childhood in which child exhibits extreme degree of withdrawal from all social contacts, 501

Autograft, skin graft from person's own body, 70, 70***f***

Autoimmune disease, disease resulting from he body's immune system attacking its own cells as if they were pathogens; examples include systemic lupus erythematosus, rheumatoid arthritis, and multiple sclerosis, 201

Autologous transfusion, procedure for collecting and storing patient's own blood several weeks prior to actual need; can then be used to replace blood lost during surgical procedure, 189

Autonomic nervous system (ANS), portion of nervous system consisting of nerves to internal organs that function involuntarily; regulates functions of glands (especially salivary, gastric, and sweat glands), adrenal medulla, heart, and smooth muscle tissue; system is divided into two parts: sympathetic and parasympathetic, 145, 418, 419–20

Axial skeleton, axial skeleton includes bones in head, spine, chest, and trunk, 89–92, 90***f***

Axillary, pertaining to armpit; there is a collection of lymph nodes in this area that drains each arm, 194***t***, 195***f***

Axon, single projection of a neuron that conducts impulse away from nerve cell body, 412, 413***f***

Azotemia, accumulation of nitrogenous waste in bloodstream; occurs when kidney fails to filter these wastes from blood, 305

B

B cells, common name for B lymphocytes, responds to foreign antigens by producing protective antibodies, 198

B lymphocytes, humoral immunity cells, which respond to foreign antigens by producing protective antibodies; simply referred to as ***B cells,*** 198

Babinski's reflex, reflex test to determine lesions and abnormalities in nervous system; Babinski reflex is present if great toe extends instead of flexes when lateral sole of foot is stroked; normal response to this stimulation would be flexion, or upward movement, of toe, 431

Bacteria, primitive, single-celled microorganisms that are present everywhere; some are capable of causing disease in humans, 197

Bacteriuria, bacteria in urine, 305

Balanic, pertaining to glans penis, 357

Balanitis, inflammation of skin covering glans penis, 359

Balanoplasty, surgical repair of glans penis, 361

Balanorrhea, discharge from glans penis, 358

Balloon angioplasty, 163***f***

Bariatric surgery, group of surgical procedures such as stomach stapling and restrictive banding to reduce size of stomach; treatment for morbid (extreme) obesity, 279

Barium (Ba), soft metallic element from earth used as radiopaque X-ray dye, 507

Barium enema (BE), 277, 277***f***

Barium swallow, 278

Barrier contraception, prevention of pregnancy using a device to prevent sperm from meeting ovum; examples include condoms, diaphragms, and cervical caps, 349

Bartholin's glands, glands located on either side of vaginal opening that secrete mucus for vaginal lubrication, 335

Basal cell carcinoma (BCC), tumor of basal cell layer of epidermis; frequent type of skin cancer that rarely metastasizes or spreads; these cancers can arise on sun-exposed skin, 63, 63***f***

Basal layer, deepest layer of epidermis; this living layer constantly multiplies and divides to supply cells to replace cells that are sloughed off skin surface, 53

Base, directional term meaning bottom or lower part, 37***t***, 224, 225***f***

Basilic vein, 150***f***

Basophil (Basos), granulocyte white blood cell that releases histamine and heparin in damaged tissues, 181***f***, 181***t***, 184

Bell jar apparatus, 226***f***

Bell's palsy, one-sided facial paralysis with unknown cause; person cannot control salivation, tearing of eyes, or expression; patient will eventually recover, 428

Benign, not cancerous; benign tumor is generally not progressive or recurring, 526

Benign prostatic hypertrophy (BPH), enlargement of prostate gland commonly seen in males over 50, 358

Beta blocker drugs, medication that treats hypertension and angina pectoris by lowering heart rate, 164

Biceps, arm muscle named for number of attachment points; ***bi***- means two and biceps have two heads attached to bone, 115

Bicuspid valve, valve between left atrium and ventricle; prevents blood from flowing

result in destruction of bronchial walls; major symptom is large amount of purulent (pus-filled) sputum; rales (bubbling chest sound) and hemoptysis may be present, 230, 234

Bronchiolar, pertaining to a bronchiole, 228

Bronchioles, narrowest air tubes in lungs; each bronchiole terminates in tiny air sacs called alveoli, 223, 223***f***, 224***f***

Bronchitis, acute or chronic inflammation of lower respiratory tract that often occurs after other childhood infections such as measles, 234

Bronchodilator, dilates or opens bronchi (airways in lungs) to improve breathing, 243

Bronchogenic carcinoma, malignant lung tumor that originates in bronchi; usually associated with history of cigarette smoking, 234, 234***f***

Bronchogram, X-ray record of lungs and bronchial tubes, 238

Bronchography, process of taking X-ray of lung after radiopaque substance has been placed into trachea or bronchial tree, 238

Bronchoplasty, surgical repair of a bronchial defect, 241

Bronchoscope, instrument to view inside a bronchus, 238, 239***f***

Bronchoscopy (Bronch), using bronchoscope to visualize bronchi; instrument can also be used to obtain tissue for biopsy and to remove foreign objects, 238, 239***f***

Bronchospasm, involuntary muscle spasm in bronchi, 230

Bronchus, distal end of trachea splits into left and right main bronchi as it enters each lung; each main bronchus is subdivided into smaller branches; smallest bronchi are bronchioles; each bronchiole ends in tiny air sacs called alveoli, 223, 223***f***

Buccal, (1) pertaining to cheeks; (2) drugs that are placed under lip or between cheek and gum, 267, 494, 496***t***

Buccolabial, pertaining to cheeks and lips, 267

Buffers, chemicals that neutralize acid, particularly stomach acid, 265

Bulbourethral gland, also called ***Cowper's gland***; these two small male reproductive system glands are located on either side of urethra just distal to prostate; secretion from these glands neutralizes acidity in urethra and vagina, 30***t***, 353***f***, 354, 354***f***, 356

Bulimia, eating disorder characterized by recurrent binge eating and then purging of food with laxatives and vomiting, 502

Bundle branch block (BBB), occurs when electrical impulse is blocked from travelling down bundle of His or bundle branches; results in ventricles beating at a different rate than atria; also called a ***heart block,*** 154

Bundle branches, part of conduction system of heart; electrical signal travels down interventricular septum, 145, 146***f***, 154

Bundle of His, bundle of His is located in interventricular septum; receives electrical impulse from atrioventricular node and distributes it through ventricular walls, causing them to contract simultaneously, 145, 146***f***, 154

Bunion, inflammation of bursa of the great toe, 105

Bunionectomy, removal of bursa at joint of great toe, 107

Burn, full-thickness burn exists when all layers are burned; also called ***third-degree burn;*** partial-thickness burn exists when first layer of skin, epidermis, is burned, and second layer of skin, dermis, is damaged; also called ***second-degree burn; first-degree burn*** damages only epidermis, 64, 64***f***

Bursa, saclike connective tissue structure found in some joints; protects moving parts from friction; some common bursa locations are elbow, knee, and shoulder joints, 96

Bursectomy, excision of a bursa, 108

Bursitis, inflammation of bursa between bony prominences and muscles or tendons; common in shoulder and knee, 96, 100

C

Cachexia, loss of weight and generalized wasting that occurs during a chronic disease, 269

Calcitonin (CT), hormone secreted by thyroid gland; stimulates deposition of calcium into bone, 381***t***, 388

Calcium (Ca^+), inorganic substance found in plasma; is important for bones, muscles, and nerves, 180, 384

Calcium channel blocker drugs, medication that treats hypertension, angina pectoris, and congestive heart failure by causing heart to beat less forcefully and less often, 164

Calcium supplements, maintaining high blood levels of calcium in association with vitamin D helps maintain bone density and treats osteomalacia, osteoporosis, and rickets, 109

Calculus, stone formed within organ by accumulation of mineral salts; found in kidney, renal pelvis, bladder, or urethra; plural is ***calculi,*** 306, 306***f***

Callus, mass of bone tissue that forms at fracture site during its healing, 100

Calyx, duct that connects renal papilla to renal pelvis; urine flows from collecting tubule through calyx and into renal pelvis, 298, 299***f***

carpal tunnel disease, which can be caused by repetitive motion such as typing, 122

Carpal tunnel syndrome (CTS), painful disorder of wrist and hand, induced by compression of median nerve as it passes under ligaments on palm side of wrist; symptoms include weakness, pain, burning, tingling, and aching in forearm, wrist, and hand, 121

Carpals, wrist bones in upper extremity, 92, 93***f*,** 94, 94***f*,** 98

Cartilage, strong, flexible connective tissue found in several locations in body, such as covering ends of bones in synovial joint, nasal septum, external ear, eustachian tube, larynx, trachea, bronchi, and intervertebral discs, 25, 86, 467***f***

Cartilaginous joints, joint that allows slight movement but holds bones firmly in place by solid piece of cartilage; public symphysis is an example of a cartilaginous joint; fetal skeleton is composed of cartilaginous tissue, 96, 96***f***

Cast, application of solid material to immobilize extremity or portion of body as a result of fracture, dislocation, or severe injury; is most often made of plaster of Paris, 109

Castration, excision of testicles in male or ovaries in female, 361

Cataract, diminished vision resulting from lens of eye becoming opaque or cloudy; treatment is usually surgical removal of cataract, 456, 456***f***

Cath, 312

Catheter (cath), flexible tube inserted into body for purpose of moving fluids into or out of body; in cardiovascular system used to place dye into blood vessels so they may be visualized on X-rays; in urinary system used to drain urine from bladder, 160, 308***f*,** 312

Catheterization, insertion of a tube through urethra and into urinary bladder for purpose of withdrawing urine or inserting dye, 312

Caudal, directional term meaning toward feet or tail, or below, 37***f*,** 37***t***

Cauterization, destruction of tissue using electric current, caustic product, or hot iron, or by freezing, 71, 523

Cecal, pertaining to the cecum, 267

Cecum, first portion of colon; is a blind pouch off beginning of large intestine; appendix grows out of end of cecum, 263, 263***f*,** 264***f***

Cell, basic unit of all living things; all tissues and organs in body are composed of cells; they perform survival functions such as reproduction, respiration, metabolism, and excretion; some cells also able to carry on specialized functions, such as contraction by muscle cells and electrical impulse transmission by nerve cells, 24

Cell membrane, outermost boundary of the cell, 24

Cell-mediated immunity, immunity resulting from activation of sensitized T lymphocytes; immune response causes antigens to be destroyed by direct action of cells; also called ***cellular immunity*,** 197

Cellular immunity, also called cell-mediated immunity; process results in production of T cells and natural killer, NK, cells that directly attach to foreign cells; immune response fights invasion by viruses, bacteria, fungi, and cancer, 197–98

Cellulitis, inflammation of cellular or connective tissues, 65

Cementum, anchors root of a tooth into socket of jaw, 260, 261, 261***f***

Central canal, canal that extends down length of spinal cord; contains cerebrospinal fluid, 417

Central fissure, 415***f***

Central nervous system (CNS), portion of nervous system consisting of brain and spinal cord; receives impulses from all over body, processes information, and then responds with action; consists of both gray and white matter, 413–17
- brain, 414–16
- meninges, 413, 417, 417***f***
- spinal cord, 416–417

Centrifuge, 179***f***

Cephalalgia, a headache, 422

Cephalic, directional term meaning toward the head, or above, 37***t*,** 39

Cephalic region, head region of the body, 33, 33***f***

Cephalic vein, 150***f***

Cerebellar, pertaining to cerebellum, 421

Cerebellitis, inflammation of cerebellum, 424

Cerebellum, second largest portion of brain, located beneath posterior portion of cerebrum; this part of brain aids in coordinating voluntary body movements and maintaining balance and equilibrium; is attached to brain stem by pons; cerebellum refines muscular movement that is initiated in cerebrum, 414, 414***f*,** 415***f***

Cerebral, pertaining to the cerebrum, 421

Cerebral aneurysm, localized abnormal dilatation of blood vessel, usually artery; result of congenital defect or weakness in wall of vessel; ruptured aneurysm is a common cause for hemorrhagic CVA, 425, 425***f***

Cerebral angiography, x-ray of blood vessels of brain after injection of radiopaque dye, 430

Cerebral contusion, bruising of brain from blow or impact; symptoms last longer than 24 hours and include unconsciousness, dizziness, vomiting, unequal pupil size, and shock, 425

laparoscope requires a small incision into abdominal cavity, 279
Cholecystic, pertaining to gallbladder, 267
Cholecystitis, inflammation of gallbladder, 275
Cholecystogram, dye given orally to patient is absorbed and enters gallbladder; X-ray is then taken, 277
Choledocholithotripsy, crushing of a gallstone in common bile duct, 279
Cholelithiasis, formation or presence of stones or calculi in gallbladder or common bile duct, 276, 276***f***
Chondrectomy, excision of cartilage, 108
Chondroma, cartilage tumor, 103
Chondromalacia, softening of cartilage, 100
Chondroplasty, surgical repair of cartilage, 108
Chorion, outer of two membranous sacs surrounding fetus; helps to form placenta, 336, 338
Chorionic, pertaining to chorion, 340
Chorionic villus sampling (CVS), removal of small piece of chorion for genetic analysis; may be done at earlier stage of pregnancy than amniocentesis, 348
Choroid, middle layer of eyeball; this layer provides blood supply for eye, 448, 448***f,*** 449
Choroid layer, 447***f***
Chronic obstructive pulmonary disease (COPD), progressive, chronic, and usually irreversible condition in which lungs have diminished capacity for inspiration (inhalation) and expiration (exhalation); person may have difficulty breathing on exertion (dyspnea) and a cough; also called ***chronic obstructive lung disease (COLD),*** 235
Chyme, semisoft mixture of food and digestive fluids that pass from stomach into small intestines, 262
Cicatrix, a scar, 65
Cilia, term for eyelashes that protect eye from foreign particles or for nasal hairs that help filter dust and bacteria out of inhaled air, 221, 451
Ciliary body, intraocular eye muscles that change shape of the lens, 448***f,*** 449
Circadian rhythm, 24-hour clock that governs our periods of wakefulness and sleepiness, 384
Circulating nurse, nurse who assists surgeon and scrub nurse by providing needed materials during procedure and by handling surgical specimen; person does not wear sterile clothing and may enter and leave operating room during procedure, 523
Circulatory system, system that transports blood to all areas of body; organs of circulatory system include heart and blood vessels (arteries, veins, and capillaries); also called ***cardiovascular system,*** 140, 140***f***
Circumcision, surgical removal of end of prepuce or foreskin of penis; generally performed on newborn male at request of parents; primary reason is for ease of hygiene; is also a ritual practice in some religions, 355, 361
Circumduction, movement in a circular direction from a central point, 118***t***
Cirrhosis, chronic disease of the liver, 276
Clamp, surgical instrument used to grasp tissue and control bleeding, 521***t***
Clavicle, also called collar bone; bone of pectoral girdle, 92, 93***f,*** 94, 94***f***, 94***t***
Clavicular, pertaining to clavicle or collar bone, 98
Clean catch specimen (CC), urine sample obtained after cleaning off urinary opening and catching or collecting a sample in midstream (halfway through urination process) to minimize contamination from genitalia, 310
Cleft lip, congenital anomaly in which upper lip fails to come together; often seen along with cleft palate; corrected with surgery, 270
Cleft palate, congenital anomaly in which roof of mouth has split or fissure; corrected with surgery, 270
clinical psychologist (PhD), diagnoses and treats mental disorders; specializes in using individual and group counseling to treat patients with mental and emotional disorders, 500
Clinical psychology, 500
Clitoris, small organ containing erectile tissue covered by labia minora; contains sensitive tissue aroused during sexual stimulation and is similar to penis in male, 332***f,*** 335–36, 335***f***
Closed fracture, simple fracture with no open skin or wound, 100, 101***f***
Clubbing, abnormal widening and thickening of ends of fingers and toes associated with chronic oxygen deficiency; seen in patients with chronic respiratory conditions or circulatory problems, 230
Coagulate, convert liquid to gel or solid, as in blood coagulation, 185
Coarctation of the aorta (CoA), severe congenital narrowing of aorta, 158
Coccygeal, pertaining to coccyx or tailbone, 98, 416***f***
Coccyx, tailbone,three to five very small vertebrae attached to the sacrum, often become fused, 89, 90***f***, 91, 92***f***, 92***t***
Cochlea, portion of labyrinth associated with hearing; is rolled in shape of snail shell; organs of Corti line cochlea, 467***f,*** 468
Cochlear, pertaining to cochlea, 471
Cochlear implant, mechanical device surgically placed under skin behind outer ear (pinna); converts sound signals into magnetic impulses

to stimulate auditory nerve; can be beneficial for those with profound sensorineural hearing loss, 475, 475***f***

Cochlear nerve, branch of vestibulocochlear nerve that carries hearing information to brain, 467, 467***f***

Cognitive disorders, deterioration of mental functions due to temporary brain or permanent brain dysfunction; includes dementia and Alzheimer's disease, 501

Coitus, 355

Cold sores, 271

Colectomy, surgical removal of colon, 279

Collagen fibers, fibers made up of insoluble fibrous protein present in connective tissue that forms flexible mat to protect skin and other parts of body, 54

Collecting tubule, portion of renal tubule, 299, 300***f,*** 302***f***

Colles' fracture, specific type of wrist fracture, 101, 101***f***

Colon, also called ***large intestine;*** functions to reabsorb most of fluid in digested food; material that remains after water reabsorption is feces; sections of colon are cecum, ascending colon, transverse colon, descending colon, and sigmoid colon, 26***f,*** 29***t,*** 35***t,*** 36***t,*** 258, 263, 264***f,***

Colonic, pertaining to colon, 267

Colonoscope, instrument to view inside colon, 278

Colonoscopy, flexible fiberscope passed through anus, rectum, and colon is used to examine upper portion of colon; polyps and small growths can be removed during procedure, 278

Color vision tests, use of polychromic (multicolored) charts to determine ability of patient to recognize color, 460, 460***f***

Colorectal, pertaining to colon and rectum, 267

Colorectal carcinoma, cancerous tumor originating in the colon or rectum, 272

Colostomy, surgical creation of opening in some portion of colon through abdominal wall to outside surface; fecal material (stool) drains into bag worn on abdomen, 280, 280***f***

Colostrum, thin fluid first secreted by breast after delivery; does not contain much protein, but is rich in antibodies, 341

Colposcope, instrument to view inside vagina, 347

Colposcopy, visual examination of cervix and vagina using colposcope or instrument with magnifying lens, 347

Coma, profound unconsciousness resulting from illness or injury, 422

Combining form, word root plus combining vowel; is always written with a / between word root and combining vowel; for example, in combining form ***cardi/o, cardi*** is word root and ***/o*** is combining vowel, 3–4

Combining vowel, vowel inserted between word parts that makes it possible to pronounce long medical terms; is usually the vowel ***o,*** 2, 3–4

Comedo, medical term for blackhead; is an accumulation of sebum in sebaceous gland that has become blackened, 58

Comminuted fracture, fracture in which bone is shattered, splintered, or crushed into many pieces or fragments; fracture is completely through bone, 101

Common bile duct (CBD), duct that carries bile from gallbladder to duodenum, 265, 265***f,*** 276***f***

Common iliac artery, 148***f***

Common iliac vein, 150***f***

Compact bone, hard exterior surface bone; also called ***cortical bone,*** 86, 87***f,*** 96***f***

Complemental air, 225***t***

Complete blood count (CBC), blood test consisting of five tests; red blood cell count (RBC), white blood count (WBC), hemoglobin (Hg), hematocrit (Hct), and white blood cell differential, 187

Compound fracture, open fracture in which skin has been broken through by fracture, 101, 101***f***

Compression fracture, fracture involving loss of height of vertebral body, 101

Computed tomography scan (CT scan, CAT), imaging technique able to produce cross-sectional view of body; X-ray pictures are taken at multiple angles through body and computer uses all images to construct composite cross-section, 508

Conception, fertilization of ovum by a sperm, 333, 334

Concussion, injury to brain resulting from blow or impact from object; can result in unconsciousness, dizziness, vomiting, unequal pupil size, and shock, 426

Conductive hearing loss, loss of hearing as a result of blocking of sound transmission in middle ear and outer ear, 469

Condyle, refers to rounded portion at end of a bone, 88, 88***f***

Cones, sensory receptors of retina that are active in bright light and see in color, 449

Confidentiality, 14

Congenital anomalies, 337

Congenital septal defect (CSD), defect, present at birth, in wall separating two chambers of heart; results in a mixture of oxygenated and deoxygenated blood being carried to surrounding tissues; there can be atrial septal defect (ASD) and ventricular septal defect (VSD), 155

Congestive heart failure (CHF), pathological condition of heart in which there is reduced outflow of blood from left side of heart; results in weakness, breathlessness, and edema, 155

Conization, surgical removal of core of cervical tissue; also refers to partial removal of cervix, 349

Conjunctiva, protective mucous membrane lining on underside of each eyelid and across anterior surface of each eyeball, 448, 448***f***, 450***f***, 451, 459

Conjunctival, pertaining to conjunctiva, 454

Conjunctivitis, also referred to as ***pinkeye*** or inflammation of conjunctiva, 459

Conjunctivoplasty, surgical repair of conjunctiva, 462

Connective tissue, supporting and protecting tissue in body structures; examples are fat or adipose tissue, cartilage, and bone, 25, 26***f***

Conscious, condition of being awake and aware of surroundings, 422

Constipation, experiencing difficulty in defecation or infrequent defecation, 269

Consultation reports, document in patient's medical record; reports given by specialists who physician has requested to evaluate patient, 12

Contracture, abnormal shortening of muscle, making it difficult to stretch muscle, 120

Contraindication, condition in which particular drug should not be used, 496

Contrast studies, radiopaque substance is injected or swallowed; X-rays are then taken that outline body structure containing radiopaque substance, 509, 509***f***

Controlled substances, drugs that have potential for being addictive (habit forming) or can be abused, 492, 492***t***

Contusion, injury caused by blow to body; causes swelling, pain, and bruising; skin is not broken, 58

Conversion reaction, somatoform disorder in which patient unconsciously substitutes physical signs or symptoms for anxiety; most common physical signs or symptoms are blindness, deafness, and paralysis, 503

Convulsions, severe involuntary muscle contractions and relaxations; these have a variety of causes, such as epilepsy, fever, and toxic conditions, 422

Corium, living layer of skin located between epidermis and subcutaneous tissue; also referred to as ***dermis,*** it contains hair follicles, sweat glands, sebaceous glands, blood vessels, lymph vessels, nerve fibers, and muscle fibers, 54

Cornea, portion of sclera that is clear and transparent and allows light to enter interior of eye; also plays role in bending light rays, 447***f***, 448, 448***f***, 452***f***

Corneal, pertaining to cornea, 454

Corneal abrasion, scraping injury to cornea; if it does not heal, it may develop into ulcer, 456

Coronal plane, vertical plane that divides body into front (anterior or ventral) and back (posterior or dorsal) sections; also called ***frontal plane,*** 32***f***, 33

Coronal section, sectional view of body produced by cut along frontal plane; also called ***frontal section,*** 33

Coronary, pertaining to heart, 147, 152

Coronary arteries, group of three arteries that branch off aorta and carry blood to myocardium, 147, 147***f***

Coronary artery bypass graft (CABG), open-heart surgery in which blood vessel is grafted to route blood around point of constriction in diseased coronary artery, 162

Coronary artery disease (CAD), insufficient blood supply to heart muscle due to obstruction of one or more coronary arteries; may be caused by atherosclerosis and may cause angina pectoris and myocardial infarction, 155, 155***f***

Corpus, body or central portion of uterus, 332***f***, 334

Corpus (uterus), 332***f***

Corpus albicans, 333***f***

Corpus luteum, 333***f***

Cortex, outer layer of organ; in endocrine system, it refers to outer layer of adrenal glands; in urinary system, outer layer of kidney, 298, 299***f***, 382, 382***f***

Cortical, pertaining to cortex, 98

Cortical bone, hard exterior surface bone; also called ***compact bone,*** 86, 87***f***

Corticosteroid cream, powerful anti-inflammatory cream, 72

Corticosteroids, general term for group of hormones secreted by adrenal contex; they include mineralocorticoid hormones, glucocorticoid hormones, and steroid sex hormones; used as medication for its strong anti-inflammatory properties, 109, 205, 243, 382, 397

Cortisol, steroid hormone secreted by adrenal cortex; regulates carbohydrate metabolism, 382

Costal, pertaining to ribs, 98

Cowper's glands, also called ***bulbourethral glands;*** these two small male reproductive system glands are located on either side of urethra just distal to prostate; secretion from these glands neutralizes acidity in urethra and vagina, 356

Cystic fibrosis (CF), hereditary condition causing exocrine glands to malfunction; patient produces very thick mucus that causes severe congestion within lungs and digestive system; through more advanced treatment, many children are now living into adulthood with this disease, 235
Cystitis, inflammation of bladder, 301, 310
Cystocele, hernia or outpouching of bladder that protrudes into vagina; may cause urinary frequency and urgency, 310, 344
Cystogram, record of bladder, 311
Cystography, process of instilling contrast material or dye into bladder by catheter to visualize urinary bladder on X-ray, 311
Cystolith, bladder stone, 306
Cystopexy, surgical fixation of bladder, 314
Cystoplasty, surgical repair of bladder, 314
Cystorrhagia, rapid bleeding from bladder, 306
Cystoscope, instrument used to visually examine bladder, 312
Cystoscopy (cysto), visual examination of urinary bladder using instrument called cystoscope, 312
Cystostomy, creation of opening through body wall and into bladder, 314
Cystotomy, incision into bladder, 314
Cytologic testing, examination of cells to determine structure and origin; pap smears are considered a form of cytologic testing, 529
Cytology, study of cells, 24, 39
Cytoplasm, watery internal environment of a cell, 24
Cytotoxic, pertaining to poisoning cells, 197, 198

D

Dacryoadenitis, inflammation of lacrimal gland, 459
Dacryocystitis, inflammation of tear sac, 459
Day surgery, type of outpatient surgery in which patient is discharged on same day he or she is admitted; also called ambulatory surgery, 523
Deafness, inability to hear or having some degree of hearing impairment, 472
Debridement, removal of foreign material and dead or damaged tissue from wound, 71, 516
Decibel (dB), measures intensity or loudness of sound; zero decibels is quietest sound measured and 120 dB is loudest sound commonly measured, 473
Deciduous teeth, 20 teeth that begin to erupt around age of 6 months; eventually pushed out by permanent teeth, 260, 261
Decongestant, substance that reduces nasal congestion and swelling, 243
Decubitus ulcer (decub), bedsore or pressure sore caused by pressure over bony prominences on body; caused by lack of blood flow, 65
Deep, directional term meaning away from surface of body, 37***t***
Deep tendon reflex (DTR), muscle contraction in response to stretch caused by striking muscle tendon with reflex hammer; test used to determine if muscles are responding properly, 122
Defecation, evacuation of feces from rectum, 263
Defibrillation, procedure that converts serious irregular heartbeats, such as fibrillation, by giving electric shocks to heart, 161, 161***f***
Delirium, state of mental confusion with lack of orientation to time and place, 423
Delivery, emergence of baby from birth canal, 338, 338***f***
Delusion, false belief held with conviction even in face of strong evidence to contrary, 503
Dementia, progressive impairment of intellectual function that interferes with performing activities of daily living; patients have little awareness of their condition; found in disorders such as Alzheimer's, 423, 501
Dendrite, branched process off a neuron that receives impulses and carries them to cell body, 412, 413***f***
Dental, pertaining to teeth 267
Dental caries, gradual decay and disintegration of teeth caused by bacteria that can result in inflamed tissue and abscessed teeth; commonly called a ***tooth cavity***, 270
Dentalgia, tooth pain, 269
Dentin, main bulk of tooth; is covered by enamel, 260, 261, 261***f***
Dentist, practitioner of dentistry, 268
Dentistry, branch of healthcare involved with prevention, diagnosis, and treatment of conditions involving teeth, jaw, and mouth; dentistry is practiced by ***dentist*** or ***oral surgeon***, 268
Denture, partial or complete set of artificial teeth that are set in plastic materials; substitute for natural teeth and related structures, 279
Deoxygenated, blood in veins that is low in oxygen content, 140
Depigmentation, loss of normal skin color or pigment, 59
Depression, downward movement, as in dropping shoulders, 88–89, 118***t***
Dermabrasion, abrasion or rubbing using wire brushes or sandpaper, 71
Dermal, pertaining to skin, 57
Dermatitis, inflammation of skin, 65

tract that can cause marked difficulty breathing, 233
Diplopia, double vision, 455
Directional/positional terms, 35, 37***f***
Discharge summary, part of patient's medical record; a comprehensive outline of patient's entire hospital stay; includes condition at time of admission, admitting diagnosis, test results, treatments and patient's response, final diagnosis, and follow-up plans, 12
Dislocation, occurs when bones in joint are displaced from their normal alignment, 105
Disorders diagnosed in infancy and childhood, mental disorders associated with childhood; include mental retardation, attention deficit disorder, and autism, 501
Dissection, surgical cutting of parts for separation and study, 523
Dissociative disorders, disorders in which severe emotional conflict is so repressed that split in personality occurs; include amnesia and multiple personality disorder, 501
Dissociative identity disorder, having two or more distinct personalities, 501
Distal, directional term meaning located farthest from point of attachment to body, 37***f***, 37***t***, 39
Distal convoluted tubule, portion of renal tubule, 299, 300***f***, 302***f***
Diuresis, abnormal secretion of large amounts of urine, 306
Diuretic, substance that increases excretion of urine, which promotes loss of water and salt from body; can assist in lowering blood pressure; therefore, these drugs are used to treat hypertension; potassium in body may be depleted with continued use of diuretics; potassium-rich foods such as bananas, kiwi, and orange juice can help correct deficiency, 164, 315
Diverticulectomy, surgical removal of diverticulum, 280
Diverticulitis, inflammation of diverticulum or sac in intestinal tract, especially in colon, 273, 273***f***
Diverticulosis, abnormal condition of having diverticula (out pouches off gut), 273
Diverticulum, 273, 273***f***
Dopaminergic drugs, group of medications to treat Parkinson's disease by either replacing dopamine that is lacking or increasing strength of dopamine that is present, 433
Doppler ultrasonography, measurement of sound-wave echos as they bounce off tissues and organs to produce image; in cardiovascular system, used to measure velocity of blood moving through blood vessels to look for blood clots, 160, 509
Dorsal, directional term meaning near or on back or spinal cord side of body, 37***f***, 37***t***, 39
Dorsal cavities, 34, 34***f***, 35***t***
Dorsiflexion, backward bending, as of hand or foot, 116***t***, 117***f***
Dorsum, refers to posterior region of back of body, 33, 33***f***
Draping, process of covering patient with sterile cloths that allow only operative site to be exposed to surgeon, 523
Drug, 491
 administration, 494, 494***t***–96***t***
 classification, 492, 492***t***
 names, 491, 491***t***
Drug Enforcement Agency (DEA), government agency that enforces regulation of controlled substances, 492
Drug interaction, occurs when effect of one drug is altered because it was taken at same time as another drug, 497
Drug tolerance, decrease in susceptibility to drug after continued use of drug, 497
Dry gangrene, late stages of gangrene characterized by affected area becoming black and leathery, 65
Dual-energy absorptiometry (DXA), measurement of bone density using low dose X-ray for purpose of detecting osteoporosis, 106
Duchenne's muscular dystrophy, 121
Duodenal, pertaining to duodenum, 267
Duodenum, first section of small intestines; digestion is completed in duodenum after chyme mixes with digestive juices from pancreas and gallbladder, 262, 262***f***, 263***f***, 264***f***, 265***f***, 272***f***, 276***f***
Dura mater, term means tough mother; is fibrous outermost meninges layer that forms a tough protective layer, 417, 417***f***, 430***f***
Dwarfism, condition of being abnormally small; may be result of hereditary condition or endocrine dysfunction, 393
Dyscrasia, general term indicating presence of disease affecting blood, 185
Dysentery, disease characterized by diarrhea, often with mucus and blood, severe abdominal pain, fever, and dehydration, 273
Dyskinesia, difficult or painful movement, 120
Dysmenorrhea, painful cramping associated with menstruation, 342
Dysorexia, abnormal appetite, 269
Dyspepsia, indigestion, 269
Dysphagia, having difficulty eating, 269
Dysphasia, impairment of speech as a result of brain lesion, 423
Dysphonia, abnormal voice, 231
Dyspnea, difficult, labored breathing, 231, 232

E

secondary sexual characteristics, 332, 333, 381***t***, 382
Ethmoid bone, cranial bone, 89, 91***t***
Eupnea, normal breathing, 231
Eustachian tube, tube or canal that connects middle ear with nasopharynx and allows for balance of pressure between outer and middle ear; infection can travel via mucous membranes of eustachian tube, resulting in middle ear infections, 222, 467***f***, 468
Eversion, directional term meaning turning outward, 117***t***, 117***f***
Ewing's sarcoma, malignant growth found in shaft of long bones that spreads through periosteum; removal is treatment of choice, as tumor will metastasize or spread to other organs, 103
Excretory urography (EU), injection of dye into bloodstream followed by taking X-ray to trace action of kidney as it excretes dye, 311
Exfoliative cytology, scraping cells from tissue and then examining them under microscope, 70
Exhalation, to breathe air out of lungs; also called expiration, 220
Exocrine, 380
Exocrine glands, glands that secrete substances into a duct; examples include tears and tear ducts, 380
Exophthalmos, condition in which eyeballs protrude, such as in Graves' disease; generally caused by overproduction of thyroid hormone, 390, 390***f***
Exostosis, bone spur, 103
Exotropia, outward turning of eye; also an example of strabismus (muscle weakness of eye), 450***f***, 459
Expectorant, substance that assists in removal of secretions from bronchopulmonary membranes, 243
Expiration, 220, 226***f***
Expiratory reserve volume (ERV), amount of air that can be forcibly exhaled after normal quiet respiration; also called ***supplemental air***, 225***t***
Exploratory laparotomy, abdominal operation for purpose of examining abdominal organs and tissues for signs of disease or other abnormalities, 280
Exploratory surgery, surgery performed for purpose of determining if there is cancer present or if known cancer has spread; biopsies are generally performed, 529
Explosive disorder, impulse control disorder in which patient is unable to control violent rages, 502
Expulsion stage, stage of labor and delivery during which baby is delivered, 338, 338***f***
Extension, movement that brings limb into or toward a straight condition, 116***t***, 116***f***
Extensor carpi, muscle named for its action, extension, 115
External auditory meatus, opening into external ear canal, 467, 467***f***, 468
External ear, outermost portion of ear; consists of auricle, auditory canal, and eardrum, 466***f***, 467***f***, 467–68, 472
External iliac artery, 148***f***, 315***f***
External iliac vein, 150***f***, 315***f***
External oblique, muscle named for direction of its fibers, on an oblique angle, 115
External respiration, exchange of oxygen and carbon dioxide that takes place in lungs, 220
External sphincter, ring of voluntary muscle that controls emptying of urine from bladder, 300, 301
Extracorporeal circulation (ECC), during open heart surgery, routing of blood to heart-lung machine so it can be oxygenated and pumped to rest of body, 161
Extracorporeal shockwave lithotripsy (ESWL), use of ultrasound waves to break up stones; process does not require surgery, 313***f***
Extraction, removing or pulling teeth, 279
Extraocular, pertaining to being outside eyeball, for example extraocular eye muscles, 454
Eye, 31***t***, 447***f***, 448***f***
  abbreviations, 464
  anatomical terms, 454
  anatomy and physiology, 448–52
  conjunctiva, 451
  diagnostic procedures, 460–61
  eyeball, 448–49
  eyelids, 448, 448***f***, 451, 459
  lacrimal apparatus, 451, 451***f***
  muscles, 450, 450***f***
  pathology, 455–59
  pharmacology, 463
  retina, 449, 449***f***, 452***f***
  terminology, 453–61
  therapeutic procedures, 462–63
  vision, 452, 452***f***
Eye muscles, there are six muscles that connect eyeball to orbit cavity; muscles allow for rotation of eyeball, 450
Eyeball, eye by itself, without any appendages such as eye muscles or tear ducts, 448–49
Eyedrops, substance placed into eye to control eye pressure in glaucoma; also used during eye examinations to dilate pupil of eye for better examination of interior of eye, 494, 496

Eyelashes, along upper and lower edges of eyelids; protect eye from foreign particles; also called ***cilia,*** 451

Eyelids, upper and lower fold of skin that provides protection from foreign particles, injury from sun and intense light, and trauma; both upper and lower edges of eyelids have small hairs or cilia; in addition, sebaceous or oil glands are located in eyelids which secrete lubricating oil, 448***f***, 451, 459

F

Facial bones, skull bones that surround mouth, nose, and eyes; muscles for chewing are attached to facial bones, 89, 91***f***, 91***t***

Facial nerve, 418***t***

Factitious disorders, intentionally feigning illness symptoms in order to gain attention such as malingering, 502

Falling test, test used to observe balance and equilibrium; patient is observed balancing on one foot, then with one foot in front of the other, and then walking forward with eyes open; same test is conducted with patient's eyes closed; swaying and falling with eyes closed can indicate ear and equilibrium malfunction, 474

Fallopian tubes, organs in female reproductive system that transport eggs from ovary to uterus, 30***t***, 35***t***, 333, 334***f***

Family and group psychotherapy, form of psychological counseling in which therapist places minimal emphasis on patient past history and strong emphasis on having patient state and discuss goals and then find a way to achieve them, 505

Farsightedness, 457, 457***f***

Fascia, connective tissue that wraps muscles; it tapers at each end of a skeletal muscle to form tendons, 114

Fascial, pertaining to fascia, 119

Fasciitis, inflammation of fascia, 121

Fasciotomy, incision into fascia, 122

Fasting blood sugar (FBS), blood test to measure amount of sugar circulating throughout body after 12-hour fast, 395

Fats, lipid molecules transported throughout body dissolved in blood, 180

Fecal occult blood test (FOBT), laboratory test on feces to determine if microscopic amounts of blood are present; also called ***hemoccult*** or ***stool guaiac,*** 276

Feces, food that cannot be digested becomes waste product and is expelled or defecated as feces, 263

Federal Drug Administration (FDA), 498

Female reproductive system, system responsible for producing eggs for reproduction and provides place for growing baby; organs include ovaries, fallopian tubes, uterus, vagina, and mammary glands, 30***t***, 331***f***, 332***f***
- abbreviations, 351
- anatomical terms, 340–41
- anatomy and physiology, 332–39
- breast, 336, 336***f***
- diagnostic procedures, 347–48
- internal genitalia, 332–35
- pathology, 342–46
- pharmacology, 351
- terminology, 339–48
- therapeutic procedures, 349–50
- vulva, 335–36

Female urethra, 301***f***

Femoral, pertaining to femur or thigh bone, 98

Femoral artery, 148***f***

Femoral vein, 150***f***

Femur, also called ***thigh bone;*** is a lower extremity bone, 85***f***, 88***f***, 92, 93***f***, 94, 95***f***, 95***t***

Fertility drug, medication that triggers ovulation; also called ***ovulation stimulant***, 351

Fertilization, also called ***impregnation;*** fusion of ova and sperm to produce embryo, 332

Fetal, pertaining to fetus, 340

Fetal monitoring, using electronic equipment placed on mother's abdomen to check baby's heart rate and strength during labor, 348

Fetus, term to describe developing newborn from end of eighth week until birth, 336, 337, 337***f***

Fever blisters, 271

Fibrillation, abnormal quivering or contractions of heart fibers; when this occurs within fibers of ventricle of heart, arrest and death can occur; emergency equipment to defibrillate, or convert heart to a normal beat, is necessary, 156

Fibrin, whitish protein formed by action of thrombin and fibrinogen, which is basis for clotting of blood, 182

Fibrinogen, blood protein that is essential for clotting to take place, 180

Fibrinous, pertaining to being fibrous, 184

Fibrocystic breast disease, benign cysts forming in breast, 345, 345***f***

Fibroid tumor, benign tumor or growth that contains fiberlike tissue; uterine fibroid tumors are most common tumors in women, 343, 343***f***

Fibromyalgia, condition with widespread aching and pain in muscles and soft tissue, 121

Fibrous joints, joint that has almost no movement because ends of bones are joined together

by thick fibrous tissue; sutures of skull are example, 95, 96, 96***f***
Fibula, one of the lower leg bones in lower extremity, 85***f,*** 92, 93***f,*** 94, 95***f***, 95***t***
Fibular, pertaining to fibula, a lower leg bone, 98
Fibular vein, 150***f***
Film, thin sheet of cellulose material coated with light-sensitive substance used in taking photographs; there is a special photographic film that is sensitive to X-rays, 507
Film badge, badge containing film that is sensitive to X-rays; is worn by all personnel in radiology to measure amount of X-rays to which they are exposed, 507
Filtration, first stage of urine production during which waste products are filtered from blood, 302, 302***f***
Fimbriae, fingerlike extensions on end of fallopian tubes; drape over each ovary in order to direct ovum into fallopian tube after it is expelled by ovary, 333, 333***f***, 334, 334***f,*** 383***f***
Fine motor skills, use of precise and coordinated movements in such activities as writing, buttoning, and cutting, 515
First-degree burn, 64, 64***f***
Fissure, deep groove or slit-type opening, 59, 59***f,*** 88, 89
Fistulectomy, excision of a fistula, 280
Fixation, procedure to stabilize fractured bone while it heals; ***external fixation*** includes casts, splints, and pins inserted through skin; ***internal fixation*** includes pins, plates, rods, screws, and wires that are applied during an ***open reduction***, 109
Flat bone, type of bone with thin flattened shape; examples include scapula, ribs, and pelvic bones, 86, 87***f***
Flexion, act of bending or being bent, 116***t***, 116***f***
Flexor carpi, muscle named for its action, flexion, 115
Floating kidney, 309
Fluorescein angiography, process of injecting dye (fluorescein) to observe movement of blood for detecting lesions in macular area of retina; used to determine if there is detachment of retina, 460
Fluorescein staining, applying dye eyedrops that are bright green fluorescent color; used to look for corneal abrasions or ulcers, 460
Fluoroscopy, x-rays strike glowing screen which can change from minute to minute, therefore able to show movement such as digestive tract moving, 509
Flutter, arrhythmia in which atria beat too rapidly, but in regular pattern, 156
Focal seizure, localized epileptic seizure often affecting one limb, 423
Follicle-stimulating hormone (FSH), hormone secreted by anterior pituitary gland; stimulates growth of eggs in females and sperm in males, 381***t***, 384, 385
Foramen, passage or opening through bone for nerves and blood vessels, 88, 89
Forceps, surgical instrument used to grasp tissues, 521***t***
Formed elements, solid, cellular portion of blood; consists of erythrocytes, leukocytes, and platelets, 180
Fossa, shallow cavity or depression within or on surface of a bone, 88, 89
Fovea capitis, 88***f***
Fovea centralis, area of retina that has sharpest vision, 448***f***, 449
Fowler position, surgical position in which patient is sitting with back positioned at 45° angle, 522***f,*** 523***t***
Fracture (FX, Fx), injury to bone that causes it to break; named to describe type of damage to bone, 100–02
Fraternal twins, twins that develop from two different ova fertilized by two different sperm; although twins, these siblings do not have identical DNA, 341
Free edge, exposed edge of a nail that is trimmed when nails become too long, 55, 55***f***
Frequency, greater than normal occurrence in urge to urinate, without increase in total daily volume of urine; frequency is indication of inflammation of bladder or urethra, 306
Frontal bone, forehead bone of skull, 89, 91***f***, 91***t***
Frontal lobe, one of four cerebral hemisphere lobes; controls motor functions, 414, 415, 415***f***
Frontal plane, vertical plane that divides body into front (anterior or ventral) and back (posterior or dorsal) sections; also called ***coronal plane,*** 32, 32***f,*** 33
Frontal section, sectional view of body produced by cut along frontal plane; also called ***coronal section,*** 32, 33
Frozen section (FS), thin piece of tissue is cut from frozen specimen for rapid examination under a microscope, 70
Full-term pregnancy, 337***f***
Functional bowel syndrome, 274
Functional residual capacity (FRC), air that remains in lungs after normal exhalation has taken place, 225***t***
Fundus, domed upper portion of organ such as stomach or uterus, 262, 262***f***
Fundus (uterus), 332***f,*** 334, 334***f,*** 337***f***
Fungal scrapings, scrapings, taken with curette or scraper, of tissue from lesions are placed on a growth medium and examined under a microscope to identify fungal growth, 70

Fungi, organisms found in Kingdom Fungi; some are capable of causing disease in humans, such as yeast infections or histoplasmosis, 196, 197

Funny bone, 88

Furuncle, staphylococcal skin abscess with redness, pain, and swelling; also called a ***boil,*** 69

G

Gait, manner of walking, 515

Gait training, assisting person to learn to walk again or how to use assistive device to walk, 516

Gallbladder (GB), small organ located just under liver; functions to store bile produced by liver; gallbladder releases bile into duodenum through common bile duct, 29***t***, 35***t***, 36***t***, 257***f***, 258, 265, 265***f***, 276***f***

Gametes, reproductive sex cells—ova and sperm, 382

Gamma globulin, protein component of blood containing antibodies that help to resist infection, 180

Ganglion, knotlike mass of nerve tissue located outside brain and spinal cord, 418

Ganglion cyst, cyst that forms on tendon sheath, usually on hand, wrist, or ankle, 121

Gangrene, necrosis of skin usually due to deficient blood supply, 65

Gastralgia, stomach pain, 269

Gastrectomy, surgical removal of stomach, 280

Gastric, pertaining to stomach, 267

Gastric carcinoma, cancerous tumor of stomach, 271

Gastric stapling, procedure that closes off large section of stomach with rows of staples; results in a much smaller stomach to assist very obese patients to lose weight, 280

Gastritis, inflammation of stomach that can result in pain, tenderness, nausea, and vomiting, 271

Gastroenteritis, inflammation of stomach and small intestines, 3, 271

Gastroenterologist, physician specialized in treating diseases and conditions of gastrointestinal tract, 268

Gastroenterology, branch of medicine specializing in conditions of gastrointestinal system, 29***t***, 40, 268

Gastroesophageal reflux disease (GERD), acid from stomach backs up into esophagus, causing inflammation and pain, 271

Gastrointestinal (GI), 29***t***

Gastrointestinal system (GI), system that digests food and absorbs nutrients; organs include mouth, pharynx, esophagus, stomach, small and large intestines, liver, gallbladder, and anus; also called digestive system, 258

Gastrointestinal tract, continuous tube that extends from mouth to anus; also called ***gut*** or ***alimentary canal,*** 258

Gastroscope, instrument to view inside stomach, 278

Gastroscopy, flexible gastroscope is passed through mouth and down esophagus in order to visualize inside stomach; used to diagnose peptic ulcers and gastric carcinoma, 278

Gastrostomy, surgical creation of gastric fistula or opening through abdominal wall; opening is used to place food into stomach when esophagus is not entirely open (esophageal stricture), 280

Gavage, using nasogastric tube to place liquid nourishment directly into stomach, 279

General anesthesia (GA), general anesthesia produces a loss of consciousness including absence of pain sensation; administered to patient by either intravenous or inhalation method; patient's vital signs are carefully monitored when using general anesthetic, 520, 521***t***

General hospital, hospitals that typically provide services to diagnose (laboratory, diagnostic imaging) and treat (surgery, medications, therapy) diseases for a short period of time; in addition, they usually provide emergency and obstetrical care; also called ***acute care hospital,*** 13

Generic name, recognized and accepted official name for a drug; each drug has only one generic name; this name is not subject to trademark, so any pharmaceutical manufacturer may use it; also called ***nonproprietary name,*** 491, 491***t***

Genital herpes, creeping skin disease that can appear like a blister or vesicle, caused by sexually transmitted virus, 359

Genital warts, growths and elevations of warts on genitalia of both males and females that can lead to cancer of cervix in females, 360

Genitalia, male and female reproductive organs, 332

Genitourinary system (GU), organs of the urinary system and female or male sexual organs, 298, 354

Gestation, length of time from conception to birth, generally nine months; calculated from first day of last menstrual period, with a range of from 259 days to 280 days, 336, 337

Gigantism, excessive development of body due to overproduction of growth hormone by pituitary gland; opposite of dwarfism, 394

Gingiva, tissue around teeth; also called ***gums,*** 258, 259***f***, 260, 261***f***
Gingival, pertaining to gums, 267
Gingivitis, inflammation of gums characterized by swelling, redness, and tendency to bleed, 270
Glands, organs of body that release secretions; exocrine glands, like sweat glands, release their secretions into ducts; endocrine glands, such as thyroid gland, release their hormones directly into blood stream, 380, 412
adrenal, 30***t***
apocrine, 56
bulbourethral, 354, 356
lymph, 194
parathyroid, 30***t***
pineal, 30***t***, 380, 384, 384***f***
pituitary, 30***t***, 380, 384–85, 385***f***, 393–94, 414***f***
prostate, 30***t***, 36***t***, 301***f***, 354, 354***f***, 356, 358–59
salivary, 29***t***, 257***f***, 258, 264, 264***f***
sebaceous, 27***t***, 52, 55, 55***f***
sudoriferous, 56
sweat, 27***t***, 52, 56
thymus, 28***t***, 30***t***, 35***t***, 193, 196, 196***f***, 379***f***, 380, 381***t***, 387, 387***f***, 394
thyroid, 30***t***, 221***f***, 379***f***, 380, 381***t***, 387–88, 388***f***, 394–95
Glans penis, larger and softer tip of penis; is protected by covering called prepuce or foreskin, 354***f***, 355
Glaucoma, increase in intraocular pressure that, if untreated, may result in atrophy (wasting away) of optic nerve and blindness; treated with medication and surger; there is increased risk of developing glaucoma in persons over 60 years of age, people of African ancestry, persons who have sustained serious eye injury, and anyone with family history of diabetes or glaucoma, 456
Globulins, one type of protein found dissolved in plasma, 180
Glomerular, 300***f***
Glomerular capsule, also called Bowman's capsule; part of renal corpuscle; is a double-walled cuplike structure that encircles glomerulus; in filtration stage of urine production, waste products filtered from blood enter Bowman's capsule as glomerular filtrate, 299, 300***f***, 302***f***
Glomerular filtrate, product of filtration stage of urine production; water, electrolytes, nutrients, wastes, and toxins that are filtered from blood passing through glomerulus; filtrate enters Bowman's capsule, 302
Glomerulonephritis, inflammation of kidney (primarily of glomerulus); since glomerular membrane is inflamed, it becomes more permeable and will allow protein and blood cells to enter filtrate; results in protein in urine (proteinuria) and hematuria, 308
Glomerulus, ball of capillaries encased by Bowman's capsule; in filtration stage of urine production, wastes filtered from blood leave glomerulus capillaries and enter Bowman's capsule, 299, 300***f***, 302***f***
Glossal, pertaining to tongue, 267
Glossopharyngeal nerve, 418***t***
Glottis, opening between vocal cords; air passes through glottis as it moves through larynx; changing tension of vocal cords changes size of opening, 222
Glucagon, hormone secreted by pancreas; stimulates liver to release glucose into blood, 359***t***, 361
Glucocorticoids, group of hormones secreted by adrenal cortex; regulate carbohydrate levels in body; cortisol is an example, 380***t***, 382
Glucose, form of sugar used by cells of body to make energy; transported to cells in blood, 180
Glucose tolerance test (GTT), test to determine blood sugar level; a measured dose of glucose is given to patient either orally or intravenously; blood samples are then drawn at certain intervals to determine ability of patient to utilize glucose; used for diabetic patients to determine their insulin response to glucose, 395
Glutamic oxaloacetic transaminase (GOT), 159
Gluteal, pertaining to buttocks, 40
Gluteal region, refers to buttock region of body, 33, 33***f***
Gluteus maximus, muscle named for its size and location; gluteus means ***rump area*** and maximus means ***large,*** 115
Glycosuria, presence of an excess of sugar in urine, 306, 390
Goiter, enlargement of thyroid gland, 394, 394***f***
Gonadotropins, common name for follicle-stimulating hormone and luteinizing hormone, 381***t***, 384, 385
Gonads, organs responsible for producing sex cells; female gonads are ovaries, and they produce ova; male gonads are testes, and they produce sperm, 382
Gonorrhea, sexually transmitted inflammation of mucous membranes of either sex; can be passed on to infant during birth process, 360
Grade, tumor can be graded from grade I through grade IV; grade is based on microscopic appearance of tumor cells; grade

H

occurs in mitral valve, but may affect any of heart valves, 156

Heart valve stenosis, cusps or flaps of heart valve are too stiff; therefore, they are unable to open fully, making it difficult for blood to flow through, or to shut tightly, allowing blood to flow backwards; condition may affect any of heart valves, 156

Heartburn, 270

Heimlich maneuver, technique for removing foreign body or food from trachea or pharynx when it is choking a person; maneuver consists of applying pressure just under diaphragm to pop obstruction out, 242

Hematemesis, to vomit blood from gastrointestinal tract, often looks like coffee grounds, 269

Hematic, pertaining to blood, 40, 184

Hematic system, system that consists of plasma and blood cells—erythrocytes, leukocytes, and platelets; responsible for transporting oxygen, protecting against pathogens, and controlling bleeding, 28***t***

Hematinic, substance that increases number of erythrocytes or amount of hemoglobin in blood, 190

Hematochezia, passing bright red blood in stools, 269

Hematocrit (Hct, Hct, crit), blood test to measure volume of red blood cells (erythrocytes) within total volume of blood, 188

Hematologist, physician who specializes in treating diseases and conditions of blood, 184

Hematology, branch of medicine specializing in conditions of hematic system, 28***t,*** 40, 184

Hematoma, swelling or mass of blood caused by break in vessel in organ or tissue, or beneath skin, 185

Hematopoiesis, process of forming blood, 180

Hematosalpinx, condition of having blood in fallopian tubes, 342

Hematuria, condition of blood in urine, 306

Hemianopia, loss of vision in half of visual field; stroke patient may suffer from this disorder, 459

Hemiparesis, weakness or loss of motion on one side of body, 423

Hemiplegia, paralysis on only one side of body, 423

Hemoccult, 276

Hemodialysis (HD), use of artificial kidney machine that filters blood of a person to remove waste products; use of this technique in patients who have defective kidneys is lifesaving, 313, 313***f***

Hemoglobin (Hgb, Hb, HGB), iron-containing pigment of red blood cells that carries oxygen from lungs to tissue, 180, 188

Hemolytic anemia, anemia that develops as result of excessive loss of erythrocytes, 186

Hemolytic disease of the newborn (HDN), condition in which antibodies in mother's blood enter fetus's blood and cause anemia, jaundice, edema, and enlargement of liver and spleen; also called ***erythroblastosis fetalis,*** 345

Hemolytic reaction, destruction of patient's erythrocytes that occurs when receiving transfusion of incompatible blood type; also called a ***transfusion reaction***, 186

Hemophilia, hereditary blood disease in which there is a prolonged blood clotting time; is transmitted by sex-linked trait from females to males; appears almost exclusively in males, 185

Hemoptysis, coughing up blood or blood-stained sputum, 231

Hemorrhage, blood flow, escape of blood from a blood vessel, 185

Hemorrhoid, varicose veins in rectum, 158, 273

Hemorrhoidectomy, surgical excision of hemorrhoids from anorectal area, 280

Hemostasis, to stop bleeding or stagnation of circulating blood, 182, 524

Hemostat, surgical instrument used to grasp blood vessels to control bleeding, 521***t***

Hemostatic agent, 189

Hemothorax, condition of having blood in chest cavity, 231

Hepatic, pertaining to liver, 268

Hepatic duct, duct that leads from liver to common bile duct; transports bile, 265, 265***f,*** 276***f***

Hepatic portal vein, 150***f***

Hepatitis, infectious, inflammatory disease of liver; hepatitis B and C types are spread by contact with blood and bodily fluids of infected person, 276

Hepatoma, liver tumor, 276

Herniated nucleus pulposus (HNP), rupture of fibrocartilage disk between two vertebrae; results in pressure on spinal nerve and causes pain, weakness, and nerve damage; also called a slipped disk, 104, 104***f***

Hernioplasty, surgical repair of a hernia; also called herniorrhaphy, 280

Herniorrhaphy, 280

Herpes labialis, infection of lip by herpes simplex virus type 1 (HSV-1); also called ***fever blisters*** or ***cold sores***, 271

Herpes zoster virus, 429

Hertz (Hz), measurement of frequency or pitch of sound; lowest pitch on audiogram is 250 Hz; measurement can go as high as 8000 Hz, which is highest pitch measured, 474

Hesitancy, decrease in force of urine stream, often with difficulty initiating flow; often a symptom of blockage along urethra, such as enlarged prostate gland, 307

Heterograft, skin graft from animal of another species (usually a pig) to a human; also called a ***xenograft,*** 71
Hiatal hernia, protrusion of stomach through diaphragm and extending into thoracic cavity; gastroesophageal reflux disease is a common symptom, 271, 271***f***
Hilum, controlled entry/exit point of an organ such as kidney or lung, 224, 298, 299***f***
Hipbone, 93***f***
Hirsutism, excessive hair growth over body, 59, 390
Histology, study of tissues, 25, 40
Histoplasma capsulatum, 235
Histoplasmosis, pulmonary disease caused by fungus found in dust in droppings of pigeons and chickens, 235
History and physical, medical record document written by admitting physician; details patient's history, results of physician's examination, initial diagnoses, and physician's plan of treatment, 11
Hives, appearance of wheals as part of allergic reaction, 62, 200
Hodgkin's disease (HD), also called Hodgkin's lymphoma; cancer of lymphatic cells found in concentration in lymph nodes, 201
Hodgkin's lymphoma, 201, 202***f***
Holter monitor, portable ECG monitor worn by patient for a period of a few hours to a few days to assess heart and pulse activity as person goes through activities of daily living, 160
Home health care, agencies that provide nursing, therapy, personal care, or housekeeping services in patient's own home, 13
Homeostasis, steady state or state of balance within body; kidneys assist in maintaining this regulatory, steady state, 301, 380
Homologous transfusion, replacement of blood by transfusion of blood received from another person, 189
Hordeolum, a ***stye*** (or sty), a small purulent inflammatory infection of a sebaceous gland of eye, treated with hot compresses and surgical incision, 459
Horizontal plane, horizontal plane that divides body into upper (superior) and lower (inferior) sections; also called ***transverse plane,*** 32, 33
Hormonal contraception, use of hormones to block ovulation and prevent contraception; may be in pill form, patch or implant under skin, or injection, 349
Hormone, chemical substance secreted by endocrine gland; enters blood stream and is carried to target tissue; hormones work to control functioning of target tissue; given to replace loss of natural hormones or to treat disease by stimulating hormonal effects, 380
Hormone replacement therapy (HRT), artificial replacement of hormones in patient who is unable to produce sufficient hormones; example is estrogen replacement in menopausal women, 351, 396
Hormone therapy, treatment of cancer with natural hormones or with chemicals that produce hormonelike effects, 529
Hospice, organized group of healthcare workers who provide supportive treatment to dying patients and their families, 13
Human growth hormone therapy, therapy with human growth hormone in order to stimulate skeletal growth; used to treat children with abnormally short stature, 397
Human immunodeficiency virus (HIV), virus that causes AIDS; also known as a retrovirus, 202, 202***f,*** 360
Human papilloma virus (HPV), 343
Humanistic psychotherapy, form of psychological counseling in which therapist does not delve into patients' past; it is believed that patients can learn how to use their own internal resources to deal with their problems, 505
Humeral, pertaining to humerus or upper arm bone, 98
Humerus, upper arm bone in upper extremity, 85***f***, 87***f***, 92, 93***f,*** 94, 94***f***, 94***t***
Humoral immunity, immunity that responds to antigens, such as bacteria and foreign agents, by producing antibodies; also called ***antibody-mediated immunity,*** 197
Humpback, 104
Hunchback, 104
Hyaline membrane disease (HMD), 235
Hydrocele, accumulation of fluid within testes, 358
Hydrocephalus, accumulation of cerebrospinal fluid within ventricles of brain, causing head to be enlarged; treated by creating artificial shunt for fluid to leave brain, 426, 426***f***
Hydrochloric acid (HCl), acid secreted by stomach lining; aids in digestion, 262
Hydronephrosis, distention of pelvis due to urine collecting in kidney resulting from obstruction, 308
Hydrotherapy, using water for treatment purposes, 517
Hymen, thin membranous tissue that covers external vaginal opening or orifice; membrane is broken during first sexual encounter of female; can also be broken prematurely by

use of tampons or during some sports activities, 335

Hymenectomy, surgical removal of hymen; performed when hymen tissue is particularly tough, 350

Hyoid bone, single, U-shaped bone suspended in neck between mandible and larynx; a point of attachment for swallowing and speech muscles, 89, 221***f***

Hypercalcemia, condition of having excessive amount of calcium in blood, 390

Hypercapnia, excessive carbon dioxide, 231

Hyperemesis, excessive vomiting, 270

Hyperemia, redness of skin caused by increased blood flow to skin, 59

Hyperesthesia, having excessive sensation, 423

Hyperglycemia, having excessive amount of glucose (sugar) in blood, 390

Hyperhidrosis, abnormal condition of excessive sweat, 59

Hyperkalemia, condition of having excessive amount of potassium in blood, 391

Hyperkinesia, excessive amount of movement, 120

Hyperlipidemia, condition of having too high a level of lipids such as cholesterol in bloodstream; risk factor for developing atherosclerosis and coronary artery disease, 185

Hyperopia, with this condition a person can see things in the distance but has trouble reading material at close vision; also known as ***farsightedness,*** 457, 457f

Hyperparathyroidism, state of excessive thyroid, 393

Hyperpigmentation, abnormal amount of pigmentation in skin, which is seen in diseases such as acromegaly and adrenal insufficiency, 59

Hyperpituitarism, state of excessive pituitary gland, 394

Hyperplasia, excessive development of normal cells within an organ, 527

Hyperpnea, excessive deep breathing, 231

Hypersecretion, excessive hormone production by endocrine gland, 391

Hypertension (HTN), high blood pressure, 158

Hyperthyroidism, condition resulting from overactivity of thyroid gland that can result in a crisis situation; also called ***Graves' disease,*** 394, 395

Hypertonia, excessive tone, 120

Hypertrophy, increase in bulk or size of a tissue or structure, 120

Hyperventilation, to breathe both fast (tachypnea) and deep (hyperpnea), 231

Hypnotic, substance used to produce sleep or hypnosis, 433

Hypocalcemia, condition of having a low calcium level in blood, 391

Hypochondria, somatoform disorder involving a preoccupation with health concerns, 503

Hypochondriac, term meaning ***pertaining to under the cartilage***, 36***t***, 40

Hypochromic anemia, anemia resulting from having insufficient hemoglobin in erythrocytes; named because hemoglobin molecule is responsible for dark red color of erythrocytes, 186

Hypodermic, pertaining to under skin, 9, 57

Hypodermis, deepest layer of skin; composed primarily of adipose, 54

Hypogastric, pertaining to below stomach; anatomical division of abdomen, middle section of bottom row, 36***t***

Hypogastric region, 36***t***

Hypoglossal, pertaining to under tongue, 268

Hypoglossal nerve, 418***t***

Hypoglycemia, condition of having low sugar level in blood, 391

Hypokinesia, insufficient movement, 120

Hyponatremia, condition of having low sodium level in blood, 391

Hypoparathyroidism, state of insufficient thyroid, 393

Hypopituitarism, state of insufficient pituitary gland, 394

Hypopnea, insufficient or shallow breathing, 231

Hyposecretion, deficient hormone production by an endocrine gland, 391

Hypospadias, congenital opening of male urethra on underside of penis, 359

Hypotension, low blood pressure, 158

Hypothalamus, portion of diencephalon that lies just below thalamus; controls body temperature, appetite, sleep, sexual desire, and emotions such as fear; also regulates release of hormones from pituitary gland and regulates parasympathetic and sympathetic nervous systems, 384, 385, 385***f***, 414, 414***f***, 415

Hypothyroidism, result of deficiency in secretion by thyroid gland; results in lowered basal metabolism rate with obesity, dry skin, slow pulse, low blood pressure, sluggishness, and goiter; treatment is replacement with synthetic thyroid hormone, 395

Hypotonia, insufficient tone, 120

Hypoventilation, to breathe both slow (bradypnea) and shallow (hypopnea), 231

Hypoxemia, deficiency of oxygen in blood, 231

Hypoxia, absence of oxygen in tissues, 231

Hysterectomy, removal of uterus, 350

Hysteropexy, surgical fixation of uterus, 350

Hysterorrhexis, rupture of uterus, 344

Hysterosalpingography (HSG), process of taking X-ray of uterus and oviducts after radiopaque material is injected into organs, 347

I

Iatrogenic, usually unfavorable response that results from taking medication, 497
Ichthyoderma, dry and scaly skin condition, 59
Ichthyosis, condition in which skin becomes dry, scaly, and keratinized, 65
Identical twins, twins that develop from splitting of one fertilized ovum; these siblings have identical DNA, 341
Idiosyncrasy, unusual or abnormal response to drug or food, 497
Ileal, pertaining to ileum, 268
Ileocecal valve, sphincter between ileum and cecum, 262, 263, 264***f***
Ileostomy, surgical creation of passage through abdominal wall into ileum, 280, 280***f***
Ileum, third portion of small intestines; joins colon at cecum; ileum and cecum are separated by ileocecal valve, 10, 262–63, 263***f***
Ileus, severe abdominal pain, inability to pass stools, vomiting, and abdominal distention as a result of intestinal blockage; may require surgery to reverse blockage, 273
Iliac, pertaining to ilium; one of pelvic bones, 98
Ilium, one of three bones that form the os coxae or innominate bone of the pelvis, 10, 5***f,*** 92, 94, 95***f,*** 95***t***
Immune response, ability of lymphocytes to respond to specific antigens, 196, 197–98
Immunity, body's ability to defend itself against pathogens, 196–98
  immune response, 196, 197–98
  standard precautions, 198
Immunization, providing protection against communicable diseases by stimulating immune system to produce antibodies against that disease; children can now be immunized for: hepatitis B, diphtheria, tetanus, pertussis, tetanus, ***Haemophilus influenzae*** type b, polio, measles, mumps, rubella, and chickenpox; also called ***vaccination,*** 196, 197, 204
Immunocompromised, having immune system unable to respond properly to pathogens, 203
Immunodeficiency disorder, 203
Immunoglobulins (Ig), antibodies secreted by B cells; all antibodies are immunoglobulins; assist in protecting body and its surfaces from invasion of bacteria; for example, immunoglobulin IgA in colostrum, first milk from mother, helps to protect newborn from infection, 199
Immunologist, physician who specializes in treating infectious diseases and other disorders of immune system, 200
Immunology, branch of medicine specializing in conditions of lymphatic and immune systems, 28***t,*** 200
Immunosuppressants, substances that block certain actions of immune system; required to prevent rejection of transplanted organ, 205
Immunotherapy, production or strengthening of patient's immune system in order to treat disease, 204, 529
Impacted fracture, fracture in which bone fragments are pushed into each other, 102
Impetigo, highly contagious staphylococcal skin infection, most commonly occurring on faces of children; begins as blisters that then rupture and dry into thick, yellow crust, 66, 66***f***
Implant, prosthetic device placed in jaw to which a tooth or denture may be anchored, 279
Implantable cardiovert-defibrillator, device implanted in heart that delivers electrical shock to restore normal heart rhythm; particularly useful for persons who experience ventricular fibrillation, 161
Impulse control disorders, inability to resist impulse to perform some act harmful to individual or others; includes kleptomania, pyromania, explosive disorder, and pathological gambling, 502
Incision and drainage (I&D), making incision to create opening for drainage of material such as pus, 71
Incisors, biting teeth in very front of mouth that function to cut food into smaller pieces; humans have eight incisors, 259***f,*** 260, 260***f***
Incus, one of three ossicles of middle ea; also called ***anvil,*** 467***f,*** 468, 468***f***
Infant respiratory distress syndrome (IRDS), lung condition most commonly found in premature infants characterized by tachypnea and respiratory grunting; also called ***hyaline membrane disease*** (HMD) and ***respiratory distress syndrome of the newborn,*** 235
Infarct, area of tissue within organ that undergoes necrosis (death) following loss of blood supply, 153
Inferior, directional term meaning toward feet or tail, or below, 34***f,*** 37***t***
Inferior vena cava, branch of vena cava that drains blood from abdomen and lower body, 142***f,*** 144, 145***f,*** 150***f,*** 157***f,*** 382***f***
Infertility, inability to produce children; generally defined as no pregnancy after properly timed intercourse for one year, 346
Inflammation, tissue response to injury from pathogens or physical agents; characterized by redness, pain, swelling, and feeling hot to touch, 200, 200***f***
Inflammatory bowel disease (IBD), 275

J

K

L

Medial, directional term meaning to middle or near middle of body or structure, 37***f,*** 37***t***
Median cubital vein, 150***f***
Median nerve, 419***f***
Median plane, when sagittal plane passes through middle of body, dividing it into equal right and left halves; also called ***midsagittal plane,*** 30, 32
Mediastinal, collection of lymph nodes located in mediastinum (central chest area) that drain chest, 194***t,*** 195***f***
Mediastinum, central region of chest cavity; contains organs between lungs, including heart, aorta, esophagus, and trachea, 34, 35***t,*** 141***f,*** 224, 225***f***
Medical record, documents details of patient's hospital stay; each health care professional that has contact with patient in any capacity completes appropriate report of that contact and adds it to medical chart; this results in permanent physical record of patient's day-to-day condition, when and what services received, and response to treatment; also called a chart, 11–12
Medical terms, interpreting, 9–10
  pronunciation, 9–10
  spelling, 10
Medication, 491
Medulla, central area of an organ; in endocrine system refers to adrenal medulla; in urinary system, refers to inner portion of kidney, 298, 299***f,*** 415***f***
Medulla oblongata, portion of brain stem that connects spinal cord with brain; contains respiratory, cardiac, and blood pressure control centers, 414, 414***f,*** 415
Medullary, pertaining to medulla of organ like kidney or to medullla oblongata, 99
Medullary cavity, large open cavity that extends length of shaft of long bone; contains yellow bone marrow, 86, 87
Melanin, black color pigment in skin; helps to prevent sun's ultraviolet rays from entering body, 53, 54
Melanocyte-stimulating hormone (MSH), hormone secreted by anterior pituitary; stimulates pigment production in skin, 381***t,*** 385
Melanocytes, special cells in basal layer of epidermis; they contain black pigment melanin that gives skin its color and protects against ultraviolet rays of sun, 53
Melanoma, also called ***malignant melanoma;*** dangerous form of skin cancer caused by overgrowth of melanin in melanocyte; may metastasize or spread; exposure to ultraviolet light is a risk factor for developing melanoma, 66, 66***f***
Melatonin, hormone secreted by pineal gland; plays a role in regulating body's circadian rhythm, 384
Melena, passage of dark tarry stools; color is result of digestive enzymes working on blood in stool, 270
Menarche, first menstrual period, 334, 335
Ménière's disease, abnormal condition within labyrinth of inner ear that can lead to progressive loss of hearing; symptoms are dizziness or vertigo, hearing loss, and tinnitus (ringing in ears), 473
Meningeal, pertaining to meninges, 421
Meninges, three connective tissue membrane layers that surround brain and spinal cord; three layers are dura mater, arachnoid layer, and pia mater; dura mater and arachnoid layer are separated by subdural space; arachnoid layer and pia mater are separated by subarachnoid space, 413, 417, 417***f,*** 429
Meningioma, slow-growing tumor in meninges of brain, 429
Meningitis, inflammation of membranes of spinal cord and brain caused by microorganism, 429
Meningocele, congenital hernia in which meninges, or membranes, protrude through opening in spinal column or brain, 427, 428***f***
Menometrorrhagia, excessive bleeding during menstrual period and at intervals between menstrual periods, 344
Menopause, cessation or ending of menstrual activity; generally between ages of 40 and 55, 334, 335
Menorrhagia, excessive bleeding during menstrual period; can be either in total number of days or amount of blood or both, 342
Menstrual cycle, 28-day fertility cycle in women; includes ovulation and sloughing off endometrium if pregnancy does not occur, 382
Menstrual period, another name for menstrual cycle, 334, 335
Menstruation, loss of blood and tissue as endometrium is shed by uterus; flow exits body through cervix and vagina; flow occurs approximately every 28 days, 334, 335
Mental health, 499–05
  abbreviations, 505
  disciplines, 500
  pathology, 500–04
  psychiatry, 500
  psychology, 500
  therapeutic procedures, 504–05
Mental retardation, disorder characterized by diminished ability to process intellectual functions, 501
Metacarpal, pertaining to hand bones, 99
Metacarpals, hand bones in upper extremity, 92, 93***f,*** 94, 94***t***

Metastacized, 194
Metastases (mets), spreading of cancerous tumor from original site to different locations of body; singular is metastasis, 526, 526***f***
Metastasis (mets), movement and spread of cancer cells from one part of body to another; metastases is plural, 528, 528***f***
Metastasize, when cancerous cells migrate away from tumor site; commonly move through lymphatic system and become trapped in lymph nodes, 194
Metatarsal, pertaining to foot bones, 99
Metatarsals, ankle bones in lower extremity, 92, 93***f,*** 94, 95***f,*** 95***t***
Metered dose inhaler (MDI), 240
Metrorrhagia, rapid (menstrual) blood flow from uterus, 342
Metrorrhea, discharge from uterus, 342
Microtia, abnormally small ears, 471
Micturition, another term for urination, 300
Midbrain, portion of brain stem, 385***f,*** 414, 414***f,*** 415–416
Middle ear, middle section of ear; contains ossicles, 466***f,*** 467, 467***f,*** 468, 469***f,*** 472
Middle ear infection, 472
Midline organs, 36***t***
Midsagittal plane, when sagittal plane passes through middle of body, dividing it into equal right and left halves, also called ***median plane***, 32
Migraine, specific type of headache characterized by severe head pain, photophobia, vertigo, and nausea, 427
Miner's lung, 234
Mineralocorticoids, group of hormones secreted by adrenal cortex; regulate electrolytes and fluid volume in body; aldosterone is an example, 380***t,*** 382
Minnesota Multiphasic Personality Inventory (MMPI), 505
Minor tranquilizers, medications that are central nervous system depressants and are prescribed for anxiety, 504
Miotic drops, substance that causes pupil to constrict, 463
Miscarriage, 346
Mitral valve, valve between left atrium and ventricle in heart; prevents blood from flowing backwards into atrium; also called bicuspid valve because it has two cusps or flaps, 142***f,*** 143, 144***f***
Mobility, state of having normal movement of all body parts, 515
Mobilization, treatments such as exercise and massage to restore movement to joints and soft tissue, 517
Moist hot packs, applying moist warmth to body part to produce slight dilation of blood vessels in skin; causes muscle relaxation in deeper regions of body and increases circulation, which aids healing, 517
Molars, large somewhat flat-topped back teeth; function to grind food; humans have up to twelve molars, 260***f,*** 261
Monoaural, referring to one ear, 471
Monochromatism, unable to perceive one color, 457
Monocytes (monos), agranulocyte white blood cell important for phagocytosis, 181***t***
Mononucleosis (Mono), acute infectious disease with large number of atypical lymphocytes; caused by Epstein–Barr virus; there may be abnormal liver function, 202
Monoparesis, weakness of one extremity, 423
Monoplegia, paralysis of one extremity, 423
Monospot, test of infectious mononucleosis in which there is nonspecific antibody called heterophile antibody, 204
Mood disorders, characterized by instability in mood; includes major depression, mania, and bipolar disorder, 502
Morbid obesity, 270
Morbidity, number that represents number of sick persons in particular population, 528
Mortality, number that represents number of deaths in particular population, 528
Motor neurons, nerves that carry activity instruction from CNS to muscles or glands out in body; also called ***efferent neurons,*** 114, 418, 419***f***
Mucolytic, substance that liquefies mucus so it is easier to cough and clear it from respiratory tract, 243
Mucous membrane, membrane that lines body passages that open directly to exterior of body, such as mouth and reproductive tract, and secretes thick substance, or mucus, 220–21
Mucus, sticky fluid secreted by mucous membrane lining of respiratory tract; assists in cleansing air by trapping dust and bacteria, 221
Multigravida, woman who has had more than one pregnancy, 341
Multipara, woman who has given birth to more than one child, 341
Multiple sclerosis (MS), inflammatory disease of central nervous system; rare in children; generally strikes adults between ages of 20 and 40; there is progressive weakness and numbness, 428
Murmur, abnormal heart sound as soft blowing sound or harsh click; may be soft and heard

only with a stethoscope, or so loud it can be heard several feet away; also called a ***bruit,*** 153
Muscle actions, 115, 116***t***–18***t***
Muscle biopsy, removal of muscle tissue for pathological examination, 122
Muscle cells, 24***f***
Muscle tissue, tissue able to contract and shorten its length, thereby producing movement; muscle tissue may be under voluntary control (attached to bones) or involuntary control (heart and digestive organs), 25, 26***f***
Muscle tissue fibers, bundles of muscle tissue that form muscle, 25, 113
Muscle wasting, 120
Muscles, bundles of parallel muscle tissue fibers; as fibers contract (shorten in length) they pull whatever they are attached to closer togethe; may move two bones closer together or make opening narrowier; muscle contraction occurs when message is transmitted from brain through nervous system to muscles, 27***t,*** 113, 412; ***see also*** Muscular system
Muscular, pertaining to muscles, 120
Muscular dystrophy (MD), inherited disease causing progressive muscle weakness and atrophy, 121
Muscular system, 111–135, 112***f***
abbreviations, 123
anatomical terms, 119
anatomy and physiology, 113–18
combining forms, 119
diagnostic procedures, 122
muscle types, 113
pathology, 120–22
pharmacology, 123
suffixes, 119
terminology, 119
terminology for muscle actions, 115, 116***t***–18***t***
therapeutic procedures, 122–23
Musculoskeletal system (MS) system providing support for body and produces movement; organs include: muscles, tendons, bones, joints, and cartilage; ***see*** Muscular system; Skeletal system
Mutation, change or transformation from original, 528
Myalgia, muscle pain, 120
Myasthenia, lack of muscle strength, 120
Myasthenia gravis, disorder causing loss of muscle strength and paralysis; autoimmune disease, 428
Mycoplasma **pneumonia,** less severe but longer lasting form of pneumonia caused by ***Mycoplasma pneumoniae*** bacteria; also called ***walking pneumonia,*** 236
Mydriatic drops, substance that causes pupil to dilate, 463
Myelin, tissue that wraps around many of nerve fibers; composed of fatty material and functions as insulator, 412, 413***f,*** 414
Myelinated, nerve fibers covered with layer of myelin, 413
Myelitis, inflammation of spinal cord, 427
Myelogram, x-ray record of spinal cord following injection of meninges with radiopaque dye, 430
Myelography, injection of radiopaque dye into spinal canal; an X-ray is taken to examine normal and abnormal outlines made by dye, 106, 431
Myeloma, malignant neoplasm originating in plasma cells in bone, 103
Myelomeningocele, hernia composed of meninges and spinal cord, 427, 428***f***
Myelonic, pertaining to spinal cord, 421
Myocardial, pertaining to heart muscle, 119, 152
Myocardial infarction (MI), condition caused by partial or complete occlusion or closing of one or more of coronary arteries; symptoms include severe chest pain or heavy pressure in middle of chest; delay in treatment could result in death; also referred to as ***MI*** or ***heart attack,*** 142, 155, 155***f,*** 156, 156***f***
Myocarditis, inflammation of heart muscle, 157
Myocardium, middle layer of muscle; thick and composed of cardiac muscle; layer produces heart contraction, 114, 142, 142***f,*** 145***f***
Myometrium, middle muscle layer of uterus, 334, 334***f***
Myoneural junction, point at which nerve contacts muscle fiber, 114
Myopathy, any disease of muscles, 121
Myopia, with this condition person can see things that are close up but distance vision is blurred; also known as ***nearsightedness,*** 458, 458***f***
Myoplasty, surgical repair of muscle, 123
Myorrhaphy, suture a muscle, 123
Myorrhexis, muscle ruptured, 121
Myotonia, muscle tone, 120
Myringectomy, excision of eardrum, 475
Myringitis, eardrum inflammation, 472
Myringoplasty, surgical reconstruction of eardrum; also called ***tympanoplasty,*** 475
Myringotomy, surgical puncture of eardrum with removal of fluid and pus from middle ear, to eliminate persistent ear infection and excessive pressure on tympanic membrane; polyethylene tube is placed in tympanic membrane to allow for drainage of middle ear cavity, 476

Myxedema, condition resulting from hypofunction of thyroid gland; symptoms can include anemia, slow speech, enlarged tongue and facial features, edematous skin, drowsiness, and mental apathy, 395

N

Nail bed, connects nail body to connective tissue underneath, 55

Nail body, flat plate of keratin that forms most of nails, 55

Nail root, base of nail; nails grow longer from root, 55

Nails, structure in integumentary system, 27***t*****,** 55, 55***f***, 63

Narcissistic personality, personality disorder characterized by abnormal sense of self-importance, 502

Narcotic analgesic, drug used to treat severe pain; has potential to be habit forming if taken for prolonged time; also called opiates, 433

Nares, external openings of nose that open into nasal cavity, 220, 221***f***

Nasal, pertaining to nose, 229

Nasal bone, facial bone, 89, 91***f*****,** 91***t***

Nasal cannula, two-pronged plastic device for delivering oxygen into nose; one prong is inserted into each naris, 240

Nasal cavity, large cavity just behind external nose that receives outside air; covered with mucous membrane to cleanse air; nasal septum divides nasal cavity into left and right halves, 29***t*****,** 219***f***, 220–221, 221***f***, 259***f*****,** 451

Nasal septum, flexible cartilage wall that divides nasal cavity into left and right halves; covered by mucous membrane, 220

Nasogastric (NG), pertaining to nose and stomach, 268

Nasogastric intubation (NG tube), flexible catheter is inserted into nose and down esophagus to stomach; may be used for feeding or to suction out stomach fluids, 279

Nasolacrimal duct, duct that collects tears from inner corner of eye socket and drains them into nasal cavity, 451, 451***f***

Nasopharyngitis, inflammation of nasal cavity and throat, 233

Nasopharynx, superior section of pharynx that receives air from nose, 221***f*****,** 222

Natural immunity, immunity not specific to particular disease and does not require prior exposure to pathogen; also called innate immunity, 197

Natural killer (NK) cells, t cells that can kill by entrapping foreign cells, tumor cells, and bacteria; also called T8 cells, 197, 198

Nausea, feeling of needing to vomit, 270

Nearsightedness, 458, 458***f***

Nebulizer, 240

Neck, narrow length of bone that connects ball of ball-and-socket joint to diaphysis of long bone, 88, 88***f***

Necrosis, dead tissue, 60

Neonate, term used to describe newborn infant during first four weeks of life, 341

Neonatologist, specialist in treatment of newborn, 342

Neonatology, study of newborn, 342

Neoplasm, abnormal growth of tissue that may be benign or malignant; also called a ***tumor,*** 528

Nephrectomy, excision of a kidney, 314

Nephritis, inflammation of kidney, 308

Nephrogram, x-ray of kidney, 311

Nephrolith, kidney stone, 307

Nephrolithiasis, presence of calculi in kidney, 309

Nephrolithotomy, incision into kidney to remove a stone, 314

Nephrologist, specialist in treatment of kidney disorders, 305

Nephrology, branch of medicine specializing in conditions of urinary system, 29***t*****,** 40, 305

Nephroma, kidney tumor, 309

Nephromalacia, softening of kidney, 307

Nephromegaly, enlarged kidney, 307

Nephron, functional or working unit of kidney that filters blood and produces urine; there are more than 1 million nephrons in adult kidney; each nephron consists of renal corpuscle and renal tubules, 298, 299, 300***f***

Nephropathy, kidney disease, 309

Nephropexy, surgical fixation of kidney, 315

Nephroptosis, drooping kidney, 309

Nephrosclerosis, hardening of kidney, 307

Nephrosis, abnormal condition (degeneration) of kidney, 309

Nephrostomy, creating new opening across body wall into kidney, 315

Nephrotic syndrome (NS), damage to glomerulus resulting in protein appearing in urine, proteinuria, and corresponding decrease in protein in bloodstream, 309

Nephrotomy, incision into kidney, 315

Nerve block, also referred to as regional anesthesia; this anesthetic interrupts patient's pain sensation in particular region of body; anesthetic is injected near nerve that will be blocked from sensation; patient usually remains conscious, 432, 521***t***

Nulligravida, woman who has never been pregnant, 341
Nullipara, woman who has never produced a viable baby, 341
Number prefixes, 6
Nurse, to breastfeed a baby, 336
Nurse anesthetist, registered nurse who has received additional training and education in administration of anesthetic medications, 520
Nurse's notes, medical record document that records patient's care throughout day; includes vital signs, treatment specifics, patient's response to treatment, and patient's condition, 12
Nursing home, facility that provides long-term care for patients who need extra time to recover from illness or accident before they return home or for persons who can no longer care for themselves; also called ***long-term care facility,*** 13
Nyctalopia, difficulty seeing in dim light; usually due to damaged rods, 455
Nystagmus, jerky-appearing involuntary eye movement, 459

O

Obesity, having abnormal amount of fat in body, 270, 391
Oblique fracture, fracture at angle to bone, 102, 102***f***
Oblique muscles, oblique means slanted; two of eye muscles are oblique muscles, 450, 450***f***
Oblique view, positioning patient so that X-rays pass through body on angle, 507
Obsessive-compulsive disorder (OCD), type of anxiety disorder in which person performs repetitive rituals in order to reduce anxiety, 501
Obstetrician, 342
Obstetrics (OB), branch of medicine that treats women during pregnancy and childbirth, and immediately after childbirth, 30***t,*** 342
Occipital bone, cranial bone, 89, 91***f,*** 91***t***
Occipital lobe, one of four cerebral hemisphere lobes; controls eyesight, 414, 415, 415***f***
Occupational Safety and Health Administration (OSHA), federal agency that issued mandatory guidelines to ensure that all employees at risk of exposure to body fluids are provided with personal protective equipment, 198
Occupational therapy (OT), assists patients to regain, develop, and improve skills that are important for independent functioning; occupational therapy personnel work with people who, because of illness, injury, developmental, or psychological impairments, require specialized training in skills that will enable them to lead independent, productive, and satisfying lives; occupational therapists instruct patients in use of adaptive equipment and techniques, body mechanics, and energy conservation; also employ modalities such as heat, cold, and therapeutic exercise, 514
Ocular, pertaining to eye, 454
Oculomotor nerve, 418***t***
Oculomycosis, condition of eye fungus, 458
Olfactory nerve, 418***t***
Oligomenorrhea, scanty menstrual flow, 342
Oligospermia, condition of having few sperm, 358
Oliguria, condition of scanty amount of urine, 307
Oncogenic, cancer causing, 528
Oncology, branch of medicine dealing with tumors, 525–30
  abbreviations, 530
  diagnostic procedures, 529
  staging tumors, 526–27, 527***t***
  therapeutic procedures, 529
  vocabulary, 527–28
Onychectomy, excision of a nail, 71
Onychia, infected nailbed, 69
Onychomalacia, softening of nails, 60
Onychomycosis, abnormal condition of nail fungus, 69
Onychophagia, nail biting, 69
Oophorectomy, removal of an ovary, 350
Oophoritis, inflammation of an ovary, 342
Open fracture, 101, 101***f***
Operative report, medical record report from surgeon detailing operation; includes pre- and postprocedure itself, and how patient tolerated procedure, 12, 520
Ophthalmalgia, eye pain, 455
Ophthalmic, pertaining to eyes, 454
Ophthalmic decongestants, over-the-counter medications that constrict arterioles of eye, reduce redness and itching of conjunctiva, 463
Ophthalmologist, physician specialized in treating conditions and diseases of eye, 455
Ophthalmology (Ophth), branch of medicine specializing in condition of eye, 31***t,*** 448, 455
Ophthalmoplegia, paralysis of eye, 455
Ophthalmorrhagia, rapid bleeding from eye, 455
Ophthalmoscope, instrument to view inside eye, 460, 461***f***
Ophthalmoscopy, examination of interior of eyes using instrument called ophthalmoscope; physician will dilate pupil in order to see cornea, lens, and retina; identifies abnormalities in blood vessels of eye and some systemic diseases, 460
Opiates, 433

Opportunistic infections, infectious diseases associated with AIDS since they occur as a result of lowered immune system and resistance of body to infections and parasites, 203

Opposition, moves thumb away from palm; ability to move thumb into contact with other fingers, 118***t***

Optic, pertaining to eye, 454

Optic disk, area of retina associated with optic nerve; also called blind spot, 449

Optic nerve, second cranial nerve that carries impulses from retinas to brain, 418***t***, 448, 448***f***, 452***f***

Optical, pertaining to eye or vision, 454

Optician, grinds and fits prescription lenses and contacts as prescribed by physician or optometrist, 455

Optometer, instrument to measure vision, 461

Optometrist (OD), doctor of optometry; provides care for eyes including examining eyes for diseases, assessing visual acuity, prescribing corrective lenses and eye treatments, and educating patients, 455

Optometry, process of measuring vision, 455

Oral, (1) pertaining to mouth; (2) administration of medication through mouth, 268, 471, 494***t***

Oral cavity, the mouth, 29***t***, 257***f***, 258–61, 259***f***

Oral contraceptive pills (OCPs), birth control medication that uses low doses of female hormones to prevent conception by blocking ovulation, 351

Oral hypoglycemic agents, medication taken by mouth that causes decrease in blood sugar; not used for insulin-dependent patients; no proof that medication will prevent long-term complications of diabetes mellitus, 397

Oral surgeon, practitioner of oral surgery, 268

Oral surgery, branch of dentistry that uses surgical means to treat dental conditions; specialist is ***oral surgeon***, 268

Orbit, 91***f***

Orchidectomy, excision of testes, 361

Orchidopexy, surgical fixation to move undescended testes into scrotum and attaching to prevent retraction, 358, 361

Orchiectomy, surgical removal of testes, 361

Orchioplasty, surgical repair of testes, 361

Orchiotomy, incision into testes, 361

Organs, group of different types of tissue coming together to perform special functions; for example, heart contains muscular fibers, nerve tissue, and blood vessels, 27, 27***t***–31***t***

Organs of Corti, sensory receptor hair cells lining cochlea; these cells change sound vibrations to electrical impulses and send impulses to brain via vestibulocochlear nerve, 468

Origin, attachment of skeletal muscle to less movable bone in joint, 115

Oropharynx, middle section of pharynx that receives food and drink from mouth, 221***f***, 222, 261

Orthodontic, pertaining to straight teeth, 261

Orthodontics, dental specialty concerned with straightening teeth, 269

Orthodontist, dental specialist in straightening teeth, 269

Orthopedic surgeon, 100

Orthopedic surgery, branch of medicine specializing in surgical treatments of musculoskeletal system, 27***t***, 100

Orthopedics (Ortho), branch of medicine specializing in diagnosis and treatment of conditions of musculoskeletal system, 27***t***, 100

Orthopedist, 100

Orthopnea, term to describe patient who needs to sit up straight in order to breathe comfortably, 232

Orthostatic hypotension, sudden drop in blood pressure person experiences when standing up suddenly, 153

Orthotics, use of equipment, such as splints and braces, to support paralyzed muscle, promote specific motion, or correct musculoskeletal deformities, 100, 515

Os coxae, also called innominate bone or hip bone; pelvis portion of lower extremity; consists of ilium, ischium, and pubis and unites with sacrum and coccyx to form pelvis, 92, 94, 95***t***

Osseous tissue, bony tissue; one of hardest tissues in body, 86

Ossicles, three small bones in middle ear; bones are incus, malleus, and stapes; ossicles amplify and conduct sound waves to inner ear, 468, 468***f***

Ossification, process of bone formation, 86

Ostealgia, bone pain, 100

Osteoarthritis (OA), noninflammatory type of arthritis resulting in degeneration of bones and joints, especially those bearing weight, 3, 105

Osteoblast, embryonic bone cell, 86

Osteochondroma, tumor composed of both cartilage and bony substance, 103

Osteoclasia, intentional breaking of bone in order to correct deformity, 108

Osteocyte, mature bone cells, 86

Osteogenic sarcoma, most common type of bone cancer; usually begins in osteocytes found at ends of long bones, 103

Osteomalacia, softening of bones caused by deficiency of phosphorus or calcium; is thought that in children cause is insufficient sunlight and vitamin D, 103

P

Palatoplasty, surgical repair of palate, 281
Palliative therapy, treatment designed to reduce intensity of painful symptoms, but not to produce a cure, 529
Pallor, abnormal paleness of skin, 60
Palpitations, pounding, racing heartbeat, 153
Palsy, temporary or permanent loss of ability to control movement, 423
Pancreas, organ in digestive system that produces digestive enzymes; also a gland in endocrine system that produces two hormones, insulin and glucagon, 29***t,*** 30***t,*** 35***t,*** 36***t,*** 257***f,*** 258, 265, 265***f,*** 276***f,*** 379***f,*** 380, 381***t,*** 383–84, 383***f,*** 392
Pancreatic, pertaining to pancreas, 268, 389
Pancreatic duct, duct carrying pancreatic juices from pancreas to duodenum, 265, 265***f***
Pancreatic enzymes, digestive enzymes produced by pancreas and added to chyme in duodenum, 265
Pancreatitis, inflammation of pancreas, 276
Pancytopenia, too few of all types of blood cells, 185
Panhypopituitarism, deficiency in all hormones secreted by pituitary gland; often recognized because of problems with glands regulated by pituitary—adrenal cortex, thyroid, ovaries, and testes, 394
Panic attacks, type of anxiety disorder characterized by sudden onset of intense apprehension, fear, terror, or impending doom often accompanied by racing heart rate, 500
Pansinusitis, inflammation of all sinuses, 232
Pap (Papanicolaou) smear, test for early detection of cancer of cervix named after developer of test, George Papanicolaou, a Greek physician; a scraping of cells is removed from cervix for examination under a microscope, 347
Papilla, 55***f***
Papilledema, swelling of optic disk, often as a result of increased intraocular pressure; also called ***choked disk,*** 455
Papule, small, solid, circular raised spot on surface of skin, often as a result of inflammation in oil gland, 61, 61***f***
Paracentesis, insertion of needle into abdominal cavity to withdraw fluid; tests to diagnose disease may be conducted on fluid, 278
Paralysis, temporary or permanent loss of function or voluntary movement, 423
Paranasal sinuses, air-filled cavities within facial bones that open into nasal cavity; act as echo chamber during sound production, 221, 221***f***
Paranoid personality disorder, personality disorder characterized by exaggerated feelings of persecution, 502
Paraplegia, paralysis of lower portion of body and both legs, 423
Parasympathetic branch, branch of autonomic nervous system; serves as counterbalance for sympathetic nerves; therefore, it causes heart rate to slow down, lower blood pressure, constrict eye pupils, and increase digestion, 419
Parathyroid glands, four small glands located on back surface of thyroid gland; parathyroid hormone secreted by these glands regulates amount of calcium in blood, 30***t,*** 378, 379***t,*** 380, 381***t***, 384, 384***f***
Parathyroid hormone (PTH), hormone secreted by parathyroid glands; the more hormone, the higher the calcium level in blood and lower the level stored in bone; low hormone level will cause tetany, 381***t,*** 384
Parenteral, route for introducing medication other than through gastrointestinal tract; most commonly involves injection into body through needle and syringe, 494, 495***t***
Parathyroidal, pertaining to parathyroid glands, 389
Parathyroidectomy, excision of one or more of parathyroid glands; performed to halt progress of hyperparathyroidism, 397
Parenteral administration of drugs, 495***t***
Paresthesia, abnormal sensation such as burning or tingling, 423
Parietal bone, cranial bone, 89, 91***f,*** 91***t***
Parietal layer, outer pleural layer around lungs; lines inside of chest cavity, 34, 35
Parietal lobe, one of four cerebral hemisphere lobes; receives and interprets nerve impulses from sensory receptors, 414, 415, 415***f***
Parietal pericardium, outer layer of pericardium surrounding heart, 142
Parietal peritoneum, outer layer of serous membrane sac lining abdominopelvic cavity, 34, 35
Parietal pleura, outer layer of serous membrane sac lining thoracic cavity, 34, 35, 224
Parkinson's disease, chronic disorder of nervous system with fine tremors, muscular weakness, rigidity, and shuffling gait, 427
Paronychia, infection around nail, 69, 69***f***
Parotid duct, 264***f***
Parotid glands, pair of salivary glands located in front of ears, 264, 264***f***
Passive acquired immunity, immunity that results when person receives protective substances produced by another human or animal; may take form of maternal antibodies crossing placenta to baby or antitoxin injection, 196, 197

Passive aggressive personality, personality disorder in which person expresses feelings or anger or hostility through indirect or covert actions, 503

Passive range of motion (PROM), therapist putting patient's joints through full range of motion without assistance from patient, 517

Patella, also called ***kneecap;*** lower extremity bone, 85, 94, 95***f,*** 95***t***

Patellar, pertaining to patella or kneecap, 99

Patent, open or unblocked, such as patent airway, 232

Patent ductus arteriosus (PDA), congenital heart anomaly in which opening between pulmonary artery and aorta fails to close at birth; condition requires surgery, 158

Pathogenic, pertaining to microscopic organisms, such as bacteria, capable of causing disease, 201

Pathogens, disease-bearing organisms, 52, 181

Pathologic fracture, fracture caused by diseased or weakened bone, 102

Pathological gambling, impulse control disorder in which patient is unable to control urge to gamble, 502

Pathologist, physician who specializes in evaluating specimens removed from living or dead patients, 527

Pathologist's report, medical record report given by pathologist who studies tissue removed from patient (for example: bone marrow, blood, or tissue biopsy), 12

Pathology, branch of medicine specializing in studying how disease affects body, 200

Pectoral girdle, consists of clavicle and scapula; functions to attach upper extremity to axial skeleton, 92, 93***f,*** 94, 94***f***

Pediculosis, infestation with lice, 67

Pedophilia, sexual disorder characterized by having sexual interest in children, 503

Pelvic, pertaining to pelvis, 99

Pelvic cavity, inferior portion of abdominopelvic cavity, 34, 34***f,*** 35***t***

Pelvic examination, physical examination of vagina and adjacent organs performed by physician placing fingers of one hand into vagina; visual examination is performed using speculum, 348

Pelvic girdle, consists ofilium, ischium, and pubis; functions to attach lower extremity to axial skeleton, 93***f,*** 95***f,*** 95***t***

Pelvic inflammatory disease (PID), any inflammation of female reproductive organs, generally bacterial in nature, 344

Pelvic region, lowest anterior region of trunk, 33, 34***f***

Pelvic ultrasonography, use of ultrasound waves to produce image or photograph of organ, such as uterus, ovaries, or fetus, 347

Pelvis, 96***f***

Penile, pertaining to penis, 357

Penis, male sex organ; composed of erectile tissue that becomes erect during sexual stimulation, allowing it to be placed within female vagina for ejaculation of semen; larger, soft tip is referred to as glans penis, 30***t,*** 353***f,*** 354, 355

Peptic ulcer disease (PUD), ulcer occurring in lower portion of esophagus, stomach, and duodenum and thought to be caused by acid of gastric juices, 272, 272***f***

Percussion, use of fingertips to tap body lightly and sharply; aids in determining size, position, and consistency of underlying body part, 242

Percutaneous diskectomy, thin catheter tube is inserted into intervertebral disk through skin and herniated or ruptured disk material is sucked out or a laser is used to vaporize it, 108

Percutaneous transhepatic cholangiography (PTC), contrast medium is injected directly into liver to visualize bile ducts; used to detect obstructions, 277

Percutaneous transluminal coronary angioplasty (PTCA), method for treating localized coronary artery narrowing; balloon catheter is inserted through skin into coronary artery and inflated to dilate narrow blood vessel, 163

Perforated ulcer, 272

Pericardial cavity, cavity formed by serous membrane sac surrounding heart, 34, 35, 35***t***

Pericarditis, inflammatory process or disease of pericardium, 10, 157

Pericardium, double-walled outer sac around heart; inner layer of pericardium is called epicardium, outer layer is heart itself; this sac contains pericardial fluid that reduces friction caused by heart beating, 141***f,*** 142, 142***f***

Perimetritis, inflammation around uterus, 344

Perimetrium, outer layer of uterus, 334, 334***f***

Perineal, pertaining to perineum, 341

Perineum, in male, external region between scrotum and anus; in female, external region between vagina and anus, 335, 336, 337***f,*** 354, 355

Periodontal disease, disease of supporting structures of teeth, including gums and bones, 271

Periodontal ligaments, small ligaments that anchor root of tooth in socket of jaw, 260, 261, 261***f***

Periodontics, branch of dentistry concerned with treating conditions involving gums and tissues surrounding teeth; specialist is a ***periodontist,*** 269

and laryngopharynx, 29***t,*** 196, 220, 221***f,*** 222, 258, 259***f***, 261, 271

Pheochromocytoma, usually benign tumor of adrenal medulla that secretes epinephrine; symptoms include anxiety, heart palpitations, dyspnea, profuse sweating, headache, and nausea, 392

Phimosis, narrowing of foreskin over glans penis that results in difficulty with hygiene; condition can lead to infection or difficulty with urination; treated with circumcision, surgical removal of foreskin, 359

Phlebitis, inflammation of a vein, 158

Phlebotomist, 188, 188***f***

Phlebotomy, creating opening into vein to withdraw blood, 188, 188***f***

Phlegm, thick mucus secreted by membranes that line respiratory tract; when phlegm is coughed through mouth, is called ***sputum;*** phlegm is examined for color, odor, and consistency, 232

Phobias, type of anxiety disorder in which person has irrational fears; example is arachnophobia, fear of spiders, 500

Phonophoresis, use of ultrasound waves to introduce medication across skin into subcutaneous tissues, 517

Photophobia, strong sensitivity to bright light, 456

Photorefractive keratectomy (PRK), use of laser to reshape cornea to correct errors of refraction, 462

Photosensitivity, condition in which skin reacts abnormally when exposed to light such as ultraviolet rays of sun, 61

Physical medicine, use of natural methods, including physical therapy, to cure diseases and disorders, 515

Physical therapy (PT), treating disorders using physical means and methods; physical therapy personnel assess joint motion, muscle strength and endurance, function of heart and lungs, and performance of activities required in daily living, along with other responsibilities; physical therapy treatment includes gait training, therapeutic exercise, massage, joint and soft tissue mobilization, thermal and cryotherapy, electrical stimulation, ultrasound, and hydrotherapy; methods strengthen muscles, improve motion and circulation, reduce pain, and increase function, 514

Physician's offices, individual or groups of physicians providing diagnostic and treatment services in arivate office setting rather than hospital, 13

Physician's orders, medical record document that contains complete list of care, medications, tests, and treatments physician orders for patient, 12

Physician's progress notes, part of patient's medical record; physician's daily record of patient's condition, results of physician's examinations, summary of test results, updated assessment and diagnoses, and further plans for patient's care, 12

Physician's Desk Reference (PDR), 492

Pia mater, term means soft mother; this thin innermost meninges layer is applied directly to surface of brain, 417, 417***f***

Pineal gland, gland in endocrine system that produces hormone called melatonin, 30***t,*** 297***f***, 397***f***, 380, 384, 384***f***

Pinealectomy, surgical removal of pineal gland, 397

Pinna, also called ***auricle;*** external ear, which functions to capture sound waves as they go past outer ear, 467, 467***f***

Pisse prophets, 298

Pituitary, pertaining to pituitary gland, 389

Pituitary anterior lobe, 381***t***

Pituitary gland, endocrine gland located behind optic nerve in brain; also called master gland since it controls functions of many other endocrine glands; is divided into two lobes: anterior and posterior; anterior pituitary gland secretes hormones that aid in controlling growth and stimulating thyroid gland, sexual glands, and adrenal cortex; posterior pituitary is responsible for antidiuretic hormone and oxytocin, 30***t,*** 379***f,*** 380, 384–86, 385***f,*** 393, 414***f***

Pituitary posterior lobe, 381***t***

Placebo, inactive, harmless substance used to satisfy patient's desire for medication; also given to control groups of patients in research studies in which another group receives drug; effect of placebo versus drug is then observed, 497

Placenta, also called afterbirth; organ attached to uterine wall composed of maternal and fetal tissues; oxygen, nutrients, carbon dioxide, and wastes are exchanged between mother and baby through placenta; baby is attached to placenta by way of umbilical cord, 336, 337, 337***f***

Placenta previa, occurs when placenta is in lower portion of uterus and thus blocks birth canal, 346, 346***f***

Placental stage, third stage of labor, which takes place after delivery of infant; uterus resumes strong contractions and placenta detaches from uterine wall and is delivered through vagina, 338, 338***f***

Plantar flexion, bend sole of foot; point toes downward, 116, 116***f***

Plaque, yellow, fatty deposit of lipids in artery, 154, 154***f,*** 155***f***

Plasma, liquid portion of blood containing 90% water; remaining 10% consists of plasma proteins (serum albumin, serum globulin, fibrinogen, and prothrombin), inorganic substances (calcium, potassium, and sodium), organic components (glucose, amino acids, cholesterol), and waste products (urea, uric acid, ammonia, and creatinine), 28***t***, 179***f***, 180

Plasma proteins, proteins that are found in plasma; includes serum albumin, serum globulin, fibrinogen, and prothrombin, 180

Plasmapheresis, method of removing plasma from body without depleting formed elements; whole blood is removed and cells and plasma are separated; cells are returned to patient along with donor plasma transfusion, 189

Plastic surgery, surgical specialty involved in repair, reconstruction, or improvement of body structures such as skin that are damaged, missing, or misshapen; physician is plastic surgeon, 58

Platelet count, blood test to determine number of platelets in given volume of blood, 188

Platelets, cells responsible for coagulation of blood; also called thrombocytes and contain no hemoglobin, 28***t***, 179***f***, 180, 182***f***

Pleura, protective double layer of serous membrane around lungs; parietal membrane is outer layer and visceral layer is inner membrane; secretes thin, watery fluid to reduce friction associated with lung movement, 34, 35, 224

Pleural, pertaining to pleura, 41

Pleural cavity, cavity formed by serous membrane sac surrounding lungs, 34, 35, 35***t***, 224

Pleural effusion, abnormal presence of fluid or gas in pleural cavity; physicians can detect presence of fluid by tapping chest (percussion) or listening with stethoscope (auscultation), 237

Pleural rub, grating sound made when two surfaces, such as pleural surfaces, rub together during respiration; caused when one of surfaces becomes thicker as result of inflammation or other disease conditions; rub can be felt through fingertips when placed on chest wall or heard through stethoscope, 232

Pleurectomy, excision of pleura, 241

Pleurisy, inflammation of pleura, 237

Pleuritis, 237

Pleurocentesis, puncture of pleura to withdraw fluid from thoracic cavity in order to diagnose disease, 241

Pleurodynia, pleural pain, 232

Plural endings, 10

Pneumoconiosis, condition resulting from inhaling environmental particles that become toxic, such as coal dust (anthracosis) or asbestos (asbestosis), 236

Pneumocystis pneumonia (PCP), Pneumonia with a nonproductive cough, very little fever, and dyspnea caused by fungus ***Pneumocystis jiroveci;*** opportunistic infection often seen in those with weakened immune systems, such as AIDS patients, 203, 236

Pneumonia, inflammatory condition of lung, which can be caused by bacterial and viral infections, diseases, and chemicals, 236

Pneumothorax, collection of air or gas in pleural cavity, which can result in collapse of lung, 237, 237***f***

Podiatrist, 100

Podiatry, healthcare profession specializing in diagnosis and treatment of disorders of feet and lower legs; healthcare professional is ***podiatrist***, 100

Poliomyelitis, acute viral disease that causes inflammation of gray matter of spinal cord, resulting in paralysis in some cases; has been brought under almost total control through vaccinations, 427

Polyarteritis, inflammation of many arteries, 158

Polycystic kidneys, formation of multiple cysts within kidney tissue; results in destruction of normal kidney tissue and uremia, 309, 309***f***

Polycythemia vera, production of too many red blood cells in bone marrow, 186

Polydipsia, condition of having excessive amount of thirst, such as in diabetes, 391

Polymyositis, disease involving muscle inflammation and weakness from unknown cause, 121

Polyneuritis, inflammation of many nerves, 429

Polyp, small tumor with pedicle or stem attachment; commonly found in vascular organs such as nose, uterus, and rectum, 274, 275***f***

Polyphagia, to eat excessively, 270

Polyposis, small tumors that contain pedicle or footlike attachment in mucous membranes of large intestine (colon), 274, 275***f***

Polysomnography, monitoring a patient while sleeping to identify sleep apnea; also called ***sleep apnea study***, 239

Polyuria, condition of having excessive urine production; can be a symptom of disease conditions such as diabetes, 307, 391

Pons, this portion of brain stem forms bridge between cerebellum and cerebrum; also where nerve fibers cross from one side of brain to control functions and movement on other side of brain, 414, 414***f***, 415, 415***f***

Pontine, pertaining to pons, 421

Popliteal artery, 148***f***

Popliteal vein, 150***f***

vaginal delivery or as result of pelvic tumors pressing down, 344
Pronation, to turn downward or backward, as with hand or foot, 118***t***, 118***f***
Prone, directional term meaning lying horizontally facing downward, 38***f***, 38***t***
Prone position, 522***f***, 523***t***
Pronunciation, of medical terms, 9–10
Prophylaxis, prevention of disease; for example, antibiotic can be used to prevent occurrence of disease, 497
Proprietary name, name a pharmaceutical company chooses as trademark or market name for its drug; also called ***brand*** or ***trade name,*** 491
Prostate cancer, slow-growing cancer that affects large number of males after age 50; PSA (prostate-specific antigen) test is used to assist in early detection of this disease, 359
Prostate gland, gland in male reproductive system that produces fluids that nourish sperm, 30***t***, 35***t***, 300***f***, 301***f***, 353***f***, 354, 354***f***, 356, 358
Prostate-specific antigen (PSA), blood test to screen for prostate cancer; elevated blood levels of PSA associated with prostate cancer, 360
Prostatectomy, surgical removal of prostate gland, 361
Prostatic, pertaining to prostate gland, 357
Prostatitis, inflamed condition of prostate gland that may be result of infection, 359
Prosthesis, artificial device used as substitute for body part either congenitally missing or absent as result of accident or disease; for instance, artificial leg or hip prosthesis, 107
Prosthetic hip joint, 108***f***
Prosthetic lens implant, use of artificial lens to replace lens removed during cataract surgery, 462
Prosthetics, artificial devices, such as limbs and joints, that replace missing body part, 100, 515
Prosthetist, 100
Protease inhibitor drugs, medications that inhibit protease, enzyme viruses need to reproduce, 205
Protein-bound iodine test (PBI), blood test to measure concentration of thyroxine (T_4) circulating in blood stream; iodine becomes bound to protein in blood and can be measured; useful in establishing thyroid function, 395
Proteinuria, protein in urine, 307
Prothrombin, protein element within blood that interacts with calcium salts to form thrombin, 182
Prothrombin time (Pro time), measurement of time it takes for sample of blood to coagulate, 188
Protocol (prot), actual plan of care, including medications, surgeries, and treatments for care of patient; often, entire healthcare team, including physician, oncologist, radiologist, nurse, and patient, will assist in designing treatment plan, 526
Proton pump inhibitor, blocks stomach's ability to secrete acid; used to treat peptic ulcers and gastroesophageal reflux disease, 281
Protozoans, single-celled organisms that can infect body, 196, 197
Proximal, directional term meaning located closest to point of attachment to body, 37***f***, 37***t***
Proximal convoluted tubule, portion of renal tubule, 299, 300***f***, 302***f***
Pruritus, severe itching, 61
Pseudocyesis, false pregnancy, 346
Pseudohypertrophic muscular dystrophy, one type of inherited muscular dystrophy in which muscle tissue is gradually replaced by fatty tissue, making muscle look strong, 121
Psoriasis, chronic inflammatory condition consisting of crusty papules forming patches with circular borders, 67, 67***f***
Psychiatric nurse, nurse with additional training in care of patients with mental, emotional, and behavioral disorders, 500
Psychiatric social work, social worker with additional training in care of patients with mental, emotional, or behavioral disorders, 500
Psychiatrist (MD or DO), physician with specialized training in diagnosing and treating mental disorders; prescribes medication and conducts counseling, 500
Psychiatry, branch of medicine that deals with the diagnosis, treatment, and prevention of mental disorders, 500
Psychoanalysis, method of obtaining a detailed account of past and present emotional and mental experiences from patient to determine source of problem and eliminate effects, 505
Psychology, study of human behavior and thought process; behavioral science is primarily concerned with understanding how human beings interact with their physical environment and with each other, 500
Psychopharmacology, study of effects of drugs on mind and particularly use of drugs in treating mental disorders; main classes of drugs for treatment of mental disorders are antipsychotic drugs, antidepressant drugs, minor tranquilizers, and lithium, 504
Psychotherapy, method of treating mental disorders by mental rather than chemical or physical means; includes psychoanalysis, humanistic therapies, and family and group therapy, 505

Pterygium, hypertrophied conjunctival tissue in inner corner of eye, 459
Puberty, beginning of menstruation and ability to reproduce; usually occurs around age 16, 334, 335
Pubic, pertaining to pubis; one of pelvic bones, 99
Pubic region, genital region of body, 33, 33***f***
Pubis, one of three bones that form os coxae or innominate bone, 94, 95***f,*** 95***t***
Pulmonary, pertaining to lung, 229
Pulmonary angiography, injecting dye into blood vessel for purpose of taking X-ray of arteries and veins of lungs, 238
Pulmonary artery, large artery that carries deoxygenated blood from right ventricle to lung, 140***f,*** 144, 145***f***
Pulmonary capillaries, network of capillaries in lungs that tightly encase each alveolus; site of gas exchange, 223
Pulmonary circulation, pulmonary circulation transports deoxygenated blood from right side of heart to lungs where oxygen and carbon dioxide are exchanged; then it carries oxygenated blood back to left side of heart, 140
Pulmonary edema, condition in which lung tissue retains excessive amount of fluid; results in labored breathing, 236
Pulmonary embolism, blood clot or air bubble in pulmonary artery or one of its branches, 236
Pulmonary fibrosis, formation of fibrous scar tissue in lungs, which leads to decreased ability to expand lungs; may be caused by infections, pneumoconiosis, autoimmune diseases, and toxin exposure, 236
Pulmonary function test (PFT), group of diagnostic tests that give information regarding air flow in and out of the lungs, lung volumes, and gas exchange between the lungs and bloodstream, 225, 225***t,*** 239
Pulmonary semilunar valve, 144***f***
Pulmonary trunk, 142***f***
Pulmonary valve, semilunar valve between right ventricle and pulmonary artery in heart; prevents blood from flowing backwards into ventricle, 142***f,*** 143, 144***f,*** 145***f***
Pulmonary vein, large vein that returns oxygenated blood from lungs to left atrium, 140***f,*** 144, 145***f***
Pulmonologist, physician specialized in treating diseases and disorders of respiratory system, 229
Pulmonology, branch of medicine specializing in conditions of respiratory system, 29***t,*** 229
Pulp cavity, hollow interior of tooth; contains soft tissue made up of blood vessels, nerves, and lymph vessels, 260, 261, 261***f***
Pulse (P), expansion and contraction produced by blood as it moves through artery; pulse can be taken at several pulse points throughout body where artery is close to surface, 149
Pupil, hole in center of iris; size of pupil is changed by iris dilating or constricting, 447***f,*** 448***f,*** 449, 452***f***
Pupillary, pertaining to pupil, 454
Purified protein derivative (PPD), 239
Purkinje fibers, part of conduction system of heart; found in ventricular myocardium, 144, 146***f***
Purpura, hemorrhages into skin and mucous membranes, 61, 61***f,***
Purulent, pus-filled sputum, which can be result of infection, 61
Pustule, raised spot on skin containing pus, 62, 62***f***
Pyelitis, inflammation of renal pelvis, 309
Pyelogram, x-ray record of the pelvis after injection of radiopaque dye, 311
Pyelonephritis, inflammation of renal pelvis and kidney; one of most common types of kidney disease; may be result of lower urinary tract infection that moved up to kidney by way of ureters; may be large quantities of white blood cells and bacteria in urine, and blood (hematuria) may even be present in urine in this condition; can occur with any untreated or persistent case of cystitis, 309
Pyeloplasty, surgical repair of renal pelvis, 315
Pyloric, pertaining to pylorus, 268
Pyloric sphincter, sphincter at distal end of stomach; controls passage of food into duodenum, 262, 262***f,*** 265***f***
Pyoderma, pus producing skin infection, 62
Pyosalpinx, condition of having pus in fallopian tubes, 343
Pyothorax, condition of having pus in chest cavity, 232, 237
Pyromania, impulse control disorder in which patient is unable to control impulse to start fires, 502
Pyrosis, heartburn, 270
Pyuria, presence of pus in urine, 307

Q

Quadriplegia, paralysis of all four extremities; same as tetraplegia, 423

R

Radial, pertaining to radius; lower arm bone, 99
Radial artery, 148***f***

Radial keratotomy, spokelike incisions around cornea that result in it becoming flatter; surgical treatment for myopia, 463
Radial nerve, 419***f***
Radial vein, 150***f***
Radiation therapy, use of X-rays to treat disease, especially cancer, 529
Radical mastectomy, surgical removal of breast tissue plus chest muscles and axillary lymph nodes, 350
Radical surgery, extensive surgery to remove as much tissue associated with tumor as possible, 529
Radiculitis, nerve root inflammation, 429
Radiculopathy, disease of nerve root, 429
Radioactive implant, embedding radioactive source directly into tissue to provide highly localized radiation dosage to damage nearby cancerous cells; also called ***brachytherapy,*** 529
Radiography, making of X-ray pictures, 106, 507
Radioimmunoassay (RIA), test used to measure levels of hormones in plasma of blood, 396
Radioisotope, radioactive form of element, 507
Radiologist, physician who practices diagnosis and treatment by use of radiant energy; responsible for interpreting X-ray films, 507
Radiology, branch of medicine that uses radioactive substances such as X-rays, isotopes, and radiation to prevent, diagnose, and treat diseases, 510
Radiolucent, structures that allow X-rays to pass through and expose photographic plate, making it appear as black area on X-ray, are termed radiolucent, 507
Radiopaque, structures impenetrable to X-rays, appearing as light area on radiograph (X-ray), 507
Radius, one of forearm bones in upper extermity, 92, 93***f,*** 94, 94***f***
Range of motion (ROM), range of movement of a joint, from maximum flexion through maximum extension; measured as degrees of a circle, 516
Raynaud's phenomenon, periodic ischemic attacks affecting extremities of body, especially fingers, toes, ears, and nose; affected extremities become cyanotic and very painful; attacks are brought on by arterial constriction due to extreme cold or emotional stress, 158
Reabsorption, second phase of urine production; substances needed by body are reabsorbed as filtrate passes through kidney tubules, 302
Recklinghausen disease, excessive production of parathyroid hormone, which results in degeneration of bones, 393
Rectal, (1) pertaining to rectum; (2) substances introduced directly into rectal cavity in form of suppositories or solution; drugs may have to be administered by this route if patient is unable to take them by mouth due to nausea, vomiting, and surgery, 268, 494, 496***t***
Rectocele, protrusion or herniation of rectum into vagina, 344
Rectum, area at end of digestive tube for storage of feces that leads to anus, 258, 263, 263***f,*** 264***f,*** 332***f,*** 335***f,*** 337***f,*** 354***f***
Rectus abdominis, muscle named for its location and direction of its fibers: rectus means straight and abdominis means abdominal, 115
Rectus muscles, rectus means straight; four of eye muscles are rectus muscles, 450, 450***f***
Red blood cell count (RBC), blood test to determine number of erythrocytes in volume of blood; decrease in red blood cells may indicate anemia; increase may indicate polycythemia, 188
Red blood cell morphology, examination of blood for abnormalities in shape (morphology) of erythrocytes; used to determine diseases like sickle-cell anemia, 188
Red blood cells (RBC), also called erythrocytes or RBCs; cells that contain hemoglobin and iron-containing pigment that binds oxygen in order to transport it to cells of body, 169***f,*** 170
Red bone marrow, tissue that manufactures most of blood cells; found in cancellous bone cavities, 86, 87
Reduction, correcting a fracture by realigning bone fragments; ***closed reduction*** is doing this without entering body; ***open reduction*** is making surgical incision at site of fracture to do reduction, often necessary where there are bony fragments to be removed, 109
Refractive error test, eye examination performed by physician to determine and correct refractive errors in eye, 461
Refracts, bending of light rays as they enter eye, 448
Regional anesthesia, regional anesthesia is also referred to as nerve block; anesthetic interrupts patient's pain sensation in a particular region of body; anesthetic is injected near nerve that will be blocked from sensation; patient usually remains conscious, 520, 521***t***
Regional ileitis, 272
Regurgitation, to flow backwards; in cardiovascular system refers to blood flowing backwards through valve; in digestive system refers to food flowing backwards from stomach to mouth, 154, 270

dioxide levels in blood, and administering breathing treatments, 225, 229

Respiratory therapy, allied health specialty that assists patients with respiratory and cardiopulmonary disorders, 229

Retina, innermost layer of eye; contains visual receptors called rods and cones; rods and cones receive light impulses and transmit them to brain via optic nerve, 447***f***, 448, 448***f***, 449, 449***f***, 452***f***

Retinal, pertaining to retina, 454

Retinal arteries, 452***f***

Retinal blood vessels, blood vessels that supply oxygen to rods and cones of retina, 449

Retinal detachment, occurs when retina becomes separated from choroid layer; separation seriously damages blood vessels and nerves, resulting in blindness, 458

Retinal veins, 452***f***

Retinitis pigmentosa, progressive disease of eye resulting in retina becoming hard (sclerosed), pigmented (colored), and atrophied (wasting away); no known cure, 458

Retinoblastoma, malignant glioma of retina, 458

Retinopathy, retinal disease, 458

Retinopexy, surgical fixation of retina, 463

Retrograde pyelogram (RP), diagnostic X-ray in which dye is inserted through urethra to outline bladder, ureters, and renal pelvis, 312, 312***f***

Retroperitoneal, pertaining to behind peritoneum; used to describe position of kidneys, which is outside of peritoneal sac alongside spine, 35, 298

Retrovirus, 202

Reverse transcriptase inhibitor drugs, medication that inhibits reverse transcriptase, enzyme needed to viruses to reproduce, 205

Reye's syndrome, brain inflammation that occurs in children following viral infection, usually flu or chickenpox; characterized by vomiting and lethargy and may lead to coma and death, 427

Rh factor, antigen marker found on erythrocytes of persons with Rh+ blood, 182–83

Rh-negative (Rh-), person with Rh– blood type; person's RBCs do not have Rh marker and will make antibodies against Rh+ blood, 183

Rh-positive (Rh+), person with Rh+ blood type; person's RBCs have Rh marker, 183

Rheumatoid arthritis (RA), chronic form of arthritis with inflammation of joints, swelling, stiffness, pain, and changes in cartilage that can result in crippling deformities, 105, 105***f***

Rhinitis, inflammation of nose, 232

Rhinomycosis, condition of having fungal infection in nose, 232

Rhinoplasty, plastic surgery of nose, 233

Rhinorrhagia, rapid and excessive flow of blood from nose, 241

Rhinorrhea, watery discharge from nose, expecially with allergies or a cold, runny nose, 232

Rhonchi, somewhat musical sound during expiration, often found in asthma or infection, and caused by spasms of bronchial tubes; also called ***wheezing,*** 232

Rhytidectomy, surgical removal of excess skin to eliminate wrinkles; commonly referred to as a ***facelift,*** 71

Rib cage, also called chest cavity; formed by curved ribs extending from vertebral column around sides and attaching to sternum; ribs are part of axial skeleton, 89, 91, 92***f***

Ribs, 90***f***, 91***f***

Rickets, deficiency in calcium and vitamin D found in early childhood that results in bone deformities, especially bowed legs, 103

Right atrium, 140***f***, 142***f***, 145***f***

Right coronary artery, 147***f***

Right hypochondriac, anatomical division of abdomen; right upper row, 36***t***

Right iliac, anatomical division of abdomen; right lower row; also called ***right inguinal,*** 36***t***

Right lower quadrant (RLQ), clinical division of abdomen; contains portions of small and large intestines, right ovary and fallopian tube, appendix, right ureter, 36***t***

Right lumbar, anatomical division of abdomen, right middle row, 36***t***

Right lymphatic duct, one of two large lymphatic ducts drains right arm and right side of neck and chest; empties lymph into right subclavian vein, 194, 195

Right upper quadrant (RUQ), clinical division of abdomen; contains right lobe of liver, gallbladder, portion of pancreas, and portions of small and large intestine, 36***t***

Right ventricle, 140***f***, 142***f***, 145***f***

Rinne and Weber tuning-fork tests, physician holds tuning fork, instrument that produces constant pitch when it is struck against or near bones on side of head; these tests assess both nerve and bone conduction of sound, 474

Rods, sensory receptors of retina that are active in dim light and do not perceive color, 449

Roentgen (r), unit for describing exposure dose of radiation, 508

Roentgenology, X-rays, 507

Root, portion of tooth below gum line, 260, 261***f***

Root canal, dental treatment involving pulp cavity of root of tooth; procedure used to save tooth

that is badly infected or abscessed, 260, 261, 261***f***, 279
Rotation, moving around a central axis, 118***t***
Rotator cuff injury, rotator cuff consists of joint capsule of shoulder joint reinforced by tendons from several shoulder muscles; at high risk for strain or tearing injuries, 122
Round window, 468***f***
Route of administration, 494
Rubella, contagious viral skin infection; commonly called ***German measles,*** 67
Rugae, prominent folds in mucosa of stomach; smooth out and almost disappear allowing stomach to expand when full of food; also found in urinary bladder, 262, 262***f,*** 300
Rule of nines, 65***f***

S

Saccule, found in inner ear; plays role in equilibrium, 468
Sacral, pertaining to sacrum, 99
Sacrum, five fused vertebrae that form large flat bone in upper buttock region, 85***f***, 89, 90***f,*** 92***t***
Sagittal plane, vertical plane that divides body into left and right sections, 32, 32***f***
Sagittal section, sectional view of body produced by cut along sagittal plane, 32
Saliva, watery fluid secreted into mouth from salivary glands; contains digestive enzymes that break down carbohydrates and lubricants that make it easier to swallow food, 258
Salivary glands, exocrine glands with ducts that open into mouth; produce saliva, which makes bolus of food easier to swallow and begins digestive process; there are three pairs of salivary glands: parotid, submandibular, and sublingual, 29***t,*** 257***f,*** 258, 264
Salpingectomy, excision of fallopian tubes, 350
Salpingitis, inflammation of fallopian tube or tubes; also, inflammation of eustachian tube, 343, 472
Salpingocyesis, tubal pregnancy, 346
Salpingotomy, incision into fallopian tubes, 476
Sanguinous, pertaining to blood, 184
Sarcoidosis, inflammatory disease of lymph system in which lesions may appear in liver, skin, lungs, lymph nodes, spleen, eyes, and small bones of hands and feet, 203
Scabies, contagious skin disease caused by egg-laying mite that causes intense itching; often seen in children, 67
Scalpel, surgical instrument used to cut and separate tissue, 521***t***
Scan, recording emission of radioactive waves on photographic plate after substance has been injected into body, 508
Scapula, also called shoulder blade; upper extremity bone, 92, 93***f,*** 94, 94***f***
Scapular, pertaining to scapula or shoulder blade, 99
Schedule I, drugs with highest potential for addiction and abuse; not accepted for medical use; examples are heroin and LSD, 492***t***
Schedule II, drugs with high potential for addiction and abuse accepted for medical use in United States; examples are codeine, cocaine, morphine, opium, and secobarbital, 492***t***
Schedule III, drugs with moderate-to-low potential for addiction and abuse; examples are butabarbital, anabolic steroids, and acetaminophen with codeine, 492***t***
Schedule IV, drugs with lower potential for addiction and abuse than Schedule III drugs; examples are chloral hydrate, phenobarbital, and diazepam, 492***t***
Schedule V, drugs with low potential for addiction and abuse; example is low-strength codeine combined with other drugs to suppress coughing, 492***t***
Schizophrenia, mental disorders characterized by distortions of reality such as delusions and hallucinations, 503
Schwann cell, 413***f***
Sciatic nerve, 419***f***
Sclera, tough protective outer layer of eyeball; commonly referred to as white of eye, 447***f,*** 448, 448***f***
Scleral, pertaining to sclera, 454
Scleral buckling, placing a band of silicone around outside of sclera to stabilize detaching retina, 463
Scleritis, inflammation of sclera, 458
Scleroderma, disorder in which skin becomes taut, thick, and leatherlike, 62
Scleromalacia, softening of sclera, 456
Sclerotomy, incision into sclera, 453
Scoliosis, abnormal lateral curvature of spine, 104***f***, 105
Scratch test, form of allergy testing in which body is exposed to allergen through light scratch in skin, 204, 204***f***
Scrotum, sac that serves as container for testes; sac, which is divided by septum, supports testicles and lies between legs and behind penis, 354, 355
Scrub nurse, surgical assistant who hands instruments to surgeon; person wears sterile clothing and maintains sterile operative field, 524
Sebaceous cyst, sac under skin filled with sebum or oil from sebaceous gland; can grow to large size and may need to be excised, 67

Sebaceous glands, also called oil glands; produce substance called sebum that lubricates skin surface, 27***t,*** 50, 55, 55***f,*** 451
Seborrhea, excessive discharge of sebum, 62
Sebum, thick, oily substance secreted by sebaceous glands that lubricates skin to prevent drying out; when sebum accumulates, it can cause congestion in sebaceous glands and whiteheads or pimples may form; when sebum becomes dark it is referred to as comedo or blackhead, 55
Second-degree burn, 64, 64***f***
Secretion, third phase of urine production; additional waste products are added to filtrate as it passes through kidney tubules, 302
Sedative, produces relaxation without causing sleep, 433
Seizure, sudden attack of severe muscular contractions associated with loss of consciousness; seen in grand mal epilepsy, 423
Self-innoculation, infection that occurs when person becomes infected in different part of body by pathogen from another part of his or her own body, such as intestinal bacteria spreading to urethra, 198
Semen, semen contains sperm and fluids secreted by male reproductive system glands; leaves body through urethra, 354
Semen analysis, procedure used when performing fertility workup to determine if male is able to produce sperm; semen is collected by patient afer abstaining from sexual intercourse for a period of three to five days; sperm in semen are analyzed for number, swimming strength, and shape; also used to determine if vasectomy has been successful; after a period of six weeks, no sperm should be present in sample from patient, 360
Semicircular canals, portion of labyrinth associated with balance and equilibrium, 467
Semiconscious, state of being aware of surroundings and responding to stimuli only part of time, 423
Semilunar valve, heart valves located between ventricles and great arteries leaving heart; pulmonary valve is located between right ventricle, and pulmonary artery and aortic valve are located between left ventricle and aorta, 143
Seminal vesicles, two male reproductive system glands located at base of bladder; secrete fluid that nourishes sperm into vas deferens; fluid plus sperm constitutes much of semen, 30***t,*** 35***t,*** 96***f,*** 353***f***, 354, 356
Seminiferous tubules, network of coiled tubes that make up bulk of testes; sperm development takes place in walls of tubules and mature sperm are released into tubule in order to leave testes, 354, 355
Sensorineural hearing loss, type of hearing loss in which sound is conducted normally through external and middle ear but there is a defect in inner ear or with cochlear nerve, resulting in inability to hear; hearing aid may help, 469
Sensory neurons, nerves that carry sensory information from sensory receptors to brain; also called ***afferent neurons,*** 418, 419***f***
Sensory receptors, nerve fibers located directly under skin surface; these receptors detect temperature, pain, touch, and pressure; messages for these sensations are conveyed to brain and spinal cord from nerve endings in skin, 52, 53***f,*** 412
Sepsis, 185
Septal, pertaining to nasal septum, 229
Septicemia, having bacteria in blood stream; commonly referred to as ***blood poisoning,*** 185
Sequential multiple analyzer computer (SMAC), machine for doing multiple blood chemistry tests automatically, 188
Serous fluid, watery secretion of serous membranes, 224
Serum, clear, sticky fluid that remains after blood has clotted, 180
Serum bilirubin, blood test to determine amount of waste product bilirubin in bloodstream; elevated levels indicate liver disease, 276
Serum lipoprotein level, laboratory test to measure amount of cholesterol and triglycerides in blood, 159
Severe acute respiratory syndrome (SARS), acute viral respiratory infection that begins like the flu but quickly progresses to severe dyspnea; high fatality rate; first appeared in China in 2003, 236
Severe combined immunodeficiency syndrome (SCIDS), disease seen in children born with nonfunctioning immune system; often forced to live in sealed sterile rooms, 203
Sex hormones, hormones secreted by gonads and adrenal cortex; estrogen and progesterone in females and testosterone in males, 332, 354
Sexual disorders, disorders include aberrant sexual activity and sexual dysfunction; includes pedophilia, masochism, voyeurism, low sex drive, and premature ejaculation, 503
Sexually transmitted disease (STD), disease usually acquired as result of sexual intercourse; formerly more commonly referred to as venereal disease, 360

response to therapy; TNM staging system is frequently used; T refers to tumor's size and invasion, N refers to lymph node involvement, and M refers to presence of metastases of tumor cells, 526–27

Staging laparotomy, surgical procedure in which abdomen is entered to determine extent and staging of tumor, 529

Staging tumors, 526–27

Standard precautions, 198

Stapedectomy, removal of stapes bone to treat otosclerosis (hardening of bone); prosthesis or artificial stapes may be implanted, 476

Stapes, one of three ossicles of middle ear; attached to oval window leading to inner ear; also called ***stirrup,*** 467***f,*** 468, 468***f***

Stent, stainless steel tube placed within blood vessel or duct to widen lumen, 162***f,*** 163

Sterility, inability to father children due to problem with spermatogenesis, 358

Sterilization, process of rendering male or female sterile or unable to conceive children, 361

Sternal, pertaining to sternum or breast bone, 99

Sternocleidomastoid, muscle named for its attachments, sternum, clavicle, and mastoid process, 115

Sternum, also called ***breast bone;*** part of axial skeleton and anterior attachment for ribs, 85***f,*** 89, 90***f***

Steroid sex hormones, class of hormones secreted by adrenal cortex; includes aldosterone, cortisol, androgens, estrogens, and progestins, 380***t,*** 382

Stethoscope, instrument for listening to body sounds, such as chest, heart, or intestines, 159

Stillbirth, viable-aged fetus dies before or at time of delivery, 346

Stirrup, 467***f,*** 468, 468***f***

Stomach, J-shaped muscular organ that acts as sac to collect, churn, digest, and store food; composed of three parts: fundus, body, and antrum; hydrochloric acid is secreted by glands in mucous membrane lining of stomach; food mixes with other gastric juices and hydrochloric acid to form semisoft mixture called chyme, which then passes into duodenum, 29***t,*** 35***t,*** 257***f,*** 258, 271, 271***f***

Stool culture, laboratory test of feces to determine if there are any pathogenic bacteria present, 277

Stool guaiac, 276

Strabismus, eye muscle weakness resulting in each eye looking in different direction at same time; may be corrected with glasses, eye exercises, and/or surgery; also called ***lazy eye*** or ***crossed eyes,*** 450, 450***f,*** 459

Strabotomy, incision into eye muscles in order to correct strabismus, 463

Strain, trauma to muscle from excessive stretching or pulling, 122

Stratified squamous epithelium, layers of flat or scalelike cells found in epidermis; ***stratified*** means multiple layers and ***squamous*** means flat, 53

Strawberry hemangioma, congenital collection of dilated blood vessels causing red birthmark that fades a few months after birth, 68, 68***f***

Stress fracture, slight fracture caused by repetitive low-impact forces, like running, rather than single forceful impact, 102

Stress testing, method for evaluating cardiovascular fitness; patient is placed on treadmill or bicycle and then subjected to steadily increasing levels of work; EKG and oxygen levels are taken while patient exercises, 160, 160***f***

Striated muscle, another name for skeletal muscle, referring to its striped appearance under microscope, 114, 114***f***

Stricture, narrowing of passageway in urinary system, 307

Stridor, harsh, high-pitched, noisy breathing sound made when there is obstruction of bronchus or larynx; found in conditions such as croup in children, 233

Stroke, 425

Stye (sty), 459

Subarachnoid space, space located between arachnoid layer and pia mater;contains cerebrospinal fluid, 417, 417***f***

Subcutaneous (SC, sc, sub-q, subcu), (1) pertaining to under skin; (2) injection of medication under skin, 54, 65, 495***f,*** 495***t,*** 521***t,*** 521***t***

Subclavian artery, 148***f***

Subclavian vein, 150***f,*** 195***f***

Subcutaneous layer, deepest layer of skin where fat is formed; layer of fatty tissue protects deeper tissues of body and acts as insulation for heat and cold, 52, 54***f***

Subdural hematoma, mass of blood forming beneath dura mater of brain, 430, 430***f***

Subdural space, space located between dura mater and arachnoid layer, 417, 417***f***

Sublingual (SL), (1) pertaining to under tongue; (2) administration of medicine by placing it under tongue, 268, 494, 494***t,*** 494***f***

Sublingual duct, 264***f***

Sublingual glands, pair of salivary glands in floor of mouth, 264, 264***f***

Subluxation, incomplete dislocation, joint alignment is disrupted, but ends of bones remain in contact, 106

U

V

W

Z